Operative Techniques and Medical Management of Liver Transplantation

Operative Techniques and Medical Management of Liver Transplantation

Editor: Duke Todd

AMERICAN
MEDICAL PUBLISHERS
www.americanmedicalpublishers.com

AMERICAN
MEDICAL PUBLISHERS
www.americanmedicalpublishers.com

Cataloging-in-Publication Data

Operative techniques and medical management of liver transplantation / edited by Duke Todd.
p. cm.
Includes bibliographical references and index.
ISBN 979-8-88740-233-8
1. Liver--Transplantation. 2. Liver--Surgery. 3. Surgery, Operative--Technique.
4. Disease management. 5. Medical care. I. Todd, Duke.
RD546 .O64 2023
617.556--dc23

American Medical Publishers,
41 Flatbush Avenue,
1st Floor, New York,
NY 11217, USA

ISBN 979-8-88740-233-8 (Hardback)

Contents

Preface

It is often said that books are a boon to mankind. They document every progress and pass on the knowledge from one generation to the other. They play a crucial role in our lives. Thus I was both excited and nervous while editing this book. I was pleased by the thought of being able to make a mark but I was also nervous to do it right because the future of students depends upon it. Hence, I took a few months to research further into the discipline, revise my knowledge and also explore some more aspects. Post this process, I begun with the editing of this book.

A liver transplant is a surgical procedure that involves the replacement of a diseased liver with a healthy liver received from a donor. It is used to treat conditions such as chronic or acute liver failure and hepatocellular carcinoma. Liver transplantation can be categorized depending on the type of donor and is broadly categorized into deceased donor liver transplants and live donor liver transplants. The most common procedure of liver transplantation is orthotopic liver transplantation (OLT). In this procedure, the original liver is removed followed by the replacement of the donor liver in the exact anatomic position. Whole organ is generally transplanted, however, segmental liver transplantation can also be done, which enables the transplantation of two recipients with a single cadaveric organ. Reduced grafts technique is commonly used for the cases having mismatch between the organ size of the recipient and the donor. This book outlines the operative techniques and medical management of liver transplantation in detail. A number of latest researches have been included to keep the readers up-to-date with the global concepts in this area of study. The book will prove to be immensely beneficial to students and researchers in this field.

I thank my publisher with all my heart for considering me worthy of this unparalleled opportunity and for showing unwavering faith in my skills. I would also like to thank the editorial team who worked closely with me at every step and contributed immensely towards the successful completion of this book. Last but not the least, I wish to thank my friends and colleagues for their support.

Editor

1

The Delivery of Multipotent Adult Progenitor Cells to Extended Criteria Human Donor Livers Using Normothermic Machine Perfusion

Richard W. Laing[1,2*†], *Samantha Stubblefield*[3], *Lorraine Wallace*[1], *Valerie D. Roobrouck*[4], *Ricky H. Bhogal*[1,2], *Andrea Schlegel*[2], *Yuri L. Boteon*[1,2], *Gary M. Reynolds*[1], *Anthony E. Ting*[3], *Darius F. Mirza*[1,2], *Philip N. Newsome*[1,2], *Hynek Mergental*[1,2†] and *Simon C. Afford*[1,2*†]

[1] NIHR Liver Biomedical Research Unit, Centre for Liver Research, College of Medical and Dental Sciences, Institute of Immunology and Immunotherapy, University of Birmingham, Birmingham, United Kingdom, [2] Liver Unit, Queen Elizabeth Hospital, University Hospitals Birmingham NHS Foundation Trust, Birmingham, United Kingdom, [3] Athersys Inc., Cleveland, OH, United States, [4] ReGenesys BVBA, Leuven, Belgium

***Correspondence:**
Richard W. Laing
richard.laing@nhs.net
Simon C. Afford
s.c.afford@bham.ac.uk

†ORCID:
Richard W. Laing
orcid.org/000000-0002-8143-4278
Hynek Mergental
orcid.org/0000-0001-5480-9380
Simon C. Afford
orcid.org/000000-0003-2858-3319

Background: Pre-clinical research with multi-potent adult progenitor cells (MAPC® cells, Multistem, Athersys Inc., Cleveland, Ohio) suggests their potential as an anti-inflammatory and immunomodulatory therapy in organ transplantation. Normothermic machine perfusion of the liver (NMP-L) has been proposed as a way of introducing therapeutic agents into the donor organ. Delivery of cellular therapy to human donor livers using this technique has not yet been described in the literature. The primary objectives of this study were to develop a technique for delivering cellular therapy to human donor livers using NMP-L and demonstrate engraftment.

Methods: Six discarded human livers were perfused for 6 h at 37°C using the Liver Assist (Organ Assist, Groningen). 50 × 106 CMPTX-labeled MAPC cells were infused directly into the right lobe via the hepatic artery (HA, $n = 3$) or portal vein (PV, $n = 3$) over 20 min at different time points during the perfusion. Perfusion parameters were recorded and central and peripheral biopsies were taken at multiple time-points from both lobes and subjected to standard histological stains and confocal microscopy. Perfusate was analyzed using a 35-plex multiplex assay and proteomic analysis.

Results: There was no detrimental effect on perfusion flow parameters on infusion of MAPC cells by either route. Three out of six livers met established criteria for organ viability. Confocal microscopy demonstrated engraftment of MAPC cells across vascular endothelium when perfused via the artery. 35-plex multiplex analysis of perfusate yielded 13 positive targets, 9 of which appeared to be related to the infusion of MAPC cells (including Interleukin's 1b, 4, 5, 6, 8, 10, MCP-1, GM-CSF, SDF-1a). Proteomic analysis revealed 295 unique proteins in the perfusate from time-points following the infusion of cellular therapy, many of which have strong links to MAPC cells and mesenchymal stem cells in the literature. Functional enrichment analysis demonstrated their immunomodulatory potential.

Conclusion: We have demonstrated that cells can be delivered directly to the target organ, prior to host immune cell population exposure and without compromising the perfusion. Transendothelial migration occurs following arterial infusion. MAPC cells appear to secrete a host of soluble factors that would have anti-inflammatory and immunomodulatory benefits in a human model of liver transplantation.

Keywords: liver transplantation, organ preservation, organ donation, mesenchymal progenitor cells, machine perfusion, stem cell therapy, immunomodulation, marginal donors

HIGHLIGHTS

- Transplant surgeons are becoming more reliant on the use of marginal donor livers
- NMP-L provides the unique opportunity to deliver therapeutics to donor livers
- MAPC cells have beneficial immunomodulatory and anti-inflammatory effects
- Infusing MAPC cells via the hepatic artery results in consistent engraftment
- MAPC cells secrete a unique beneficial proteome that may improve outcomes.

INTRODUCTION

The demand for donor livers overwhelms supply and in the UK, 19% of patients die or are removed from the list whilst waiting for a transplant (1). Strategies to improve the quality of high risk donor livers [531 rejected in the UK last year (1)] would increase the pool of transplantable livers and improve patient outcomes.

Multipotent adult progenitor cells (MAPC®) have been proposed as an immune-active treatment for a wide variety of conditions (2). They belong to the family of mesenchymal stem cells (MSC) but show a higher proliferative capacity and a broader differentiation potential (3). A distinct bone-marrow derived cellular population, they meet the formal criteria for designation as stromal stem cells in that they are plastic-adherent and express CD73, CD90, and CD105, in the absence of the hematopoietic markers CD14, CD34, CD45, and HLA-DR (4). They differ from MSC based on cellular phenotype (negative for CD140a, CD140b, alkaline phosphatase and express major histocompatibility complex class I at lower levels), size, transcriptional profile, and expansion capacity (5). Proof of concept of their efficacy has been demonstrated in animal models for the treatment of different conditions including graft versus host disease and in a porcine and human lung model of machine perfusion (6–11). Not only can they impair the induction of CD8+ cytotoxic T-lymphocyte function and supress T-lymphocyte proliferation (12), but MAPC cells and related mesenchymal stem cells (MSC) have been shown to reduce ischaemia reperfusion injury (IRI) and reduce the inflammatory response in solid organs (2, 10, 13, 14). These preclinical studies suggest that MAPC cells could exert their beneficial effects in a solid organ transplant model through immunomodulation by promoting immunological tolerance (9, 15–17).

Transplantation is the only curative option for patients with end-stage liver disease and the global shortage of suitable donor livers has been extensively reported (18, 19). The UK transplant activity data over the past decade (2008–2018) demonstrates a 54% increase in transplant activity (657 to 1014) (1). The increase in donor numbers over this period has been achieved through a 58% increase in livers donated following brain death (DBD) and a 257% increase in those donated following circulatory death (DCD) (20). Our own data shows a pre-transplant on-list mortality rate for priority patients of up to 40% (unpublished data). It is widely accepted that whilst the use of extended criteria DCD or marginal DBD liver grafts may provide additional organs for transplantation they are known to be associated with additional challenges (21–23). Given the significant clinical impact of these factors, there is an urgent clinical need to attempt to modulate the inflammatory and immune responses they induce.

Normothermic machine perfusion of the liver (NMP-L) is a novel technique whereby a donor liver graft is perfused at physiological temperature and pressure with a complex solution containing an oxygen carrier and other constituents (including colloid, electrolytes etc.) that aims to preserve the graft under physiological conditions *ex-situ*. It has been shown to be a superior to static cold storage as a method of organ preservation (24, 25), it also provides the unique opportunity to assess organ viability prior to transplantation (26–29). The potential use of NMP-L as a method of delivering cell-based and novel small molecule therapies aimed at improving the condition of extended criteria livers has been proposed (30) and is steadily gaining credence within the transplant community as experimental proof that concept data is emerging (31, 32). Despite examples in animal models, delivery of cellular therapy using machine has not been demonstrated in a human liver model (33–35).

The aims of this study were to (a) develop and demonstrate feasibility of NMP-L as a technique for delivering cellular therapy to extended criteria human donor livers; (b) determine the best vascular route for delivery and confirm the presence of cellular engraftment and (c) determine parameters that may reflect biologically functional activity imparted by the presence of the therapeutically administered MAPC cells.

Abbreviations: CD, cluster of differentiation; DBD, donation following brain death; DCD, donation following circulatory death; HA, hepatic artery; ICAM-1, intercellular adhesion molecule-1; IRI, ischaemia reperfusion injury; MAPC cells, multipotent adult progenitor cells; MSC, mesenchymal stem cells; NHS, National Health Service; NHSBT, National Health Service Blood and Transplant; NMP-L, normothermic machine perfusion of the liver; PV, portal vein.

MATERIALS AND METHODS

Preparation of MAPC Cells

MAPC cells were provided by Athersys Inc. (Cleveland, Ohio, USA). The isolation and cultivation of these MAPC cells have been previously described (36). Cryovials containing $\sim 10 \times 10^6$ cells labeled with CellTracker™ Red CMTPX dye (Thermo Fisher Scientific Inc.) were thawed and prepared according to clinical protocols immediately prior to infusion into the donor liver (see supplementary information for protocols). Cellular concentrations and viability were determined using trypan blue dye exclusion and 50×10^6 cells were made up to a final volume of 50 ml with 0.9% normal saline ready for infusion. Calculations of number of cells were based on clinical studies where cells were delivered systemically (150–600 million) and this was scaled down due to infusion into the target organ and in this case the right lobe of the liver (16).

Source of Discarded Human Livers

The six donor livers included in this study were offered, accepted and retrieved with the initial intention to use them for clinical transplantation. They were procured by one of the UK's National Organ Retrieval Service teams using nationally agreed surgical protocols (National standards for organ retrieval from deceased donors (joint with NHSBT). Available from: http://www.bts.org.uk). Following assessment by either the retrieval or transplanting surgeon, the livers were declined by all UK transplant centers and consent-permitting, subsequently offered for research by the NHSBT co-ordinating office. Ethical approval for the study was granted by the National Research Ethics Service committee in London-Surrey Borders (reference number 13/LO/1928). Consent for the use of donor tissues for research was obtained by the specialist nurses in organ donation from the designated donor's next of kin.

Preparation of the Donor Liver for NMP-L and MAPC Cell Infusion

On receipt of the donor liver, its preparation for NMP-L was initially analogous to clinical transplantation. A polyethylene Leadercath Arterial catheter [Vygon [UK] Ltd] was placed to permit infusion of cellular therapy into the right lobe either via the hepatic artery or portal vein. For arterial infusion the guidewire was passed through the gastroduodenal arterial stump and gently directed into the main branch of the right hepatic artery. For portal venous infusion the needle supplied was used to puncture the portal vein proximal to the bifurcation and the wire passed down the right portal venous branch. The catheter was then guided over the wire and into the appropriate vessel and secured using 5-0 prolene sutures. Cells were infused directly into the right lobe via either the right hepatic arterial branch or

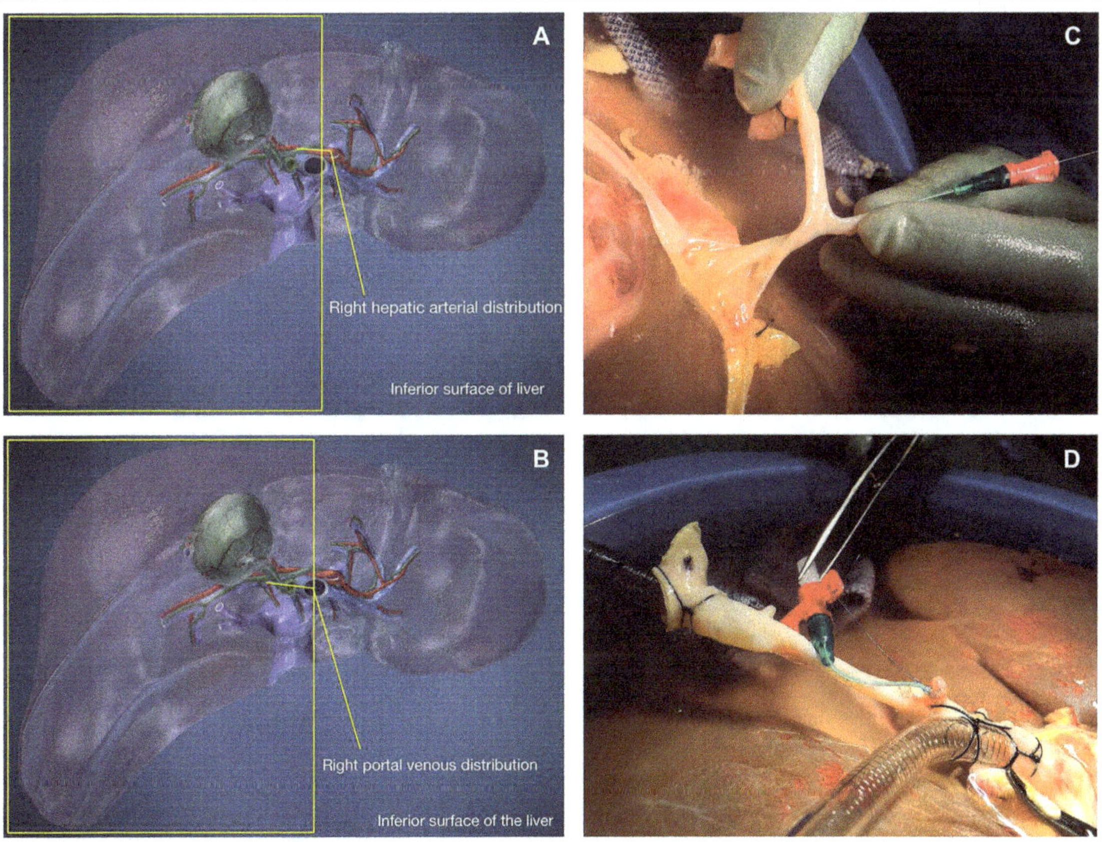

FIGURE 1 | Cells were infused via the gastroduodenal arterial stump **(C,D)** into the right hepatic arterial branch **(A)** or directly into the right portal venous branch **(B)**.

the right portal vein branch to create an internal control and gain information on engraftment of recirculating cells. A 3-way tap was attached to the catheter, flushed with 2 ml of Ringer's solution and set to the closed position. The distal end of the catheter was always placed in the main trunk of the right arterial or portal venous branch (**Figure 1**). Following insertion and securing of cannulae, The liver was placed into the machine reservoir and connected to a Liver Assist device (CE marked; Organ Assist, Groningen, The Netherlands) as previously described (29, 37).

Infusion of MAPC Cells

MAPC cells were infused via syringe driver attached to the Vygon Leadercath catheter over 20 min into the right lobe via the hepatic artery (HA, $n = 3$; HA1, HA2, HA3 [1 DBD and 2 DCD]) or portal vein (PV, $n = 3$; PV1, PV2, PV3 [1 DBD and 2 DCD]) during the perfusion. The cells were infused as described initially after 4 h of perfusion ($n = 2$, first HA and PV infusion). Vascular flow characteristics were unaffected by the infusion, therefore subsequent infusions were performed after 1 h ($n = 4$, 2 HA, and PV infusions).

Assessment of Physiology and Sample Collection Protocol

Flow rates, pressures, resistances and temperatures in the hepatic arterial and portal venous circuits were recorded every 30 min and specifically before, during and after cell infusions. Arterial and hepatic venous perfusion fluid was sampled every 30 min and immediately assessed using a Cobas b 221 point of care system (Roche Diagnostics, USA). Samples were also processed to permit the freezing of perfusate at −80°C. Livers that metabolized lactate to below 2.5 mmol/L within 2 h were termed "viable" as it is predicted that these livers have the metabolic capacity to function sufficiently following transplantation (28)—a hypothesis that was tested during the clinical pilot study as well as in the VITTAL trial (Viability Testing and Transplantation of Marginal Livers) which is now closed to recruitment (27, 38).

Histological Assessment

Liver biopsies were taken from both the left and right lobes; on the back bench prior to the start of NMP-L, pre-cell infusion and at the end of the 6-h perfusion. Biopsies were fixed in formalin, embedded in paraffin and sections cut at 4 μm. The MAPC cells were identified by the CellTracker™ Red CMTPX dye and their biodistribution—related to their route of administration assessed using confocal microscopy. Three-color confocal microscopy (4',6-diamidino-2-phenylindole [DAPI] on the blue channel, CMTPX Red on the red channel and CD31 on the green channel (to identify vascular endothelium)) was used to demonstrate the presence and location of MAPC cells. The creation of virtual slides through imaging of whole tissue mounts was achieved using the ZEISS AxioScanZ.1 slide scanner and confocal microscopy was performed using the ZEISS LSM780 confocal microscope.

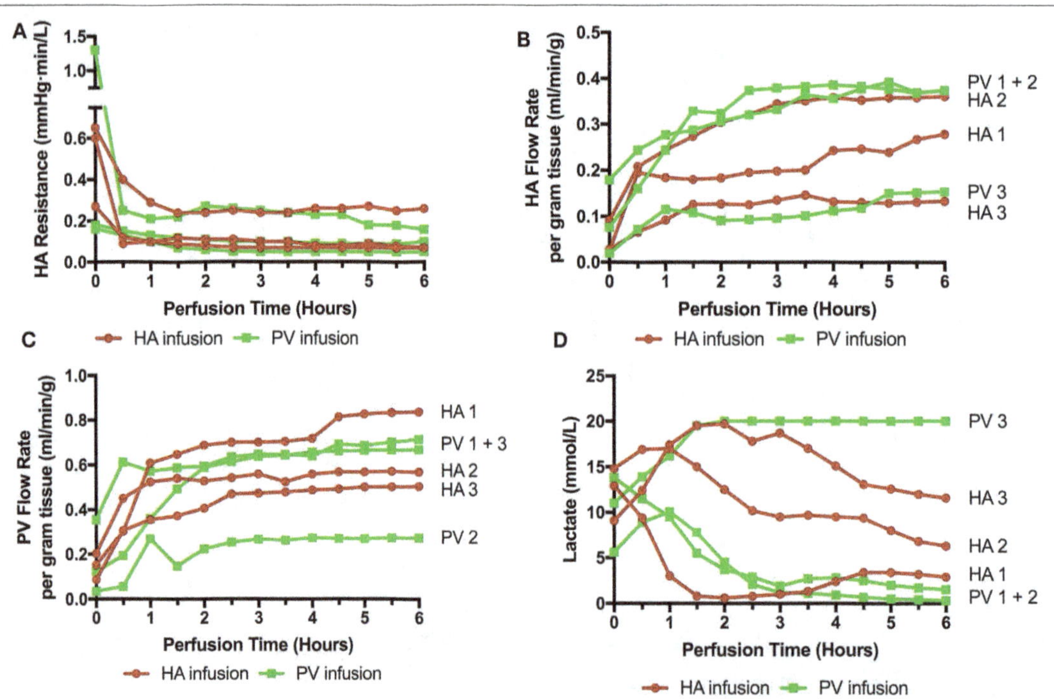

FIGURE 2 | Perfusion parameters during 6 perfusions (HA1-3 cells infused via right hepatic artery. PV1-3 cells infused via right portal venous branch). **(A)** HA resistance; **(B)** HA flow rate adjusted for liver weight; **(C)** PV flow rate; **(D)** Lactate level over the course of the perfusion. 3 livers met viability criteria according to our Birmingham Machine Perfusion Group Viability Criteria. Two of the non-viable livers HA3 and PV3 also have very low arterial flow rates due to high intrinsic arterial resistances.

Assessment of Soluble Markers in Perfusate Samples

Cytokine and Chemokine Analysis Using Multiplex Array

Perfusate samples from all perfusions at 4 time-points were analyzed using the 34-Plex Human ProcartaPlex™ Panel 1A multiplex kit (ThermoFisher Scientific Ltd.). The target list included Eotaxin/CCL11; GM-CSF; GRO alpha/CXCL1; IFN alpha; IFN gamma; IL-1 beta; IL-1 alpha; IL-1RA; IL-2; IL-4; IL-5; IL-6; IL-7; IL-8/CXCL8; IL-9; IL-10; IL-12 p70; IL-13; IL-15; IL-17A; IL-18; IL-21; IL-22; IL-23; IL-27; IL-31; Interferon gamma-induced protein 10 (IP-10/CXCL10); Monocyte chemoattractant protein-1(MCP-1/CCL2); Macrophage inflammatory protein-1 alpha (MIP-1 alpha/CCL3); MIP-1 beta/CCL4; RANTES/CCL5; Stromal cell-derived factor-1 (SDF1 alpha/CXCL12); TNF alpha; TNF beta/LTA. A "viable" liver that had not received MAPC cells and was transplanted as part of the clinical pilot study was used as a control. The multiplex assay was performed according to the manufacturers guidelines and run on a Luminex® 100™ System. Raw data were analyzed using Prism 8.0 for Mac OS X.

Proteomic Analysis of the Perfusate

Proteomic analysis of individual perfusate samples from four time-points was performed for each liver and compared to results from all other livers ($n = 8$) previously perfused with standard perfusate that had not received cellular therapy. This was to maximize the probability of identifying unique proteins in the MAPC cell perfused livers. Hemoglobin depletion of haemolysed samples using Hemoglobind (BioTech Support Group LLC, Monmouth Junction, NJ) was followed by trypsin-based liquid digestion, peptide cleaning, gradient separation and elution into a Linear Trap Quadropole (LTQ) Orbitrap Elite mass spectrometer for liquid chromatography (LC-MS/MS). Scan results were searched against Uniprot database. Protein-protein interactions (PPI's) and functional enrichments (FE's) were determined using the String© database 2017 (https://string-db.org, String Consortium 2020) and Cytoscape© (Cystoscape Consortium (39–41).

RESULTS

Donor Demographics and Perfusion Parameters

Six livers were perfused (2 DBD and 4 DCD) with a median donor age of 52.5 (35–71), cold ischemic time of 500 min (453–754), and donor risk index of 2.41 (1.58–3.22). Three received cells via the right hepatic artery and 3 via the right portal vein (1 DBD and 2 DCD in each group). The timing of infusions

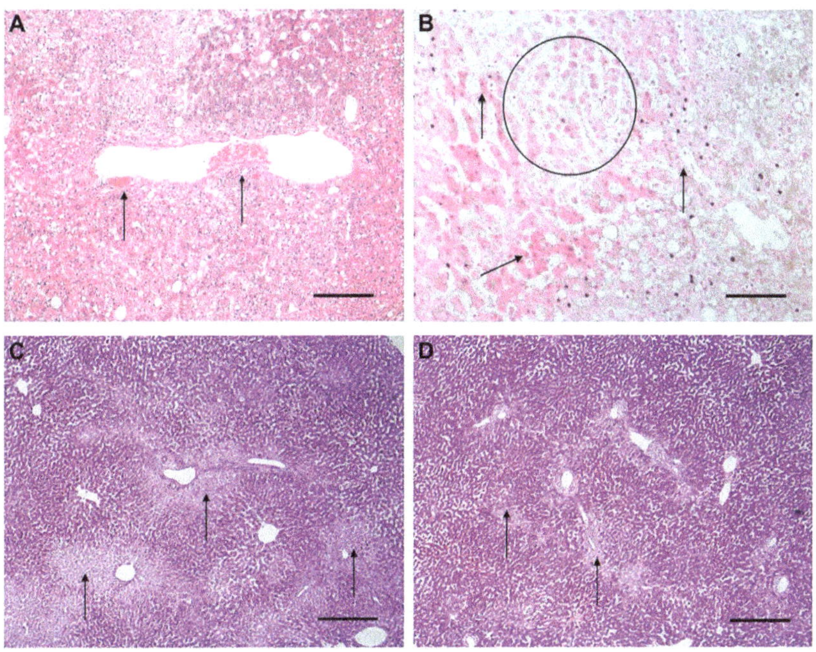

FIGURE 3 | Light microscopy images of H&E **(A,B)** and periodic acid Schiff stains **(C,D)**. **(A,B)** are H&E stained sections from early NMP-Ls showing some histological abnormalities. Architecture of the liver parenchyma was well-maintained in those livers that were deemed viable. Liver PV3 **(B)** was severely steatotic and H&E stained sections demonstrated large droplet macrovescicular steatosis and loss of cohesion between hepatocytes in liver cell plates suggesting endothelial disruption. In those livers that met viability criteria, increases in glycogen storage were observed (**Figures 3C,D**). In HA3 (slide **A**), portal microvessels (arrows) are seen plugged by disintegrating red cells. Original objective × 10, Original objective × 10, scale = 100 μm. **(B)** 1 h after commencement of perfusion number PV3, loss of cohesion between hepatocytes in liver cell plates is observed (circle). Normal liver cell plates are arrowed. Original objective × 20, scale = 50 μm. **(C,D)** are periodic acid Schiff stained sections of liver PV1. **(C)** PV1 before NMP-L. **(D)** PV1 After 4 h of NMP-L. Glycogen stains as dark pink, arrows highlight pale glycogen depleted areas. It can be seen that there is less glycogen depleted pale areas after perfusion indicating that the hepatocytes have taken up glucose from the perfusate and metabolize it to glycogen. Original objective × 5 for both, scale = 200 μm

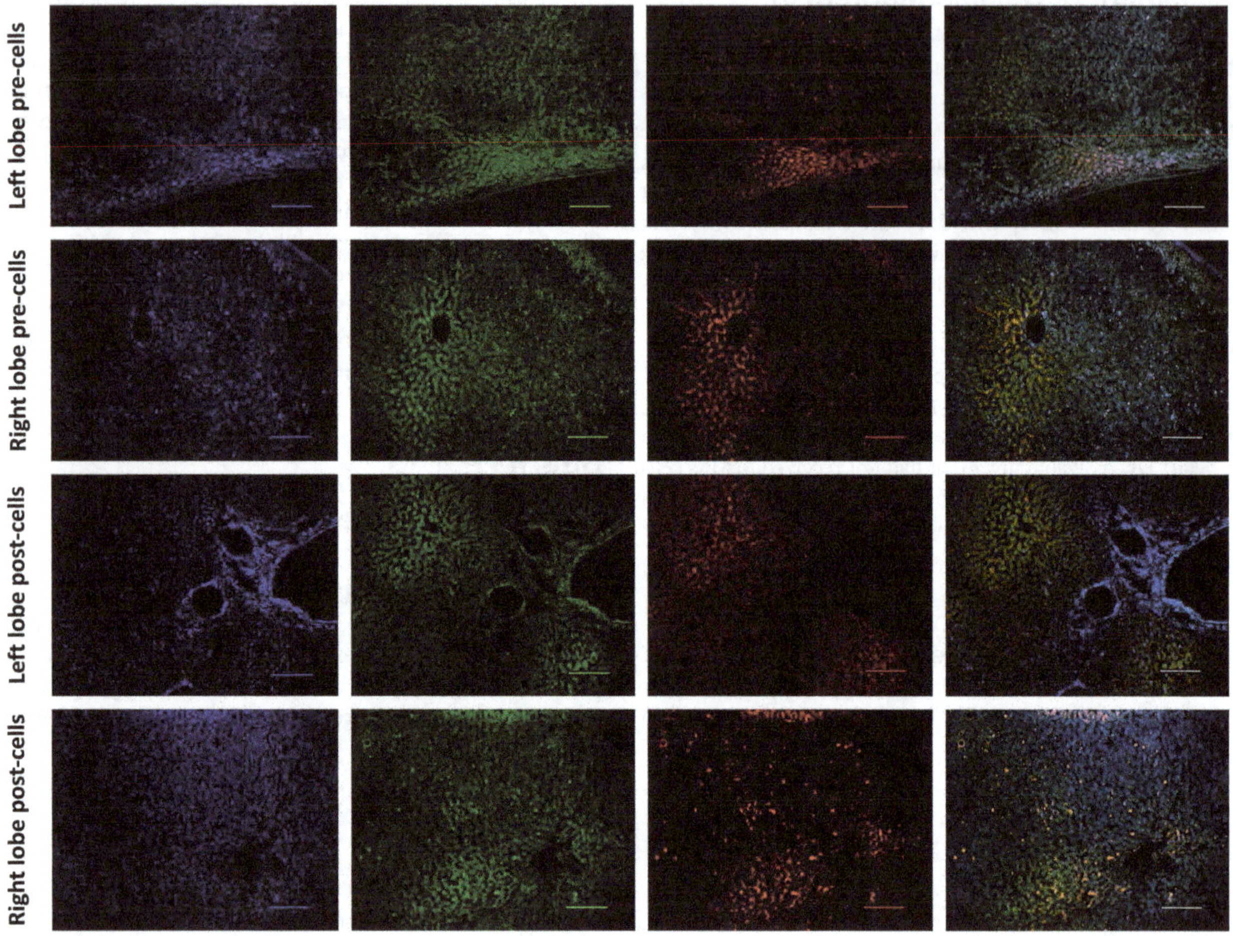

FIGURE 4 | Confocal microscopy images showing representative tissue sections (as labeled) of livers infused with MAPC cells. Blue channel (Nucleic acid probe DAPI 345nm) (4′,6-diamidino-2-phenylindole), Red channel (615 nm) CMTPX Red and green channel (FITC 495 nm). Four confocal microscopy panels (blue channel, green channel, red channel, and composite) of representative images of the left lobe **(A)** and right lobe **(B)** prior to MAPC cell administration and left lobe **(C)** and right lobe **(D)** 4 h after MAPC cell administration via the right hepatic artery. The cells are clearly seen in **(D)** fluorescing in the red and green channels and visible as orange cells in the composite image. Cells were never seen in any of the left lobe biopsies at 1 or 4 h after MAPC cell administration. A-D Objective × 10, scale =100 μm.

varied also. HA1 and PV1 received cells toward the end of the perfusion (infusions started at 4 h 40 mins and ran over 20 min, cells delivered with 1 h perfusion remaining) and in the remaining four livers (HA2, 3, and PV2, 3) the cells were infused after 40 min of perfusion and were delivered fully with 5 h of perfusion remaining. There were no significant detrimental effects on the perfusion parameters during cellular infusion and neither resistances or flow rates were adversely affected. Of interest, flow rates in the artery transiently increased by ~30% during all 3 arterial infusions but flows returned to normal shortly after stopping the infusions (data not shown). Arterial resistance and flow, portal flow and lactate can be seen in **Figure 2**.

Histology and Confocal Microscopy

Histological features were in keeping with efficacy of perfusion and liver quality. Architecture of the liver parenchyma was well-maintained in those livers that were deemed viable (**Figure 3A**). Liver PV3 was severely steatotic and H&E stained sections demonstrated large droplet macrovescicular steatosis and loss of cohesion between hepatocytes in liver cell plates suggesting endothelial disruption (**Figure 3B**). In those livers that met viability criteria, increases in glycogen storage were observed (**Figures 3C,D**). Three-color confocal microscopy (4′,6-diamidino-2-phenylindole [DAPI] on the blue channel, CMTPX Red and CD31 on the green channel (to identify vascular endothelium) was used to demonstrate the presence and location of MAPC cells. Cells were visualized in the right lobe of all 6 livers. MAPC cells were visualized in every low power field of view in central and peripheral biopsies of the right lobe (5 random biopsies each of central and peripheral tissue) and were visualized 1 h after infusion and 5 h after infusion [**Figures 4**, **5**, **6**, **7** show confocal images comparing right and left lobes pre and post-infusion (4), low power HA vs. PV infusion (5), and high power post HA infusion (6) and post PV infusion (7)]. MAPC cells were never visualized

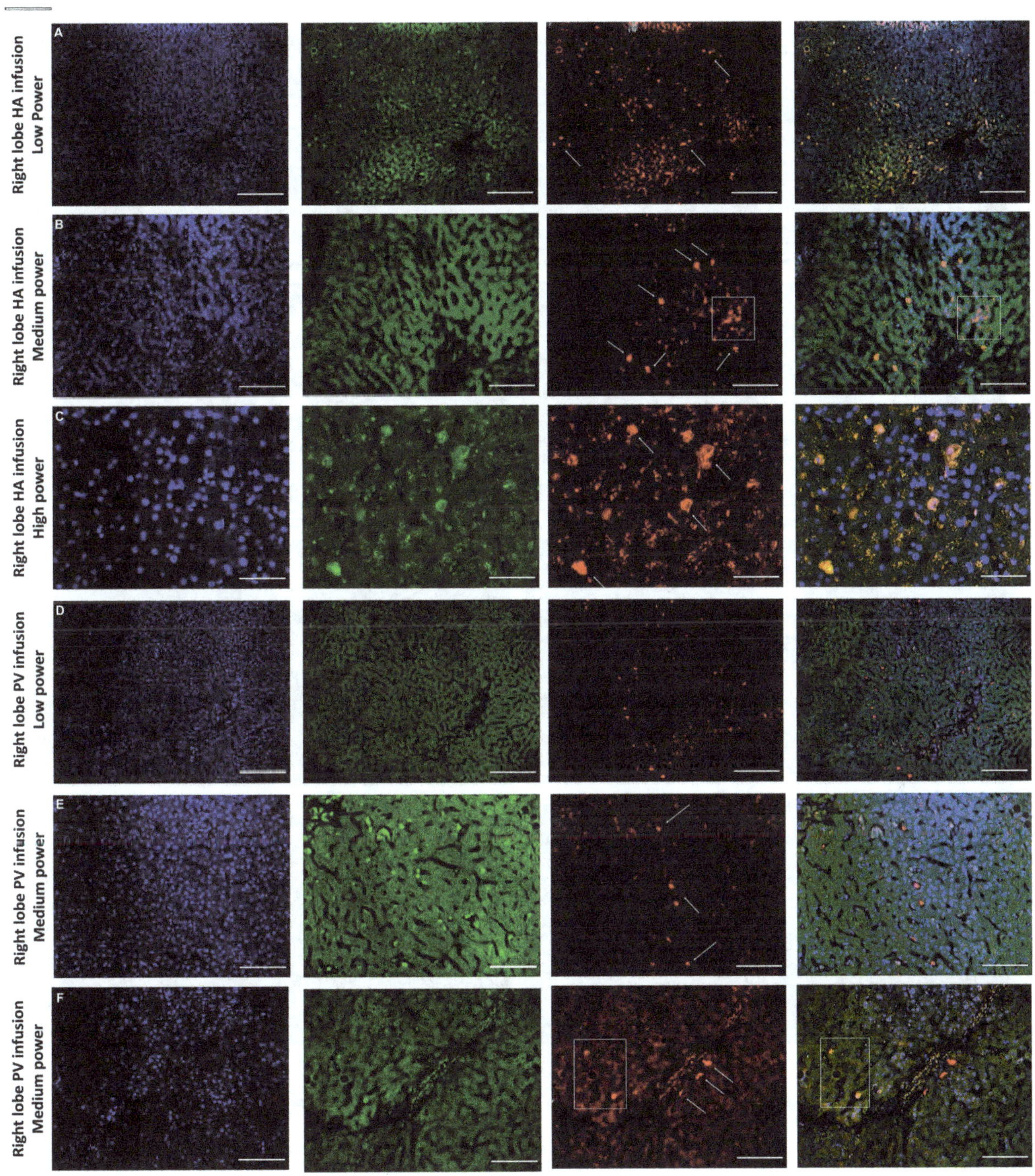

FIGURE 5 | Confocal microscopy images showing representative tissue sections (as labeled) of livers infused with MAPC cells. Blue channel (Nucleic acid probe DAPI 345nm) (4′,6-diamidino-2-phenylindole), Red channel (615 nm) CMTPX Red and green channel (FITC 495 nm). Six confocal microscopy **(A–F)** (blue channel, green channel, red channel, and composite) of representative images of the right lobe comparing route of delivery of the MAPC cells. **(A)** HA low power; **(B)** HA medium power; **(C)** HA high power; **(D)** PV low power; **(E)** PV medium power; **(F)** PV high power. **(A–C)** Demonstrate widespread delivery of MAPC cells which are visible (arrows) in both the green and red channel images suggesting a possible conformational change following engraftment which is more clearly demonstrated in **Figures 6**, **7**. The square annotation in **(B)** shows the autofluorescence commonly seen in the red channel in liver tissue, however the granular pattern is clearly different to the solid appearance of the cells that fluoresce due to the CMTPX stain. **(C–E)** Demonstrate cells arrested within the sinusoids of the liver following administration via the right portal vein. These are much brighter in the red channel and they clearly reside within the vascular channels. In **(F)** there are two cells which appear similar to those in **(A–C)** suggesting that they may have started to engraft within the parenchyma, although many remain in the sinusoids. **(A,D)** — × 10 objective, scale = 100 μm; **(B,E)** — × 20 objective, scale = 50 μm; **(C,F)** × 40 objective, scale = 25 μm.

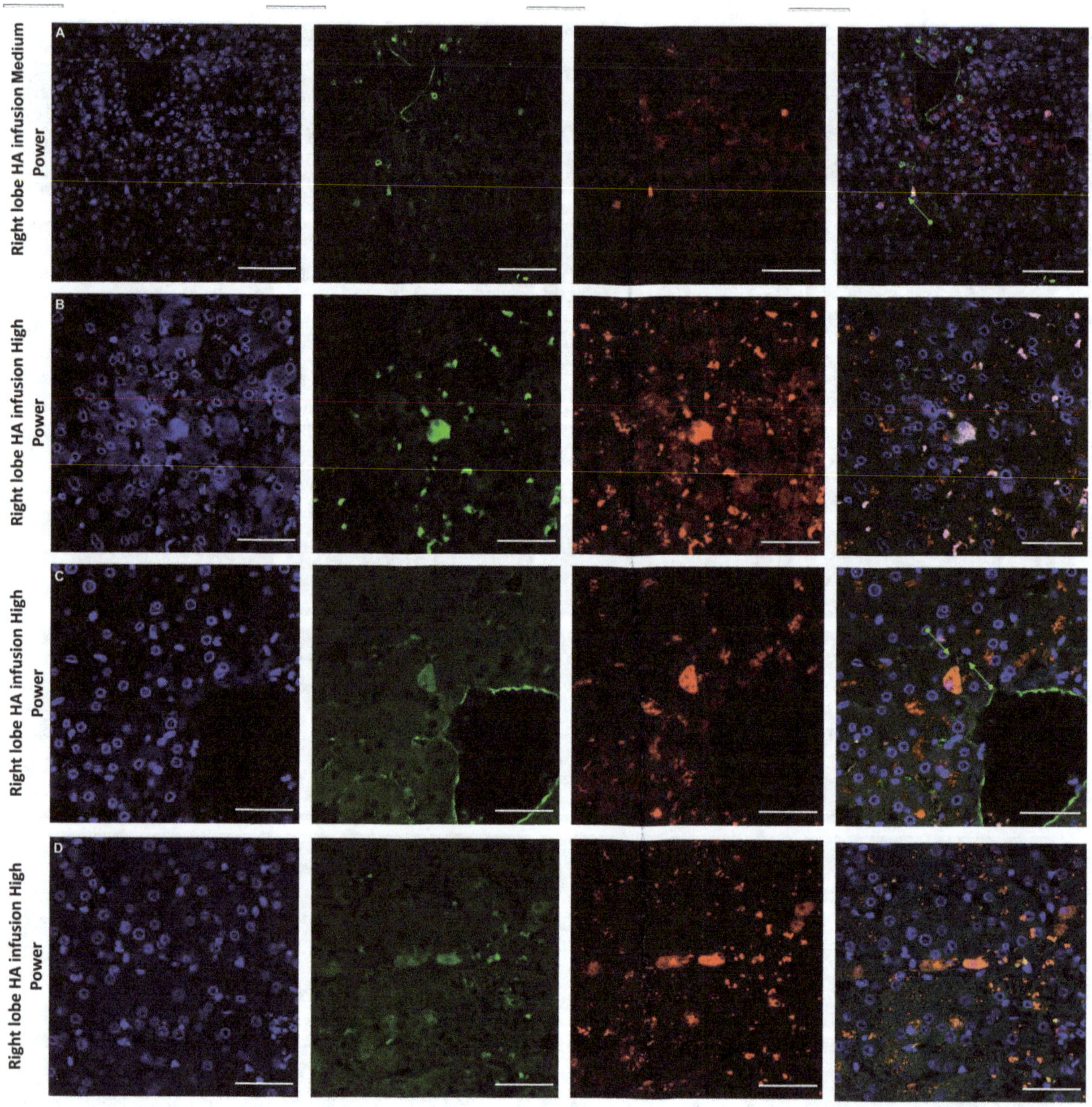

FIGURE 6 | Confocal microscopy images showing representative tissue sections (as labeled) of livers infused with MAPC cells. Blue channel (Nucleic acid probe DAPI 345nm) (4′,6-diamidino-2-phenylindole), Red channel (615 nm) CMTPX Red and green channel (FITC 495 nm). Four confocal microscopy panels (blue channel, green channel, red channel, and composite) of representative images of the right lobes of 3 livers infused with MAPC cells via the right hepatic artery after 1 h (**A**—medium power) and 4 h (**B–D**—high power). Here the green arrows in **(A,C)** demonstrate the vascular endothelium stained with CD31 and cells that appear to lie out with the vasculature between the parenchymal cells. These cells also fluoresce in the FITC channel and this may be because they have undergone some form of conformation change during the engraftment process. A × 20 objective, scale = 50 μm; **(B–D)** × 40 objective, scale = 25 μm.

in the left lobe. Arterially infused cells appeared to cross the CD31 stained vascular endothelium and migrate to within the parenchyma. These cells also appear to undergo some form of conformational change as they are also expressed in the green channel in addition to the red channel as opposed to those cells that remain in the vascular channels and are visible in the red channel only.

Cytokine and Chemokine Analysis of Perfusate Using Luminex

From the 34-plex multiplex analysis, the concentrations of 13 out of 34 targets were shown to increase over the course of the perfusion: IL-1RA, IL-1beta, IL4, 5, 6, 8, 10, 18, IFN-gamma, TNF-alpha, MCP-1, GM-CSF, SDF-1 alpha. The results are displayed in **Figure 8** (median values with

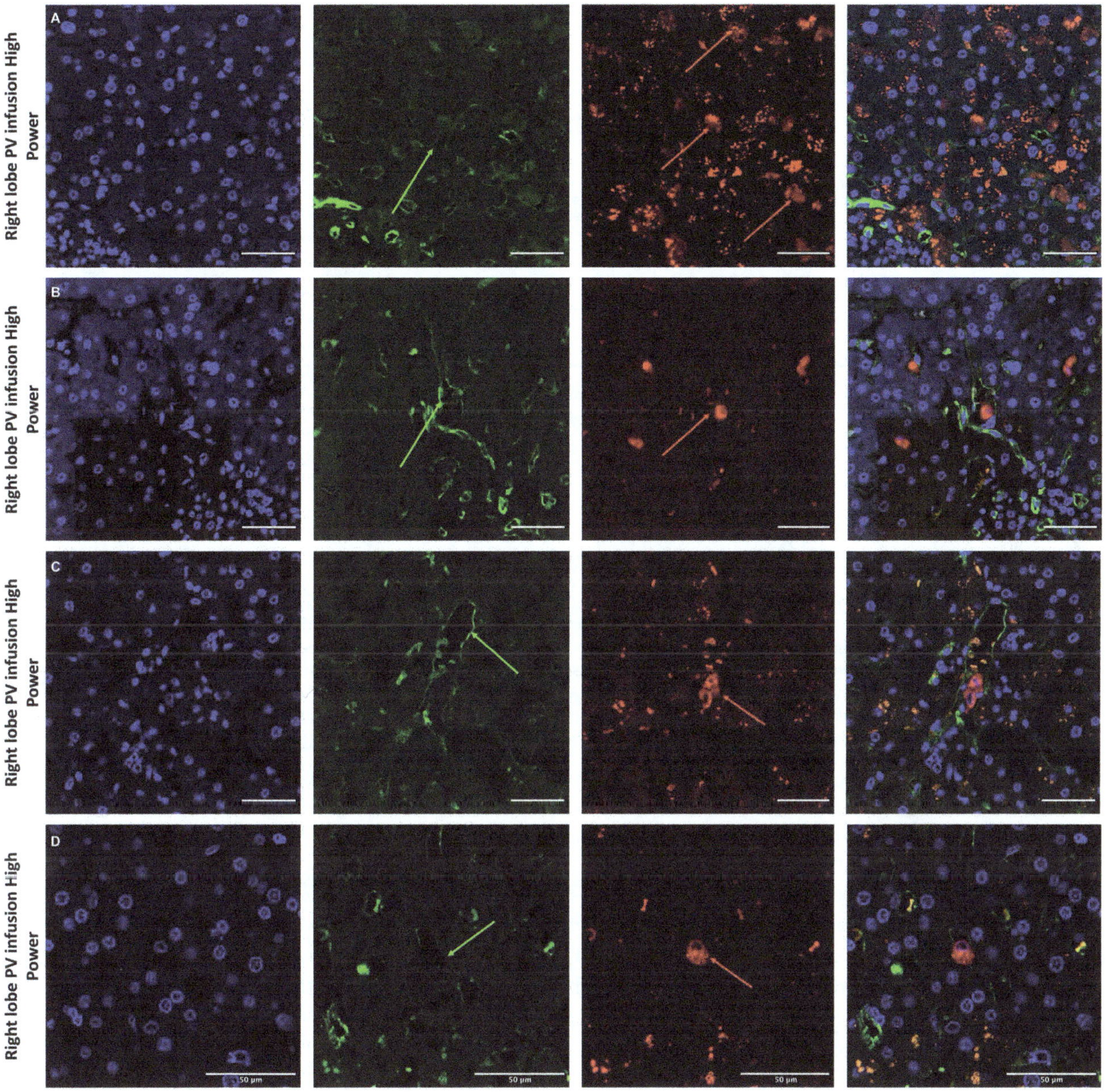

FIGURE 7 | Confocal microscopy images showing representative tissue sections (as labeled) of livers infused with MAPC cells. Blue channel (Nucleic acid probe DAPI 345nm) (4',6-diamidino-2-phenylindole), Red channel (615 nm) CMTPX Red and green channel (FITC 495 nm). Four confocal microscopy panels (blue channel, green channel, red channel, and composite) of representative images of the right lobes of 3 livers infused with MAPC cells via the right portal vein after 1 h (**A**—high power) and 4 h (**B–D**—high power). In this series, the green arrows again demonstrate the vascular endothelium using the CD31 stain but here the MAPC cells are barely visible in the FITC channel and are clearly fluorescing in the red channel suggesting that that are yet to undergo the changes seen in **Figure 6**. **(A–D)** × 40 objective, scale = 25 μm.

range), with the six livers split into two groups—group 1 ($n = 2$) cells infused after 5 h and group 2 ($n = 4$) cells infused after 1 h. A transplanted control which underwent perfusion was also analyzed at 2 time points (0 and 6 h). The changes in concentration of nine targets (**Figure 8A**) – IL4, 5, 6, 8, 10, MCP-1, SDF-1 alpha, IL-1 beta, and GM-CSF appeared related to the presence of MAPC cells, as they were only detected after their infusion. The levels of the remaining four targets (**Figure 8B**) TNF-alpha, IFN-gamma, IL-18, and IL-1RA appeared unrelated to the presence of MAPC cells.

Proteomic Analysis of Perfusates

Analysis of perfusates from the 6 donor livers identified a total of 1,300 unique proteins of which 48 were present in every sample. Of interest these included alcohol dehydrogenase

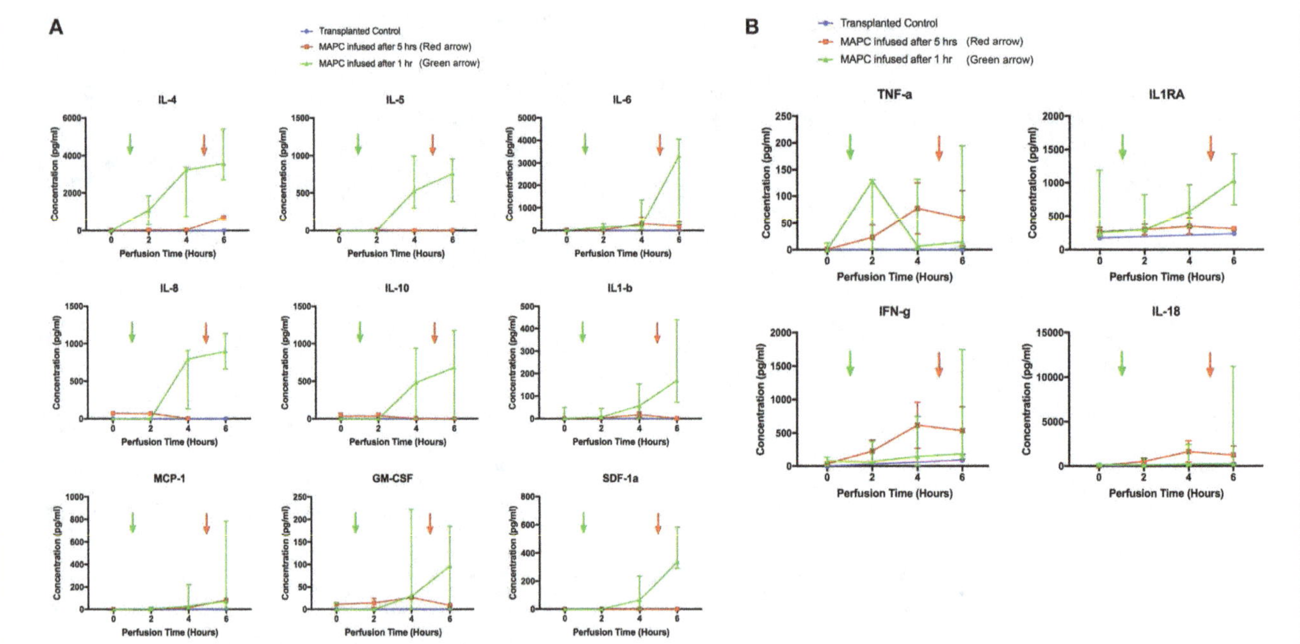

FIGURE 8 | Perfusate analysis using Luminex platform. Pattern of nine targets appear related to cellular perfusion **(A)**, with concentrations increasing in perfusates of livers after the infusion of MAPC cells. Four targets **(B)** appear unrelated to the infusion of MAPC cells. **(A)** shows nine targets that had an apparent increase in concentration within the perfusate samples following MAPC cell administration. IL4 appeared to increase shortly after cell administration—increasing in the final hour of the perfusion after MAPC administration—whereas the remaining targets required longer to increase. As can be seen in the legend the green arrow denotes the administration of MAPC cells at 1 h and the red arrow at 5 h. **(B)** Shows four targets (TFN-alpha, IL1RA, Interferon-gamma, and IL-18) that increased their concentrations during the perfusion and appear unrelated to MAPC cell administration but more likely linked with levels of inflammation within the marginal livers.

Ib and 4, superoxide dismutase 1, aldehyde dehydrogenase, complement component 3, apolipoproteins A-II, B and H, glyceraldehyde-3-phosphate dehydrogenase, serpin peptidase inhibitor clade G member 1, kininogen 1 and inter-alpha-trypsin inhibitor heavy chain family, member 4. When the results from these perfusions were compared to a group of 8 contemporaneous perfusions with similar demographics and characteristics that had not received therapeutic intervention, 295 unique proteins were identified in the perfusate from time-points following the infusion of cellular therapy (i.e., after 5 h for HA1 and PV1 and after 1 h in HA2 and 3 and PV2 and 3). The network edges were set to high confidence (>0.700 interaction score) which yielded a PPI enrichment p-value of 1.05e−05 showing that it was highly likely that this group of proteins were biologically connected. Unconnected nodes were removed and 191 proteins were imported to Cytoscape for further functional enrichment and network analyses. These proteins (**Figure 9**), through functional enrichment analysis, were shown to be involved with 549 gene ontology processes (GO:Processes) [false discovery rate [FDR] <0.05]. These are grouped and depicted in **Figure 10**. Seventeen of these proteins were also identified as having strong links to MAPC cells and MSC in the literature (**Figure 11**)—with 14 of 17 in the top 50 most connected proteins in terms of "node degree" or PPI (**Supplementary Table 1**). Many of these had strong tissue associations with the bone marrow and the liver (**Supplementary Table 3**). The descriptions of these proteins can be found in **Table 1** whilst the functional enrichment data can be seen in **Supplementary Tables 1–3**.

DISCUSSION

This is the first study to demonstrate the feasibility and potential advantages of using NMP-L to deliver stem cell therapy to marginal human donor livers. Our data demonstrate that delivery of MAPC cells to human donor livers is feasible, has no detrimental effect on flow or resistance, cells infused via the artery appear to undergo transendothelial migration and there is evidence of beneficial biological activity.

MAPC cells are a distinct bone-marrow derived cellular population that share properties associated with MSC. Unlike standard MSC culture conditions however, they prefer hypoxic conditions in media supplemented with epidermal growth factor and platelet-derived growth factor. MAPC cells have been shown to be non-immunogenic and exert strong immunosuppressive effects on T-cells *in vitro* and may also supress an ongoing immune response (12, 42). These findings paved the way for the use of MAPC cells in models of graft-versus host disease and as an anti-inflammatory therapeutic treatment in models of transplantation. MAPC cells were chosen for this study because they share many of the positive properties of MSC, and a clinical grade version of MAPC cells, MultiStem® cells, have been evaluated in several clinical trials and are easily scalable for use in future NMP-L clinical trials (43–45).

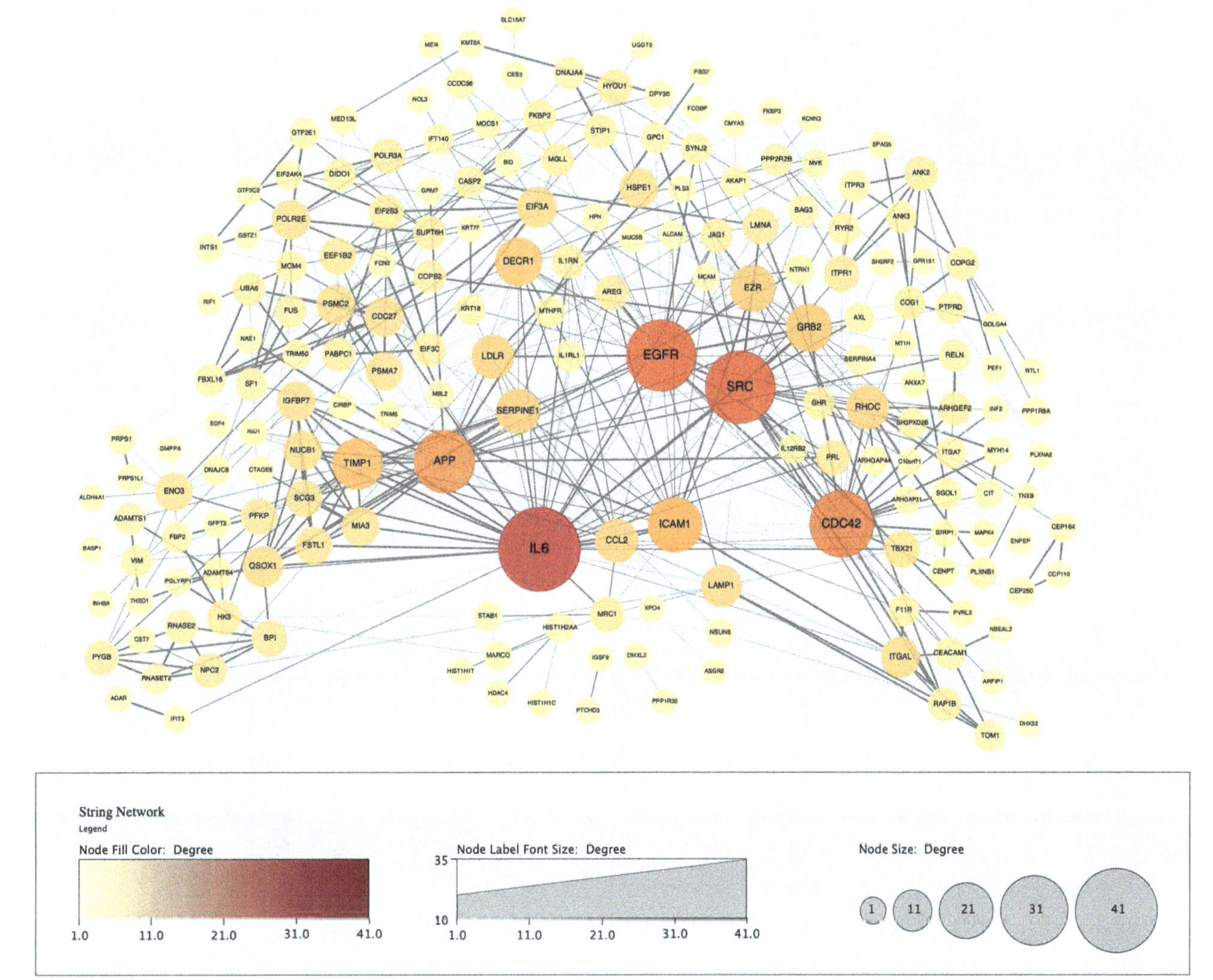

FIGURE 9 | Protein-protein interaction (PPI) network demonstrating 191 unique proteins (nodes) identified in the perfusate of livers infused with MAPC cells during NMP-L. Node size and color is proportional to the number of Interactions associated with said protein. "Edges" or Interactions are based on high confidence of interaction (String database confidence score > 0.700).

Most animal studies using stem cells in models of liver transplantation deliver the cells either systemically intravenously (where most cells are trapped in the lungs) or via the portal vein—a route that was used for a safety and feasibility study in human subjects (16). Indeed, the portal venous route is also the preferred route for islet cell infusion for the treatment of Type-I diabetes although increased portal venous resistance has been demonstrated (46). The argument for systemic infusion is that the cells appear to exert effects through paracrine mechanisms and soluble mediators (47). Despite this, their effects appear to be strengthened when cell-cell contact is present (42). This points to the presence of cell contact-dependent suppressive activity or suggests that the interaction of immune cells to MAPC cells upregulates their suppressive function through other soluble factors. The process of machine perfusion provides a valuable window of opportunity to deliver cellular therapy directly into the target donor organ, ensuring the presence of the anti-inflammatory therapy before the onset of the immune response during organ reperfusion at clinical transplantation. In this study, there was no evidence of increased resistance or reduced flows when cells were infused via either vascular route. The transient increases in arterial flow are addressed later in the discussion.

Cells were easily identified using fluorescence microscopy, although cells never appeared in the left lobe suggesting that cells became trapped in the disposable circuit if they did not engraft on the first pass. There appeared to be a difference in MAPC cell homing depending on route of infusion with cells infused via the portal vein "arresting" within the sinusoidal channels (localization) whereas arterially-infused cells transmigrated across the vascular endothelium (homing) (**Figures 5, 6, 7**). These cells also appeared to undergo some

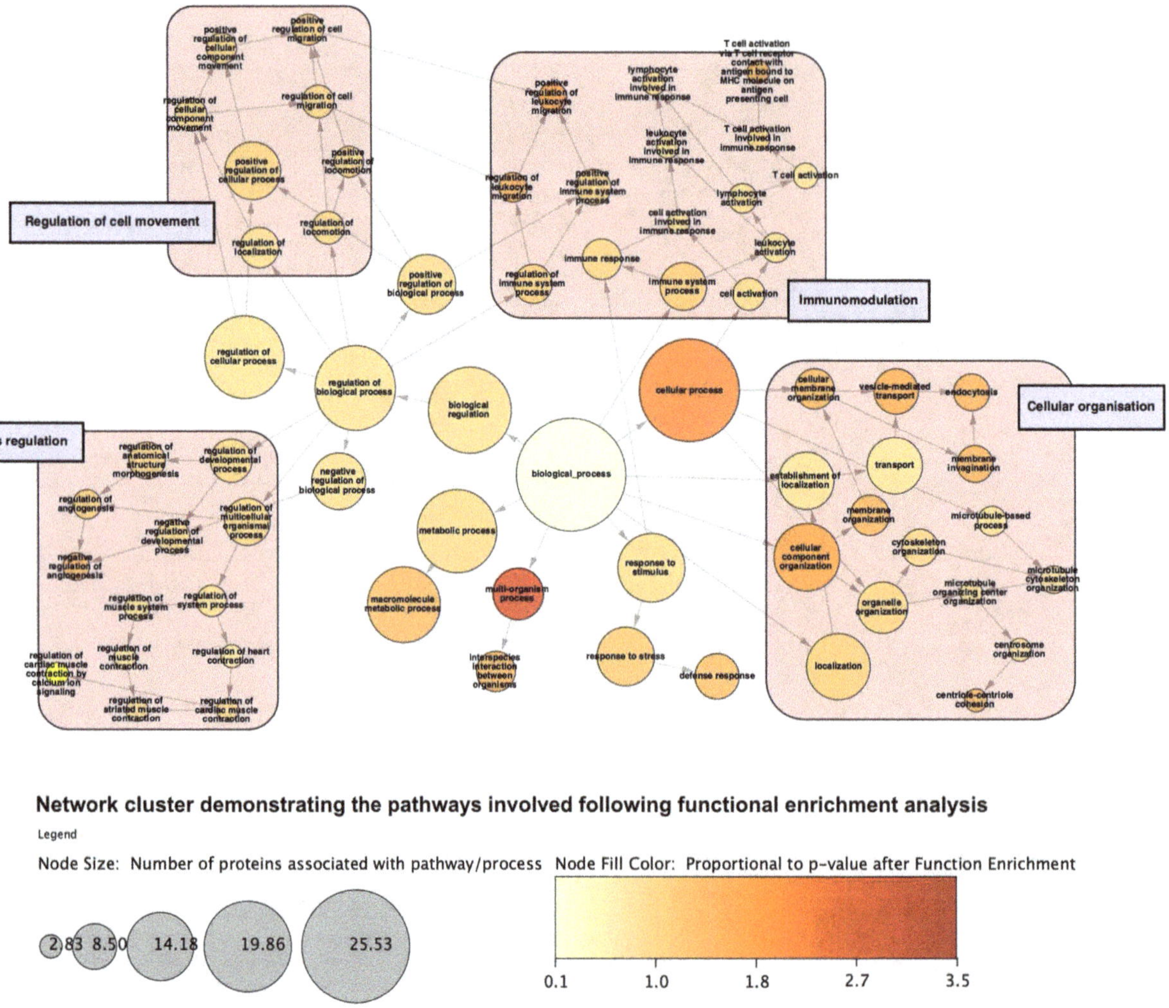

FIGURE 10 | Network cluster demonstrating categories of gene ontology processes that the proteins are involved with following function enrichment analysis. Proteins are grossly involved with regulation of a range of biological a cellular processes, immunomodulation, cellular movement, and compartment organization. Node size is proportional to the number of proteins involved with said process.

form of conformational change possibly through "inside-out" signaling or changes in integrin conformation (48). They fluoresce in the green channel as well as the red after crossing the vascular endothelium to reside within the parenchyma (**Figure 7**). This observation is similar to that seen in flow assays when migrated cells go from phase light to phase dark and may well influence fluorescent spectral overlap during confocal microscopy.

Hepatic sinusoidal endothelium differs from vascular endothelium in terms of structure and adhesion molecule expression. Despite hepatic sinusoidal endothelium having increased expression of intercellular adhesion molecule-1 (ICAM-1), the absence of cell-cell junctions and reduction in p- and e-selectin expression may reduce the chances of MAPC transmigration across sinusoidal endothelium when infused via the portal route. Cells infused via the artery must pass through a narrow pre- or inter-sinusoidal confluence which may improve their changes of retention within the tissue. The arterial system also supplies the bile ducts and presence of cells near the bile ducts may help ameliorate the bile duct endothelial damage that can occur at reperfusion.

When looking for evidence of MAPC cell functional activity, Luminex analysis of perfusates from different time points yielded some interesting results. Of the 35 intended targets, 13 were detectable in the perfusate. Four of these appeared to be related to graft quality and not the presence of cells although TNF-a, IFN-gamma, and IL1-RA have been shown to upregulate the immunomodulatory effects of stem cells. TNF-a and IFN-gamma, which drive inflammatory and immune mediated responses via activation of macrophages and induction of MHC-II molecules, increased over the course of the perfusion. In combination, they have been shown to increase the immunosuppressive effects of MAPC cells through indoleamine 2,3 dioxygenase activation (49, 50). IL-1RA has also been shown

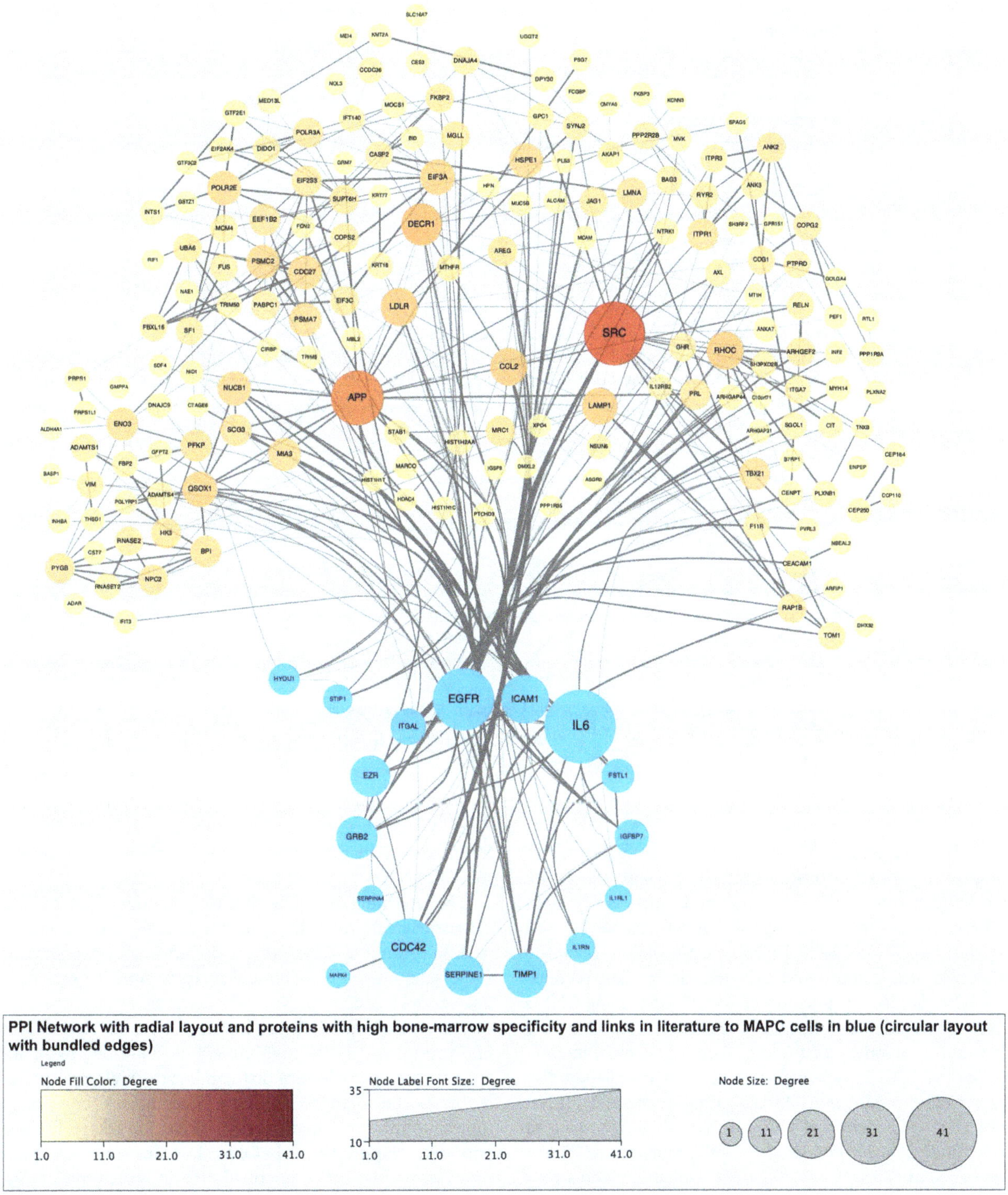

FIGURE 11 | Protein-protein interaction (PPI) network highlighting proteins with evidential links to MAPC cells and MSC in the literature (blue nodes). Of note, these proteins are some of those with the largest number of interactions and roles in biological processes.

to be an effective anti-inflammatory mediator when used in combination with MSC in models of acute liver failure (51). As mentioned, the concentrations of 9 targets appeared to be related to the timing of MAPC cell infusion. IL4 has been shown to suppresses liver TNF-a mRNA expression, neutrophil accumulation and liver injury (52) whilst IL-10 has been

TABLE 1 | Descriptions of proteins identified unique to perfusate following MAPC cells administration with links in the literature to MAPC cell and MSC activity.

Protein	Description
IL6	B-cell stimulatory factor 2; Cytokine with a wide variety of biological functions. It is a potent inducer of the acute phase response.
EGFR	Receptor tyrosine kinase binding ligands of the EGF family and activating several signaling cascades to convert extracellular cues into appropriate cellular responses.
CDC42	Cell division control protein 42 homolog; Plasma membrane-associated small GTPase which cycles between an active GTP-bound and an inactive GDP-bound state.
ICAM1	Intercellular adhesion molecule 1; ICAM proteins are ligands for the leukocyte adhesion protein LFA-1 (integrin alpha-L/beta-2).
TIMP1	Tissue inhibitor of metalloproteinases 1; Metalloproteinase inhibitor that functions by forming one to one complexes with target metalloproteinases.
GRB2	Growth factor receptor-bound protein 2; Adapter protein that provides a critical link between cell surface growth factor receptors and the Ras signaling pathway.
EZR	Cytovillin; Probably involved in connections of major cytoskeletal structures to the plasma membrane.
SERPINE1	Serpin peptidase inhibitor, clade E (nexin, plasminogen activator inhibitor type 1), member 1; Serine protease inhibitor. This inhibitor acts as "'bait" for tissue plasminogen activator, urokinase, protein C and matriptase-3/TMPRSS7.
ITGAL	Leukocyte function-associated molecule 1 alpha chain; Integrin alpha-L/beta-2 is a receptor for ICAM1, ICAM2, ICAM3, and ICAM4.
IGFBP7	Insulin-like growth factor binding protein 7; Binds IGF-I and IGF-II with a relatively low affinity. Stimulates prostacyclin (PGI2) production. Stimulates cell adhesion.
FSTL1	Follistatin-related protein 1; May modulate the action of some growth factors on cell proliferation and differentiation.
HYOU1	Hypoxia up-regulated 1. Has a pivotal role in cytoprotective cellular mechanisms triggered by oxygen deprivation. May play a role as a molecular chaperone and participate in protein folding.
IL1RN	Interleukin-1 receptor antagonist protein; Inhibits the activity of interleukin-1 by binding to receptor IL1R1 and preventing its association with the coreceptor IL1RAP for signaling.
STIP1	Transformation-sensitive protein IEF SSP 3521; Acts as a co-chaperone for HSP90AA1. Mediates the association of the molecular chaperones HSPA8/HSC70 and HSP90.
IL1RL1	Interleukin 1 receptor-like 1; Receptor for interleukin-33 (IL-33). Its stimulation recruits MYD88, IRAK1, IRAK4, and TRAF6, followed by phosphorylation of MAPK3/ERK1 and/or MAPK1/ERK2, MAPK14, and MAPK8.
SERPINA4	Serpin peptidase inhibitor, clade A (alpha-1 antiproteinase, antitrypsin), member 4; Inhibits human amidolytic and kininogenase activities of tissue kallikrein.
MAPK4	Extracellular signal-regulated kinase 4; Atypical MAPK protein. Phosphorylates microtubule- associated protein 2 (MAP2) and MAPKAPK5. May promote entry in the cell cycle.

shown to protect against hepatic ischemia-reperfusion injury by suppressing NFkB activation and subsequent expression of pro-inflammatory mediators (53) and importantly both have been shown to be upregulated following MAPC cell administration (54, 55). MCP-1 (CCL2) expression appeared to correlate with cell infusion and has been shown to be secreted by MAPC cells (56). Stimulation of MAPC cells using TNF-a and IFN-g increases expression of chemokine receptor type 2 and promotes migration of the cells to areas of inflammation where MCP-1 (CCL2) is being secreted. This stimulation also increases transcription of iNOS and cyclooxygenase-2 mRNA which leads to production of NO and PGE which are involved mechanistically in the suppression of T-cell proliferation (57, 58). The presence of NO in the MAPC cells-containing media may explain the transient increase in arterial flow and decreased vascular resistance when cells were infused into the right lobe, which subsided within 10 min of the infusion stopping (59). The precise mechanistic relevance of these observations are not clear at present and remain the subject of ongoing research in our group. However, a potential explanation is that the anti-inflammatory response may be liver centric and attempting to reduce the extent of parenchymal injury whilst the increase in inflammatory markers is allowing the potential influx of immune cells that are required for later liver injury resolution (60, 61).

To determine the presence of potentially unique MAPC cell-associated proteins, proteomic analysis of the individual perfusate samples taken after cell infusion was compared to those samples pre-infusion and to eight similar livers that did not receive cellular therapy. The analysis as described in the results section would suggest that MAPC cells, in the presence of a pro-inflammatory environment as confirmed by multiplex analysis, secrete molecules that regulate the biological activity of the extracellular matrix as well as chemokines, cytokines, and molecules that participate in and regulate a variety of biological pathways (**Figure 10** and **Table 1**). Many of these proteins have previously been described in the secretome of MAPC cells and could play an important role in a pro-inflammatory environment, during for example, ischemia-reperfusion (62). The expression of HYOU1 suggests that MAPC cells may be involved in the enhancing the cytoprotective mechanisms within the liver during NMP-L (63). In addition MAPC cells increase the expression of known cell cycle proteins such as GRB2, MAPK4 and the growth factor EGFR. Furthermore, proteins involved in tissue injury resolution such as TIMP-1 and STIP1 are also upregulated suggesting that MAPC cells may regulate this part of the IRI process too (64). The expression of ITGAL and ICAM-1 suggests a potential immuo-modulatory role for MAPC cells although this needs further experimental clarification (65).

We are aware of several limitations in this study, in particular the number of livers included, the timings of the infusions and the different routes of delivery, all of which in combination impact upon the statistical power of the study. We spent a long time considering how best to carry out this research in a cohort of organs that are scarce and generally very heterogenous in nature. Importantly it is precisely such organs that may benefit from this type of therapeutic approach in future. In terms of research, livers obviously differ to kidneys in terms of blood supply and the number in the body. The use of discarded kidneys affords the researcher the opportunity to use one for the intervention and one as a control. Nor is there the need to consider the blood supply to use for delivery of the therapy. In contrast in livers, we must consider the optimal route for delivery and also try to create some form of internal control as discarded human livers are too heterogenous to be able to draw robust statistical conclusions given the limited numbers offered for scientific research. We were also unable to comment on the effect of MAPC cell delivery on overall organ "viability" or the ability of the MAPC cells to "rescue" an organ currently deemed untransplantable. In this regard, multiple factors are at play in terms of overall organ viability. It is likely that the mechanisms at play may not significantly impact upon gross organ viability but are more likely to attenuate the inflammatory and immune responses at a cellular level and this would hopefully translate into improved outcomes following *in-situ* reperfusion.

This research, as stated in the aims was a pilot study that set out to (a) develop a technique for infusion and demonstrate the feasibility of NMP-L to deliver cellular therapy to extended criteria human donor livers; (b) determine the best vascular route for delivery and confirm the presence of cellular engraftment and (c) determine parameters that may reflect biologically functional activity imparted by the presence of the therapeutically administered MAPC cells. Whilst we recognize that the comparatively small n-numbers and differences of timing of infusion of the cells were potential limitations to our study, we nevertheless believe that the techniques and the data obtained are sufficiently robust to permit cautious but valid analysis and conclusions.

CONCLUSION

This is the first study to investigate the feasibility of using machine perfusion to deliver cellular therapy to human donor livers. We have demonstrated that cells can be delivered directly to the target organ without compromising the perfusion. This not only overcomes the disadvantages associated with systemic infusion, but ensures the cells are present before ingress of the recipient immune cell population. The arterial route of infusion appears to result in more effective cellular engraftment. MAPC cells secrete a host of soluble factors that are known to have anti-inflammatory and immunomodulatory effects that would be especially beneficial for extended criteria donor livers.

AUTHOR CONTRIBUTIONS

RL: conception and design, collection and/or assembly of data, data analysis and interpretation, manuscript writing, final approval of manuscript. SS: conception and design, administrative support, collection and/or assembly of data, data analysis, and interpretation, manuscript writing. LW: collection and/or assembly of data, data analysis, and interpretation. VR: provision of study material or patients, data analysis, and interpretation, manuscript writing. RB: data analysis and interpretation, manuscript writing. AS: data analysis and interpretation, manuscript writing. YB: collection and/or assembly of data. GR: collection and/or assembly of data, data analysis, and interpretation. AT: conception and design, manuscript writing, final approval of manuscript. DM: conception and design, manuscript writing. PN: conception and design, manuscript writing. HM: collection and/or assembly of data, provision of study material or patients. SA: conception and design, manuscript writing, final approval of manuscript. All authors contributed to the article and approved the submitted version.

ACKNOWLEDGMENTS

We gratefully acknowledge the generous project support provided by all the team members of the Liver Unit at Queen Elizabeth Hospital Birmingham. We thank Mr. Barney Stephenson for his help during the initial perfusions. We would also like to thank Ms. Bridget Gunson for her assistance in obtaining the regulatory approval for the study. Finally, we would like to thank our organ donors, their families and the NHSBT network for allowing us to perform this work. This paper presents independent research supported by the NIHR Birmingham Liver Biomedical Research Unit and the views expressed are those of the authors and not necessarily those of the NHS, the NIHR, or the Department of Health.

REFERENCES

1. NHS Blood and Transplant. *Organ Donation and Transplantation Activity Report*. NHSBT (2016).
2. Mays RW, van't Hof W, Ting AE, Perry R, Deans R. Development of adult pluripotent stem cell therapies for ischemic injury and disease. *Exp Opin Biol Ther.* (2007) 7:173–84. doi: 10.1517/14712598.7.2.173
3. Jiang Y, Jahagirdar BN, Reinhardt RL, Schwartz RE, Keene CD, Ortiz-Gonzalez XR, et al. Pluripotency of mesenchymal stem cells derived from adult marrow. *Nature.* (2002) 418:41–9. doi: 10.1038/nature00870
4. Dominici M, Le Blanc K, Mueller I, Slaper-Cortenbach I, Marini F, Krause D, et al. Minimal criteria for defining multipotent mesenchymal stromal cells. The International Society for Cellular Therapy position statement. *Cytotherapy.* (2006) 8:315–7. doi: 10.1080/14653240600855905
5. Roobrouck VD, Clavel C, Jacobs SA, Ulloa-Montoya F, Crippa S, Sohni A,

et al. Differentiation potential of human postnatal mesenchymal stem cells, mesoangioblasts, and multipotent adult progenitor cells reflected in their transcriptome and partially influenced by the culture conditions. *Stem Cells.* (2011) 29:871–82. doi: 10.1002/stem.633

6. Walker PA, Bedi SS, Shah SK, Jimenez F, Xue H, Hamilton JA, et al. Intravenous multipotent adult progenitor cell therapy after traumatic brain injury: modulation of the resident microglia population. *J Neuroinflamm.* (2012) 9:228. doi: 10.1186/1742-2094-9-228
7. DePaul MA, Palmer M, Lang BT, Cutrone R, Tran AP, Madalena KM, et al. Intravenous multipotent adult progenitor cell treatment decreases inflammation leading to functional recovery following spinal cord injury. *Sci Rep.* (2015) 5:16795. doi: 10.1038/srep16795
8. Medicetty S, Wiktor D, Lehman N, Raber A, Popovic ZB, Deans R, et al. Percutaneous adventitial delivery of allogeneic bone marrow-derived stem cells via infarct-related artery improves long-term ventricular function in acute myocardial infarction. *Cell Transplant.* (2012) 21:1109–20. doi: 10.3727/096368911X603657
9. Eggenhofer E, Popp FC, Mendicino M, Silber P, Van't Hof W, Renner P, et al. Heart grafts tolerized through third-party multipotent adult progenitor cells can be retransplanted to secondary hosts with no immunosuppression. *Stem Cells Transl Med.* (2013) 2:595–606. doi: 10.5966/sctm.2012-0166
10. La Francesca Sea. Multipotent adult progenitor cells decrease cold ischemic injury in *ex vivo* perfused human lungs: an initial pilot and feasibility study. *Transplant Res.* (2014) 3:19. doi: 10.1186/2047-1440-3-19
11. Martens A, Ordies S, Vanaudenaerde BM, Verleden SE, Vos R, Van Raemdonck DE, et al. Immunoregulatory effects of multipotent adult progenitor cells in a porcine *ex vivo* lung perfusion model. *Stem Cell Res Ther.* (2017) 8:159. doi: 10.1186/s13287-017-0603-5
12. Plessers J, Dekimpe E, Van Woensel M, Roobrouck VD, Bullens DM, Pinxteren J, et al. Clinical-Grade human multipotent adult progenitor cells block CD8+ cytotoxic T lymphocytes. *Stem Cells Transl Med.* (2016) 5:1607–19. doi: 10.5966/sctm.2016-0030
13. Ting AE, Sherman W. Allogeneic stem cell transplantation for ischemic myocardial dysfunction. *Curr Opin Organ Transplant.* (2012) 17:675–80. doi: 10.1097/MOT.0b013e32835a66a1
14. Ryu JC, Davidson BP, Xie A, Qi Y, Zha D, Belcik JT, et al. Molecular imaging of the paracrine proangiogenic effects of progenitor cell therapy in limb ischemia. *Circulation.* (2013) 127:710–9. doi: 10.1161/CIRCULATIONAHA.112.116103
15. Casiraghi F, Azzollini N, Cassis P, Imberti B, Morigi M, Cugini D, et al. Pretransplant infusion of mesenchymal stem cells prolongs the survival of a semiallogeneic heart transplant through the generation of regulatory T cells. *J Immunol.* (2008) 181:3933–46. doi: 10.4049/jimmunol.181.6.3933
16. Popp FC, Fillenberg B, Eggenhofer E, Renner P, Dillmann J, Benseler V, et al. Safety and feasibility of third-party multipotent adult progenitor cells for immunomodulation therapy after liver transplantation–a phase I study (MISOT-I). *J Transl Med.* (2011) 9:124. doi: 10.1186/1479-5876-9-124
17. Soeder Y, Loss M, Johnson CL, Hutchinson JA, Haarer J, Ahrens N, et al. First-in-Human case study: multipotent adult progenitor cells for immunomodulation after liver transplantation. *Stem Cells Transl Med.* (2015) 4:899–904. doi: 10.5966/sctm.2015-0002
18. Johnson RJ, Bradbury LL, Martin K, Neuberger J, Registry UKT. Organ donation and transplantation in the UK-the last decade: a report from the UK national transplant registry. *Transplantation.* (2014) 97(Suppl. 1):S1–27. doi: 10.1097/01.TP.0000438215.16737.68
19. Renz JF. A critical analysis of liver allograft utilization from the US deceased donor pool. *Liver Transpl.* (2010) 16:543–7. doi: 10.1002/lt.22040
20. NHSBT. *Organ Donation and Transplantation Activity Report 2007/2008.* NHSBT (2007).
21. Abt PL, Desai NM, Crawford MD, Forman LM, Markmann JW, Olthoff KM, et al. Survival following liver transplantation from non-heart-beating donors. *Ann Surg.* (2004) 239:87–92. doi: 10.1097/01.sla.0000103063.82181.2c
22. Mateo R, Cho Y, Singh G, Stapfer M, Donovan J, Kahn J, et al. Risk factors for graft survival after liver transplantation from donation after cardiac death donors: an analysis of OPTN/UNOS data. *Am J Transplant.* (2006) 6:791–6. doi: 10.1111/j.1600-6143.2006.01243.x
23. Laing RW, Scalera I, Isaac J, Mergental H, Mirza DF, Hodson J, et al. Liver transplantation using grafts from donors after circulatory death: a propensity score-matched study from a single center. *Am J Transplant.* (2016) 16:1795–804. doi: 10.1111/ajt.13699
24. Imber CJ, St Peter SD, Lopez de Cenarruzabeitia I, Pigott D, James T, Taylor R, et al. Advantages of normothermic perfusion over cold storage in liver preservation. *Transplantation.* (2002) 73:701–9. doi: 10.1097/00007890-200203150-00008
25. Nasralla D, Coussios CC, Mergental H, Akhtar MZ, Butler AJ, Ceresa CDL, et al. A randomized trial of normothermic preservation in liver transplantation. *Nature.* (2018) 557:50–6. doi: 10.1038/s41586-018-0047-9
26. Sutton ME, op den Dries S, Karimian N, Weeder PD, de Boer MT, Wiersema-Buist J, et al. Criteria for viability assessment of discarded human donor livers during *ex vivo* normothermic machine perfusion. *PLoS ONE.* (2014) 9:e110642. doi: 10.1371/journal.pone.0110642
27. Mergental H, Perera MT, Laing RW, Muiesan P, Isaac JR, Smith A, et al. Transplantation of declined liver allografts following normothermic *ex-situ* evaluation. *Am J Transplant.* (2016) 11:3235–45. doi: 10.1111/ajt.13875
28. Laing RW, Mergental H, Yap C, Kirkham A, Whilku M, Barton D, et al. Viability testing and transplantation of marginal livers (VITTAL) using normothermic machine perfusion: study protocol for an open-label, non-randomised, prospective, single-arm trial. *BMJ Open.* (2017) 7:e017733. doi: 10.1136/bmjopen-2017-017733
29. Mergental H, Stephenson BTF, Laing RW, Kirkham AJ, Neil DAH, Wallace LL, et al. Development of clinical criteria for functional assessment to predict primary nonfunction of high-risk livers using normothermic machine perfusion. *Liver Transpl.* (2018) 24:1453–69. doi: 10.1002/lt.25291
30. Van Raemdonck D, Neyrinck A, Rega F, Devos T, Pirenne J. Machine perfusion in organ transplantation: a tool for *ex-vivo* graft conditioning with mesenchymal stem cells? *Curr Opin Organ Transplant.* (2013) 18:24–33. doi: 10.1097/MOT.0b013e32835c494f
31. Nystedt J, Anderson H, Tikkanen J, Pietila M, Hirvonen T, Takalo R, et al. Cell surface structures influence lung clearance rate of systemically infused mesenchymal stromal cells. *Stem Cells.* (2013) 31:317–26. doi: 10.1002/stem.1271
32. Moll G, Rasmusson-Duprez I, von Bahr L, Connolly-Andersen AM, Elgue G, Funke L, et al. Are therapeutic human mesenchymal stromal cells compatible with human blood? *Stem Cells.* (2012) 30:1565–74. doi: 10.1002/stem.1111
33. Gregorini M, Corradetti V, Pattonieri EF, Rocca C, Milanesi S, Peloso A, et al. Perfusion of isolated rat kidney with mesenchymal stromal cells/extracellular vesicles prevents ischaemic injury. *J Cell Mol Med.* (2017) 21:3381–93. doi: 10.1111/jcmm.13249
34. Rigo F, De Stefano N, Navarro-Tableros V, David E, Rizza G, Catalano G, et al. Extracellular vesicles from human liver stem cells reduce injury in an *ex vivo* normothermic hypoxic rat liver perfusion model. *Transplantation.* (2018) 102:e205–10. doi: 10.1097/TP.0000000000002123
35. Verstegen MMA, Mezzanotte L, Ridwan RY, Wang K, de Haan J, Schurink IJ, et al. First report on *ex vivo* delivery of paracrine active human mesenchymal stromal cells to liver grafts during machine perfusion. *Transplantation.* (2020) 104:e5–7. doi: 10.1097/TP.0000000000002986
36. Boozer S, Lehman N, Lakshmipathy U, Love B, Raber A, Maitra A, et al. Global characterization and genomic stability of human multistem, a multipotent adult progenitor cell. *J Stem Cells.* (2009) 4:17–28.
37. Laing RW, Bhogal RH, Wallace L, Boteon Y, Neil DAH, Smith A, et al. The Use of an acellular oxygen carrier in a human liver model of normothermic machine perfusion. *Transplantation.* (2017) 101:2746–56. doi: 10.1097/TP.0000000000001821
38. ClinicalTrials.gov *Viability Testing and Transplantation of Marginal Livers (VITTAL).* (2016) Available online at: https://clinicaltrials.gov/ct2/show/NCT02740608 (accessed May 27, 2020).
39. Shannon P, Markiel A, Ozier O, Baliga NS, Wang JT, Ramage D, et al. Cytoscape: a software environment for integrated models of biomolecular interaction networks. *Genome Res.* (2003) 13:2498–504. doi: 10.1101/gr.1239303
40. Bell GW, Lewitter F. Visualizing networks. *Methods Enzymol.* (2006) 411:408–21. doi: 10.1016/S0076-6879(06)11022-8
41. Szklarczyk D, Morris JH, Cook H, Kuhn M, Wyder S, Simonovic M, et al. The STRING database in 2017: quality-controlled protein-protein association networks, made broadly accessible. *Nucleic Acids Res.* (2017) 45:D362–8. doi: 10.1093/nar/gkw937
42. Jacobs SA, Pinxteren J, Roobrouck VD, Luyckx A, van't Hof W, Deans R, et al. Human multipotent adult progenitor cells are nonimmunogenic and exert potent immunomodulatory effects on alloreactive T-cell

responses. *Cell Transplant.* (2013) 22:1915–28. doi: 10.3727/096368912X657369

43. Maziarz RT, Devos T, Bachier CR, Goldstein SC, Leis JF, Devine SM, et al. Single and multiple dose multistem (multipotent adult progenitor cell) therapy prophylaxis of acute graft-versus-host disease in myeloablative allogeneic hematopoietic cell transplantation: a phase 1 trial. *Biol Blood Marrow Transplant.* (2015) 21:720–8. doi: 10.1007/978-3-319-13832-9
44. Penn MS, Ellis S, Gandhi S, Greenbaum A, Hodes Z, Mendelsohn FO, et al. Adventitial delivery of an allogeneic bone marrow-derived adherent stem cell in acute myocardial infarction: phase I clinical study. *Circ Res.* (2012) 110:304–11. doi: 10.1161/CIRCRESAHA.111.253427
45. Hess DC, Wechsler LR, Clark WM, Savitz SI, Ford GA, Chiu D, et al. Safety and efficacy of multipotent adult progenitor cells in acute ischaemic stroke (MASTERS): a randomised, double-blind, placebo-controlled, phase 2 trial. *Lancet Neurol.* (2017) 16:360–8. doi: 10.1016/S1474-4422(17)30046-7
46. Wang W, Liu S, Zheng W, Gao F, Hawthorne WJ, Yi S. Hepatic artery vs. portal vein infusion of microbeads: a large animal pre-clinical model evaluating the intrahepatic capacity for cell infusion and imaging. *Xenotransplantation.* (2010) 17:207–14. doi: 10.1111/j.1399-3089.2010.00580.x
47. Liang X, Ding Y, Zhang Y, Tse HF, Lian Q. Paracrine mechanisms of mesenchymal stem cell-based therapy: current status and perspectives. *Cell Transplant.* (2014) 23:1045–59. doi: 10.3727/096368913X667709
48. Zarbock A, Ley K. Mechanisms and consequences of neutrophil interaction with the endothelium. *Am J Pathol.* (2008) 172:1–7. doi: 10.2353/ajpath.2008.070502
49. Reading JL, Yang JH, Sabbah S, Skowera A, Knight RR, Pinxteren J, et al. Clinical-grade multipotent adult progenitor cells durably control pathogenic T cell responses in human models of transplantation and autoimmunity. *J Immunol.* (2013) 190:4542–52. doi: 10.4049/jimmunol.1202710
50. Prasanna SJ, Gopalakrishnan D, Shankar SR, Vasandan AB. Pro-inflammatory cytokines, IFNgamma and TNFalpha, influence immune properties of human bone marrow and Wharton jelly mesenchymal stem cells differentially. *PLoS ONE.* (2010) 5:e9016. doi: 10.1371/journal.pone.0009016
51. Shi XL, Zhu W, Tan JJ, Xiao JQ, Zhang L, Xu Q, et al. Effect evaluation of interleukin-1 receptor antagonist nanoparticles for mesenchymal stem cell transplantation. *World J Gastroenterol.* (2013) 19:1984–91. doi: 10.3748/wjg.v19.i12.1984
52. Kato A, Yoshidome H, Edwards MJ, Lentsch AB. Reduced hepatic ischemia/reperfusion injury by IL-4: potential anti-inflammatory role of STAT6. *Inflamm Res.* (2000) 49:275–9. doi: 10.1007/PL00000207
53. Yoshidome H, Kato A, Edwards MJ, Lentsch AB. Interleukin-10 suppresses hepatic ischemia/reperfusion injury in mice: implications of a central role for nuclear factor kappaB. *Hepatology.* (1999) 30:203–8. doi: 10.1002/hep.510300120
54. Walker PA, Shah SK, Jimenez F, Gerber MH, Xue H, Cutrone R, et al. Intravenous multipotent adult progenitor cell therapy for traumatic brain injury: preserving the blood brain barrier via an interaction with splenocytes. *Exp Neurol.* (2010) 225:341–52. doi: 10.1016/j.expneurol.2010.07.005
55. Yang B, Hamilton JA, Valenzuela KS, Bogaerts A, Xi X, Aronowski J, et al. Multipotent adult progenitor cells enhance recovery after stroke by modulating the immune response from the spleen. *Stem Cells.* (2017) 35:1290–302. doi: 10.1002/stem.2600
56. Aranguren XL, Pelacho B, Penuelas I, Abizanda G, Uriz M, Ecay M, et al. MAPC transplantation confers a more durable benefit than AC133+ cell transplantation in severe hind limb ischemia. *Cell Transplant.* (2011) 20:259–69. doi: 10.3727/096368910X516592
57. Ravanidis S, Bogie JF, Donders R, Craeye D, Mays RW, Deans R, et al. Neuroinflammatory signals enhance the immunomodulatory and neuroprotective properties of multipotent adult progenitor cells. *Stem Cell Res Ther.* (2015) 6:176. doi: 10.1186/s13287-015-0169-z
58. English K, Barry FP, Field-Corbett CP, Mahon BP. IFN-gamma and TNF-alpha differentially regulate immunomodulation by murine mesenchymal stem cells. *Immunol Lett.* (2007) 110:91–100. doi: 10.1016/j.imlet.2007.04.001
59. Patel KM, Crisostomo P, Lahm T, Markel T, Herring C, Wang M, et al. Mesenchymal stem cells attenuate hypoxic pulmonary vasoconstriction by a paracrine mechanism. *J Surg Res.* (2007) 143:281–5. doi: 10.1016/j.jss.2006.11.006
60. Ko YE, Yoon SY, Ly SY, Kim JH, Sohn KY, Kim JW. 1-palmitoyl-2-linoleoyl-3-acetyl-rac-glycerol (PLAG) reduces hepatic injury in concanavalin A-treated mice. *J Cell Biochem.* (2018) 119:1392–405. doi: 10.1002/jcb.26299
61. Calvente CJ, Tameda M, Johnson CD, Del Pilar H, Lin YC, Adronikou N, et al. Neutrophils contribute to spontaneous resolution of liver inflammation and fibrosis via microRNA-223. *J Clin Invest.* (2019) 130:4091–109. doi: 10.1172/JCI122258
62. Burrows GG, Van't Hof W, Newell LF, Reddy A, Wilmarth PA, David LL, et al. Dissection of the human multipotent adult progenitor cell secretome by proteomic analysis. *Stem Cells Transl Med.* (2013) 2:745–57. doi: 10.5966/sctm.2013-0031
63. Ruan L, Huang HS, Jin WX, Chen HM, Li XJ, Gong QJ. Tetrandrine attenuated cerebral ischemia/reperfusion injury and induced differential proteomic changes in a MCAO mice model using 2-D DIGE. *Neurochem Res.* (2013) 38:1871–9. doi: 10.1007/s11064-013-1093-1
64. Duarte S, Hamada T, Kuriyama N, Busuttil RW, Coito AJ. TIMP-1 deficiency leads to lethal partial hepatic ischemia and reperfusion injury. *Hepatology.* (2012) 56:1074–85. doi: 10.1002/hep.25710
65. Wang HW, Babic AM, Mitchell HA, Liu K, Wagner DD. Elevated soluble ICAM-1 levels induce immune deficiency and increase adiposity in mice. *FASEB J.* (2005) 19:1018–20. doi: 10.1096/fj.04-3094fje

2

Induction Phase of Spontaneous Liver Transplant Tolerance

Geoffrey W. McCaughan [1,2*], *David G. Bowen* [2,3] *and Patrick J. Bertolino* [2,3]

[1] *Liver Injury and Cancer Program, The Centenary Institute, University of Sydney and Royal Prince Alfred Hospital, Sydney, NSW, Australia,* [2] *AW Morrow Gastroenterology and Liver Centre, University of Sydney and Royal Prince Alfred Hospital, Sydney, NSW, Australia,* [3] *Liver Immunology Program, The Centenary Institute, University of Sydney and Royal Prince Alfred Hospital, Sydney, NSW, Australia*

Correspondence:
Geoffrey W. McCaughan
g.mccaughan@centenary.org.au

The liver has long been known to possess tolerogenic properties. Early experiments in liver transplantation demonstrated that in animal models, hepatic allografts could be accepted across MHC-mismatch without the use of immunosuppression, and that transplantation of livers from the same donor was capable of inducing tolerance to other solid organs that would normally otherwise be rejected. Although this phenomenon is less pronounced in human liver transplantation, lower levels of immunosuppression are nevertheless required for graft acceptance than for other solid organs, and in a minority of individuals immunosuppression can be discontinued in the longer term. The mechanisms underlying this unique hepatic property have not yet been fully delineated, however it is clear that immunological events in the early period post-liver transplant are key to generation of hepatic allograft tolerance. Both the hepatic parenchyma and the large number of donor passenger leukocytes contained within the liver allograft have been demonstrated to contribute to the generation of donor-specific tolerance in the early post-transplant phase. In particular, the unique nature of hepatic-leukocyte interactions appears to play a crucial role in the ability of the liver to silence the recipient alloimmune response. In this review, we will summarize the evidence regarding the potential mechanisms that mediate the critical early phase in the generation of hepatic allograft tolerance.

Keywords: Transplantation, liver allograft, tolerance, hepatocytes, passenger leucocytes, suicidal emperipolesis, high antigen load, T cells

THE SPONTANEOUS "LIVER TOLERANCE EFFECT"

It was first recognized over 50 years ago that outbred pigs could spontaneously accept liver allografts indefinitely without any immunosuppressive treatment (1). This finding has since been confirmed in wild type mice (2), as well as in many inbred mouse (3) and rat (4) strains. In a series of elegant experiments in outbred rats, recipients of liver allografts also accepted subsequent skin or heart transplants from the same donor strain while rejecting third party grafts [reviewed in (5)]. These experiments formally demonstrated that the liver, in addition to being spontaneously accepted, can also induce donor strain-specific tolerance to subsequent transplants of other tissues. Furthermore, a liver transplant (LT) is able to reverse severe on-going graft rejection of a previous organ transplant from the same donor strain, including heart, pancreas and skin, thus conferring donor specific immunity.

When liver transplantation became accepted clinical practice in the early 1980s, it was expected that this so-called "liver tolerance effect" would also be seen in humans. Indeed, patients who receive liver allografts do require less immunosuppression than recipients of other organs, and successful weaning off immunosuppressive therapy, either intentional or forced by lympho-proliferative disorders or life-threatening infections, has been reported (6). However, this has been observed in only in a small subset of patients (to be discussed later).

When considering LT tolerance, regardless of whether it is in an experimental or clinical setting, it is worth splitting it conceptually into two distinct periods: induction and maintenance phases. This review will concentrate on the former but will contrast it to the latter.

THE INDUCTION PHASE—EARLY STUDIES

Following the seminal observation by Sir Roy Calne in 1969 that pig liver allografts are spontaneously accepted (1), most studies in LT have been performed using rat models. LT in rats is technically easier than in mice, as their vessels are 8 times larger and more readily manipulated. This reduces hepatic ischemic time during surgery and increases the success rate of this procedure. In addition, the outcome of rat liver transplantation is genetically determined by the donor and recipient strain: while some strain combinations result in liver allograft acceptance, others lead to rejection. This not only recapitulates the two possible outcomes in clinical LT, but also allows side by side comparisons to be made between accepting and rejecting strain combinations. In their original experiments in rats, Kamada et al. (4) made several important mechanistic discoveries. Firstly, during the first days after LT there was little difference in liver injury between rats that would ultimately accept their liver allograft and recipients who subsequently rejected their liver transplant, as assessed by liver enzyme levels and intrahepatic cellular infiltrates. However, while liver enzyme elevation and cellular infiltrates were transient and returned to normal within a few weeks in tolerant animals, they progressively increased in non-tolerant rats leading ultimately to allograft rejection by day 18 in the absence of immunosuppression. The mechanisms underlying these intriguing findings were further explored in subsequent studies (7) that tracked anti-donor cytotoxic T cells in different compartments of tolerant animals. These studies revealed that the thoracic duct that ultimately drained the tolerant liver was significantly depleted of anti-donor cytotoxic T cell reactivity; rather, this reactivity accumulated in the liver allograft at early time points (7). This paradoxical observation was surprising at the time, as the intrahepatic accumulation of potentially harmful T cells did not lead to graft rejection, but was instead associated with tolerance induction and graft acceptance. The most plausible explanation for these findings was that alloreactive CD8 T cells were retained in the liver, resulting in their systemic depletion in the recipient (see below), and were subsequently silenced *in situ* within the tolerated liver allograft. To determine whether T cells were silenced early by regulatory T cells (termed suppressor T cells at that time), splenic cells harvested from tolerant LT animals within the first 30 days post-transplant were adoptively transferred into recipients of irradiated livers that would usually undergo rejection in the same strain. Such treatment failed to reliably induce tolerance of irradiated liver allografts (8). Whether antibodies mediated LT tolerance in the rat was investigated by serum transfer from tolerant LT recipients, which also failed to induce tolerance in the majority of recipients [reviewed in (5)]. These studies indicated that the T cell silencing mechanisms that regulate spontaneous acceptance of liver allografts were not mediated solely by circulating anti-donor antibodies or regulatory T cells but involved other mechanisms. These findings suggested that these non-regulatory mechanisms occurred at an early time point, within the first few days post-surgery, within the liver allograft itself.

THE INDUCTION PHASE—SUBSEQUENT STUDIES IN RATS

In some of our early studies, we used a combination of immunohistology and quantitative PCR methods to analyze and compare the intrahepatic responses in tolerant and rejecting animals at days 3–5 post-LT (9). To our surprise, but consistent with the histological and biochemical observations previously made by Kamada and colleagues, tolerant and rejecting livers expressed similar levels of CD4, CD8, CD3 cells and IL-2, interferon-γ, IL-4, and IL-10 mRNA (9). However, our subsequent experiments revealed increased intrahepatic lymphocyte apoptosis in the tolerant liver, suggesting that T cells retained in the liver died or were cleared *in situ* (10). Fas-FasL mediated T cell death of CD8 T cells after rat liver transplantation was also reported by Dresske et al. (11).

At approximately the same time, Starzl et al. provided evidence for early migration of donor, or passenger, lymphocytes (PLs) from the hepatic allograft into systemic lymphoid tissues, and demonstrated that the lymphoid tissues of recipients accepting a liver allograft contained donor cells that survived months after liver transplantation (12). Based on this observation, they suggested that chimerism was the tolerance mechanism driving liver allograft acceptance. They hypothesized that tolerance resulted from an equilibrium between two limited antagonistic graft-versus-host and host-vs.-graft responses that would stabilize over months (12). One of the major criticisms of this model is that it remains unclear whether the survival of donor PL in the recipient is a consequence rather than the cause of tolerance in the recipient. Furthermore, although microchimerism is observed in some LT patients, it does not explain why some LT patients accepted their liver allografts without any sign of microchimerism (13). Despite these concerns, this model has profoundly influenced the LT field by inspiring subsequent studies that investigated the potential key role of PLs in tolerance [reviewed in more detail by (14)].

Although our experiments in rats confirming PL migration within 24 h post-LT, we were unable to identify persistence of donor cells, indicating that they failed to establish microchimerism. Our studies also indicated that the degree of donor cell migration was the same in tolerant vs. rejecting strain combinations (15). Our cytokine studies subsequently revealed a significant but important paradox. Rather than finding increased level of immune activation cytokine mRNA in the lymph nodes and spleen of rejecting animals, our findings revealed the opposite: IL-2 and interferon-γ mRNA expression levels were significantly higher in lymphoid tissues of tolerant vs. rejecting recipients (15). Cytokine levels peaked at 24 h post-transplant (15) and their main source were donor CD4 T cells. Subsequent studies showed that high cytokine levels were associated with increased lymphocyte apoptosis (10). In contrast to IL-2 and interferon-γ, TGF-β, IL-6, TNF-α, and IL-10 mRNA levels were similar between tolerant and rejecting animals (15). Supporting a key role for donor passenger leucocytes in inducing LT tolerance, irradiation of the donor livers before transplantation, which results in depletion of intrahepatic leukocytes, abrogated spontaneous acceptance of the donor liver, resulting in rejection (16). Furthermore, acceptance of irradiated livers was restored when large numbers of donor splenocytes were adoptively transferred into recipients or the irradiated donor liver was "parked" for 24 h allowing re-constitution of the original intrahepatic leucocyte population (16). These findings were notable, as this was the first time that spontaneous LT tolerance in the rat model had been abrogated. By comparing three different rat transplantation models without immunosuppression (small bowel, liver and liver/small bowel transplantation), Meyer et al. (17) showed that donor cell numbers persisting in the spleen 100 days after transplantation were not significantly different during rejection and tolerance. They concluded that "the allograft determines the presence of peripheral donor cells rather than being influenced itself by their existence." However, the same study demonstrated that tolerance was associated with persistence of donor cells identified as DCs and KCs in the allograft itself. This graft chimerism seems to be unique to the liver and might explain the unique tolerance inducing properties of this organ.

In a seminal study, Calne et al. (18) performed a series of elegant experiments in rats in which they assessed the role of the parenchyma and donor PLs in tolerance induced by liver allografts. To assess the role of donor PL, they performed "parking" experiments in which they transplanted donor livers into allogeneic recipients to reconstitute the donor liver with recipient leucocytes. After 20 days, liver grafts were removed and transplanted into second recipients, thus allowing analysis of the role of donor liver parenchyma vs. PLs in LT tolerance. Recipients of a chimeric liver containing PLs syngeneic with transplanted skin but parenchyma syngeneic with the recipient subsequently rejected skin grafts (18), suggesting that expression of donor MHC restricted to donor PLs was not sufficient to induce tolerance, and that the liver parenchyma itself was necessary for the induction of spontaneous LT tolerance. Similar findings were obtained in other studies (11, 19, 20). By generating bone marrow radiation chimeras in which the liver contains hematopoietic antigen-presenting cells of a different genotype than the parenchymal tissue, Kreisel et al. showed that although PL influenced the tempo of rat liver graft rejection and were important for inducing liver tolerance, this immunological unresponsiveness was not dependent on the presence of antigen-presenting cells of donor type (20).

The findings by Kamada et al. that immune infiltration occurred in both tolerant and rejecting strain combinations, and that donor effector cells were reduced systemically but detected in the tolerant liver, also suggested that recipient T cells underwent cell death after interacting with the donor hepatic parenchyma itself. However, the exact cellular interactions, immune pathways, and mode of cell death were yet to be discovered. The use of transgenic mouse models deepened our understanding of early events after LT and provided further mechanistic insight into these processes.

THE INDUCTION PHASE—KNOWLEDGE GAINED FROM MORE RECENT MOUSE STUDIES

Rationale for Using Transgenic Mouse Models in LT Studies

Characterization of the molecular and cellular basis of LT tolerance requires assessing the activation, phenotype, function, and fate of alloreactive T cells in the recipient. This is challenging with regard to the polyclonal alloresponse studied in rat models, as graft-reactive T cells represent a heterogenous population recognizing often uncharacterized epitopes with varying affinities, and comprise only 1–10% of total T cells diluted within a large pool of non-alloreactive recipient T cells. Thus, while rat models have considerably advanced our knowledge of immune responses in LT, the complex polyclonal response and the limited availability of tools and reagents to analyze this response have significantly hindered progress.

Although LT in the mouse is a technical "tour de force," only successfully achieved by a handful of surgeons worldwide, the large number of reagents as well as transgenic, knock out, knock in, and reporter mouse lines available offer unparalleled tools for analysis of the immune response that is simply not feasible in rats. TCR transgenic mice in which all CD8 or CD4 T cells express a monoclonal T cell receptor recognizing a specific alloantigen are particularly useful tools, as all T cells in the mouse recognize the same ligand with the same affinity. This response is thus monoclonal, homogenous, and thus easier to interpret. Importantly, TCR transgenic T cells can also be labeled with a cellular dye or via the expression a transgenic fluorescent reporter protein before being adoptively transferred into mice undergoing transplantation. This allows their identification and tracking in the host, and thus the assessment of cell numbers, dynamics, and fate in the recipient. Several studies have used this approach to characterize the function and fate of T cells activated by their cognate antigen in an intact liver in great detail. These studies have revealed previously unreported properties of the liver that have significant consequences for LT.

Recognition of Cognate Antigen in the Liver by Effector and Naïve CD8 T Cells

Early studies investigating the fate of *in vitro* activated CD8 and CD4 T cells adoptively transferred into syngeneic recipient mice reported efficient intrahepatic trapping of donor CD8 T cells. As T cells retained in the liver were apoptotic, these investigators suggested that the liver was a disposal site for terminally differentiated mature CD8 T cells (21) or for the active killing of effector cells (22), and that this process was linked to tolerance in this organ (23). Although this "graveyard model" gained some traction, it failed to explain how a non-antigen dependent passive process could drive antigen-specific tolerance. Apoptosis of CD8 T cells upon secondary activation in the liver would also preclude the generation of effector or memory T cell responses, and would be difficult to reconcile with clinical observations: in particular, the effective clearance of hepatotropic pathogens such as the hepatitis A virus, which undergoes universal clearance, and the hepatitis B and C viruses, where infection resolves in 90 and 30% of individuals, respectively (24). Additionally, this model is inconsistent with the high numbers of functional effector memory T cells detected in this organ (25–27). Recent studies have provided some insight into the fate of activated T cells in the liver. *In vitro* activated CD8 T cells adoptively transferred into non-antigen expressing recipient mice survive and differentiate into liver resident memory T cells (T_{RM}) (28), a recently described memory T cell subset that plays a key role in intrahepatic immunity characterized in one of our recent studies (25). Our studies suggest that the fate of adoptively transferred CD8 T cells recognizing hepatically-expressed antigen depends on the intrahepatic antigen load. While a low number of antigen-expressing hepatocytes were cleared, allowing the survival of transferred CD8 T cells, expression of cognate antigen by a high number of hepatocytes led to the silencing of these CD8 T cells by inducing death or functional exhaustion associated with high expression of PD-1 (29). This latter scenario would be the one encountered in liver transplantation.

Fate of Naive CD8 T Cell Activated Within the Liver

Naïve alloreactive T cells continuously recirculate via blood and lymph, and most are found in lymph nodes and spleen where they transit for several hours before exiting and rejoining the circulation. This recirculation pattern allows naïve T cells to be exposed to antigen presenting cells in both lymph nodes and spleen, but also within the hepatic sinusoids [reviewed in (30)]. Although prior dogma held that activation of naïve T cells is restricted to lymphoid organs and cannot occur in extra-lymphatic tissues, the unusual interactions between the liver and activated T cells, as well as a series of early *in vitro* studies showing that hepatocytes could function effectively as antigen-presenting cells (31–33), prompted us and others to test whether this paradigm applied to the liver.

The fate of naïve CD8 T cells expressing a transgenic TCR recognizing an allo-MHC molecule or antigen expressed in the liver was investigated by several groups. While some groups focused on liver sinusoidal endothelial cells (LSECs) or stellate cells, our studies focused on hepatocytes as they are the selective target of prevalent liver pathogens, including the major human hepatitis viruses and malaria. Our early *in vitro* studies demonstrated that hepatocytes are efficient antigen presenting cells able to activate naïve CD8 T cells (31–33). However, T cells activated by hepatocytes underwent a differentiation program distinct from that triggered by dendritic cells (DCs), the major professional antigen presenting cell population: while naïve CD8 T cells activated by DCs became potent cytotoxic T cells that survived for up to 5 days in culture, naïve transgenic CD8 T cells activated by hepatocytes transiently became CTLs, but died prematurely within three days following primary activation (32) due to insufficient costimulation, and failure to express adequate levels of IL-2 and the survival gene bcl-x_L (33). To assess whether naïve CD8 T cells could be directly activated by hepatocytes *in vivo*, naïve TCR transgenic CD8 T cells recognizing the allo-MHC molecule H-2K^b were transferred into recipient mice expressing H-2K^b as a transgene under the control of the sheep metallothionein or mouse albumin promoters, restricting expression to hepatocytes. CD8 T cells were rapidly retained in the liver after adoptive transfer, and underwent subsequent activation and proliferation (34, 35). Retention and activation were antigen-specific, as T cells were not retained in a non-antigen expressing liver (34). Restriction of H2-K^b expression to hepatocytes excluded T cell activation in lymphoid tissues, suggesting that hepatocytes activated naïve CD8 T cells independently of secondary lymphoid tissues (34, 35). Electron microscopy studies provided visual evidence of these interactions, and showed that they occurred through the fenestrae of liver sinusoidal endothelial cells (36). This was the first report of primary T cell activation outside secondary lymphoid tissues. By tracking hepatocyte-activated transgenic CD8 T cells in the recipient, we demonstrated that intrahepatic activation by hepatocytes promoted antigen-specific tolerance, whereas effective immunity to hepatically expressed antigen required primary activation of CD8 T cells in the secondary lymphoid organs (35). These results highlighted the role of the site of primary activation in determining the outcome of the CD8 T cell response for the first time, a phenomenon potentially acting as a key mechanism driving tolerance after liver transplantation. The potential mechanisms determining the hepatic silencing of the CD8 T cell response will be detailed below.

By generating bone marrow irradiated chimeras in which H-2K^b expression was restricted to bone marrow-derived cells, we showed that bone marrow-derived cells were sufficient for intrahepatic retention of CD8 T cells (37). As Kupffer cells (KCs) are the main sinusoidal cell derived from bone marrow in radiation-induced chimeric models, these results suggest that antigen expressing KCs could also activate naïve CD8 T cells.

Liver sinusoidal endothelial cells (LSECs) and hepatic stellate cells have also been demonstrated to be capable of activating naïve CD8 T cells (38, 39). LSECs have been the subject of several studies, as they are scavenger cells able to process antigen via the direct presentation pathway for presentation in the context of MHC class I, but are also able to cross-present antigen (40), a property largely restricted to certain subsets of dendritic cells. Unlike hepatocytes, these cells express low levels of MHC class II in addition to MHC class I, and could therefore act as antigen presenting cells for CD4 T cells (41). The role of LSEC and other liver cells in presenting antigen has been the subject of several previous reviews (12–44).

Collectively, these results suggest that a variety of cell types can activate naïve CD8 T cells within the hepatic sinusoids.

To our knowledge, the liver is the only non-lymphoid organ that supports primary CD8 T cell activation. The liver owes this property to its unique architecture, being comprised of a myriad of narrow sinusoids lined with perforated endothelium and harboring liver resident macrophages within their lumens. When combined, these features create a unique environment in which the blood flow is slower than in other capillary beds, allowing selectin-independent recruitment of leucocytes within the liver (30), and direct contact with a range of potential antigen presenting cells not possible in other non-lymphoid organs with continuous endothelium and higher capillary flow rates. This property may be critical for understanding immunity in this organ and tolerance after LT.

Studies in LT Using Transgenic Mouse Models

Liver transplantation creates altered conditions for the recipient immune system that are expected to have a profound effect on T cell activation:

1. *The inflamed microenvironment related to surgery*: Inflammation associated with surgery and ischemia-reperfusion injury alters expression of molecules that regulate T cell activation (MHC, adhesion, and costimulatory molecules and cytokines) (45). These changes might promote bystander activation of non-graft reactive T cells or recruit T cells that would not contribute to a physiological response under uninflamed conditions, i.e., those recognizing low affinity ligands. To assess whether procedural associated inflammation alters intrahepatic T cell activation, we have recently developed a mouse LT model in which labeled naïve TCR transgenic CD8 T cells recognizing the allo-MHC molecule H-2K^b can be easily identified after adoptive transfer into recipient mice receiving syngeneic or allogeneic H-2K^b expressing liver grafts (46). By assessing early immune events in this model, we have shown that naïve T cells are retained and activated in the liver allograft with similar kinetics to that observed in a non-transplant setting (46). Importantly, naive alloreactive CD8 T cells were not retained or activated in syngeneic liver grafts (46), providing convincing evidence that retention of alloreactive CD8 T cells in the transplanted liver is antigen-dependent and is not altered by the surgery. These results confirm similar observations made by Kamada in the rat (7).

2. *Disruption of T cell activation in lymphoid tissues by PL*: In a physiological setting, liver antigen would be processed by two different pathways leading to presentation by different cells in distinct compartments. While antigen processing via the direct pathway of MHC class I presentation leads to presentation by hepatic cells in the liver, antigens captured and cross-presented by dendritic cells are presented in lymphoid tissues (29). Although these two pathways contribute after liver transplantation, PL migration to lymphoid tissues allows a large cohort of cells that are not specialized in antigen presentation to migrate to areas dedicated to antigen presentation normally initiated by a low number of dendritic cells. This enables a third unphysiological T cell activation pathway, which disrupts physiological antigen presentation in lymphoid tissues.

The impact of PL migration in lymphoid tissues was recently investigated in our mouse LT model (46). Our results confirmed that PL migration occurred almost as soon as the recipient blood starts flowing into the graft and continues to occur within the first hours after transplantation (46). By dissecting migration patterns of different PL cell subsets, we showed that preferential migration to recipient spleen or lymph nodes resulted in differences in PL composition between these two compartments that reflected the physiological composition of these compartments: for example, while recipient spleens contained mostly donor B cells, recipient lymph nodes contained mostly donor T cells. Although most cells migrated out of grafts, most NK T cells and a significant proportion of NK cells stayed within liver allografts. The remaining NK cells circulated via the blood and were not detected in lymphoid organs. Intrahepatic retention of NKT cells confirms their tissue residency, and is consistent with findings from parabiotic experiments (47). Most importantly, migration of PLs was initially very similar in syngeneic and allogeneic recipients; (46) however, a difference between syngeneic and allogeneic two recipients was observed after 2 days, as PLs numbers dropped in the allograft recipients, reflecting their killing by alloreactive recipient CTLs (46).

Activation of alloreactive TCR transgenic CD8 T cells in recipient lymphoid tissues was a very early event, being detected at 5 h post-transplant (46). By transplanting liver allografts ubiquitously expressing a reporter protein into recipient mice harboring labeled transgenic alloreactive CD8 T cells, we were able to visualize interactions between most alloreactive transgenic CD8 T cells and PL in lymphoid tissues as soon as 5 h after the surgery, suggesting that the observed activation of alloreactive CD8 T cells was directly initiated by PLs (46). Furthermore, all alloreactive transgenic T cells contained in lymph nodes and spleen were activated, suggesting that they were recruited at once, a result that is not entirely surprising considering the large number of PLs contained in a liver allograft.

As PL-mediated T cell activation is such a prominent immune event during the first days after liver transplantation, PLs were initially considered the main cell driving T cell activation after transplantation, and their role was examined in most early studies in rat models (48). The seminal report by Starzl et al. describing PL-mediated microchimerism (12) influenced the field and reinforced this trend. As mentioned earlier a role of PL mediated activation in tolerance is supported by our early study showing that (i) adoptive transfer of large numbers of donor splenic or liver leucocytes immediately after transplantation converted rat liver allograft rejection to long term acceptance and prolonged the survival of rat kidney allografts; (49) (ii) irradiation of rat liver allograft before transplantation promoted rejection in normally tolerant strain combinations; (16) and (iii) "parking" of irradiated livers in syngeneic hosts prior to allotransplantation reconstituted tolerance (16). These findings raise some key questions: firstly, how do PL mediate tolerance? Secondly, if PL mediate tolerance after liver transplantation, why do PL from other solid organs fail to induce tolerance after transplantation?

It has long been observed that transfusing the recipient with blood from the graft donor prior to transplantation prolongs allograft survival. This effect, first described by Medawar in 1946 (50), has become known as "the blood transfusion effect," and it was initially suggested that tolerance induced by liver allografts resulted in similar fashion due to the high number of PLs transplanted along with this large organ. High PL numbers might create "high dose tolerance," promoting activation-induced cell death (AICD) of alloreactive CD8 T cells (48). AICD describes cell death occurring when activated T cells re-crosslink their TCR in the presence of IL-2 (51). As they are activated, T cells co-express death molecules and their ligands on their cell surface. If T cells are in close contact with each other, they trigger the death receptor pathway of other cells, resulting in apoptosis (51). T cells are highly sensitive to AICD during the first 2–3 days after primary activation, but as they start to overexpress FLIP (FLICE inhibitory protein) between 24 and 48 h, they become resistant after 48 h (52). While AICD of CD4 T cells is mediated by FasL, AICD of CD8 T cells involves TNFRII (53). However, AICD is a phenomenon observed *in vitro*, and it remains unclear whether it occurs after transplantation *in vivo*. Nevertheless, the timeframe during which allograft reactive T cell death is observed after LT, within the first 2–3 days post-surgery, coincides with the period in which T cells have been found to be sensitive to AICD *in vitro*. Thus, early PL-mediated apoptosis of recipient alloreactive CD4 and CD8 T cells in recipient lymphoid tissues after LT might occur in association with this, or a closely related, process.

It must be noted that although PL have been demonstrated to induce tolerance or prolong graft survival in rat models, transfer of large numbers of donor-derived splenocytes or intrahepatic lymphocytes do not lead to tolerance of rat kidney and heart allografts (54), suggesting that the spontaneous acceptance of liver allografts is not solely mediated by PL.

3. The non-physiological expression of alloantigen by all cells of the liver allograft: As naïve CD8 T cells can undergo primary activation in the intact liver, they might also be activated by hepatic cells in liver allografts. We confirmed that this was the case by tracking graft-reactive CD8 T cells in the recipient of a liver allograft: naïve allograft-specific CD8 T cells underwent activation in the spleen and lymph nodes, but were also concomitantly retained and activated within the liver allograft, although not within the livers of syngeneic graft recipients (46). As primary CD8 T cell activation in the livers of intact animals has been shown to promote tolerance (35), this pathway might also be a key mechanism promoting tolerance after LT. The fate of T cells activated within the liver allograft, and the relative contributions of this pathway vs. the PL-mediated activation pathway occurring in recipient lymphoid tissues, have not yet been delineated. However, studies performed in intact livers do yield some clues. To investigate a setting relevant to liver transplantation in which donor MHC molecules are expressed by all liver cells including leucocytes, donor transgenic CD8 T cells were adoptively transferred into recipient mice ubiquitously expressing their cognate antigen, the alloantigen H-2K^b. We made the surprising finding that 80–90% of T cells undergoing primary activation within the liver were rapidly eliminated by a non-apoptotic mechanism (55). Deletion resulted from T cell invasion of hepatocytes, a process leading to their rapid destruction in LAMP-1$^+$ lysosomal compartments. Cell-in-cell structures can arise by "emperipolesis" (56), a process long observed in liver sections in autoimmune hepatitis and viral hepatitis induced by HBV, HCV, and Epstein-Barr virus infections. To distinguish our findings from the classical form of emperipolesis that does not imply destruction of the invading cell, we have termed this non-apoptotic death *suicidal emperipolesis* (55). Although most liver-activated alloreactive CD8 T cells disappeared by suicidal emperipolesis, 10–20% of H-2K^b-specific CD8 T cells survived this process. These residual cells displayed poor effector function, expressed high levels of the pro-apoptotic molecule Bim, and underwent premature cell death via apoptosis, thus limiting their ability to induce liver damage (57). Although these two processes of CD8 T cell death eliminated most donor T cells, a small population of residual H-2K^b T cells persisted at later time points. However, these cells expressed high levels of PD-1, and were not functional, suggesting that they were exhausted (29). Thus, our results strongly suggest that CD8 T cells activated within the liver are tolerized by at least 3 mechanisms: death by suicidal emperipolesis, Bim-mediated apoptotic cell death, and functional exhaustion. We hypothesize that similar mechanisms operate in the hepatic allograft after LT, with PL also inducing parallel activation leading to apoptosis of graft-reactive CD8 T cells within the recipient lymphoid tissues (58). This model is supported by previous findings by Qian et al. (59). suggesting that T cell deletion is the most important mechanism mediating tolerance after mouse liver transplantation. It is also consistent with reports suggesting that both the hepatic parenchyma and PLs contribute to tolerance induction after rat LT (18) and that human liver transplantation is associated with deletion of T cells bearing specific TCR beta sequences (60). Tolerance to liver allografts is consistent with our studies showing that persisting high levels of intrahepatic antigen expression, a situation akin to that associated with organ transplantation, are generally associated with tolerance (29). In contrast, low levels of intrahepatic antigen expression, for example where antigen is expressed by low numbers of hepatocytes or via transient intrahepatic antigen presentation following administration of exogenous peptide, promote functional responses, antigen clearance and T cell survival (29). The multiple pathways occurring in the early tolerance phase post-LT are summarized in **Figure 1** and **Table 1**.

THE INDUCTION PHASE—HUMAN STUDIES

Only a few studies have examined the induction phase of tolerance in human liver transplant recipients. We described an increase in interferon γ producing peripheral blood mononuclear cells in patients who did not have a subsequent early episode of allograft rejection (61). This was consistent with studies in experimental animals showing tolerance was associated with an early immune activation phenotype (15). However, such studies are confounded by the relatively early introduction of

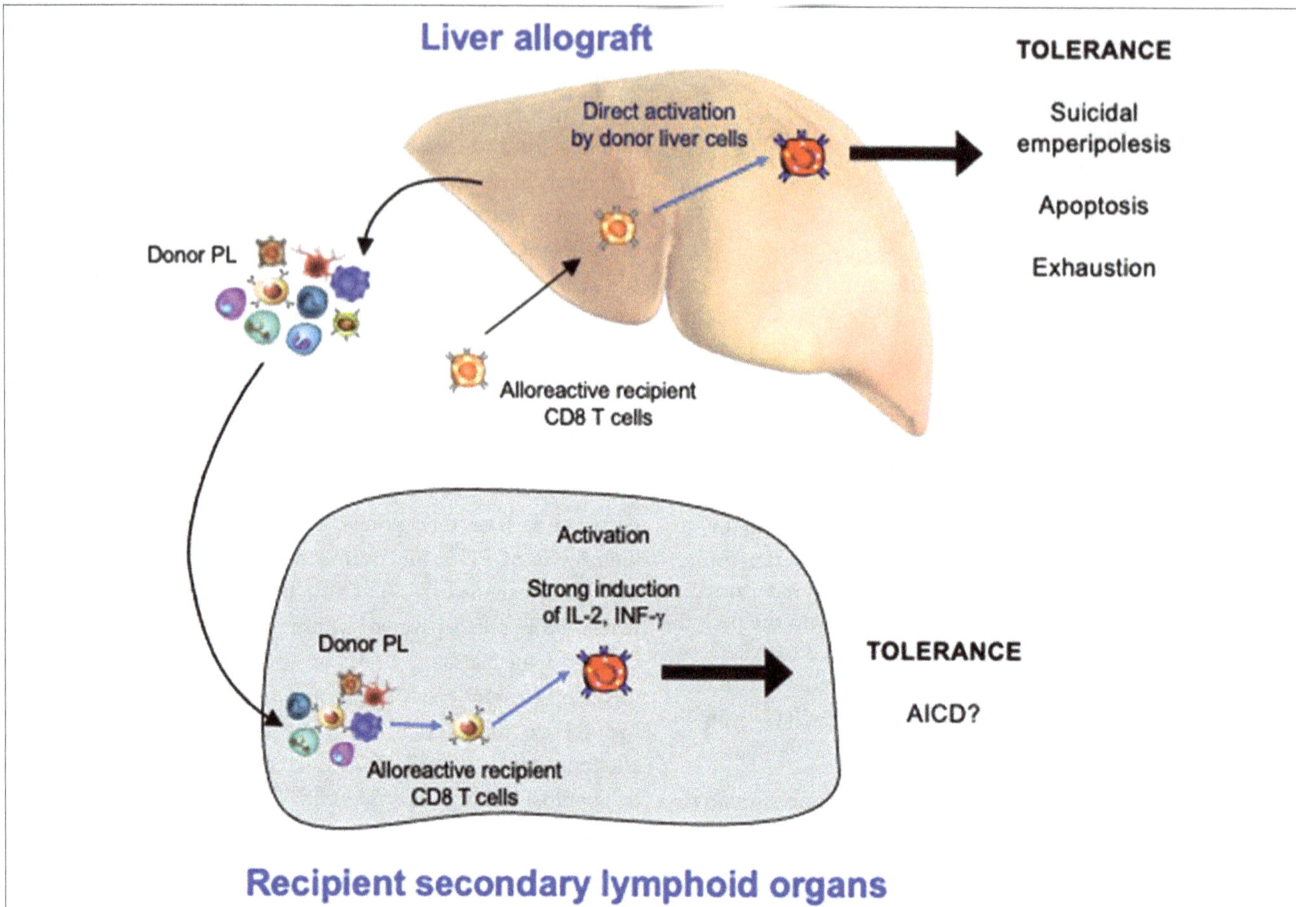

FIGURE 1 | The induction phase of liver transplant tolerance: pathways of alloreactive CD8 T cell silencing in recipient secondary lymphoid organs and within the hepatic allograft. PL, passenger leukocytes; AICD, activation induced cell death.

immunosuppressive therapy in human transplantation which may blunt or inhibit such a phenotype, as discussed below.

One of the controversies regarding the induction of LT tolerance has been the role played by regulatory T cells (Tregs). Depletion of recipient $CD25^+CD4^+$ T cells at 100 days post liver transplantation (62) or before transplantation (63) using anti-CD25 mAb induced acute liver allograft rejection suggesting that $CD25^+$ $CD4^+$ Tregs were critical in maintaining tolerance. Some studies have shown that CD8 T cells expressing CD103 and Foxp3 with regulatory function were increased in recipients spontaneously accepting liver grafts suggesting that they might also contribute to the induction of tolerance (64). Kamada et al. described two phases of *in vitro* immunosuppressive activity of splenocytes harvested from tolerant rat recipients of LT, with splenocytes harvested from days 5–28 and from >20 weeks able to suppress mixed lymphocyte reactions, however those obtained during the intervening period lacked such activity (65). More recent studies have demonstrated that splenocytes from long term tolerant animals were able to induce liver transplant tolerance, however transfer of splenocytes harvested at 30 days did not (8). Thus, the appearance of early Tregs and any role that they may play in the induction of spontaneous tolerance has been under significant scrutiny.

An important role for early Treg induction in liver tolerance has been suggested by the success of a novel protocol used by Todo and colleagues in human live donation LT (66, 67). This protocol involved the generation of donor Tregs *in vitro*, followed by their transfer to the recipient at day 13 post-transplant. Successful withdrawal of immunosuppression in 7 of 10 patients without any rejection suggested that tolerance had indeed been induced (operational tolerance). However, whether such cells were acting to induce tolerance during the early induction phase or at later time points cannot be ascertained. Furthermore, it is unclear whether immunological events following transfer of *in vitro* generated Tregs mirror those developing in the early phase post-LT in the absence of administration of such cellular therapy.

It should also be pointed out that in humans immune-ablative induction protocols followed by early cessation of immunosuppression have not been successful in tolerance induction. Indeed, in one study a significant increase in allograft rejection was seen and the study was prematurely terminated (68). Such results support the concept that some form of immune

TABLE 1 | Summarizing the main features of the induction phase of liver transplant tolerance.

Time after liver transplantation	Events occurring in SLOs	Events occurring in the liver
0–12 h	• The large bulk of PL enter SLOs within the first few hours after the surgery • PL activate alloreactive CD8 T cells located in SLOs	• Most PLs rapidly leave the liver except for NKT cells and some NK cells • Primary CD8 T cell activation by liver cells • Clearance of activated CD8 T cells by Suicidal emperipolesis?
12–24 h	• PL activated alloreactive CD8 T cells express cytokines (IL-2, IFN-γ) and start to proliferate	• CD8 T cells not cleared by suicidal emperipolesis express cytokines (IL-2, IFNγ)
24–48 h	• PL activated alloreactive CD8 T cells express cytokines (IL-2, IFN-γ) die by AICD	• CD8 T cells that were not cleared by suicidal emperipolesis fail to survive and die by neglect
After 48 h	• Some T cells survive AICD and leave SLOs	• T cells survive AICD in SLOs enter the liver but become rapidly exhausted and silenced
After 30 days		• Regulatory T cells start to be generated and maintain tolerance

activation is also required for human liver tolerance, and that protocols that allow for this may be necessary to manipulate the balance of tolerance/rejection at an early stage.

The Induction Phase—Comparison With the Maintenance Phase in Animals

Although there is no evidence that Tregs can induce LT tolerance, it has been well demonstrated in animal models that once tolerance is established Treg cells can transfer tolerance and prevent rejection (45). This usually takes about 70–100 days post LT to uniformly occur.

The Induction Phase—Comparison With the Maintenance Phase in Humans

As mentioned previously, the induction phase in humans has been sparsely investigated, and studies have been complicated by early immunosuppression used extensively in human transplantation. In contrast, several studies of functional tolerance, or so called "operational tolerance," have been undertaken. This is defined as a subgroup of patients who, upon withdrawal of immunosuppression, do not reject their liver allografts. It is rather uncommon if the frequency is defined from the time of transplant itself, occurring in probably around 5% of patients. However, if patients are carefully selected by criteria including long duration post-transplant, already on minimal immunosuppression, pediatric recipients, and no autoimmune disease then between 20 and 40% of long term LT patients can be successfully withdrawn from immunosuppression (69). More recently, the use of liver biopsy, in particular the finding of normal histology (70) and absence of donor specific antibodies are also thought to be important predictors, although the later factor remains less well delineated (71).

Patients under study for predictors of operational tolerance have displayed various molecular and cellular signals associated with peripheral blood leucocytes and with the liver itself. Predictive biomarkers of liver transplant tolerance associated operational tolerance with an increase in peripheral blood Tregs, NK cells, or γδ T cells (72) as well as genes expressed by these cell types such as sentrin-specific peptidase 6 (SENP6) and Fem-1 homolog C (FEM1C) (73, 74). In one study an increase in gene expression associated with iron metabolism was seen in the liver (75). However, the findings of such studies have been inconsistent, and there is currently an immunosuppression withdrawal trial underway using one particular molecular marker subset as a starting point for withdrawal (76). It is likely that Treg cells will be important for successful withdrawal of immunosuppression in this phase, although this still remains to be defined. Some data suggest that long term use of mTOR inhibitors may favor the emergence of Tregs thus potentially promoting the maintenance phase of tolerance (77). The exact details of these approaches are outlined in other article(s) of in this edition.

CONCLUSION

Experimentally, it is clear that the induction phase post-LT is associated with, and probably causative of, LT tolerance via immune activation events. If the same applies in humans, then current practices of early use of high dose immunosuppression in clinical LT may inhibit the induction of such early immune activation processes and thus be detrimental to tolerance induction. This concern is supported by the failure of at least one human trial of early immunosuppression withdrawal after ablative immune induction.

In conclusion, animal models have enabled us to understand the induction phase of liver tolerance, whilst new studies in humans have revealed significant insights into the maintenance phase. The challenge is to understand how these are linked, so that we may identify potential tolerant patients much earlier in their post-transplant course and modify immunosuppression accordingly. This would have the maximum benefit of decreasing immunosuppression related comorbidities, rather than waiting for many years, after which such co morbidities may not be reversible.

AUTHOR CONTRIBUTIONS

All authors listed have made a substantial, direct and intellectual contribution to the work, and approved it for publication.

REFERENCES

1. Calne RY, Sells RA, Pena JR, Davis DR, Millard PR, Herbertson BM, et al. Induction of immunological tolerance by porcine liver allografts. *Nature*. (1969) 223:472–6. doi: 10.1038/223472a0

2. Sugioka A, Morita M, Fujita J, Hasumi A, and Shiroishi T. Graft acceptance and tolerance induction in mouse liver transplantation using wild mice. *Transplant Proc.* (2001) 33:137–9. doi: 10.1016/S0041-1345(00)01942-4
3. Houssin D, Gigou M, Franco D, Bismuth H, Charpentier B, Lang P, et al. Specific transplantation tolerance induced by spontaneously tolerated liver allograft in inbred strains of rats. *Transplantation.* (1980) 29:418–9. doi: 10.1097/00007890-198005000-00015
4. Kamada N, Brons G, Davies HS. Fully allogeneic liver grafting in rats induces a state of systemic nonreactivity to donor transplantation antigens. *Transplantation.* (1980) 29:429–31. doi: 10.1097/00007890-198005000-00021
5. Kamada N. The immunology of experimental liver transplantation in the rat. *Immunology.* (1985) 55:369–89.
6. Perry I, Neuberger J. Immunosuppression: towards a logical approach in liver transplantation. *Clin Exp Immunol.* (2005) 139:2–10. doi: 10.1111/j.1365-2249.2005.02662.x
7. Kamada N. Cellular basis of transplantation tolerance induced by liver grafting in the rat. Extent of clonal deletion among thoracic duct lymphocytes, spleen and lymph node cells. *Transplantation.* (1988) 46:165–7. doi: 10.1097/00007890-198807000-00034
8. Asakura H, Ku G, Kataoka M, Flye MW. Regulatory cells develop after the spontaneous acceptance of rat liver allografts. *Surgery.* (2004) 136:532–6. doi: 10.1016/j.surg.2004.05.036
9. Sun J, Matsumoto Y, McCaughan GW, Gallagher ND, Sheil AG, Bishop GA. Levels of cytokine expression in rat liver allograft rejection compared to allograft tolerance. *Transplant Proc.* (1992) 5:2309.
10. Sharland A, Shastry S, Wang C, Rokahr K, Sun J, Sheil AG, et al. Kinetics of intragraft cytokine expression, cellular infiltration, and cell death in rejection of renal allografts compared with acceptance of liver allografts in a rat model: early activation and apoptosis is associated with liver graft acceptance. *Transplantation.* (1998) 65:1370–7. doi: 10.1097/00007890-199805270-00015
11. Dresske B, Lin X, Huang DS, Zhou X, Fandrich F. Spontaneous tolerance: experience with the rat liver transplant model. *Hum Immunol.* (2002) 63:853–61. doi: 10.1016/S0198-8859(02)00448-2
12. Starzl TE, Ramos H, Zeevi A, Ricordi C, Ildstad S, Murase N, et al. Systemic chimerism in human female recipients of male livers. *Lancet.* (1992) 340:876–7. doi: 10.1016/0140-6736(92)93286-V
13. Wood K, Sachs DH. Chimerism and transplantation tolerance: cause and effect. *Immunol Today.* (1996) 17:584–7; discussion 588. doi: 10.1016/S0167-5699(96)10069-4
14. Dai H, Zheng Y, Thomson AW, Rogers NM. Transplant Tolerance Induction: Insights From the Liver. *Front Immunol.* (2020) 11:1044. doi: 10.3389/fimmu.2020.01044
15. Bishop GA, Sun J, DeCruz DJ, Rokahr KL, Sedgwick JD, Sheil AG, et al. Tolerance to rat liver allografts. III Donor cell migration and tolerance-associated cytokine production in peripheral lymphoid tissues. *J Immunol.* (1996) 156:4925–31.
16. Sun J, McCaughan GW, Gallagher ND, Sheil AG, Bishop GA. Deletion of spontaneous rat liver allograft acceptance by donor irradiation. *Transplantation.* (1995) 60:233–6. doi: 10.1097/00007890-199508000-00004
17. Meyer D, Loffeler S, Otto C, Czub S, Gassel HJ, Timmermann W, et al. Donor-derived alloantigen-presenting cells persist in the liver allograft during tolerance induction. *Transpl Int.* (2000) 13:12–20. doi: 10.1111/j.1432-2277.2000.tb01030.x
18. Sriwatanawongsa V, Davies HS, Calne RY. The essential roles of parenchymal tissues and passenger leukocytes in the tolerance induced by liver grafting in rats. *Nat Med.* (1995) 1:428–32. doi: 10.1038/nm0595-428
19. Chiba S, Goto S, Shimizu Y, Vari F, Lord R, Edwards-Smith C, et al. The characterization of reconstituted passenger leukocytes on the induction of tolerance in rat liver transplantation. *Trans Int.* (1997) 10:350–6. doi: 10.1111/j.1432-2277.1997.tb00928.x
20. Kreisel D, Petrowsky H, Krasinskas AM, Krupnick AS, Szeto WY, McLean AD, et al. The role of passenger leukocyte genotype in rejection and acceptance of rat liver allografts. *Transplantation.* (2002) 73:1501–7. doi: 10.1097/00007890-200205150-00022
21. Huang L, Soldevila G, Leeker M, Flavell R, Crispe IN. The liver eliminates T cells undergoing antigen-triggered apoptosis *in vivo*. *Immunity.* (1994) 1:741–9. doi: 10.1016/S1074-7613(94)80016-2
22. Crispe IN, Dao T, Klugewitz K, Mehal WZ, Metz DP. The liver as a site of T-cell apoptosis: graveyard, or killing field? *Immunol Rev.* (2000) 174:47–62. doi: 10.1034/j.1600-0528.2002.017412.x
23. O'Farrelly C, Crispe IN. Prometheus through the looking glass: reflections on the hepatic immune system. *Immunol Today.* (1999) 20:394–8. doi: 10.1016/S0167-5699(99)01518-2
24. Bowen DG, McCaughan GW, Bertolino P. Intrahepatic immunity: a tale of two sites? *Trends Immunol.* (2005) 26:512–7. doi: 10.1016/j.it.2005.08.005
25. Fernandez-Ruiz D, Ng WY, Holz LE, Ma JZ, Zaid A, Wong YC, et al. Liver-resident memory CD8(+) T cells form a front-line defense against malaria liver-stage infection. *Immunity.* (2016) 45:889–902. doi: 10.1016/j.immuni.2016.08.011
26. Keating R, Yue W, Rutigliano JA, So J, Olivas E, Thomas PG, et al. Virus-specific CD8+ T cells in the liver: armed and ready to kill. *J Immunol.* (2007) 178:2737–45. doi: 10.4049/jimmunol.178.5.2737
27. Polakos NK, Klein I, Richter MV, Zaiss DM, Giannandrea M, Crispe IN, et al. Early intrahepatic accumulation of CD8+ T cells provides a source of effectors for nonhepatic immune responses. *J Immunol.* (2007) 179:201–10. doi: 10.4049/jimmunol.179.1.201
28. Holz LE, Prier JE, Freestone D, Steiner TM, English K, Johnson DN, et al. CD8(+) T cell activation leads to constitutive formation of liver tissue-resident memory T cells that seed a large and flexible niche in the liver. *Cell Rep.* (2018) 25:68–79 e64. doi: 10.1016/j.celrep.2018.08.094
29. Tay SS, Wong YC, McDonald DM, Wood NA, Roediger B, Sierro F, et al. Antigen expression level threshold tunes the fate of CD8 T cells during primary hepatic immune responses. *Proc Natl Acad Sci USA.* (2014) 111:E2540–2549. doi: 10.1073/pnas.1406674111
30. Bertolino P, McCaughan GW, Bowen DG. Role of primary intrahepatic T-cell activation in the 'liver tolerance effect'. *Immunol Cell Biol.* (2002) 80:84–92. doi: 10.1046/j.0818-9641.2001.01048.x
31. Bertolino P, Heath WR, Hardy CL, Morahan G, Miller JF. Peripheral deletion of autoreactive CD8+ T cells in transgenic mice expressing H-2Kb in the liver. *Eur J Immunol.* (1995) 25:1932–42. doi: 10.1002/eji.1830250721
32. Bertolino P, Trescol-Biémont MC, Rabourdin-Combe C. Hepatocytes induce functional activation of naive CD8^{+} T lymphocytes but fail to promote survival. *Eur J Immunol.* (1998) 28:221–236. doi: 10.1002/(SICI)1521-4141(199801)28:01<221::AID-IMMU221>3.0.CO;2-F
33. Bertolino P, Trescol-Biemont MC, Thomas J, Fazekas de St Groth B, Pihlgren M, Marvel J, et al. Death by neglect as a deletional mechanism of peripheral tolerance. *Int Immunol.* (1999) 11:1225–38. doi: 10.1093/intimm/11.8.1225
34. Bertolino P, Bowen DG, McCaughan GW, Fazekas De St Groth B. Antigen-specific primary activation of CD8+ T cells within the liver. *J Immunol.* (2001) 166:5430–8. doi: 10.4049/jimmunol.166.9.5430
35. Bowen DG, Zen M, Holz L, Davis T, McCaughan GW, Bertolino P. The site of primary T cell activation is a determinant of the balance between intrahepatic tolerance and immunity. *J Clin Invest.* (2004) 114:701–12. doi: 10.1172/JCI200421593
36. Warren A, Le Couteur DG, Fraser R, Bowen DG, McCaughan GW, Bertolino P. T lymphocytes interact with hepatocytes through fenestrations in murine liver sinusoidal endothelial cells. *Hepatology.* (2006) 44:1182–90. doi: 10.1002/hep.21378
37. Holz LE, Benseler V, Vo M, McGuffog C, Van Rooijen N, McCaughan GW, et al. Naive CD8 T cell activation by liver bone marrow-derived cells leads to a "neglected" IL-2(low) Bim(high) phenotype, poor CTL function and cell death. *J Hepatol.* (2012) 57:830–6. doi: 10.1016/j.jhep.2012.05.015
38. Lohse AW, Knolle PA, Bilo K, Uhrig A, Waldmann C, Ibe M, et al. Antigen-presenting function and B7 expression of murine sinusoidal endothelial cells and Kupffer cells. *Gastroenterology.* (1996) 110:1175–81. doi: 10.1053/gast.1996.v110.pm8613007
39. Winau F, Hegasy G, Weiskirchen R, Weber S, Cassan C, Sieling PA, et al. Ito cells are liver-resident antigen-presenting cells for activating T cell responses. *Immunity.* (2007) 26:117–29. doi: 10.1016/j.immuni.2006.11.011
40. Limmer A, Ohl J, Kurts C, Ljunggren H-G, Reiss Y, Groettrup M, et al. Efficient presentation of exogenous antigen by liver endothelial cells to CD8^{+} T cells results in antigen-specific T-cell tolerance. *Nat Med.* (2000) 6:1348–54. doi: 10.1038/82161

41. Knolle PA, Schmitt E, Jin S, Germann T, Duchmann R, Hegenbarth S, et al. Induction of cytokine production in naive CD4(+) T cells by antigen-presenting murine liver sinusoidal endothelial cells but failure to induce differentiation toward Th1 cells. *Gastroenterology.* (1999) 116:1428–40. doi: 10.1016/S0016-5085(99)70508-1
42. Elvevold K, Smedsrod B, Martinez I. The liver sinusoidal endothelial cell: a cell type of controversial and confusing identity. *Am J Physiol Gastrointest Liver Physiol.* (2008) 294:G391–400. doi: 10.1152/ajpgi.00167.2007
43. Knolle PA, Limmer A. Neighborhood politics: the immunoregulatory function of organ-resident liver endothelial cells. *Trends Immunol.* (2001) 22:432–7. doi: 10.1016/S1471-4906(01)01957-3
44. Thomson AW, Knolle PA. Antigen-presenting cell function in the tolerogenic liver environment. *Nat Rev Immunol.* (2010) 10:753–66. doi: 10.1038/nri2858
45. Benseler V, McCaughan GW, Schlitt HJ, Bishop GA, Bowen DG, Bertolino P. The liver: a special case in transplantation tolerance. *Sem Liver Dis.* (2007) 27:194–213. doi: 10.1055/s-2007-979471
46. Tay SS, Lu B, Sierro F, Benseler V, McGuffog CM, Bishop GA, et al. Differential migration of passenger leukocytes and rapid deletion of naive alloreactive CD8 T cells after mouse liver transplantation. *Liver Transpl.* (2013) 19:1224–35. doi: 10.1002/lt.23720
47. Thomas SY, Scanlon ST, Griewank KG, Constantinides MG, Savage AK, Barr KA, et al. PLZF induces an intravascular surveillance program mediated by long-lived LFA-1-ICAM-1 interactions. *J Exp Med.* (2011) 208:1179–88. doi: 10.1084/jem.20102630
48. Bishop GA, Sun J, Sheil AG, McCaughan GW. High-dose/activation-associated tolerance: a mechanism for allograft tolerance. *Transplantation.* (1997) 64:1377–82. doi: 10.1097/00007890-199711270-00001
49. Yan Y, Shastry S, Richards C, Wang C, Bowen DG, Sharland AF, et al. Posttransplant administration of donor leukocytes induces long-term acceptance of kidney or liver transplants by an activation-associated immune mechanism. *J Immunol.* (2001) 166:5258–64. doi: 10.4049/jimmunol.166.8.5258
50. Medawar PB. Immunity to homologous grafted skin; the relationship between the antigens of blood and skin. *Br J Exp Pathol.* (1946) 27:15–24.
51. Lenardo MJ. Interleukin-2 programs mouse alpha beta T lymphocytes for apoptosis. *Nature.* (1991) 353:858–61. doi: 10.1038/353858a0
52. Inaba M, Kurasawa K, Mamura M, Kumano K, Saito Y, Iwamoto I. Primed T cells are more resistant to Fas-mediated activation-induced cell death than naive T cells. *J Immunol.* (1999) 163:1315–20.
53. Zheng L, Fisher G, Miller RE, Peschon J, Lynch DH, Lenardo MJ. Induction of apoptosis in mature T cells by tumour necrosis factor. *Nature.* (1995) 377:348–51. doi: 10.1038/377348a0
54. Sun J, Sheil AG, Wang C, Wang L, Rokahr K, Sharland A, et al. Tolerance to rat liver allografts: IV. Acceptance depends on the quantity of donor tissue and on donor leukocytes. *Transplantation.* (1996) 62:1725–30. doi: 10.1097/00007890-199612270-00005
55. Benseler V, Warren A, Vo M, Holz LE, Tay SS, Le Couteur DG, et al. Hepatocyte entry leads to degradation of autoreactive CD8 T cells. *Proc Natl Acad Sci USA.* (2011) 108:16735–40. doi: 10.1073/pnas.1112251108
56. Sierro F, Tay SS, Warren A, Le Couteur DG, McCaughan GW, Bowen DG, et al. Suicidal emperipolesis: a process leading to cell-in-cell structures, T cell clearance and immune homeostasis. *Curr Mol Med.* (2015) 15:819–27. doi: 10.2174/1566524015666151026102143
57. Holz LE, Benseler V, Bowen DG, Bouillet P, Strasser A, O'Reilly L, et al. Intrahepatic murine CD8 T-cell activation associates with a distinct phenotype leading to Bim-dependent death. *Gastroenterology.* (2008) 135:989–97. doi: 10.1053/j.gastro.2008.05.078
58. Benseler V, Tay SS, Bowen DG, Bertolino P. Role of the hepatic parenchyma in liver transplant tolerance: a paradigm revisited. *Dig Dis.* (2011) 29:391–401. doi: 10.1159/000329802
59. Qian S, Lu L, Fu F, Li Y, Li W, Starzl TE, et al. Apoptosis within spontaneously accepted mouse liver allografts: evidence for deletion of cytotoxic T cells and implications for tolerance induction. *J Immunol.* (1997) 158:4654–61.
60. Savage TM, Shonts BA, Lau S, Obradovic A, Robins H, Shaked A, et al. Deletion of donor-reactive T cell clones after human liver transplant. *Am J Transplant.* (2020) 20:538–45. doi: 10.1111/ajt.15592
61. Jonsson JR, Gu W, Vanags DM, Bishop GA, McCaughan GW, Fawcett J, et al. Increased mononuclear cell activation and apoptosis early after human liver transplantation is associated with a reduced frequency of acute rejection. *Liver Transpl.* (2004) 10:397–403. doi: 10.1002/lt.20084
62. Li W, Kuhr CS, Zheng XX, Carper K, Thomson AW, Reyes JD, et al. New insights into mechanisms of spontaneous liver transplant tolerance: the role of Foxp3-expressing CD25+CD4+ regulatory T cells. *Am J Transplant.* (2008) 8:1639–51. doi: 10.1111/j.1600-6143.2008.02300.x
63. Jiang X, Morita M, Sugioka A, Harada M, Kojo S, Wakao H, et al. The importance of CD25+ CD4+ regulatory T cells in mouse hepatic allograft tolerance. *Liver Transpl.* (2006) 12:1112–8. doi: 10.1002/lt.20787
64. Lu L, Yu Y, Li G, Pu L, Zhang F, Zheng S, et al. CD8(+)CD103(+) regulatory T cells in spontaneous tolerance of liver allografts. *Int Immunopharmacol.* (2009) 9:546–8. doi: 10.1016/j.intimp.2009.01.021
65. Yoshimura S, Gotoh S, Kamada N. Immunological tolerance induced by liver grafting in the rat: splenic macrophages and T cells mediate distinct phases of immunosuppressive activity. *Clin Exp Immunol.* (1991) 85:121–7. doi: 10.1111/j.1365-2249.1991.tb05692.x
66. Todo S, Yamashita K. Anti-donor regulatory T cell therapy in liver transplantation. *Hum Immunol.* (2018) 79:288–93. doi: 10.1016/j.humimm.2017.12.010
67. Todo S, Yamashita K, Goto R, Zaitsu M, Nagatsu A, Oura T, et al. A pilot study of operational tolerance with a regulatory T-cell-based cell therapy in living donor liver transplantation. *Hepatology.* (2016) 64:632–43. doi: 10.1002/hep.28459
68. Benitez CE, Puig-Pey I, Lopez M, Martinez-Llordella M, Lozano JJ, Bohne F, et al. ATG-Fresenius treatment and low-dose tacrolimus: results of a randomized controlled trial in liver transplantation. *Am J Transplant.* (2010) 10:2296–304. doi: 10.1111/j.1600-6143.2010.03164.x
69. Alex Bishop G, Bertolino PD, Bowen DG, McCaughan GW. Tolerance in liver transplantation. *Best Pract Res Clin Gastroenterol.* (2012) 26:73–84. doi: 10.1016/j.bpg.2012.01.003
70. Feng S, Bucuvalas J. Tolerance after liver transplantation: where are we? *Liver Transpl.* (2017) 23:1601–14. doi: 10.1002/lt.24845
71. Feng S, Demetris AJ, Spain KM, Kanaparthi S, Burrell BE, Ekong UD, et al. Five-year histological and serological follow-up of operationally tolerant pediatric liver transplant recipients enrolled in WISP-R. *Hepatology.* (2017) 65:647–60. doi: 10.1002/hep.28681
72. Martinez-Llordella M, Lozano JJ, Puig-Pey I, Orlando G, Tisone G, Lerut J, et al. Using transcriptional profiling to develop a diagnostic test of operational tolerance in liver transplant recipients. *J Clin Invest.* (2008) 118:2845–57. doi: 10.1172/JCI35342
73. Perez-Sanz F, Revilla-Nuin B, Martinez-Alarcon L, Herrero JI, Ramirez P, Pons JA, et al. Tolerance biomarkers in liver transplantation: independent external validation of the predictive strength of SENP6 and FEM1C gene expression. *Transplantation.* (2019) 103:1887–92. doi: 10.1097/TP.0000000000002587
74. Li L, Wozniak LJ, Rodder S, Heish S, Talisetti A, Wang Q, et al. A common peripheral blood gene set for diagnosis of operational tolerance in pediatric and adult liver transplantation. *Am J Transplant.* (2012) 12:1218–28. doi: 10.1111/j.1600-6143.2011.03928.x
75. Bohne F, Martinez-Llordella M, Lozano JJ, Miquel R, Benitez C, Londono MC, et al. Intra-graft expression of genes involved in iron homeostasis predicts the development of operational tolerance in human liver transplantation. *J Clin Invest.* (2012) 122:368–82. doi: 10.1172/JCI59411
76. Tran L, Humar A. Tolerance studies in liver transplantation: are we fooling ourselves? *Curr Opin Organ Transplant.* (2020) 25:151–7. doi: 10.1097/MOT.0000000000000738
77. Ghazal K, Stenard F, Dahlqvist G, Barjon C, Aoudjehane L, Scatton O, et al. Treatment with mTOR inhibitors after liver transplantation enables a sustained increase in regulatory T-cells while preserving their suppressive capacity. *Clin Res Hepatol Gastroenterol.* (2018) 42:237–44. doi: 10.1016/j.clinre.2017.10.001

3

The Future of Regulatory T Cell Therapy: Promises and Challenges of Implementing CAR Technology

Yasmin R. Mohseni[1], Sim L. Tung[1], Caroline Dudreuilh[1], Robert I. Lechler[1], Gilbert O. Fruhwirth[2] and Giovanna Lombardi[1*]*

[1] Peter Gorer Department of Immunobiology, MRC Centre for Transplantation, School of Immunology and Microbial Science, King's College London (KCL), Guy's Hospital, London, United Kingdom, [2] Imaging Therapies and Cancer Group, Department of Imaging Chemistry and Biology, School of Biomedical Engineering and Imaging Sciences, King's College London, London, United Kingdom

***Correspondence:**
Yasmin R. Mohseni
yasmin.mohseni@kcl.ac.uk
Giovanna Lombardi
giovanna.lombardi@kcl.ac.uk

Cell therapy with polyclonal regulatory T cells (Tregs) has been translated into the clinic and is currently being tested in transplant recipients and patients suffering from autoimmune diseases. Moreover, building on animal models, it has been widely reported that antigen-specific Tregs are functionally superior to polyclonal Tregs. Among various options to confer target specificity to Tregs, genetic engineering is a particularly timely one as has been demonstrated in the treatment of hematological malignancies where it is in routine clinical use. Genetic engineering can be exploited to express chimeric antigen receptors (CAR) in Tregs, and this has been successfully demonstrated to be robust in preclinical studies across various animal disease models. However, there are several caveats and a number of strategies should be considered to further improve on targeting, efficacy and to understand the *in vivo* distribution and fate of CAR-Tregs. Here, we review the differing approaches to confer antigen specificity to Tregs with emphasis on CAR-Tregs. This includes an overview and discussion of the various approaches to improve CAR-Treg specificity and therapeutic efficacy as well as addressing potential safety concerns. We also discuss different imaging approaches to understand the *in vivo* biodistribution of administered Tregs. Preclinical research as well as suitability of methodologies for clinical translation are discussed.

Keywords: Tregs (regulatory T cells), transplantation, CAR (chimeric antigen receptor), cell therapy, autoimmunity, regulatory, antigen specific

INTRODUCTION

Regulatory T cells (Tregs) are a subset of T cells that function to maintain homeostasis and prevent autoimmunity (1). Tregs make up 5–10% of the $CD4^+$ T cell population (2) and are characterized by co-expression of CD4, CD25, the transcription factor Forkhead box protein 3 (FOXP3) and low levels of CD127. Although conventional human T cells (Tconv) can transiently express FOXP3, high FOXP3 levels and demethylation of the Treg specific demethylated region (TSDR), a conserved region within the *FOXP3* gene, are distinct features of Tregs (3). The importance of FOXP3 in Tregs is supported by the evidence that mutations in the *FOXP3* locus lead to Treg dysfunction and severe autoimmunity, as was first identified in *Scurfy* mutant mice (4) and the immunodysregulation polyendocrinopathy enteropathy X-linked syndrome (IPEX) in humans (5).

Tregs are divided in thymus-derived (tTregs) and peripheral-derived Tregs (pTregs) (6). During T cell development, those naïve $CD4^+$ T cells receiving an intermediate TCR signal are driven to differentiate into Tregs—the quantitative difference in strength of such signal is thought to determine Tconv cell or Treg lineage commitment (7). Peripheral Tregs develop when $FOXP3^-$ Tconv encounter repeated stimulation to non-self antigens or receive inadequate co-stimulation, as well as exposure to IL-10 and TGF-β (8).

Tregs suppress the immune system by different mechanisms including contact-dependent mechanisms, through CTLA-4 engagement for example, and contact-independent, such as the release of cytokines e.g., IL-35 or IL-10 [reviewed in (9)]. Given their proven role in preventing autoimmune diseases, Tregs have obvious potential in the promotion of tolerance. Although human Tregs constitute a small proportion of circulating $CD4^+$ T cells, they are attractive candidates for immunotherapeutic purposes given that they can be isolated, manipulated and expanded in large numbers *in vitro*. Tregs can be applied in the treatment of autoimmune diseases and in the prevention of transplant rejection and graft vs. host disease (GvHD).

ADOPTIVE TREG THERAPY: FROM POLYCLONAL TO ANTIGEN SPECIFIC

The first phase I clinical trials investigating the safety of adoptive transfer of Tregs were in the treatment of bone marrow patients to prevent GvHD, NCT00602693 (10–12). These trials demonstrated the safety and efficacy of Treg therapy. Autologous polyclonal Tregs have been infused in patients with type 1 diabetes (T1D) as well, demonstrating again the safety and feasibility of adoptive Treg therapy in this disease setting [ISRCTN06128462, (13) and NCT02691247, (14)]. Treg therapy has reached the organ transplant arena as well (UMIN-000015789 and NCT02088931) (15, 16). We have demonstrated the safety of adoptively transferred Tregs in two phase I clinical trials in liver (ThRIL, NCT02166177) and kidney (ONE study, NCT02129881) transplant patients (17, 18).

However, whilst the above clinical studies have shown the potential of polyclonally expanded Tregs, we and others have demonstrated the superiority of antigen-specific Tregs compared to polyclonal Tregs in animal models. Tang et al. successfully isolated and expanded Tregs from a transgenic mouse expressing a TCR specific for an islet antigen, and showed that antigen-specific Tregs prevented and even reversed diabetes in non-obese diabetic mice (19, 20). More recently, human Tregs were modified *in vitro* to generate Tregs specific for donor antigens, by co-culturing Tregs with donor-derived dendritic cells (DCs) or B cells (21, 22). The superiority of donor-specific human Tregs compared to polyclonal Tregs was demonstrated *in vitro* and *in vivo* in a humanized mouse model of human skin transplant (21, 22). Similar results were obtained *in vitro* by Zheng et al. as they demonstrated that mature B cells were better stimulants than immature DCs in generating Tregs expressing higher levels of FOXP3 and CD25, and with superior suppressive capacity (23). Already as part of the ONE Study (NCT02129881) kidney transplant patients have been treated with donor-specific Tregs and additional clinical trials in transplant patients are investigating the use of donor-reactive Tregs [reviewed by (9)].

Evolving from the use of APCs to generate Tregs with specificity for the target antigen, research has shifted toward gene transfer. Wright et al. transduced Tregs with a TCR specific for ovalbumin (OVA) and restricted by the MHC-class II A^b. These Tregs transferred *in vivo* were able to inhibit a well-established antigen induced arthritis in which mice were immunized with methylated BSA (mBSA) followed by intra-articular knee re-challenge with mBSA to induce T cell-mediated tissue damage. The OVA-specific Tregs were able to decrease inflammation to the knee but only when OVA was present (24). In the same study a similar effect was obtained with $CD4^+$ Tconv transduced with the same TCR and FOXP3; engineering $CD4^+$ Tconvs to express FOXP3 endows them with a suppressive function (24). We generated Tregs from C56BL/6 recipient mice specific for donor BALB/c antigen by retroviral transduction of a TCR specific for a peptide derived from MHC-class I K^d and presented by MHC-class II A^b. We demonstrated that Tregs with this specificity contributed to the indefinite survival of BALB/c heart transplants into B6 (25). Brusko et al. transduced human Tregs with a TCR specific for the melanoma antigen tyrosinase and restricted by HLA-A*0201. Tregs were expanded *in vitro* and administered *in vivo* in a tumor model. They were able to inhibit effector T cells leading to tumor growth (26). Hull et al. transduced Tregs with two TCRs isolated from islet-specific and influenza-specific $CD4^+$ T cell clones. The authors showed that the ability of the islet antigen-specific TCRs to induce Treg mediate antigen-specific suppression *in vitro* was significantly lower when compared to what was achieved using TCRs with specificity for viral antigens (27). More recently, Kim et al. transduced Tregs with a TCR specific for myelin basic protein (MBP) isolated from a T cell clone derived from a multiple sclerosis patient (28). These Tregs suppressed MBP-specific T effector *in vitro* and *in vivo* they ameliorated experimental autoimmune encephalitis (EAE) (28).

As an alternative to the use of Tregs as cell therapy, several studies have looked at generating Tregs by manipulating $CD4^+$ Tconv cells to express FOXP3. In hemophilia, up to one third of patients receiving therapeutic factor VIII (FVIII) infusions develop neutralizing antibodies. Herzog et al. transduced $CD4^+$ Tconv with FOXP3 and FVIII. Following administration of these cells to hemophilia A mice, the formation of neutralizing antibodies to FVIII was suppressed (29). In an animal model of type 1 diabetes, Jaeckel et al. transduced islet-specific $CD4^+$ Tconv with FOXP3. These cells were activated in the pancreatic lymph nodes and reversed recent-onset diabetes (30). Beavis et al. showed that the ectopic expression of FOXP3 in pathogenic synovial T cells from rheumatoid arthritis patients attenuated their function (31). Loser et al. showed the efficacy of FOXP3-transduced Tconv in suppressing contact hypersensitivity responses in mice. Moreover, these cells diminished autoimmune dermatitis in CD40L transgenic mice and cleared antinuclear antibodies (32). These studies are seminal demonstrating the acquisition by Tconvs of a suppressive profile, equally research within immunoregulation has lately been more focused toward enhancing Tregs for cell therapy.

An alternative method to confer specificity to Tregs is by transducing these cells with chimeric antigen receptors (CAR). CAR technology offers some advantages over TCR engineering. These include bypassing HLA restriction upon activation of T cells expressing CARs, increased specificity through the requirement of co-receptor signaling, and the targeting flexibility of CARs (any soluble or surface multivalent antigen can serve as target). In the following sections we focus on CARs to enhance Treg therapy.

CHIMERIC ANTIGEN RECEPTORS: LESSONS FROM CANCER THERAPY

CARs have been developed and by now clinically implemented in oncology to treat certain cancers. They represent an approach to fine-tune adoptively transferred therapeutic T cells to target specific antigens by-passing MHC-restriction and thereby enable these therapeutic cells to attack the cancer. CARs are artifical molecules engineered into target cells. They are composed of an extracellular target-recognition domain (e.g., a scFv specific for the target antigen), hinge and transmembrane domains, and intracellular signaling domains to propagate activation signals as a consequence of extracellular target engagement. CARs are less sensitive in response than TCRs due in part to the number of molecules involved in the TCR machinery, i.e., CD4/CD8 co-receptors, immunoreceptor tyrosinase-rich activation motifs (ITAMs), and subunits within the receptor complex (CARs require 100–10,000 molecules per target cell while TCRs need <10 molecules per target cell) but bind with higher affinity than the TCR; although studies have investigated increasing CAR sensitivity by incorporating lower affinity single-chain variable fragment [scFv; (33, 34)].

From CAR-T Cells in Oncology to CAR-Tregs

The first CAR was composed of a CD3ζ chain of the TCR/CD3ζ complex, but T cell activation was neither persistent *in vivo*, nor sustained and the T cells did not proliferate sufficiently (35, 36). Second generation CARs contain an additional intracellular feature, a co-stimulatory domain, which has the purpose to potentiate the signaling response of the CAR. Several co-stimulatory domains including those from CD28, 4-1BB (CD137) and OX40 (CD134) molecules have been explored in CAR-T cell therapy. Third generation CARs are composed of two different co-stimulatory molecules. Indeed it were second generation CARs that led to the breakthrough in cell-based cancer immunotherapy. In 2017, the FDA approved the first clinical products, tisagenlecleucel and axicabtagene ciloleucel—trademarked as Kymriah® and Yescarta—which are autologous CD19b-targeted CAR-T-cell immunotherapies for the treatment of B-cell acute lymphoblastic leukemia and B-cell lymphoma, respectively (37–39). CAR-T immunotherapies have the potential to be curative, but so far not all patients have responded and sometimes the effects were only temporary (39–41). CAR-T cell therapy has been also associated with severe/life-threatening side-effects and fatalities during clinical trials (42, 43). Research into CARs specific for tumor-related antigens in hematological malignancies paved the way for the application of CARs in immunoregulation. CAR-T cells have been already applied to treat autoimmune disease. In an animal model of pemphigus vulgaris, which is a rare severe autoimmune disease in which blisters of varying sizes break out on the skin and mucous membranes, chimeric auto-antibody receptor (CAAR)-T cells were generated with specificity for the keratinocyte adhesion protein Dsg3 (44). The CAAR-T cells exhibited specific cytotoxicity to anti-Dsg B cells *in vivo* without off-target toxicity (44). Although engineering CAAR-T cells may be effective in inhibiting some autoimmune diseases, Tregs can also be applied due to their powerful immunosuppressive and tolerance-promoting properties.

Tregs have been transduced to express CARs and tested in pre-clinical models of autoimmunity, GvHD and transplantation as well as colitis. Elinav et al. generated a transgenic mouse whose T cells including the Tregs expressed a CAR specific for 2,4,6-trinitrophenol. The adoptive transfer of CAR-Tregs to wild-type mice suffering 2,4,6-trinitrobenzenesulfonic acid-induced colitis was associated with significant amelioration of colitis and improved survival (45). The same group generated Tregs expressing a CAR specific for the human carcinoembryonic antigen (CEA). These Tregs markedly suppressed the severity of colitis in the CEA transgenic mouse, CEABAC, where colitis was induced by transfer of effector T cells specific for CEA (46). Another study used a CEA transgenic mouse to show that CEA-specific CAR-Tregs can inhibit allergic airway inflammation (47). More recently, Tenspolde et al. generated CAR-Tregs specific for insulin but despite them proliferating in response to insulin and being suppressive *in vitro*, these CAR-Tregs did not prevent spontaenous diabetes in mice; interestingly these cells persisted up to 4 months post adoptive transfer (48). Furthermore, in a mouse model of hemophilia A, Zhang et al. created Tregs expressing a B cell-targeting antibody receptor (BAR) containing the immunodominant FVIII C2 or A2 domains. The BAR-Tregs completely prevented anti-FVIII antibody development in FVIII-immunized mice. They also demonstrated a direct effect on FVIII-specific B cells (49).

In transplantation, we and others have generated Tregs expressing an HLA-A2-specific CAR (A2-CAR-Tregs) (50–52). We have shown that A2-CAR-Tregs were functionally superior compared to polyclonal Tregs *in vitro* and *in vivo* in a humanized mouse model of BRG mice bearing a human skin transplant reconstituted with 5:1 PBMCs to CAR-Tregs, assessed by histological analysis 5 weeks post adoptive transfer (51). Noyan et al. also demonstrated the efficacy of an A2-CAR-Tregs in inducing indefinite survival of allogeneic human skin transplants in a humanized mouse model of NRG mice injected intraperitoneally with 7.5:1 PBMCs to A2-CAR-Tregs and graft survival was assessed (52). Similar $A2^+$CAR-Tregs were also shown to ameliorate xenogeneic GvHD (50). Lately, the Levings group produced a panel of humanized HLA-A2 CAR-Tregs and developed a method to map the specificity of CARs, showing that humanization reduced HLA-A cross-reactivity (53). Recently, the same group also investigated the ability of murine HLA-A2 CAR-Tregs to prevent allograft rejection in immunocompetent mice (54). The results showed that these Tregs prolonged skin allograft survival and humural alloresponses but not in presensitised mice, suggesting HLA-A2 CAR-Tregs are unable to inhibit memory T or B cell responses (54).

In the following sections we review the challenges for CAR-Treg therapy and discuss ways to improve CAR-Treg function, safety and specificity for clinical applications.

CAR Co-stimulatory Endodomain Functions in T Cells

Past studies have focused on optimizing the CAR co-stimulatory endodomain design to provide robust CAR-T cells for fighting cancer (55) of which a wide variety had been tested. For example, CAR co-stimulatory endodomains tested in T cells in addition to CD28 include 4-1BB, OX40, inducible T cell co-stimulator (ICOS) and CD27. Zhang et al. reported that 4-1BB co-stimulation plays an important role for memory $CD8^+$ T cell proliferation *ex vivo* and is superior to CD28 co-stimulation in terms of generating antigen-specific $CD8^+$ T cell (56). Transduction of $CD4^+$ (57) and of a mixture of $CD4^+$ and $CD8^+$ (1:1 ratio) (58) T cells with a CAR construct incorporating 4-1BB resulted in augmented T cell longevity. This was due to 4-1BB co-stimulation via the CAR decreasing the exhaustion rate of T cells induced by tonic CAR signaling (57). In another study, Li et al. showed that CAR $CD4^+$ and $CD8^+$ T cells with 4-1BB co-stimulatory endodomain improved T cell function via the NF-κB signaling pathway. Compared to the CD28 co-stimulatory domain, 4-1BB was more associated with the upregulation of anti-apoptotic proteins, which might explain their function in prolonging T cell longevity (59). Whilst OX40 activity enhanced $CD4^+$ and $CD8^+$ T cell expansion and survival, it also blocked thymic $CD4^+$ Treg activity and antagonized the generation of inducible $CD4^+$ Tregs (60–62). However, OX40 activity upregulated anti-apoptotic Bcl-2 family members including Bcl-xL, Bcl-2 and Bfl-l and molecules involved in the cell cycle such as survivin and aurora B kinase (63–65). Additionally, Hombach et al. found that $CD4^+$ T cells transduced with a CAR containing an OX40 endodomain abrogated IL-10 secretion, even in conjunction with a CD28 co-stimulation domain, without impairing the other Teff functions, tipping the balance against suppression in cancer (66). Prior to that, the authors investigated the effect of OX40, 4-1BB, and CD28 CAR endodomains in $CD4^+$ and $CD8^+$ T cells, and determined that CD28 was the most potent at initiating a T cell response, and OX40 and 4-1BB sustained the response with OX40 outperforming the other two for the most prolonged time (67). Another co-stimulatory molecule expressed by T cells is ICOS, which is essential for T cell activation and proliferation (68). ICOS has a significant homology to CD28 and CTLA-4 (69, 70) but is not constitutively expressed on resting T cells but upregulated upon TCR and/or CD28 engagement (69, 71). Guedan et al. demonstrated that ICOS expression via CAR $CD4^+$ and $CD8^+$ T cells enhanced anti-tumor activity and promoted cell survival longer than 4-1BB or CD28 CAR-T cells (72). CD27 is essential for $CD4^+$ T cell functions such as promoting antigen-specific cell expansion of naïve T cells and the generation of memory T cells (73). CD27 co-stimulation via CAR $CD4^+$ and $CD8^+$ T cells upregulates anti-apoptotic Bcl-XL protein expression and resistance to antigen-induced apoptosis, leading to increased numerical expansion although it underwent equal cell division without CD27 (CD3ζ alone). CD27 CAR-T cells may be better than CD28 CAR-T cells due to enhanced survival and accumulation thus quantitatively increased response (74).

However, whether expression of these co-stimulatory endodomains via CARs on Tregs enhances their function in a similar manner to those found in CAR-T cells is still to be elucidated.

CLINICAL PRODUCTS OF CAR-T

Engineering CAR-Tregs destined for the clinic involves different stages in the GMP facility that need to be optimized. Currently, GMP protocols rely on either magnetic isolation of total $CD4^+CD25^+$ Treg populations, or fluorescence-activated cell sorted (FACS) (75). It is advisable that for the generation of CAR-Tregs the Tregs need to be highly pure to avoid any expansion of "contaminating" Teff. Delivering the CAR to the Tregs involves viral-based transfer (i.e., lentivirus or retrovirus) and although to date no safety concerns have been reported with genetically engineered T cells, using non-viral vehicles have been gaining traction, such as transposon/transposases (i.e., Sleeping beauty, *piggyBac* transposon) or gene-editing tools which will also be discussed (76). With respect to expansion, protocols already developed for polyclonal Treg infusion can be employed for CAR-Tregs. Alternatively, semi-automatic systems employed in CAR-T cell development such as rocking-motion bioreactors and static culture bags can be optimized for CAR Treg expansion (77). The number of Tregs needed for therapy remains unclear and the doses of administered Tregs varied in different trials. We have injected polyclonal Tregs ranging from 10^5 to 10^7 cells/kg bodyweight in the ThRIL and the ONE Studies (17, 18) The prediction is that fewer numbers of CAR-Tregs would be needed, although solid organ transplant trials employing antigen-specific Tregs have ranged up to 9×10^8 cells [for more details please refer to (9)].

ENHANCING CAR-TREGS

Engineering CAR-Tregs for clinical applications include boosting their potency, persistence, and safety. Given that CARs are composed of building blocks, modifying the scFv targeting moiety, or the intracellular co-stimulatory signaling domain has been a focus, and will be discussed herein. Additional payloads to the construct such as including safety switches or *in vivo* tracking modalities like imaging tracers are also discussed.

Like conventional T cells, Tregs express an array of different stimulatory and inhibitory receptors (78). However, the function of each of these receptors in Tregs may be different compared to conventional T cells. Due to the various properties of different co-stimulatory molecules, it is unlikely that one particular co-stimulatory molecule can serve all therapeutically required purposes for CAR-Treg therapy. Therefore, it is likely that for optimal function and persistence of therapeutic CAR-Tregs will be different, perhaps simultaneous co-stimulation signals are required, and possibly at different time points.

Optimizing CAR-Tregs for Universal Recognition and Function

Most of the available studies in pre-clinical models of diseases have been focusing on mono-specific CAR-Tregs. Increasing the specificity of CAR-Tregs could boost their therapeutic efficacy, coined with the added advantage of Tregs functioning indirectly through bystander suppression. Different methods of implementing universal recognition of CAR-Tregs are reviewed.

The first option is to infuse a pool of CAR-Tregs with different specificities (**Figure 1A**). This has been tested by pooling monospecific CAR-T cells targeting CD19/CD123 for B-ALL and human epidermal growth factor receptor-2 (HER2)/IL-13Rα2 for glioblastoma (79–81). However, this is logistically challenging, as expansion of autologous CAR-Tregs specific for different target antigens would be limited by the number of autologous Tregs available and the high numbers of antigens to target. Therefore, combinatorial antigen strategies or dual CAR-T cells have been developed (**Figure 1B**) using cells transduced with two different CARs with different antigen specificities and signaling domains (79, 80, 82, 83). The dual CAR-T cells were more efficient than pooled CAR-T cells in preventing antigen escape and demonstrated increased anti-tumor efficacy (79). Bi-specific CARs (or Tandem CAR) targeting two different antigens can also be used (**Figure 1C**) (81, 84, 85), but limitations include mouse scFv immunogenicity, the cross-pairing of the variable light and heavy chains between different scFvs and limited viral vector package size (86). Developing a modular or universal CAR (UniCAR; **Figure 1D**) where the CAR utilizes a soluble connecting molecule to engage the antigen of interest is also another strategy (87). Cells of interest are indirectly connected to the UniCAR through a distinct targeting module, called CAR-adaptors [*cf.* (88)]. Therefore, a tailored control of the Treg activity is possible, as the activation of the UniCAR-Tregs is strictly dependent of the targeting module and changing the targeting module opens to universal applications. Koristka et al. showed that Tregs derived from patients with autoimmune conditions were successfully engineered with UniCARs with 4-1BB/CD3ζ intracellular domains and these UniCAR-Tregs were able to suppress patient-derived effector cell functions, as determined by luciferase-expressing PC3-PSCA cancer cells (87). A FITC-CAR-Treg has been described by Pierini et al., which allows the combination of any monoclonal antibody to the FITC-CAR, facilitating a customisable approach to targeting antigens. The efficacy of the FITC-CAR-Tregs was demonstrated by showing that the injection of H-2D^d-mAbCAR-Tregs into B6 mice increased the survival of BALB/c skin and islet allograft as compared to isotype-mAbCAR-Tregs (89). These last approaches are quite promising and it is the first step toward off-the shelf therapies, which could help improving the deliverability and cost associated with these treatments.

CAR Co-stimulatory Endodomain Function in Tregs

Different co-stimulatory molecules provide different functions. Thus, it is unlikely that one particular co-stimulatory molecule can serve all therapeutic purposes required for CAR-Treg therapy. Therefore, it is likely that for optimal function and persistence of therapeutic CAR-Tregs, a particular co-stimulatory endodomain is chosen and used for the disease or health indication context that best benefits from this co-stimulatory endodomain. In addition, perhaps a combination of co-stimulation signals are required, and possibly at different time points to achieve a robust or efficient CAR-Treg therapy for patients.

The importance of the CD28 co-stimulatory domain in CAR-Tregs has been demonstrated by various groups. MacDonald et al. demonstrated that alloantigen-specific HLA-A2-specific CD28 CAR-Tregs were superior to non-targeted CAR-Tregs at preventing xenogeneic Graft vs. Host disease (GvHD) (50). We used a CAR specific for HLA-A2 that did not have an endodomain signaling component (ΔCAR) but still contained the targeting domain (i.e., ScFV specific for HLA-A2) and showed that although they were less efficient compared to fully functional CD28 CAR-Tregs *in vitro*, in a humanized mouse model of human skin transplant, ΔCAR-Tregs offered greater graft protection than polyclonal Tregs but less than CD28 CAR-Tregs. We concluded that CAR-Treg localization and activation via the TCR are important feature for their immunosuppressive capacity (51). Similarly, Noyan et al. showed that HLA-A2 specific CD28 CAR-Tregs prevented skin allograft rejection in a human skin transplant mouse model (52).

However, other co-stimulatory molecules expressed by Tregs could potentially enhance their function, stability (avoiding conversion to effector cells) and survival. To this end, Boroughs et al. performed a side-by-side comparison of CAR-Tregs expressing CARs encoding CD28 or 4-1BB endodomains. They found that CAR-Tregs with the CD28 endodomain maintained their inhibitory function whereas CAR-Tregs with the 4-1BB endodomain did not. Furthermore, only CD28 CAR-Tregs and not 4-1BB CAR-Tregs were effective suppressors of T-effector cells *in vivo* and were the most effective at inhibiting EGFR-CAR Teff mediated damage on EGFR$^+$ skin transplant (90). This is in contrast with what has been published with CAR-T cells, in which the 4-1BB endodomain but not the CD28 endodomain reduced CAR-T cell exhaustion resulting in enhanced CAR-T cell persistence and longevity (57, 91). Despite several recent successes, the overall understanding of the mechanisms governing Treg stimulation remains somewhat limited. While the evidence base is rapidly increasing, more work will be required to gain insight into these precise mechanisms to generate optimized potent and long-term stable therapeutic Tregs.

ENGINEERING BEYOND THE CAR

Enhancing the Safety Profile of CAR-Tregs

In clinical trials patient safety is of the highest priority. With cellular therapy at the clinical trial phase it is not certain

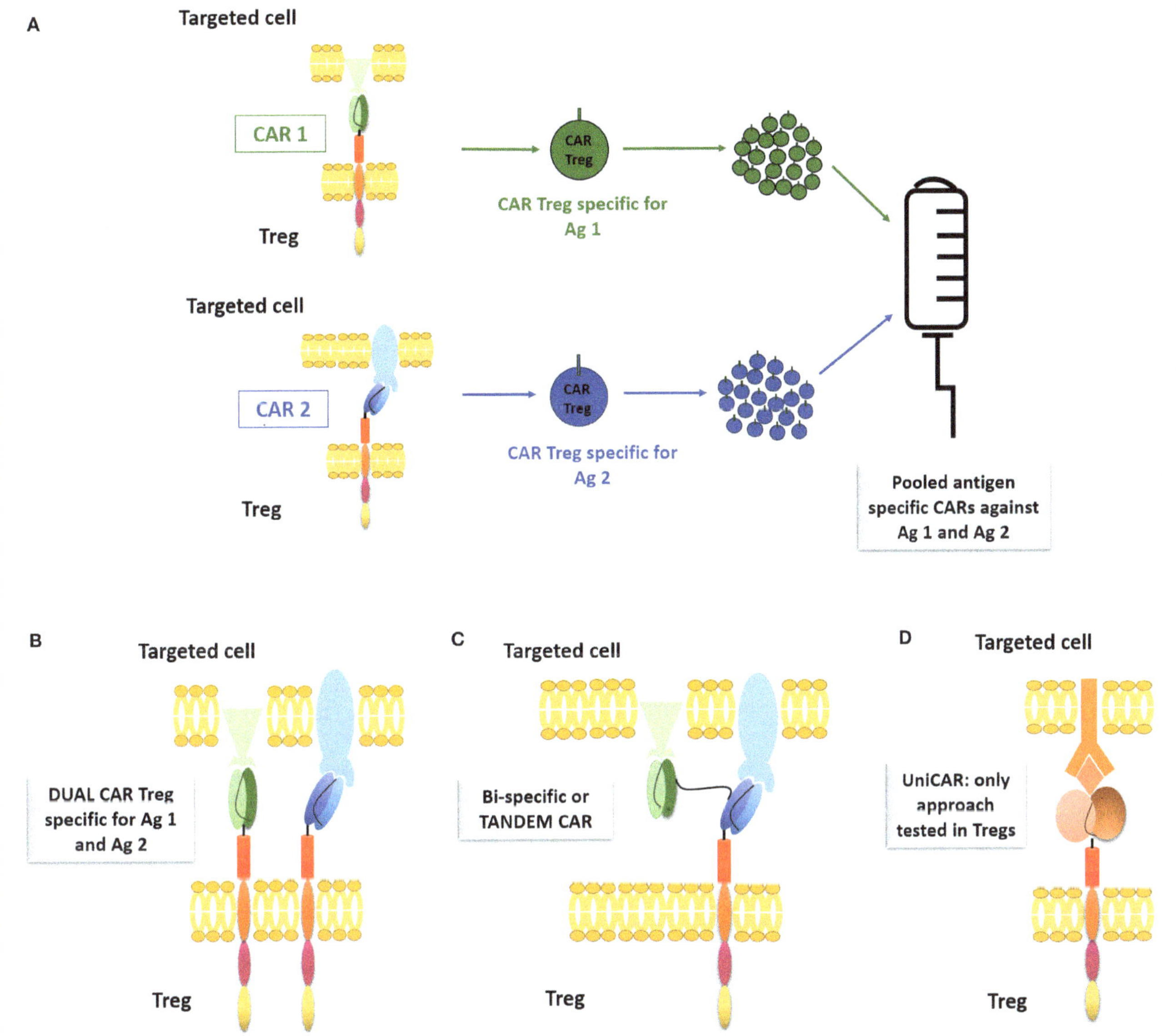

FIGURE 1 | Alternatives to CAR monospecificity. **(A)** Pooled antigen specific CARs against two different antigens. CAR1 targeting Antigen 1 (Ag1), displaying an anti-Ag1 scFV, a CD28 extracellular region, a CD28 transmembrane domain, a CD28 signaling domain and a CD3ζ signaling domain, CAR2 targeting antigen 2 (Ag 2), with anti-Ag2 scFv. **(B)** Dual CAR—two different CARS connecting molecule to interact with the cell of interest. **(C)** Bi-specific or Tandem CAR—CAR able to interact with two different antigens. **(D)** Uni-CAR—using a connecting molecule to interact with the cell of interest. The CAR is displaying an anti-connecting molecule ScFv and the targeted cell has a receptor for the connecting molecule. Only approach tested with Tregs.

whether the therapeutic cells will reach their intended destination within the patient's body and thus off-target effects may occur (92–94). In the context of CAR-Tregs, if it were to function off-target it could ensue a situation in which the patient experiences pan-immunosuppression which leads to a reduced appropriate immune response against opportunistic infections and possibly cancer development. One way to control the life of these injected therapeutic cells in the patient is to include a suicide gene feature within these genetically modified therapeutic cells before injecting them back into the patient. Suicide genes are like a "safety switch" that permits selective death on expressing cells in the event of elevated toxicity by administration of an activating soluble pharmaceutical agent in the patient (92–94). Examples of suicide genes include surface proteins such as RQR8 (93) and huEGFRt (92) which can be recognized by monoclonal antibodies (mAbs). A potential drawback of mAbs-mediated suicide genes is that the concentrations required for efficient elimination may not be easily achieved due to accessibility of the mAbs to desired tissues.

Other suicide genes can be activated by small molecules such as the herpes simplex virus thymidine kinase (HSV1-*tk*) and inducible caspase 9 (iCasp9) systems (94). HSV1-*tk* is a non-toxic enzymatic protein that converts pyrimidine and acycloguanosine nucleoside analogs for example ganciclovir into phosphorylated compounds that are toxic metabolites that presents as chain terminators and specifically kill transduced cells. This technology is widely used for cancer therapy (95). iCasp9 is a fusion of a modified human FK506 binding protein-12 (FKBP12) with the catalytic domain of human caspase 9, and its conditional dimerization allows for its activity. iCasp9 has low potential immunogenicity and its function upon activation is specific to the transduced cells. Furthermore, iCasp9 maintains function in T cells overexpressing anti-apoptotic molecules (94). These properties could promote the choice for iCasp9 as a safety feature element in CAR-Tregs amongst other human T cell therapies. Di Stasi et al. published a study which enrolled five patients who had undergone stem-cell transplant for relapsed acute leukemia and treated with iCasp9-expressing T cells. With a single dose of the dimerising drug it eliminated more than 90% of the iCasp9-expressing T cells (96). The iCasp9 safety switch has been incorporated in second generation CAR-T cells used in clinical trials targeting GD2 for cancer treatment (NCT01822652, NCT02439788) (59). Another clinical trial using fourth generation CAR-T cell therapy also employed the iCasp9 technology (NCT02992210) (59).

Overall, it could be envisioned that the ideal CAR-Treg product would be armored with an array of efficient co-stimulatory domains and suicide genes.

Reporters for Spatiotemporal *in vivo* Tracking

The administration of live cell therapeutics including CAR-Tregs raises several important questions pertaining to cell therapy localization and relocalization over time, sites of activity and overall fate of administered cells. The existence of adoptively transferred cells can be demonstrated with highly sensitive methods based on blood samples. Cytotoxic T-cells have been shown by qPCR to be present years after administration in some patients (97). Administered Tregs have also been demonstrated to be present for a long time in the circulation of patients using a stable isotope labeling approach based on deuterium; polyclonal Tregs labeled with [6,6-$^2H_2$]glucose were detected in the circulation of Type I diabetes patients for up to 1 year (14). Importantly, these methodologies suffer from not providing answers to questions relating to spatial localization, activity, and fate of the therapeutic cells at target sites. Non-invasive whole-body imaging would be a highly beneficial tool to answer all these questions in a spatiotemporal manner.

The field of *in vivo* cell tracking has re-gained new momentum through the development of adoptive cell therapies. The various cell tracking methodologies including a variety of experimental design considerations and caveats have recently been comprehensively reviewed (98), also in the context of tracking T cell therapies (99). Fundamentally, cells require labeling to visualize them *in vivo* using technologies with exquisite sensitivities. Non-invasive radionuclide imaging by single photon emission computed tomography (SPECT) or positron emission tomography (PET) offers excellent sensitivity with absolute quantification and true 3D information while being translatable to the clinic. Labels can be introduced into cells via two fundamentally different methodologies, direct and indirect cell labeling (98).

So-called "direct cell labeling" employs ready-to-use contrast agents (e.g., organic fluorophores, quantum dots, iron oxide nanoparticles, ^{19}F-fluorinated contrast agents, chelated radiometals etc.), which are introduced into cells either due to the contrast agents being cell permeant, or through assisted uptake (e.g., by transfection or internalization). We previously showed that direct radiolabeling of polyclonal murine $CD4^+$ T cells with ^{99m}Tc-hexamethylpropyleneamine oxime did not affect cell viability, but the radiolabeled cells could only be tracked for up to 24 h due to the short half-life of the radiolabel [half-life of ^{99m}Tc is 6.01h; (100)]. This enabled the assessment of Treg biodistribution within a day of administration but precluded long-term tracking of Tregs. Longer half-life isotopes could provide this opportunity, albeit are not free of caveats. The SPECT isotope ^{111}In has been used clinically to follow directly labeled white blood cells for decades (101), but due to its decay properties it has also been associated with significant radiodamage (102). ^{89}Zr has a similar half-life as ^{111}In and was used to track cells for up to 2 weeks (103, 104). With clinical PET being more sensitive than SPECT, not least through the very recent development of total-body PET, which has been shown to be another 40-times more sensitive than conventional PET (105), ^{89}Zr-labeling would result in the use of less radioactivity to achieve the same tracking results. However, radio-damage as a consequence of radioisotope incorporation into cells must be assessed, particularly in cell types such as T cells that are routinely ablated using radiation. Therefore, careful dosimetry considerations are required to assess both the preclinical and clinical feasibility of Treg tracking via this route [for caveats see (98)].

The alternative is "indirect cell labeling," whereby a genetically encoded reporter is ectopically introduced into the cells mostly by viral transduction to ensure genomic integration and thus stable long-term expression; transposon and gene editing represent alternative methodologies (106, 107). Reporter genes have critical advantages over direct labeling for cell tracking (99, 108). First, the observation period is independent of the contrast agent, for example, not affected by the half-life of a radioisotope. Second, genetic encoding avoids label dilution phenomena, which are limiting observation times in the case of fast-growing cells (e.g., expanding T cells). Third, genetic encoding circumvents complex direct cell labeling procedures and potential associated cell toxicities. A drawback of the indirect cell labeling approach is that it requires genetic engineering. However, this is not a concern for preclinical experimentation and not a concern for adoptive cell therapies that require genetic engineering to confer targeting specificity and/or efficacy, such as CAR-Treg therapy. Treg *in vivo* dynamics has been assessed preclinically using bioluminescence reporters (109, 110). Dawson et al. tracked HLA-A2 CAR-Tregs *in vivo* using bioluminescence and found that the peak of CAR-Treg infiltration to $A2^+$ skin graft was 7 days post infusion (53). However, this imaging modality is not clinically translatable because of the non-human nature of luciferases, and the added disadvantages of optical imaging at depth (absorption, scatter) precluding reliable quantification. As foreign reporters can elicit an immune response and result in immune destruction of the administered therapeutic cells, a host-compatible reporter is preferable in this context. Host reporters are from the same species but endogenously expressed in only a very limited number of host tissues, and ideally at low levels to ensure favorable contrast (99). The most promising host reporters available for the purpose of Treg tracking in skin transplant models are the human sodium iodide symporter (NIS) (111) and the human prostate-specific membrane antigen (PSMA) (112), as neither of them is expressed in human or mouse dermis or epidermis. NIS offers the advantage of a generator-produced radiotracer ($[^{99m}Tc]TcO_4^-$) for SPECT imaging avoiding complex synthesis on each imaging day. Notably, there is also a clinical PET tracer available for NIS ($[^{18}F]BF_4^-$), which is accessible via an automated synthesis protocol (113, 114). Notably, Volpe et al. have also demonstrated that NIS expression and use for imaging did not result in radiodamage-related negative effects in CAR-T cells (115). In a proof-of-principle study employing retroviral transduction methodology, we demonstrated *ex vivo* engineering of murine Tregs to express a radionuclide imaging reporter and detected them 24 h post administration by SPECT imaging (116). However, so far long-term tracking of human Tregs has not been addressed using clinically translatable imaging technologies and remains an important area of future research to aid the development and clinical translation of adoptive Treg therapy.

TRANSLATING CAR-TREGS TO THE CLINIC

The quick evolution of CAR-T cells into clinic has informed the scientific community of the pitfalls and hurdles associated with delivering an effective, safe and reproducible treatment; applying the lessons to CAR-Treg therapy should accelerate their use in clinic. Fritsche et al. extensively reviewed optimized methods in manufacturing GMP-grade CAR-Tregs (117) but factors including generating "off-the-shelf" products, increasing *in vivo* persistence and eliminating CAR-associated toxicities are a few examples of hurdles to overcome and will be discussed next.

Developing next-generation, or "off-the-shelf," products is a focal point for clinical translation of CAR-T cells and, equally, must be considered for CAR-Treg therapy. Currently, the manufacturing process of autologous CAR-T cells for cancer patients incur a few paramount disadvantages, such as possible failure during manufacturing, and critically, the 3 week long process of developing the treatment which is a setback in highly proliferative malignancies [reviewed in (118)]. Time critical treatment delivery is not as big of a concern for CAR-Tregs in autoimmunity and solid organ transplant rejection. However, risk of failure due to low absolute numbers or functionally defective Tregs because of the disease, or interference from adjunct immunosuppressive medications need to be considered. Most importantly, the high cost incurred of manufacturing and delivery patient derived CAR-T cells has been a challenge for health care systems and needs to be considered if CAR-Treg therapy is to be translated into clinic. Previously, allogeneic CAR-T cells generated from "healthy donors" have been considered as a fast, scaled-up and decreased cost method of which high numbers of CAR-T cells can be produced per donor, with the added advantage of cryopreserving large batches, ready for treatment immediately. However, this gave rise to GvHD or clearance by the host's immune system (119). Different strategies have looked at generating manipulated "off the shelf" CAR-T cell products.

The use of gene editing as a tool for generating off the shelf CAR-T cells is very promising and can be translated to CAR-Treg therapy. This can be achieved by using transcription-activator-like effector nucleases (TALENs) to knock out the TCRα chain (TRAC) or β2 microglobulin of the MHC molecule, to prevent alloreactive T cells from inducing GvHD (120). CRISPR-Cas9 is another tool to replace the TCRαβ with the CAR in the TRAC locus or β2 microglobulin of the MHC molecule to minimize immunogenicity avoiding GvHD (121, 122).

Concerns surrounding candidate patients who are on immunosuppressive regiments may also interfere or crosstalk with CAR-Treg efficacy. Drug such as antithymocyte globulin (ATG), cyclosporin, anti-CD25 and rapamycin are administered to transplant recipients and have an impact on Treg numbers and function. ATG reduces the absolute number of Tregs and high doses has been linked to impaired thymic Treg development in allogeneic HSCT (123). Cyclosporin and other calcineurin inhibitors (e.g., tacrolimus) suppress Treg activation and decrease FOXP3 expression but this can be restored by administration of IL-2 (124). We have shown in the ThRIL study the efficacy of Treg therapy in patients on immunosuppressive regimens including ATG and tacrolimus, which is encouraging for future CAR-Treg trials (17). In contrast, drugs such as sirolimus or everolimus, (rapamycin) inhibitors of the mTOR pathway may have a beneficial effect as used in combination with Tregs in the treatment of transplant patients as rapamycin is routinely used in the *ex vivo* expansion of Tregs and promote Tconv outgrowth (125).

CONCLUDING REMARKS

CAR-Tregs are the logical extension of polyclonal Treg therapy to enhance their efficacy by conferring antigen-specificity. It is an emerging area with not an insignificant amount of research required to develop and adapt existing CAR-Treg concepts and optimize them for successful clinical translation. As reviewed here the application of CAR-Tregs to the clinic needs further refinement. There is a need to maximize their suppressive function, their stability and understand better their homing capacity and longevity i.e., preventing CAR-Treg exhaustion. Such cell products raise another concern and this is the cost (126). Currently, treating a patient with anti-cancer CAR-T cell therapy costs $400,000 without the ancillary costs

(127). Furthermore, the critical rate needed to manufacture personalized products, the failure to achieve the targeted cell numbers in some patients, and the heterogeneity of the cell products generated need to be overcome. However, the safety demonstrated with the clinical application of polyclonal Tregs and the pre-clinical data with CAR-Tregs has now generated investment in CAR-Treg therapy and several start-up companies have been funded, with the aim of applying CAR-Tregs to cure autoimmune diseases and induce transplantation tolerance. The first CAR-Treg clinical trial has been granted by UK MHRA authorization in a phase I/II clinical trial (STEADFAST) for kidney transplant patients. Progress in our understanding of the biology of Tregs, the ability of functional enhancements through genetic engineering, contribute to the excitement of this field of research.

AUTHOR CONTRIBUTIONS

YM participated in manuscript writing, editing and coordination of its submission. ST and CD contributed to manuscript writing. RL, GF, and GL contributed to manuscript writing and editing. All authors contributed to the article and approved the submitted version.

REFERENCES

1. Sakaguchi S, Yamaguchi T, Nomura T, Ono M. Regulatory T cells and immune tolerance. *Cell.* (2008) 133:775–87. doi: 10.1016/j.cell.2008.05.009
2. Itoh M, Takahashi T, Sakaguchi N, Kuniyasu Y, Shimizu J, Otsuka F, et al. Thymus and autoimmunity: production of CD25+CD4+ naturally anergic and suppressive T cells as a key function of the thymus in maintaining immunologic self-tolerance. *J Immunol.* (1999) 162:5317–26.
3. Polansky JK, Kretschmer K, Freyer J, Floess S, Garbe A, Baron U, et al. DNA methylation controls Foxp3 gene expression. *Eur J Immunol.* (2008) 38:1654–63. doi: 10.1002/eji.200838105
4. Lyon MF, Peters J, Glenister PH, Ball S, Wright E. The scurfy mouse mutant has previously unrecognized hematological abnormalities and resembles wiskott-aldrich syndrome. *Proc Natl Acad Sci USA.* (1990) 87:2433–7. doi: 10.1073/pnas.87.7.2433
5. Vandenbark AA, Offner H. Critical evaluation of regulatory T cells in autoimmunity: are the most potent regulatory specificities being ignored? *Immunology.* (2008) 125:1–13. doi: 10.1111/j.1365-2567.2008.02900.x
6. Abbas AK, Benoist C, Bluestone JA, Campbell DJ, Ghosh S, Hori S, et al. Regulatory T cells: recommendations to simplify the nomenclature. *Nat Immunol.* (2013) 14:307–8. doi: 10.1038/ni.2554
7. Singer A, Adoro S, Park JH. Lineage fate and intense debate: myths, models and mechanisms of CD4- versus CD8-lineage choice. *Nat Rev Immunol.* (2008) 8:788–801. doi: 10.1038/nri2416
8. Kretschmer K, Apostolou I, Hawiger D, Khazaie K, Nussenzweig MC, von Boehmer H. Inducing and expanding regulatory T cell populations by foreign antigen. *Nat Immunol.* (2005) 6:1219–27. doi: 10.1038/ni1265
9. Romano M, Fanelli G, Albany CJ, Giganti G, Lombardi G. Past, present, and future of regulatory T cell therapy in transplantation and autoimmunity. *Front Immunol.* (2019) 10:43. doi: 10.3389/fimmu.2019.00043
10. Brunstein CG, Miller JS, Cao Q, McKenna DH, Hippen KL, Curtsinger J, et al. Infusion of *ex vivo* expanded T regulatory cells in adults transplanted with umbilical cord blood: safety profile and detection kinetics. *Blood.* (2011) 117:1061–70. doi: 10.1182/blood-2010-07-293795
11. Martelli MF, Di Ianni M, Ruggeri L, Falzetti F, Carotti A, Terenzi A, et al. HLA-haploidentical transplantation with regulatory and conventional T-cell adoptive immunotherapy prevents acute leukemia relapse. *Blood.* (2014) 124:638–44. doi: 10.1182/blood-2014-03-564401
12. Trzonkowski P, Dukat-Mazurek A, Bieniaszewska M, Marek-Trzonkowska N, Dobyszuk A, Juscinska J, et al. Treatment of graft-versus-host disease with naturally occurring T regulatory cells. *Biodrugs.* (2013) 27:605–14. doi: 10.1007/s40259-013-0050-5
13. Marek-Trzonkowska N, Mysliwiec M, Dobyszuk A, Grabowska M, Derkowska I, Juscinska J, et al. Therapy of type 1 diabetes with CD4(+)CD25(high)CD127-regulatory T cells prolongs survival of pancreatic islets - results of one year follow-up. *Clin Immunol.* (2014) 153:23–30. doi: 10.1016/j.clim.2014.03.016
14. Bluestone JA, Buckner JH, Fitch M, Gitelman SE, Gupta S, Hellerstein M, et al. Type 1 diabetes immunotherapy using polyclonal regulatory T cells. *Sci Transl Med.* (2015) 7:315ra189. doi: 10.1126/scitranslmed.aad4134
15. Todo S, Yamashita K, Goto R, Zaitsu M, Nagatsu A, Oura T, et al. A pilot study of operational tolerance with a regulatory T-cell-based cell therapy in living donor liver transplantation. *Hepatology.* (2016) 64:632–43. doi: 10.1002/hep.28459
16. Chandran S, Tang Q, Sarwal M, Laszik ZG, Putnam AL, Lee K, et al. Polyclonal regulatory T cell therapy for control of inflammation in kidney transplants. *Am J Transplant.* (2017) 17:2945–54. doi: 10.1111/ajt.14415
17. Sanchez-Fueyo A, Whitehouse G, Grageda N, Cramp ME, Lim TY, Romano M, et al. Applicability, safety, and biological activity of regulatory T cell therapy in liver transplantation. *Am J Transplant.* (2019) 20:1125–36. doi: 10.1111/ajt.15700
18. Sawitzki B, Harden PN, Reinke P, Moreau A, Hutchinson JA, Game DS, et al. Regulatory cell therapy in kidney transplantation (the ONE study): a harmonised design and analysis of seven non-randomised, single-arm, phase 1/2A trials. *Lancet.* (2020) 395:1627–39. doi: 10.1016/S0140-6736(20)30167-7
19. Tang Q, Henriksen KJ, Bi M, Finger EB, Szot G, Ye J, et al. *In vitro*-expanded antigen-specific regulatory T cells suppress autoimmune diabetes. *J Exp Med.* (2004) 199:1455–65. doi: 10.1084/jem.20040139
20. Tarbell KV, Yamazaki S, Olson K, Toy P, Steinman RM. CD25+ CD4+ T cells, expanded with dendritic cells presenting a single autoantigenic peptide, suppress autoimmune diabetes. *J Exp Med.* (2004) 199:1467–77. doi: 10.1084/jem.20040180
21. Sagoo P, Ali N, Garg G, Nestle FO, Lechler RI, Lombardi G. Human regulatory T cells with alloantigen specificity are more potent inhibitors of alloimmune skin graft damage than polyclonal regulatory T cells. *Sci Transl Med.* (2011) 3:83ra42. doi: 10.1126/scitranslmed.3002076
22. Putnam AL, Safinia N, Medvec A, Laszkowska M, Wray M, Mintz MA, et al. Clinical grade manufacturing of human alloantigen-reactive regulatory T cells for use in transplantation. *Am J Transplant.* (2013) 13:3010–20. doi: 10.1111/ajt.12433
23. Zheng J, Liu Y, Lau YL, Tu W. CD40-activated B cells are more potent than immature dendritic cells to induce and expand CD4(+) regulatory T cells. *Cell Mol Immunol.* (2010) 7:44–50. doi: 10.1038/cmi.2009.103
24. Wright GP, Notley CA, Xue SA, Bendle GM, Holler A, Schumacher TN, et al. Adoptive therapy with redirected primary regulatory T cells results in antigen-specific suppression of arthritis. *Proc Natl Acad Sci USA.* (2009) 106:19078–83. doi: 10.1073/pnas.0907396106
25. Tsang JY, Tanriver Y, Jiang S, Xue SA, Ratnasothy K, Chen D, et al. Conferring indirect allospecificity on CD4+CD25+ tregs by TCR gene transfer favors transplantation tolerance in mice. *J Clin Invest.* (2008) 118:3619–28. doi: 10.1172/JCI33185
26. Brusko TM, Koya RC, Zhu S, Lee MR, Putnam AL, McClymont SA, et al. Human antigen-specific regulatory T cells generated by T cell receptor gene transfer. *PLoS ONE.* (2010) 5:e11726. doi: 10.1371/journal.pone.0011726
27. Hull CM, Nickolay LE, Estorninho M, Richardson MW, Riley JL, Peakman M, et al. Generation of human islet-specific regulatory T cells by TCR gene transfer. *J Autoimmun.* (2017) 79:63–73. doi: 10.1016/j.jaut.2017.01.001
28. Kim YC, Zhang AH, Yoon J, Culp WE, Lees JR, Wucherpfennig KW, et al. Engineered MBP-specific human tregs ameliorate MOG-induced EAE through IL-2-triggered inhibition of effector T cells. *J Autoimmun.* (2018) 92:77–86. doi: 10.1016/j.jaut.2018.05.003

29. Herzog RW, Kuteyeva V, Saboungi R, Terhorst C, Biswas M. Reprogrammed CD4(+) T cells that express FoxP3(+) control inhibitory antibody formation in hemophilia A mice. *Front Immunol.* (2019) 10:274. doi: 10.3389/fimmu.2019.00274
30. Jaeckel E, von Boehmer H, Manns MP. Antigen-specific FoxP3-transduced T-cells can control established type 1 diabetes. *Diabetes.* (2005) 54:306–10. doi: 10.2337/diabetes.54.2.306
31. Beavis PA, Gregory B, Green P, Cribbs AP, Kennedy A, Amjadi P, et al. Resistance to regulatory T cell-mediated suppression in rheumatoid arthritis can be bypassed by ectopic foxp3 expression in pathogenic synovial T cells. *Proc Natl Acad Sci USA.* (2011) 108:16717–22. doi: 10.1073/pnas.1112722108
32. Loser K, Hansen W, Apelt J, Balkow S, Buer J, Beissert S. *In vitro*-generated regulatory T cells induced by Foxp3-retrovirus infection control murine contact allergy and systemic autoimmunity. *Gene Ther.* (2005) 12:1294–304. doi: 10.1038/sj.gt.3302567
33. Caruso HG, Hurton LV, Najjar A, Rushworth D, Ang S, Olivares S, et al. Tuning sensitivity of CAR to EGFR density limits recognition of normal tissue while maintaining potent antitumor activity. *Cancer Res.* (2015) 75:3505–18. doi: 10.1158/0008-5472.CAN-15-0139
34. Liu X, Jiang S, Fang C, Yang S, Olalere D, Pequignot EC, et al. Affinity-tuned ErbB2 or EGFR chimeric antigen receptor T cells exhibit an increased therapeutic index against tumors in mice. *Cancer Res.* (2015) 75:3596–607. doi: 10.1158/0008-5472.CAN-15-0159
35. Kershaw MH, Westwood JA, Parker LL, Wang G, Eshhar Z, Mavroukakis SA, et al. A phase I study on adoptive immunotherapy using gene-modified T cells for ovarian cancer. *Clin Cancer Res.* (2006) 12:6106–15. doi: 10.1158/1078-0432.CCR-06-1183
36. Bridgeman JS, Hawkins RE, Bagley S, Blaylock M, Holland M, Gilham DE. The optimal antigen response of chimeric antigen receptors harboring the CD3zeta transmembrane domain is dependent upon incorporation of the receptor into the endogenous TCR/CD3 complex. *J Immunol.* (2010) 184:6938–49. doi: 10.4049/jimmunol.0901766
37. US Food and Drug Administration. *FDA approves CAR-T cell therapy to treat adults with certain types of large B-cell lymphoma.* Silver Spring, MD: US Food and Drug Administration. (2017).
38. Maude SL, Teachey DT, Porter DL, Grupp SA. CD19-targeted chimeric antigen receptor T-cell therapy for acute lymphoblastic leukemia. *Blood*. (2015) 125:4017–23. doi: 10.1182/blood-2014-12-580068
39. Neelapu SS, Locke FL, Bartlett NL, Lekakis LJ, Miklos DB, Jacobson CA, et al. Axicabtagene ciloleucel CAR T-cell therapy in refractory large B-cell lymphoma. *N Engl J Med.* (2017) 377:2531–44. doi: 10.1056/NEJMoa1707447
40. Maude SL, Laetsch TW, Buechner J, Rives S, Boyer M, Bittencourt H, et al. Tisagenlecleucel in children and young adults with B-cell lymphoblastic leukemia. *N Engl J Med.* (2018) 378:439–48. doi: 10.1056/NEJMoa1709866
41. Schuster SJ, Svoboda J, Chong EA, Nasta SD, Mato AR, Anak O, et al. Chimeric antigen receptor T cells in refractory B-cell lymphomas. *N Engl J Med.* (2017) 377:2545–54. doi: 10.1056/NEJMoa1708566
42. Linette GP, Stadtmauer EA, Maus MV, Rapoport AP, Levine BL, Emery L, et al. Cardiovascular toxicity and titin cross-reactivity of affinity-enhanced T cells in myeloma and melanoma. *Blood.* (2013) 122:863–71. doi: 10.1182/blood-2013-03-490565
43. Saudemont A, Jespers L, Clay T. Current status of gene engineering cell therapeutics. *Front Immunol.* (2018) 9:153. doi: 10.3389/fimmu.2018.00153
44. Ellebrecht CT, Bhoj VG, Nace A, Choi EJ, Mao X, Cho MJ, et al. Reengineering chimeric antigen receptor T cells for targeted therapy of autoimmune disease. *Science.* (2016) 353:179–84. doi: 10.1126/science.aaf6756
45. Elinav E, Adam N, Waks T, Eshhar Z. Amelioration of colitis by genetically engineered murine regulatory T cells redirected by antigen-specific chimeric receptor. *Gastroenterology.* (2009) 136:1721–31. doi: 10.1053/j.gastro.2009.01.049
46. Blat D, Zigmond E, Alteber Z, Waks T, Eshhar Z. Suppression of murine colitis and its associated cancer by carcinoembryonic antigen-specific regulatory T cells. *Mol Ther.* (2014) 22:1018–28. doi: 10.1038/mt.2014.41
47. Skuljec J, Chmielewski M, Happle C, Habener A, Busse M, Abken H, et al. Chimeric antigen receptor-redirected regulatory T cells suppress experimental allergic airway inflammation, a model of asthma. *Front Immunol.* (2017) 8:1125. doi: 10.3389/fimmu.2017.01125
48. Tenspolde M, Zimmermann K, Weber LC, Hapke M, Lieber M, Dywicki J, et al. Regulatory T cells engineered with a novel insulin-specific chimeric antigen receptor as a candidate immunotherapy for type 1 diabetes. *J Autoimmun.* (2019) 103:102289. doi: 10.1016/j.jaut.2019.05.017
49. Zhang AH, Yoon J, Kim YC, Scott DW. Targeting antigen-specific B cells using antigen-expressing transduced regulatory T cells. *J Immunol.* (2018) 201:1434–41. doi: 10.4049/jimmunol.1701800
50. MacDonald KG, Hoeppli RE, Huang Q, Gillies J, Luciani DS, Orban PC, et al. Alloantigen-specific regulatory T cells generated with a chimeric antigen receptor. *J Clin Invest.* (2016) 126:1413–24. doi: 10.1172/JCI82771
51. Boardman DA, Philippeos C, Fruhwirth GO, Ibrahim MA, Hannen RF, Cooper D, et al. Expression of a chimeric antigen receptor specific for donor HLA class I enhances the potency of human regulatory T cells in preventing human skin transplant rejection. *Am J Transplant.* (2017) 17:931–43. doi: 10.1111/ajt.14185
52. Noyan F, Zimmermann K, Hardtke-Wolenski M, Knoefel A, Schulde E, Geffers R, et al. Prevention of allograft rejection by use of regulatory T cells with an MHC-specific chimeric antigen receptor. *Am J Transplant.* (2017) 17:917–30. doi: 10.1111/ajt.14175
53. Dawson NA, Lamarche C, Hoeppli RE, Bergqvist P, Fung VC, McIver E, et al. Systematic testing and specificity mapping of alloantigen-specific chimeric antigen receptors in regulatory T cells. *JCI Insight.* (2019) 4:10.1172/jci.insight.123672. doi: 10.1172/jci.insight.123672
54. Sicard A, Lamarche C, Speck M, Wong M, Rosado-Sanchez I, Blois, et al. Donor-specific chimeric antigen receptor tregs limit rejection in naive but not sensitized allograft recipients. *Am J Transplant.* (2020) 20:1562–73. doi: 10.1111/ajt.15787
55. Sadelain M, Brentjens R, Riviere I. The basic principles of chimeric antigen receptor design. *Cancer Discov.* (2013) 3:388–98. doi: 10.1158/2159-8290.CD-12-0548
56. Zhang P, Gao F, Wang Q, Wang X, Zhu F, Ma C, et al. Agonistic anti-4-1BB antibody promotes the expansion of natural regulatory T cells while maintaining Foxp3 expression. *Scand J Immunol.* (2007) 66:435–40. doi: 10.1111/j.1365-3083.2007.01994.x
57. Long AH, Haso WM, Shern JF, Wanhainen KM, Murgai M, Ingaramo M, et al. 4-1BB co-stimulation ameliorates T cell exhaustion induced by tonic signaling of chimeric antigen receptors. *Nat Med.* (2015) 21:581–90. doi: 10.1038/nm.3838
58. Song DG, Ye Q, Carpenito C, Poussin M, Wang LP, Ji C, et al. *in vivo* persistence, tumor localization, and antitumor activity of CAR-engineered T cells is enhanced by co-stimulatory signaling through CD137 (4-1BB). *Cancer Res.* (2011) 71:4617–27. doi: 10.1158/0008-5472.CAN-11-0422
59. Li G, Boucher JC, Kotani H, Park K, Zhang Y, Shrestha B, et al. 4-1BB enhancement of CAR T function requires NF-kappaB and TRAFs. *JCI Insight.* (2018) 3:10.1172/jci.insight.121322. doi: 10.1172/jci.insight.121322
60. Ito T, Wang YH, Duramad O, Hanabuchi S, Perng OA, Gilliet M, et al. OX40 ligand shuts down IL-10-producing regulatory T cells. *Proc Natl Acad Sci USA.* (2006) 103:13138–43. doi: 10.1073/pnas.0603107103
61. Vu MD, Xiao X, Gao W, Degauque N, Chen M, Kroemer A, et al. OX40 costimulation turns off Foxp3+ tregs. *Blood.* (2007) 110:2501–10. doi: 10.1182/blood-2007-01-070748
62. So T, Croft M. Cutting edge: OX40 inhibits TGF-beta- and antigen-driven conversion of naive CD4 T cells into CD25+Foxp3+ T cells. *J Immunol.* (2007) 179:1427–30. doi: 10.4049/jimmunol.179.3.1427
63. Rogers PR, Song J, Gramaglia I, Killeen N, Croft M. OX40 promotes bcl-xL and bcl-2 expression and is essential for long-term survival of CD4 T cells. *Immunity.* (2001) 15:445–55. doi: 10.1016/S1074-7613(01)00191-1
64. Song J, Salek-Ardakani S, Rogers PR, Cheng M, Van Parijs L, Croft M. The co-stimulation-regulated duration of PKB activation controls T cell longevity. *Nat Immunol.* (2004) 5:150–8. doi: 10.1038/ni1030
65. Song A, Tang X, Harms KM, Croft M. OX40 and bcl-xL promote the persistence of CD8 T cells to recall tumor-associated antigen. *J Immunol.* (2005) 175:3534–41. doi: 10.4049/jimmunol.175.6.3534
66. Hombach AA, Heiders J, Foppe M, Chmielewski M, Abken H. OX40 co-stimulation by a chimeric antigen receptor abrogates CD28 and IL-2 induced IL-10 secretion by redirected CD4(+) T cells. *Oncoimmunology.* (2012) 1:458–66. doi: 10.4161/onci.19855

67. Hombach AA, Abken H. Co-stimulation by chimeric antigen receptors revisited the T cell antitumor response benefits from combined CD28-OX40 signalling. *Int J Cancer*. (2011) 129:2935–44. doi: 10.1002/ijc.25960
68. Dong C, Juedes AE, Temann UA, Shresta S, Allison JP, Ruddle NH, et al. ICOS co-stimulatory receptor is essential for T-cell activation and function. *Nature*. (2001) 409:97–101. doi: 10.1038/35051100
69. Hutloff A, Dittrich AM, Beier KC, Eljaschewitsch B, Kraft R, Anagnostopoulos I, et al. ICOS is an inducible T-cell co-stimulator structurally and functionally related to CD28. *Nature*. (1999) 397:263–6. doi: 10.1038/16717
70. Rudd CE, Schneider H. Unifying concepts in CD28, ICOS and CTLA4 co-receptor signalling. *Nat Rev Immunol*. (2003) 3:544–56. doi: 10.1038/nri1131
71. McAdam AJ, Chang TT, Lumelsky AE, Greenfield EA, Boussiotis VA, Duke-Cohan JS, et al. Mouse inducible co-stimulatory molecule (ICOS) expression is enhanced by CD28 co-stimulation and regulates differentiation of CD4+ T cells. *J Immunol*. (2000) 165:5035–40. doi: 10.4049/jimmunol.165.9.5035
72. Guedan S, Chen X, Madar A, Carpenito C, McGettigan SE, Frigault MJ, et al. ICOS-based chimeric antigen receptors program bipolar TH17/TH1 cells. *Blood*. (2014) 124:1070–80. doi: 10.1182/blood-2013-10-535245
73. Hendriks J, Gravestein LA, Tesselaar K, van Lier RA, Schumacher TN, Borst J. CD27 is required for generation and long-term maintenance of T cell immunity. *Nat Immunol*. (2000) 1:433–40. doi: 10.1038/80877
74. Song DG, Powell DJ. Pro-survival signaling via CD27 costimulation drives effective CAR T-cell therapy. *Oncoimmunology*. (2012) 1:547–49. doi: 10.4161/onci.19458
75. Arroyo Hornero R, Betts GJ, Sawitzki B, Vogt K, Harden PN, Wood KJ. CD45RA distinguishes CD4+CD25+CD127-/low TSDR demethylated regulatory T cell subpopulations with differential stability and susceptibility to tacrolimus-mediated inhibition of suppression. *Transplantation*. (2017) 101:302–9. doi: 10.1097/TP.0000000000001278
76. Monjezi R, Miskey C, Gogishvili T, Schleef M, Schmeer M, Einsele H, et al. Enhanced CAR T-cell engineering using non-viral sleeping beauty transposition from minicircle vectors. *Leukemia*. (2017) 31:186–94. doi: 10.1038/leu.2016.180
77. Vormittag P, Gunn R, Ghorashian S, Veraitch FS. A guide to manufacturing CAR T cell therapies. *Curr Opin Biotechnol Biotechnol*. (2018) 53:164–81. doi: 10.1016/j.copbio.2018.01.025
78. Kumar P, Bhattacharya P, Prabhakar BS. A comprehensive review on the role of co-signaling receptors and treg homeostasis in autoimmunity and tumor immunity. *J Autoimmun*. (2018) 95:77–99. doi: 10.1016/j.jaut.2018.08.007
79. Hegde M, Corder A, Chow KK, Mukherjee M, Ashoori A, Kew Y, et al. Combinational targeting offsets antigen escape and enhances effector functions of adoptively transferred T cells in glioblastoma. *Mol Ther*. (2013) 21:2087–101. doi: 10.1038/mt.2013.185
80. Ruella M, Barrett DM, Kenderian SS, Shestova O, Hofmann TJ, Perazzelli J, et al. Dual CD19 and CD123 targeting prevents antigen-loss relapses after CD19-directed immunotherapies. *J Clin Invest*. (2016) 126:3814–26. doi: 10.1172/JCI87366
81. Zah E, Lin MY, Silva-Benedict A, Jensen MC, Chen YY. T cells expressing CD19/CD20 bispecific chimeric antigen receptors prevent antigen escape by malignant B cells. *Cancer Immunol Res*. (2016) 4:498–508. doi: 10.1158/2326-6066.CIR-15-0231
82. Kloss CC, Condomines M, Cartellieri M, Bachmann M, Sadelain M. Combinatorial antigen recognition with balanced signaling promotes selective tumor eradication by engineered T cells. *Nat Biotechnol*. (2013) 31:71–5. doi: 10.1038/nbt.2459
83. Roybal KT, Rupp LJ, Morsut L, Walker WJ, McNally KA, Park JS, et al. Precision tumor recognition by T cells with combinatorial antigen-sensing circuits. *Cell*. (2016) 164:770–9. doi: 10.1016/j.cell.2016.01.011
84. Grada Z, Hegde M, Byrd T, Shaffer DR, Ghazi A, Brawley VS, et al. TanCAR: A novel bispecific chimeric antigen receptor for cancer immunotherapy. *Mol Ther Nucleic Acids*. (2013) 2:e105. doi: 10.1038/mtna.2013.32
85. Jia H, Wang Z, Wang Y, Liu Y, Dai H, Tong C, et al. Haploidentical CD19/CD22 bispecific CAR-T cells induced MRD-negative remission in a patient with relapsed and refractory adult B-ALL after haploidentical hematopoietic stem cell transplantation. *J Hematol Onco*. (2019) 12:57-019-0741-6. doi: 10.1186/s13045-019-0741-6
86. Jensen MC, Riddell SR. Design and implementation of adoptive therapy with chimeric antigen receptor-modified T cells. *Immunol Rev*. (2014) 257:127–44. doi: 10.1111/imr.12139
87. Koristka S, Kegler A, Bergmann R, Arndt C, Feldmann A, Albert S, et al. Engrafting human regulatory T cells with a flexible modular chimeric antigen receptor technology. *J Autoimmun*. (2018) 90:116–31. doi: 10.1016/j.jaut.2018.02.006
88. Darowski D, Kobold S, Jost C, Klein C. Combining the best of two worlds: highly flexible chimeric antigen receptor adaptor molecules (CAR-adaptors) for the recruitment of chimeric antigen receptor T cells. *Mabs*. (2019) 11:621–31. doi: 10.1080/19420862.2019.1596511
89. Pierini A, Iliopoulou BP, Peiris H, Perez-Cruz M, Baker J, Hsu K, et al. T cells expressing chimeric antigen receptor promote immune tolerance. *JCI Insight*. (2017) 2:10.1172/jci.insight.92865. doi: 10.1172/jci.insight.92865
90. Boroughs AC, Larson RC, Choi BD, Bouffard AA, Riley LS, Schiferle E, et al. Chimeric antigen receptor co-stimulation domains modulate human regulatory T cell function. *JCI Insight*. (2019) 5:10.1172/jci.insight.126194. doi: 10.1172/jci.insight.126194
91. Quintarelli C, Orlando D, Boffa I, Guercio M, Polito VA, Petretto A, et al. Choice of co-stimulatory domains and of cytokines determines CAR T-cell activity in neuroblastoma. *Oncoimmunology*. (2018) 7:e1433518. doi: 10.1080/2162402X.2018.1433518
92. Wang X, Chang WC, Wong CW, Colcher D, Sherman M, Ostberg JR, et al. A transgene-encoded cell surface polypeptide for selection, *in vivo* tracking, and ablation of engineered cells. *Blood*. (2011) 118:1255–63. doi: 10.1182/blood-2011-02-337360
93. Philip B, Kokalaki E, Mekkaoui L, Thomas S, Straathof K, Flutter B, et al. A highly compact epitope-based marker/suicide gene for easier and safer T-cell therapy. *Blood*. (2014) 124:1277–87. doi: 10.1182/blood-2014-01-545020
94. Straathof KC, Pule MA, Yotnda P, Dotti G, Vanin EF, Brenner MK, et al. An inducible caspase 9 safety switch for T-cell therapy. *Blood*. (2005) 105:4247–54. doi: 10.1182/blood-2004-11-4564
95. Caruso M, Panis Y, Gagandeep S, Houssin D, Salzmann JL, Klatzmann D. Regression of established macroscopic liver metastases after in situ transduction of a suicide gene. *Proc Natl Acad Sci USA*. (1993) 90:7024–8. doi: 10.1073/pnas.90.15.7024
96. Di Stasi A, Tey SK, Dotti G, Fujita Y, Kennedy-Nasser A, Martinez C, et al. Inducible apoptosis as a safety switch for adoptive cell therapy. *N Engl J Med*. (2011) 365:1673–83. doi: 10.1056/NEJMoa1106152
97. Juno JA, van Bockel D, Kent SJ, Kelleher AD, Zaunders JJ, Munier CM. Cytotoxic CD4 T cells-friend or foe during viral infection? *Front Immunol*. (2017) 8:19. doi: 10.3389/fimmu.2017.00019
98. Iafrate M, Fruhwirth GO. How non-invasive *in vivo* cell tracking supports the development and translation of cancer immunotherapies. *Front Physiol*. (2020) 11:154. doi: 10.3389/fphys.2020.00154
99. Ashmore-Harris C, Iafrate M, Saleem A, Fruhwirth GO. Non-invasive reporter gene imaging of cell therapies, including T cells and stem cells. *Mol Ther*. (2020) 28:1392–416. doi: 10.1016/j.ymthe.2020.03.016
100. Sharif-Paghaleh E, Leech J, Sunassee K, Ali N, Sagoo P, Lechler RI, et al. Monitoring the efficacy of dendritic cell vaccination by early detection of (99m) tc-HMPAO-labeled CD4(+) T cells. *Eur J Immunol*. (2014) 44:2188–91. doi: 10.1002/eji.201344337
101. Love C, Palestro CJ. Radionuclide imaging of infection. *J Nucl Med Technol* (2004) 32:47–57; quiz 58–9. Available online at: http://tech.snmjournals.org/content/32/2/47.long
102. Roca M, de Vries EF, Jamar F, Israel O, Signore A. Guidelines for the labeling of leucocytes with (111)in-oxine. Inflammation/Infection taskgroup of the european association of nuclear medicine. *Eur J Nucl Med Mol Imaging*. (2010) 37:835–41. doi: 10.1007/s00259-010-1393-5
103. Charoenphun P, Meszaros LK, Chuamsaamarkkee K, Sharif-Paghaleh E, Ballinger JR, Ferris TJ, et al. (89)zr]oxinate4 for long-term *in vivo* cell tracking by positron emission tomography. *Eur J Nucl Med Mol Imaging*. (2015) 42:278–87. doi: 10.1007/s00259-014-2945-x
104. Sato N, Wu H, Asiedu KO, Szajek LP, Griffiths GL, Choyke PL. (89)zr-oxine complex PET cell imaging in monitoring cell-based therapies. *Radiology*. (2015) 275:490–500. doi: 10.1148/radiol.15142849
105. Cherry SR, Jones T, Karp JS, Qi J, Moses WW, et al. Total-body PET: maximizing sensitivity to create new opportunities for clinical research and patient care. *J Nucl Med*. (2018) 59:3–12. doi: 10.2967/jnumed.116.184028
106. Li W, Prazak L, Chatterjee N, Gruninger S, Krug L, Theodorou D, et al. Activation of transposable elements during aging and neuronal decline in drosophila. *Nat Neurosci*. (2013) 16:529–31. doi: 10.1038/nn.3368

107. Bressan RB, Dewari PS, Kalantzaki M, Gangoso E, Matjusaitis M, Garcia-Diaz C, et al. Efficient CRISPR/Cas9-assisted gene targeting enables rapid and precise genetic manipulation of mammalian neural stem cells. *Development.* (2017) 144:635–648. doi: 10.1242/dev.140855
108. Volpe A, Kurtys E, Fruhwirth GO. Cousins at work: how combining medical with optical imaging enhances *in vivo* cell trackin. *Int J Biochem Cell Biol.* (2018) 102:40–50. doi: 10.1016/j.biocel.2018.06.008
109. Nguyen VH, Zeiser R, Dasilva DL, Chang DS, Beilhack A, Contag CH, et al. *in vivo* dynamics of regulatory T-cell trafficking and survival predict effective strategies to control graft-versus-host disease following allogeneic transplantation. *Blood.* (2007) 109:2649–56. doi: 10.1182/blood-2006-08-044529
110. Suffner J, Hochweller K, Kuhnle MC, Li X, Kroczek RA, Garbi N, et al. Dendritic cells support homeostatic expansion of Foxp3+ regulatory T cells in Foxp3.LuciDTR mice. *J Immunol.* (2010) 184:1810–20. doi: 10.4049/jimmunol.0902420
111. Portulano C, Paroder-Belenitsky M, Carrasco N. The Na+/I- symporter (NIS): mechanism and medical impact. *Endocr Rev.* (2014) 35:106–49. doi: 10.1210/er.2012-1036
112. Minn I, Huss DJ, Ahn HH, Chinn TM, Park A, Jones J, et al. Imaging CAR T cell therapy with PSMA-targeted positron emission tomography. *Sci Adv.* (2019) 5:eaaw5096. doi: 10.1126/sciadv.aaw5096
113. O'Doherty J, Jauregui-Osoro M, Brothwood T, Szyszko T, Marsden PK, O'Doherty MJ, et al. ^{18}F-tetrafluoroborate, a PET probe for imaging Sodium/Iodide symporter expression: Whole-body biodistribution, safety, and radiation dosimetry in thyroid cancer patients. *J Nucl Med.* (2017) 58:1666–71. doi: 10.2967/jnumed.117.192252
114. Volpe A, Man F, Lim L, Khoshnevisan A, Blower J, Blower PJ, et al. Radionuclide-fluorescence reporter gene imaging to track tumor progression in rodent tumor models. *J Vis Exp.* (2018) 133:57088. doi: 10.3791/57088
115. Volpe A, Lang C, Lim L, Man F, Kurtys E, Ashmore-Harris C. et al. Spatiotemporal PET Imaging Reveals Differences in CAR-T Tumor Retention in Triple-Negative Breast Cancer Models. *Mol Ther.* (2020) 28. doi: 10.1016/j.ymthe.2020.06.028
116. Sharif-Paghaleh E, Sunassee K, Tavare R, Ratnasothy K, Koers A, Ali N, et al. *in vivo* SPECT reporter gene imaging of regulatory T cells. *PLoS ONE.* (2011) 6:e25857. doi: 10.1371/journal.pone.0025857
117. Fritsche E, Volk HD, Reinke P, Abou-El-Enein M. Toward an optimized process for clinical manufacturing of CAR-treg cell therapy. *Trends Biotechnol.* (2020). doi: 10.1016/j.tibtech.2019.12.009. [Epub ahead of print].
118. Kohl U, Arsenieva S, Holzinger A, Abken H. CAR T cells in trials: Recent achievements and challenges that remain in the production of modified T cells for clinical applications. *Hum Gene Ther.* (2018) 29:559–68. doi: 10.1089/hum.2017.254
119. Butler CL, Valenzuela NM, Thomas KA, Reed EF. Not all antibodies are created equal: Factors that influence antibody mediated rejection. *J Immunol Res.* (2017) 2017:7903471. doi: 10.1155/2017/7903471
120. Poirot L, Philip B, Schiffer-Mannioui C, Le Clerre D, Chion-Sotinel I, Derniame S, et al. Multiplex genome-edited T-cell manufacturing platform for "off-the-shelf" adoptive T-cell immunotherapies. *Cancer Res.* (2015) 75:3853–64. doi: 10.1158/0008-5472.CAN-14-3321
121. Eyquem J, Mansilla-Soto J, Giavridis T, van der Stegen SJ, Hamieh M, Cunanan KM, et al. Targeting a CAR to the TRAC locus with CRISPR/Cas9 enhances tumour rejection. *Nature.* (2017) 543:113–7. doi: 10.1038/nature21405
122. Liu X, Ranganathan R, Jiang S, Fang C, Sun J, Kim S, et al. A chimeric switch-receptor targeting PD1 augments the efficacy of second-generation CAR T cells in advanced solid tumors. *Cancer Res.* (2016) 76:1578–90. doi: 10.1158/0008-5472.CAN-15-2524
123. Gurkan S, Luan Y, Dhillon N, Allam SR, Montague T, Bromberg JS, et al. Immune reconstitution following rabbit antithymocyte globulin. *Am J Transplant.* (2010) 10:2132–41. doi: 10.1111/j.1600-6143.2010.03210.x
124. Satake A, Schmidt AM, Archambault A, Leichner TM, Wu GF, Kambayashi T. Differential targeting of IL-2 and T cell receptor signaling pathways selectively expands regulatory T cells while inhibiting conventional T cells. *J Autoimmun.* (2013) 44:13–20. doi: 10.1016/j.jaut.2013.06.009
125. Scotta C, Esposito M, Fazekasova H, Fanelli G, Edozie FC, Ali N, et al. Differential effects of rapamycin and retinoic acid on expansion, stability and suppressive qualities of human CD4(+)CD25(+)FOXP3(+) T regulatory cell subpopulations. *Haematologica.* (2013) 98:1291–9. doi: 10.3324/haematol.2012.074088
126. Ruella M, Kenderian SS. Next-generation chimeric antigen receptor T-cell therapy: going off the shelf. *Biodrugs.* (2017) 31:473–81. doi: 10.1007/s40259-017-0247-0
127. Bach PB. National coverage analysis of CAR-T therapies - policy, evidence, and payment. *N Engl J Med.* (2018) 379:1396–8. doi: 10.1056/NEJMp1807382

4

The Role of Diverse Liver Cells in Liver Transplantation Tolerance

Yanzhi Jiang [1,2†], *Weitao Que* [1†], *Ping Zhu* [2*] *and Xiao-Kang Li* [1*]

[1] *Division of Transplantation Immunology, National Research Institute for Child Health and Development, Tokyo, Japan,*
[2] *Guangdong Cardiovascular Institute, Guangdong Provincial People's Hospital, Guangdong Academy of Medical Sciences, Guangzhou, China*

Correspondence:
Ping Zhu
tanganqier@163.com
Xiao-Kang Li
ri-k@ncchd.go.jp

† These authors have contributed equally to this work

Liver transplantation is the ideal treatment approach for a variety of end-stage liver diseases. However, life-long, systemic immunosuppressive treatment after transplantation is required to prevent rejection and graft loss, which is associated with severe side effects, although liver allograft is considered more tolerogenic. Therefore, understanding the mechanism underlying the unique immunologically privileged liver organ is valuable for transplantation management and autoimmune disease treatment. The unique hepatic acinus anatomy and a complex cellular network constitute the immunosuppressive hepatic microenvironment, which are responsible for the tolerogenic properties of the liver. The hepatic microenvironment contains a variety of hepatic-resident immobile non-professional antigen-presenting cells, including hepatocytes, liver sinusoidal endothelial cells, Kupffer cells, and hepatic stellate cells, that are insufficient to optimally prime T cells locally and lead to the removal of alloreactive T cells due to the low expression of major histocompatibility complex (MHC) molecules, costimulatory molecules and proinflammatory cytokines but a rather high expression of coinhibitory molecules and anti-inflammatory cytokines. Hepatic dendritic cells (DCs) are generally immature and less immunogenic than splenic DCs and are also ineffective in priming naïve allogeneic T cells via the direct recognition pathway in recipient secondary lymphoid organs. Although natural killer cells and natural killer T cells are reportedly associated with liver tolerance, their roles in liver transplantation are multifaceted and need to be further clarified. Under these circumstances, T cells are prone to clonal deletion, clonal anergy and exhaustion, eventually leading to tolerance. Other proposed liver tolerance mechanisms, such as soluble donor MHC class I molecules, passenger leukocytes theory and a high-load antigen effect, have also been addressed. We herein comprehensively review the current evidence implicating the tolerogenic properties of diverse liver cells in liver transplantation tolerance.

Keywords: allograft, hepatic microenvironment, liver transplantation, T cell, tolerance

INTRODUCTION

Liver transplantation is the ideal therapeutic approach for a variety of end-stage liver diseases. However, life-long, systemic immunosuppressive treatment is required after transplantation to prevent rejection and graft loss, which is associated with high costs and severe side effects, including infections and malignancy (1, 2). From an immunological standpoint, a liver allograft is more tolerogenic than such grafts for other solid organs, like the heart, kidney, and lung. Spontaneous liver allograft acceptance without the need for immunosuppression has been observed in multiple experimental animal transplantation models (3–5). In clinical practice, liver allografts show a lower rejection rate than such grafts of other solid organs, and around half of carefully selected liver transplant recipients are able to be completely weaned from immunosuppression, which rarely occurs in cases of other organ transplantation (5–7). Furthermore, liver allografts are associated with tolerance induction for other simultaneous or sequentially transplanted organs in human and animal models, indicating that the liver can induce systemic tolerance (8–12). Therefore, understanding the mechanisms underlying the unique immunologically privileged liver organs is valuable for transplantation management and autoimmune disease treatment.

The liver is the central metabolic organ responsible for metabolism, nutrient storage and detoxification and also functions as an immunological organ. To fulfill its multifaceted functions, the liver comprises repetitive functional units formed by a myriad of cell types. The functional unit, known as the hepatic acinus, consists of an irregular-shaped, roughly ellipsoidal mass of parenchymal cells grouped around the terminal branches of hepatic arterioles and portal venules just as they anastomose into sinusoids (13, 14). The liver sinusoids are lined by a thin layer of fenestrated liver sinusoidal endothelial cells (LSECs) and lack organized basal lamina, which facilitate the passage of blood plasma to the underlying hepatocytes. Microvilli of hepatocytes extend into the space of Disse, existing between sinusoids and hepatocytes and exerting metabolic functions.

The liver receives a dual blood supply from the hepatic artery and portal vein. The arterial blood is oxygenated, while the venous blood is rich in pathogens, toxins and harmless dietary antigens from the gut; the liver therefore faces constant immunologic challenges. The arterial and portal-venous blood undergoes confluence and runs through the liver sinusoids toward the central vein or terminal hepatic venules at a low speed, which facilitates the uptake of gut-derived content by liver cells. As an important barrier between the gut and the circulation, the liver interstitium is highly enriched in both innate and adaptive immune cells, such as LSECs, Kupffer cells (KCs), dendritic cells (DCs), hepatic stellate cells (HSCs), natural killer (NK) cells, natural killer T (NKT) cells, and T cells. These cells contribute to the formation of a local tolerogenic milieu that ignores most harmless self and foreign antigens while retaining immunity to pathogens in order to maintain immune system homeostasis. The overall tolerogenic properties of the liver are markedly manifested in the era of transplantation.

We herein comprehensively review the current evidence implicating the tolerogenic properties of diverse liver cells in liver transplantation tolerance (**Figure 1**).

HEPATIC PARENCHYMA MEDIATED TOLERANCE EFFECTS

Role of Hepatocytes

Approximately 60–80% of the total liver cell population is composed of parenchymal hepatocytes, which robustly express and secrete large amounts of proteins involved in metabolism, glycogen synthesis and toxin decomposition (15, 16). There is growing evidence showing that hepatocytes are involved in immunity by expressing immune receptors, such as pattern recognition receptors, major histocompatibility complex (MHC) and adhesion molecules (16–18). The special physiological and immunological functions of hepatocytes and their complex interaction with non-substantive cells of the liver have a significant impact on the host's immune system and can promote immune tolerance in cases of liver transplantation.

The microvilli of hepatocytes can make contact with the filamentous pseudopodia of T cells across the endothelial fenestrations, thereby presenting antigens to T cells (19, 20). Hepatocytes continuously express MHC class I and are capable of presenting antigens to $CD8^+$ T cells to trigger $CD8^+$ T cell activation and proliferation (21). Hepatocytes can alternatively present antigens to $CD8^+$ T cells through cross-presentation, which is controlled by a specific molecular chaperone called collectrin in the endoplasmic reticulum-Golgi intermediate chamber (22). However, due to the lack of necessary survival factors, $CD8^+$ T cells activated by hepatocytes quickly undergo apoptosis through BCL-2-interacting mediator (bim)- and caspase-dependent apoptosis after transient proliferation and cytotoxic T lymphocyte (CTL) function (20, 23). Hepatocytes can also actively induce $CD8^+$ T cell apoptosis via the FAS or TNF pathway (24). Furthermore, hepatocytes primed $CD8^+$ T cells produce abundant amounts of interleukin (IL)-10 in the absence of IFN-β-producing NKT cells co-activated by the same hepatocytes, thus exerting immunosuppressive function (25). When confronted with an inflammatory response, hepatocytes can be induced to express MHC class II and present antigens to $CD4^+$ T cells (26, 27). Hepatocytes were found to mediate the Th2 differentiation of uncommitted $CD4^+$ T cells and abrogate the capacity of established Th1 cells to secrete IFN-γ (28). Interestingly, hepatocytes promote the conversion of $CD4^+$ T cells into $CD4^+CD25^+Foxp3^+$ regulatory T (Treg) cells and thus induce immune tolerance through the Notch signal pathway (29). Moreover, exosomes or paracrine factors secreted by hepatocytes can also be involved in immune tolerance by interacting with lymphocytes (30, 31).

In brief, hepatocytes regulate immune tolerance in liver transplantation directly and indirectly, and more studies in

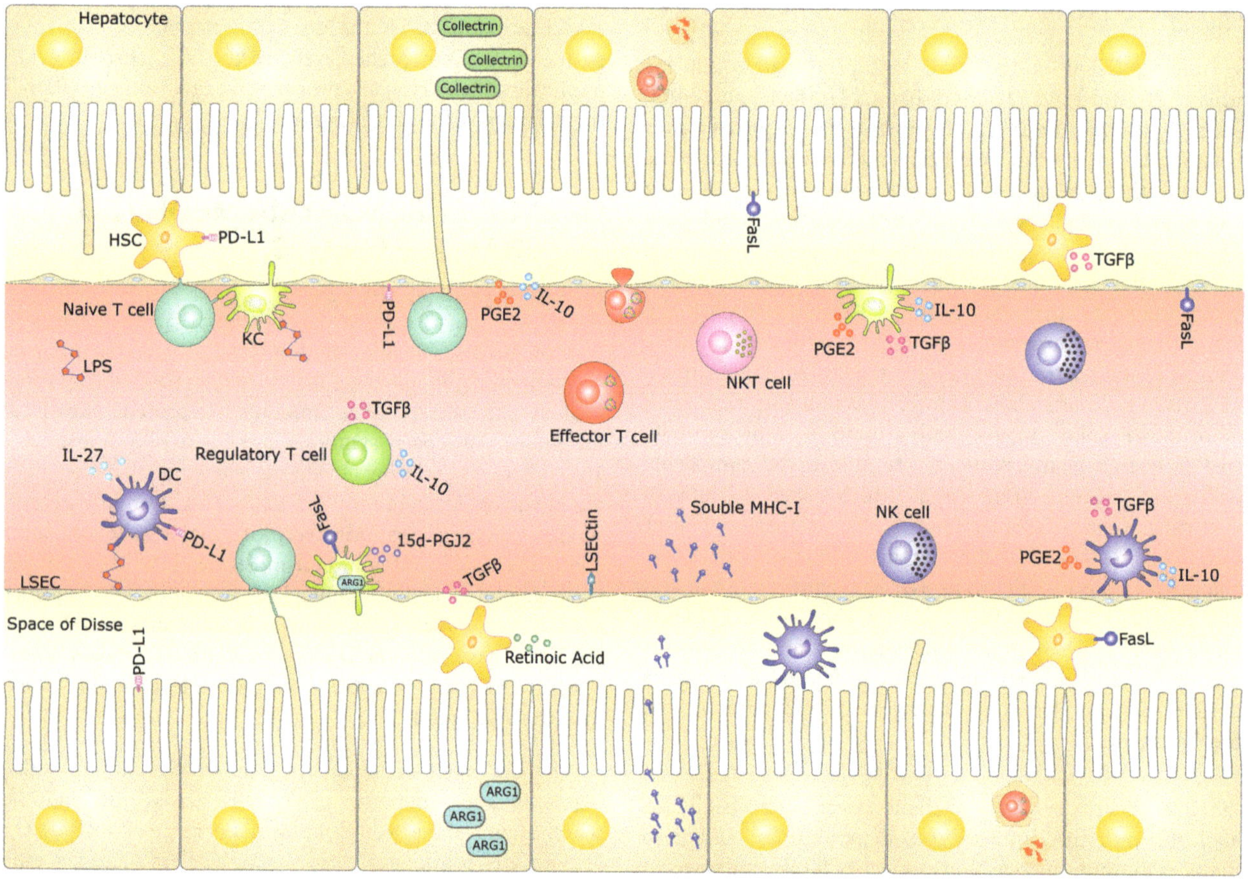

FIGURE 1 | Mechanisms of tolerogenic hepatic microenvironment. The liver sinusoids are lined by a thin layer of fenestrated LSECs and lack organized basal lamina, which facilitate the passage of blood plasma to the underlying hepatocytes. Microvilli of hepatocytes extend into the space of Disse, existing between sinusoids and hepatocytes. The oxygenated arterial and nutrient- rich portal-venous blood undergoes confluence and runs through the liver sinusoids, carrying pathogens, toxins and harmless dietary antigens from the gut. The liver is highly enriched in both innate and adaptive immune cells, such as LSECs, KCs, DCs, HSCs, NK cells, NKT cells, and T cells. The unique liver microenvironment, with its slow blood flow and fenestrated endothelium in the narrow hepatic sinusoids, permits the continuous functional interaction between circulating naive T cells and the diverse hepatic-resident immobile non-professional APCs, such as hepatocytes, LSECs, KCs, DCs, and HSCs. This makes the liver the only non-lymphoid organ that can prime naïve T cell locally. These cells contribute to the liver tolerance through direct cell-cell interaction signaling by surface inhibitory molecules, as well as immunosuppressive milieu through secretory factors. The hepatocytes could also release massive amounts of soluble MHC class I molecules and destroy activated $CD8^+$ T cells through "suicidal emperipolesis" mechanism. HSC, hepatic stellate cell; LSEC, liver sinusoidal endothelial cell; DC, dendritic cell; NK, natural killer cell; NKT, natural killer T cell; KC, Kupffer cell; IL-10, interleukin (IL)-10; TGF-β, transforming growth factor (TGF)-β; LSECtin, LSEC C-type lectin; MHC-I, major histocompatibility complex class I; PD-L1, programmed death ligand 1; FasL, Fas ligand; LPS, lipopolysaccharide; IL-27, interleukin (IL)-27; 15d-PGJ2, 15-Deoxy-Delta-12,14-prostaglandin J2; ARG1, Arginase-1; APC, Antigen-presenting cell; PGE2, Prostaglandin E2.

the future are needed to clarify the mechanism underlying hepatocyte-mediated immune tolerance.

THE INNATE IMMUNE TOLERANCE MECHANISMS

Role of LSECs

LSECs constitute about 50% of non-parenchymal cells in the liver and line the hepatic sinusoids (16). Due to the special structure and abundant blood supply of hepatic sinusoids, LSECs filter out antigens in the blood and play a vital role in maintaining the homeostasis of the hepatic immune microenvironment (32). LSECs express a variety of recognition receptors and scavenger receptors to clear away pathogens in a non-specific manner thus to maintain immune homeostasis of the liver (33–36). In addition, LSECs express MHC class I and II to present antigens to $CD8^+$ and $CD4^+$ T cells, acting as important hepatic resident non-professional APCs (32, 34, 37, 38). On the other hand, LSECs collect MHC class I molecules from their neighbor cells for cross-presentation to $CD8^+$ T cell (39).

LESCs primed naïve $CD4^+$ T cells toward Treg differentiation and suppressed the Thl and Th17 function via IL-10 and PD-1 signaling (33, 38, 40). Studies have shown that LSECs promote the growth of IL-4-expressing Th2 cells and induce a mass of IL-10 secretion through the Notch pathway, thereby creating an immunosuppressive environment within the liver

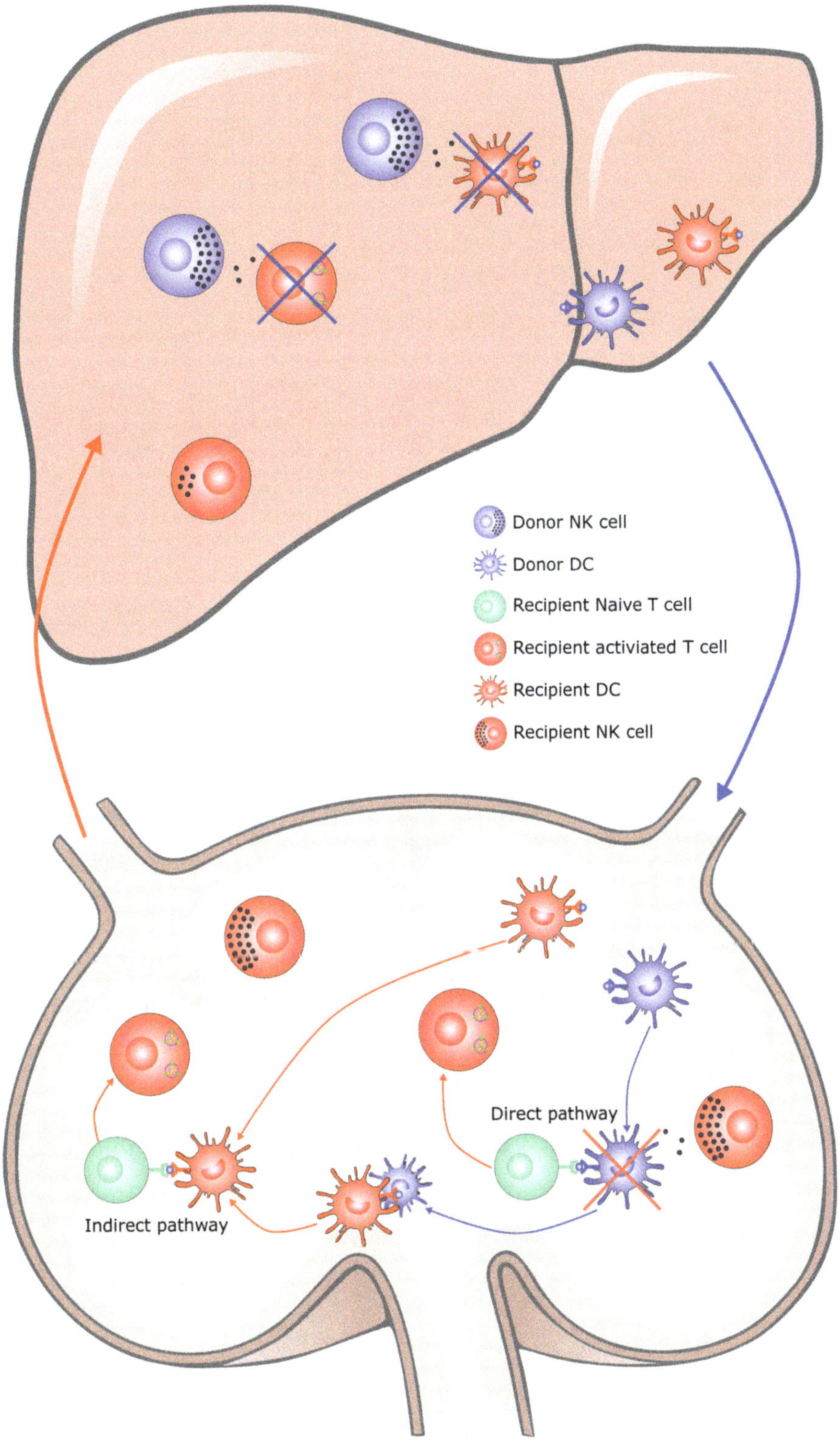

FIGURE 2 | The hypothesis of NK cells in liver transplantation tolerance. In the liver, donor hepatic NK cells promote tolerance, possibly by directly killing recipient immune cells including activated T cells and recipient immature DCs recruited to the allograft, which limited the immune rejection responses. Recipient NK cells would switch to a tolerant phenotype in the tolerogenic hepatic microenvironment. In the secondary lymphoid organs, recipient NK cells kill donor passenger DCs, thereby limiting the activation of T cells by the direct pathway, but favoring the indirect pathway-primed alloreactive T cell response, which contributes to tolerance induction. DC, dendritic cell; NK, natural killer cell; APC, Antigen-presenting cell.

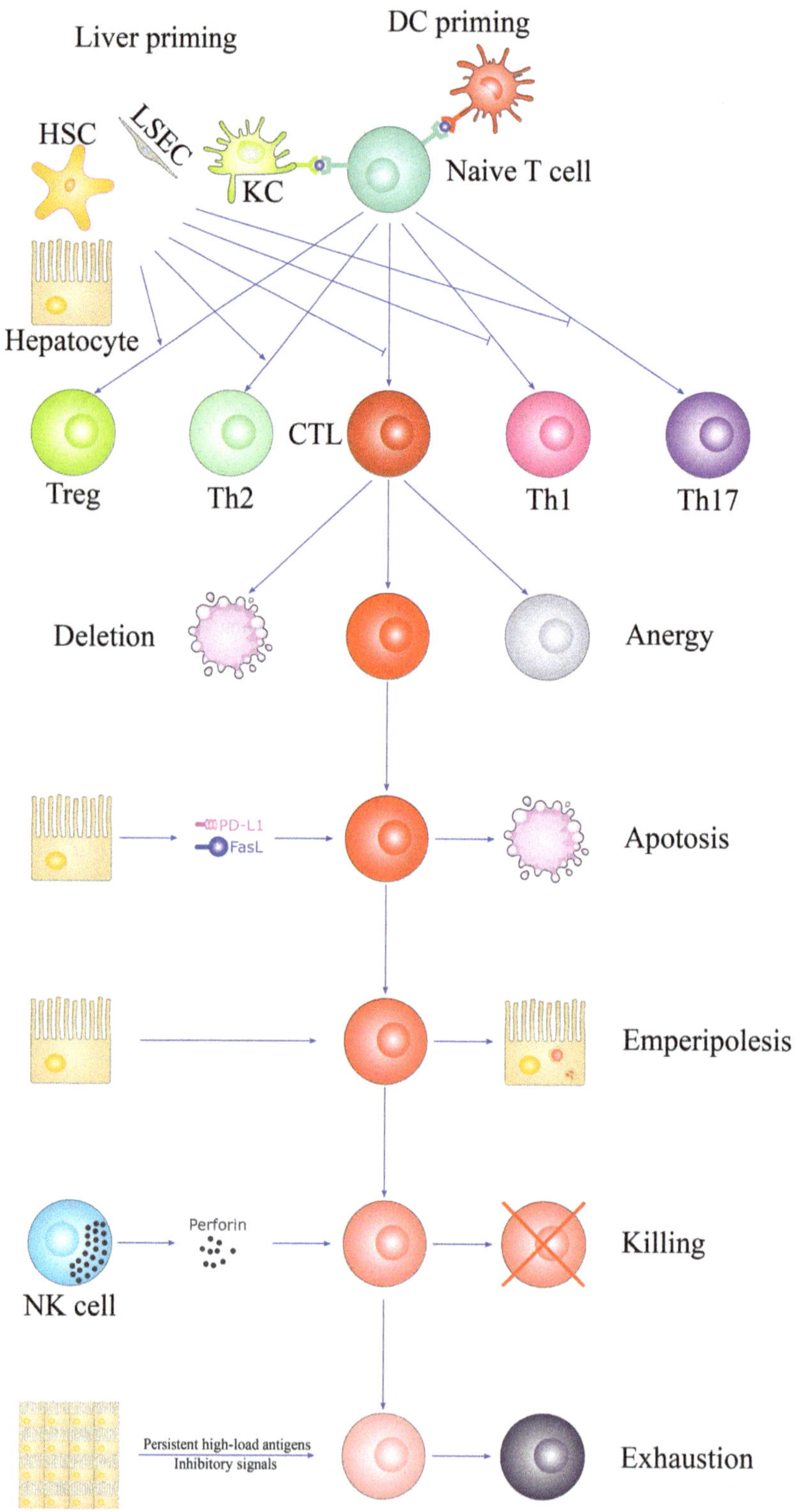

FIGURE 3 | The fate of T cells in liver tolerance. The unique liver microenvironment determines the fate of T cells after activation. T cells were primed by DCs in secondary lymphoid organs or diverse hepatic-resident immobile non-professional APCs in the liver, such as hepatocytes, LSECs, KCs, and HSCs. They are insufficient to optimally prime T cells, which lead to the removal of alloreactive CTLs and suppress the differentiation of proinflammatory Th1 and Th17 cells but favor the skewing of immunosuppressive Th2 and Tregs. The liver is also referred as the graveyard of T cells, suggesting the specific ability of the liver to destroys T cells.

(Continued)

FIGURE 3 | Activated T cells would largely eliminate through clonal deletion, clonal anergy, apoptosis, "suicidal emperipolesis," NK cell killing and T cell exhaustion, thus leading to liver tolerance. HSC, hepatic stellate cell; LSEC, liver sinusoidal endothelial cell; DC, dendritic cell; NK, natural killer cell; CTL, cytotoxic T lymphocyte; KC, Kupffer cell; Th1, T helper cell 1; Th2, T helper cell 2; Th17, T helper cell 17; Treg, Regulatory T cell; PD-L1, programmed death ligand 1; FasL, Fas ligand; APC, Antigen-presenting cell.

(41). Furthermore, LSECs are able to induce $CD4^+$ T cells apoptosis via the Fas/FasL pathway (42). LSECs-mediated $CD8^+$ T cell tolerance is antigen-dose-dependent, meaning that low-dose cross-presenting antigens induces immune tolerance, while high-dose induces effector T cells (43). $CD8^+$ T cells activated by LSECs may exhibit a distinctive phenotype of $CD25^{low}CD44^{high}$ $CD62L^{high}$, which fails to show specific cytotoxicity *in vivo* (44). The interaction of LSECs with naïve $CD8^+$ T cells would in turn promote the tolerogenic maturation of LSECs, characterized by increased expression of MHC class I and programmed death ligand 1 (PD-L1). LSECs can also induced $CD8^+$ T cells apoptosis in a PD-L1 -dependent manner (44). Besides, researchers found that LSEC C-type lectin secreted by LSECs negatively regulates the immune response by specifically recognizing activated T cells via CD44 (45, 46).

Role of KCs

KCs are liver-resident macrophages and account for one-third of the non-parenchymal cells in the liver and almost 90% of all residential macrophages in the body (47). Under physiological conditions, KCs are maintained by self-renewal from local precursors, whereas in response to inflammation, KCs are differentiated from infiltrated bone marrow-derived monocytes. KCs predominantly reside in the periportal region of the sinusoidal lumen, where they are optimally located to respond to systemic or gut-derived antigens and circulating immune cell populations. KCs are equipped with an array of scavenger receptors, Toll-like receptors, complement receptors and Fc receptors through which they detect, bind and internalize pathogens, accompanied by the production of cytokines and chemokines, such as tumor necrosis factor-α (TNF-α), IL-1β, IL-6, IL-12, and IL-18 (37, 48, 49). Under steady-state conditions, KCs also serve as tolerogenic APCs by expressing low levels of MHC class II molecules and costimulatory molecules and secrete anti-inflammatory mediators, such as IL-10, transforming growth factor (TGF)-β1, nitric oxide, or prostaglandin E2, which can suppress antigen-specific T cells activation (50–53). KCs also strongly express the coinhibitory molecules programmed death (PD-1) and PD-L1, which can also inhibit the proliferation and functions of T cells by directly contacting them (54, 55). Furthermore, the interplay between KCs and hepatic Tregs is critical for IL-10 production and the induction of systemic T cell tolerance to hepatocyte-derived antigens (56). The role of KCs in organ transplantation induction has long been implicated in animal transplantation model (57–59). Early studies reported that KCs could contribute to absorption and subsequent clearance of alloreactive antibodies (60, 61). More recently, Chen et al. demonstrated that the deletion of graft KCs using gadolinium trichloride prevented the apoptosis of recipient T cells and consequently spontaneous graft acceptance in a rat liver transplantation model. The apoptosis of T cells induced by KCs was related to nuclear factor kappa B (NF-κB) activity and the Fas/FasL pathway, which was associated with spontaneous liver tolerance (62). However, when this approach was examined in a mouse liver transplantation model, the deletion of graft KCs using clodronate liposomes retained liver allograft acceptance (63). It is also worth to note that in the setting of transplantation, a large proportion of donor-derived KCs are being substituted by recipient-derived macrophages over time after transplantation. The recipient-derived macrophages are thought to be more immunogenic and thus able to promote graft pathology (55, 64, 65).

Role of Liver DCs

DCs are professional APCs that play critical roles in the instigation and regulation of immune responses (66, 67). The general ontogeny, function and classification have been well-described elsewhere (68, 69). The liver harbors more interstitial DCs than any other non-lymphoid organs, including classical myeloid DCs (mDCs) and plasmacytoid DCs (pDCs) (70). They predominantly reside around the portal triad and central vein, with a few cells scattered interstitially between hepatocytes. Due to continuous *in situ* exposure to gut-derived factors, freshly isolated murine hepatic DCs are resistant to lipopolysaccharide (LPS) mediated maturation, which is termed the endotoxin tolerance phenomenon and is also observed in macrophages/monocytes (71, 72). Compared with secondary lymphoid tissue DCs, freshly isolated hepatic DCs are immature and less immunogenic, express low levels of MHC class II and costimulatory molecules (CD80 and CD86) and secrete low levels of IL-12 (73–76). They prefer to produce IL-10 and IL-27 in response to LPS (77) and are less effective in priming naïve allogeneic T cells and Th1 skewing while favoring Th2 cell polarization (71, 73, 78, 79). Human hepatic DCs favor the generation of Th2 cells and Tregs through an IL-10-dependent mechanism (80, 81). The liver is particularly enriched in pDCs, which can suppress effector T cells through IL-27/Stat3 pathway-dependent PD-L1 expression and induce IL-10-producing Tregs via inducible costimulatory ligand (ICOS-L) expression (82, 83).

DCs were thought to be key mediators in spontaneous hepatic allograft tolerance due to their central roles in regulating the immune response. The trigger of allograft immunity relies on three antigen recognition pathways: the direct pathway, indirect pathway, and semi-direct pathway (84, 85). Donor hepatic DCs quickly migrate to the recipient graft-draining lymphoid tissues as passenger leukocytes, where they directly present intact, donor (allogeneic) MHC molecules to alloreactive T cells. The direct allorecognition pathway is considered the dominant pathway of acute rejection. Although this phenomenon exists in almost all types of organ transplantation, the phenotype and function of donor DCs determines the fate of alloreactive T cells, resulting in either graft tolerance or graft rejection. The tolerogenic properties of hepatic DCs may tilt the balance toward graft tolerance. Liver allografts were acutely rejected when donor hepatic DCs were depleted using a CD11c-DTR mouse model before transplantation (86). However, when the interstitial DC quantity was significantly increased by FMS-like tyrosine kinase 3 ligand (Flt3L) treatment of the donor, liver allografts were also rejected acutely (87, 88). Acute rejection is associated with a marked IL-12 reduction by donor DCs. IL-12 neutralization enhanced the apoptotic death of T cells within both the grafts and the spleen and prolonged the survival of grafts from Flt3L-treated donors. Donor grafts from DAP12$^{-/-}$ mice, whose mDCs exhibit a more mature phenotype than that of naïve mice with enhanced migratory and T cell allostimulatory abilities, failed to induce tolerance and were rejected acutely (89).

Following transplantation, donor-derived hepatic DCs were quickly diminished and replaced by recipient DCs, which peaked on post-operative day 7 and persisted indefinitely. These recipient DCs acquired and expressed intact donor MHC molecules via cell-cell contact or extracellular vesicles and were thus termed cross-dressed DCs (90–94). Interestingly, around 60% of host DCs in liver grafts are cross-dressed DCs. They express high levels of PD-L1 and IL-10, subvert the host anti-donor T cell responses and promote liver transplantation tolerance (95). In contrast, the non-cross-dressed DCs show a minimal suppressor function.

Although the role of DCs in spontaneous hepatic allograft tolerance remains to be further investigated, the manipulation of DCs, such as by *in situ* targeting or infusion after *ex vivo* generation, has been shown to be a promising approach for promoting donor-specific tolerance. The *ex vivo* generation of regulatory DCs can be achieved by culturing DC progenitors using low concentrations of granulocyte-macrophage colony-stimulating factor (GM-CSF) ± IL-4, with the addition of one or more pharmacological agents, such as IL-10, dexamethasone, Vitamin D3, or rapamycin (96–98). The *in situ* manipulation of DCs, such as by the delivery of immunomodulatory factors targeting DCs to regulate alloreactive T cell responses, is an alternative approach to achieve donor-specific transplantation tolerance (99). In experimental transplantation models, the manipulation of DCs showed encouraging efficacy and safety in organ-specific tolerance induction (99–101). Several early-phase clinical trials of *ex vivo*-generated DCs in living-donor liver transplantation have recently been initiated (clinicaltrials.gov identifier: NCT03164265 and NCT04208919) (99, 102).

Role of HSCs

HSCs account for about 5–8% of liver non-parenchymal cells (103). HSCs are distributed in the space of Disse, in which the cytoplasm is rich in retinoid lipid droplets and vitamin A and regulate the blood flow in the sinusoids of the liver. HSCs undergo activation in response to liver injury and inflammatory events (104, 105). Activated HSCs secrete cytokines, chemokines and extracellular matrix to participate in the pathogenesis of liver fibrogenesis.

The HSCs are potent liver-resident APCs that have the ability of tolerizing T cells. They can induce T cells apoptosis through the PD-L1, B7-H4, and the Fas/FasL signaling pathways and veto the activation of CD8^{+} T cells through a CD54-dependent pathway, thereby suppressing the T cell immune response and maintaining homeostasis and tolerance in the liver (106–111). In a mouse islet transplantation model, co-transplantation of HSCs and islet cells reduced the rejection rate and prolonged the survival of the graft through TRAIL-mediated T cell apoptosis and reduced immune cell infiltration in the graft (112, 113). Activated HSCs induce the conversion of mature monocytes into myeloid-derived suppressor cells (MDSCs), which may contribute to liver immunosuppression (114, 115). In addition, HSCs also participate in immune tolerance by secreting the immunosuppressive factors TGF-β1 and *all-trans* retinoic acid, thereby promoting the differentiation and proliferation of Foxp3^{+} Tregs (116–119). In liver transplantation models, activated HSCs induced immune tolerance by inducing T cell apoptosis and stimulating IL-10 and TGF-β1 production (110). Activated HSCs also promote transplantation tolerance by inducing selective expansion of allogeneic Tregs and reducing inflammation and alloimmunity (117).

Role of NK and NKT Cells

NK cells and NKT cells are innate lymphocytes particularly enriched in the liver. Following transplantation, NK cells and NKT cells persist in the liver and blood, unlike donor T cells, B cells, and DCs, which migrate into secondary lymphoid organs and are rejected rapidly. This phenomenon suggests that these cells are resistant to rejection and may contribute to liver tolerance (120). NK cells represent ~30–50% of total lymphocytes in the liver, with constitutive cytolytic functions that are responsible for exogenous pathogen clearance and tumor immunity (121–123). The function of NK cells is controlled by the balance of a series of activatory and inhibitory signals receptors constitutively expressed on the cell surface. NK cells can readily recognize allogeneic cells via a unique self-non-self recognition system, termed "missing self" or "missing ligand" recognition, as MHC-incompatible allogeneic cells lack self MHC class I molecules to engage NK inhibitory receptors (124, 125). However, the exact role of NK cells remains unclear. There is evidence that NK cells contribute to both allograft rejection and tolerance in liver transplantation.

Donor-derived NK cells play a major role in liver tolerance, while recipient-derived NK cells are inclined to reject allografts (126). Following transplantation, donor-derived NK cells migrate from liver grafts into the recipient circulation and sustained for ~2 weeks (127). While some of them may persist within the liver graft for decades (128). Donor hepatic NK cells promote tolerance, possibly by directly killing recipient immune cells including activated T cells, as suggested by an *in vitro* study in which alloantigen-activated T cells express stress-induced NKG2D ligands via the ATM/ATR pathway and became susceptible to autologous NK cell lysis (129). Alternatively, hepatic NK cells may kill recipient immature dendritic cells recruited to the allograft, as suggested by the fact that NK cells lyse immature DCs at sites of inflammation (130). However, there is no clear *in vivo* evidence of the above hypothesis (**Figure 2**). Infusion of donor liver NK cells could attenuate liver allograft acute rejection and prolong graft survival in rats (131). Although recipient NK cells can mediate rejection by directly lysing allogeneic liver cells, they become phenotypically distinct and functionally less responsive after migrating to the liver, due to the hepatic microenvironment (132). Recently, Jamil et al. reported that recipient NK cells switched to a tolerant phenotype, as reflected by reduced activating receptor expression, cytotoxicity and cytokine production (133). The tolerance of recipient NK cells occurs upstream of the MHC class I-mediated education via perturbation of the IL-12/STAT4 signaling pathway. Outside of the liver, recipient NK cells kill donor passenger DCs, thereby limiting the activation of T cells by the direct pathway, but favoring the indirect pathway-primed alloreactive T cell response, which contributes to tolerance induction (134–137). In addition, clinical data also showed the correlation of NK cells with allograft tolerance in liver transplantation, but information regarding the origin of the NK cells (from the recipient or donor) was lacking (130, 138, 139).

NKT cells are liver-resident lymphocytes that actively patrol the liver. They share features of both NK and T cells and recognize the lipid antigens from either the host or a microbe presented by the non-classical MHC class I-like molecule CD1. NKT cells contribute to most of the immune responses in the liver and play diverse roles in acute liver injury, liver fibrosis and tolerance. NKT cells are believed to promote liver tolerance induction (140). NKT (Jα281) knockout in the donor liver graft was associated with extensive lymphocytic infiltration of portal triads and bile duct epithelium and significantly impaired the graft survival in mouse liver transplantation models (141).

THE ADAPTIVE IMMUNE TOLERANCE MECHANISMS

The Fate of T Cells

T cells are the major executor of transplantation rejection, doing so by directly destroying allograft cells. The fate of T cells after their activation determines the outcome of transplantation: either allograft tolerance or rejection. Naïve T cells usually lack permission to enter the parenchyma of most organs, due to the lack of the adhesion molecules and chemokine receptors required for adhesion to endothelial cells or subsequent transendothelial migration (142). Naïve T cells circulate in the blood and migrate into secondary lymphoid organs, where they are activated by interacting with DCs. The T cell activation results in adhesion molecule and chemokine receptor upregulation, which allows them to migrate and infiltrate tissues. In the liver, however, the situation is different. The unique liver microenvironment, with its slow blood flow and fenestrated endothelium in the narrow hepatic sinusoids, permits the continuous functional interaction between circulating naive T cells and the diverse hepatic-resident immobile non-professional APCs, as mentioned above. This makes the liver the only non-lymphoid organ that can prime naïve T cells locally independently of DCs and secondary lymphoid organs (143). These non-professional APCs are generally tolerogenic, as reflected in their low expression of MHC molecules, costimulatory molecules and proinflammatory cytokines but rather high expression of coinhibitory molecules and anti-inflammatory cytokines (43, 44, 51, 52, 108, 144–148). They are insufficient to optimally prime the T cells, which leads to the removal of alloreactive T cells, thus promoting tolerance (49, 149–151).

A classic theory refers to the liver as the graveyard of T cells, suggesting the specific ability of the liver to retain and eliminate activated T cells (152, 153). The liver destroys T cells undergoing apoptosis or activated T cells recognizing their antigen *in situ* by clonal deletion, clonal anergy and T cell exhaustion. Activated $CD8^+$ T cells perfused through the liver are selectively retained primarily by ICAM-1-expressing hepatocytes, LESCs and KCs and subsequently undergo apoptosis (154). Another important mechanism involved in liver tolerance is the phenomenon that liver-activated T cells may be rapidly destroyed by endosomal/lysosomal-depended degradation following an active invasion of hepatocytes expressing the recognition of their cognate antigens (155). This unique mechanism of peripheral deletion was termed "suicidal emperipolesis" and results in the deletion of at least 75% of antigen-specific $CD8^+$ T cells within the first 24 h following activation in the liver.

Other hepatic non-professional APCs, such as LESCs, KCs, and HSCs, also play an important role in liver tolerance through clonal anergy or the deletion of T cells within the hepatic microenvironment. In mouse liver transplantation models, activated $CD8^+$ T cells infiltrating the liver allograft were eliminated by locally induced apoptotic cell death (156). Thus, the systemic administration of mouse IL-2, which rescued $CD8^+$ T cells from apoptosis, induces acute graft rejection (156, 157). In human liver allografts, prominent T cell apoptosis in the sinusoids was also evident in biopsy specimens (158). Even if some activated $CD8^+$ T cells survive these early depletion processes, they may progress to a functionally defective state, known as exhaustion. T cell exhaustion is another pattern of T cell dysfunction that has been frequently studied in the era of chronic viral infection and antitumor immunity (159). T cells become exhausted when encountering a persistent high load of antigens or receiving inhibitory signals, and this condition is characterized by a progressive loss of effector functions and proliferative capacity (160–164). This would most likely happen in the setting of liver transplantation, where the allograft is a large-sized mass and the immunosuppressive microenvironment has an abundant amount of inhibitory signals. Direct evidence of alloreactive $CD8^+$ T cell exhaustion was observed following the rapid and extensive activation of T cells early after transplantation in mice (165). However, the contribution of T cell exhaustion to spontaneous liver tolerance needs to be further explored.

$CD4^+$ T cells help coordinate immune responses primarily by secreting cytokines that target other immune cells to orchestrate a synchronized immune response (166). After activation, naive

$CD4^+$ T cells differentiate into distinct T helper cell lineages, including IFN-γ-producing Th1 cells, IL-4-producing Th2 cells, IL-17-producing Th17 cells, and Tregs (167). The cytokine environment dictates the differentiation and conversion of $CD4^+$ T cells. The profile of the hepatic microenvironment suppresses the differentiation of proinflammatory Th1 and Th17 cells but favors the skewing of immunosuppressive Th2 and Tregs, which promote allograft tolerance. Tregs are the most well-known suppressor T cells and play an important role in both transplantation tolerance induction and maintenance (168–170). The frequency of Tregs was shown to be increased in liver grafts and host spleens after transplantation (171). The depletion of host Tregs enhanced the T cell response and reduced apoptosis, thereby abrogating spontaneous liver allograft acceptance in a mouse model (171, 172).

OTHER PROPOSED LIVER TOLERANCE MECHANISMS

Role of Soluble Donor MHC-I Molecules

Liver allografts release massive amounts of soluble MHC class I molecules that persist in the recipient circulation at high concentrations (173), which may act as a plausible mechanism of liver transplantation tolerance. The activation of T cells requires the first signal to be provided by the MHC/antigen-peptide complex and the second signal to be provided by the co-stimulatory signal. Stimulation of T cell receptors in the absence of a co-stimulatory signal induces T cells apoptosis (174). Due to the lack of costimulatory molecules, the binding of soluble MHC molecules to T cells leads to tolerance of antigen-specific T cells and is widely used in the study of allogeneic transplantation. A large number of soluble MHC class I molecules are released into the circulatory system in liver transplantation and are involved in inducing immune tolerance and promoting the graft survival (173, 175–178).

Although earlier studies reported that MHC class I-deficient liver allografts were still accepted indefinitely (179), the low immunogenicity due to MHC-deficient makes these studies difficult to interpret. Other studies have shown that soluble MHC molecules inhibit transplant rejection and prolong the graft survival by inhibiting allergic T cells and inducing CTL apoptosis in a dose-dependent manner (180–185). The advent of MHC/antigen-peptide multimer technology has provided T-cell receptor (TCR) with a relatively high-affinity ligand and an effective way of regulating the activation and function of T cells. Soluble MHC class I molecules can also neutralize antibodies by binding to alloantibodies, thereby preventing alloantibody-mediated rejection (175). Furthermore, researchers constructed a mouse soluble MHC dimer and found that it was able to bind to TCR specifically and regulate the TCR expression and phosphorylation, thereby inhibiting the activation and cytotoxicity of T cells (186, 187). Fried et al. reported in 2005 that rat RT1.A-Fc dimers were able to prolong the survival time of heart grafts, suggesting the utility of soluble MHC dimers for inhibiting transplant rejection. pMHC dimer may therefore be useful for inhibiting transplant rejection (188).

Role of Passenger Leukocytes and Microchimerism

Passenger leukocytes are donor leukocytes that circulate in the recipient's lymphatic tissue after transplantation (189, 190). Microchimerism refers to the persistently low levels of donor cells (<1 per 10^4 or 10^5 cells) within the peripheral circulation of the transplant recipient (191). The role of passenger leukocytes and microchimerism in organ transplantation has been controversial. Studies have found that passenger leukocytes are important factors for promoting graft rejection in skin, lung and kidney transplants (192–194). However, in liver transplantation, passenger leukocytes and microchimerism can induce transplant immune tolerance.

Liver passenger leukocytes include B cells, T cells, NK cells, NKT cells, and DCs, which quickly enter the recipient's peripheral circulation and then enter the secondary lymphoid organs after transplantation (120). Previous studies detected a large number of donor passenger leukocytes in recipient secondary lymphoid organs or peripheral blood after liver transplantation in rat, mouse and human models (4, 189, 195). Starzl et al. proposed that liver allografts induced tolerance by the lymphocyte balance between the host and the passenger leukocytes (i.e., the ability to reach a stable chimeric state) (191). Subsequent studies have shown that passenger leukocytes interact with allogeneic $CD8^+$ T cells in secondary lymphoid organs, which is an early event in spontaneous liver tolerance (120, 196). Removal of passenger leukocytes by irradiating the donor graft before transplantation results in acute rejection of the graft (196, 197). However, tolerance can be restored by supplementation of liver passenger leukocytes or spleen lymphocytes (196–198). Further research found elevated IL-2 and IFN-γ mRNA levels and apoptotic T cells in transplant-tolerant recipients' secondary lymphoid organs (195, 199). However, other researchers have also suggested that microchimerism is not a major factor in spontaneous liver tolerance, as it fails to predict patients who are suitable for the discontinuation of immunosuppressive therapy (200, 201). Therefore, microchimerism may be the result of tolerance rather than the cause (202). In summary, more research is needed on the role of passenger leukocytes and microchimerism in immune tolerance in liver transplantation.

Role of the High-Load Antigen Effect

The liver is the largest internal solid organ in the body, which may favor allograft tolerance due to its large tissue mass and high-load alloantigens (MHC molecules). The high-load alloantigens dilutes the finite T cell clones and cytokine levels, leading to a low density of alloreactive T cells and insufficient cytokines, and thus potentially result in exhaustion of T cells and subsequent tolerance. This hypothesis was supported by the results of animal transplantation experiments, which showed that larger skin grafts extended the survival (203, 204), as did multiple organ transplantation (205). In contrast, small grafts have higher rejection rates in rat liver transplant models (206–208). In the reduced-volume liver transplantation model, the recipient's tolerance to the graft increased as did the antigen load, which is consistent with other findings (209). In clinical studies, combined liver-kidney transplantation has been associated with a weaker immune response, lower rejection rate and higher survival rate (9, 10, 210). These findings suggested that a high antigen load may partially account for liver tolerance, although the mechanism remains unclear. Some researchers have proposed plausible explanations for liver tolerance: first, the liver's large size dilutes alloreactive T cells and cytokines, which lower the alloimmune responses (211, 212); second, the liver allograft harbors a large number of passenger leukocytes that may contribute to tolerance as discussed above; last, the high-load antigens favor T cell exhaustion (213).

CONCLUDING REMARKS

The unique tolerogenic hepatic microenvironment is due to the hepatic acinus anatomy and the complex cellular network, thus enabling the local activation of naïve T cells by interacting with diverse hepatic-resident immobile non-professional APCs and resulting in the dysfunction and depletion of T alloreactive T cells. Outside the liver graft, passenger hepatic DCs and recipient NK cells also limit the priming of alloreactive T cells. In addition, soluble donor MHC I molecules, the passenger leukocyte theory and the high-load antigen effect may also be important for achieving liver tolerance. These tolerogenic mechanisms determine the fate of T cells toward clonal deletion, clonal anergy and exhaustion, which eventually leads to tolerance (**Figure 3**). However, other critical mechanisms may exist, so further studies are yet needed. Understanding the mechanisms underlying the unique immunologically privileged liver organ is valuable for transplantation management and autoimmune disease treatment.

AUTHOR CONTRIBUTIONS

All authors listed have made a substantial, direct and intellectual contribution to the work, and approved it for publication.

REFERENCES

1. Watt KDS, Pedersen RA, Kremers WK, Heimbach JK, Charlton MR. Evolution of causes and risk factors for mortality post-liver transplant: results of the NIDDK long-term follow-up study. *Am J Transplant.* (2010) 10:1420–7. doi: 10.1111/j.1600-6143.2010.03126.x
2. Feng S, Bucuvalas J. Tolerance after liver transplantation: where are we? *Liver Transpl.* (2017) 23:1601–14. doi: 10.1002/lt.24845
3. Zimmermann FA, Davies HS, Knoll PP, Gokel JM, Schmidt T. Orthotopic liver allografts in the rat. The influence of strain combination on the fate of the graft. *Transplantation.* (1984) 37:406–10. doi: 10.1097/00007890-198404000-00019
4. Qian S, Demetris AJ, Murase N, Rao AS, Fung JJ, Starzl TE. Murine liver allograft transplantation: tolerance and donor cell chimerism. *Hepatology.* (1994) 19:916–24. doi: 10.1002/hep.1840190418
5. Calne RY, Sells RA, Pena JR, Davis DR, Millard PR, Herbertson BM, et al. L. Induction of immunological tolerance by porcine liver allografts. *Nature.* (1969) 223:472–6. doi: 10.1038/223472a0
6. Benítez C, Londoño MC, Miquel R, Manzia TM, Abraldes JG, Lozano JJ, et al. Prospective multicenter clinical trial of immunosuppressive drug withdrawal in stable adult liver transplant recipients. *Hepatology.* (2013) 58:1824–35. doi: 10.1002/hep.26426
7. Feng S, Ekong UD, Lobritto SJ, Demetris AJ, Roberts JP, Rosenthal P, et al. Complete immunosuppression withdrawal and subsequent allograft function among pediatric recipients of parental living donor liver transplants. *JAMA.* (2012) 307:283–93. doi: 10.1001/jama.2011.2014
8. Opelz G, Margreiter R, Döhler B. Prolongation of long-term kidney graft survival by a simultaneous liver transplant: the liver does it, and the heart does it too. *Transplantation.* (2002) 74:1390–4. doi: 10.1097/00007890-200211270-00008
9. Rasmussen A, Davies HF, Jamieson NV, Evans DB, Calne RY. Combined transplantation of liver and kidney from the same donor protects the kidney from rejection and improves kidney graft survival. *Transplantation.* (1995) 59:919–21. doi: 10.1097/00007890-199503000-00025
10. Creput C, Durrbach A, Samuel D, Eschwege P, Amor M, Kriaa F, et al. Incidence of renal and liver rejection and patient survival rate following combined liver and kidney transplantation. *Am J Transplant.* (2003) 3:348–56. doi: 10.1034/j.1600-6143.2003.00050.x
11. Sawada T, Asanuma Y, Furuya T, Shibata S, Yasui O, Sato T, et al. Induction of systemic tolerance in islet allograft by liver transplantation. *Transplant Proc.* (2001) 33:2995–9. doi: 10.1016/S0041-1345(01)02285-0
12. Qian S, Fung JJ, Sun H, Demetris AJ, Starzl TE. Transplantation unresponsiveness induced by liver allografts in mouse strains with various histocompatibility disparities. *Transplant Proc.* (1992) 24:1605–6.
13. Lautt WW, Greenway CV. Conceptual review of the hepatic vascular bed. *Hepatology.* (1987) 7:952–63. doi: 10.1002/hep.1840070527
14. Rappaport AM. The microcirculatory hepatic unit. *Microvasc Res.* (1973) 6:212–28. doi: 10.1016/0026-2862(73)90021-6
15. Seki E, Brenner DA. Toll-like receptors and adaptor molecules in liver disease: update. *Hepatology.* (2008) 48:322–35. doi: 10.1002/hep.22306
16. Racanelli V, Rehermann B. The liver as an immunological organ. *Hepatology.* (2006) 43:S54–62. doi: 10.1002/hep.21060
17. Liu S, Gallo DJ, Green AM, Williams DL, Gong X, Shapiro RA, et al. Role of toll-like receptors in changes in gene expression and NF-kappa B activation in mouse hepatocytes stimulated with lipopolysaccharide. *Infect Immun.* (2002) 70:3433–42. doi: 10.1128/IAI.70.7.3433-3442.2002
18. Kubes P, Jenne C. Immune Responses in the Liver. *Ann Rev Immunol.* (2018) 36:247–77. doi: 10.1146/annurev-immunol-051116-052415
19. Warren A, Le Couteur DG, Fraser R, Bowen DG, McCaughan GW, Bertolino P. T lymphocytes interact with hepatocytes through fenestrations in murine liver sinusoidal endothelial cells. *Hepatology.* (2006) 44:1182–90. doi: 10.1002/hep.21378
20. Bertolino P, Trescol-Biémont MC, Rabourdin-Combe C. Hepatocytes induce functional activation of naive $CD8^+$ T lymphocytes but fail to promote survival. *Eur J Immunol.* (1998) 28:221–36. doi: 10.1002/(SICI)1521-4141(199801)28:01<221::AID-IMMU221>3.0.CO;2-F
21. Holz LE, Warren A, Le Couteur DG, Bowen DG, Bertolino P. $CD8^+$ T cell tolerance following antigen recognition on hepatocytes. *J Autoimmun.* (2010) 34:15–22. doi: 10.1016/j.jaut.2009.08.005
22. Dolina JS, Cechova S, Rudy CK, Sung SSJ, Tang WW, Lee J, et al. Cross-Presentation of soluble and cell-associated antigen by murine hepatocytes is enhanced by collectrin expression. *J Immunol.* (2017) 198:2341–51. doi: 10.4049/jimmunol.1502234
23. Holz LE, Benseler V, Bowen DG, Bouillet P, Strasser A, O'Reilly L, et al. Intrahepatic murine CD8 T-cell activation associates with a distinct phenotype leading to Bim-dependent death. *Gastroenterology.* (2008) 135:989–97. doi: 10.1053/j.gastro.2008.05.078
24. Crispe IN. Hepatic T cells and liver tolerance. *Nat Rev Immunol.* (2003) 3:51–62. doi: 10.1038/nri981
25. Wahl C, Bochtler P, Schirmbeck R, Reimann J. Type I IFN-producing CD4 Valpha14i NKT cells facilitate priming of IL-10-producing CD8 T cells by hepatocytes. *J Immunol.* (2007) 178:2083–93. doi: 10.4049/jimmunol.178.4.2083
26. Herkel J, Jagemann B, Wiegard C, Lazaro JFG, Lueth S, Kanzler S, et al. MHC class II expressing hepatocytes function as antigen-presenting cells and activate specific CD4 T lymphocyutes. *Hepatology.* (2003) 37:1079–85. doi: 10.1053/jhep.2003.50191

27. DeTemple DE, Oldhafer F, Falk CS, Chen-Wacker C, Figueiredo C, Kleine M, et al. Hepatocyte-induced CD4+ T cell alloresponse is associated with major histocompatibility complex class II up-regulation on hepatocytes and suppressible by regulatory T cells. *Liver Transpl.* (2018) 24:407–19. doi: 10.1002/lt.25019
28. Wiegard C, Wolint P, Frenzel C, Cheruti U, Schmitt E, Oxenius A, et al. Defective T helper response of hepatocyte-stimulated CD4 T cells impairs antiviral CD8 response and viral clearance. *Gastroenterology.* (2007) 133:2010–8. doi: 10.1053/j.gastro.2007.09.007
29. Burghardt S, Claass B, Erhardt A, Karimi K, Tiegs G. Hepatocytes induce Foxp3+ regulatory T cells by notch signaling. *J Leukocyte Biol.* (2014) 96:571–7. doi: 10.1189/jlb.2AB0613-342RR
30. Holman NS, Church RJ, Nautiyal M, Rose KA, Thacker SE, Otieno MA, et al. Hepatocyte-derived exosomes promote liver immune tolerance: possible implications for idiosyncratic drug-induced liver injury. *Toxicol Sci.* (2019) 170:499–508. doi: 10.1093/toxsci/kfz112
31. Sierro F, Tay SS, Warren A, Le Couteur DG, McCaughan GW, Bowen DG, et al. Suicidal emperipolesis: a process leading to cell-in-cell structures, T cell clearance and immune homeostasis. *Curr Mol Med.* (2015) 15:819–27. doi: 10.2174/1566524015666151026102143
32. Sørensen KK, Simon-Santamaria J, McCuskey RS, Smedsrød B. Liver sinusoidal endothelial cells. *Comp Physiol.* (2015) 5:1751–74. doi: 10.1002/cphy.c140078
33. Carambia A, Frenzel C, Bruns OT, Schwinge D, Reimer R, Hohenberg H, et al. Inhibition of inflammatory CD4 T cell activity by murine liver sinusoidal endothelial cells. *J Hepatol.* (2013) 58:112–8. doi: 10.1016/j.jhep.2012.09.008
34. Limmer A, Ohl J, Wingender G, Berg M, Jüngerkes F, Schumak B, et al. Cross-presentation of oral antigens by liver sinusoidal endothelial cells leads to CD8 T cell tolerance. *Eur J Immunol.* (2005) 35:2970–81. doi: 10.1002/eji.200526034
35. Rubinstein D, Roska AK, Lipsky PE. Liver sinusoidal lining cells express class II major histocompatibility antigens but are poor stimulators of fresh allogeneic T lymphocytes. *J Immunol.* (1986) 137:1803–10.
36. Knolle PA, Gerken G. Local control of the immune response in the liver *Immunol Rev.* (2000) 174:21–34. doi: 10.1034/j.1600-0528.2002.017408.x
37. Crispe IN. The liver as a lymphoid organ. *Annu Rev Immunol.* (2009) 27:147–63. doi: 10.1146/annurev.immunol.021908.132629
38. Knolle PA, Schmitt E, Jin S, Germann T, Duchmann R, Hegenbarth S, et al. Induction of cytokine production in naive CD4(+) T cells by antigen-presenting murine liver sinusoidal endothelial cells but failure to induce differentiation toward Th1 cells. *Gastroenterology.* (1999) 116:1428–40. doi: 10.1016/S0016-5085(99)70508-1
39. Schölzel K, Schildberg FA, Welz M, Börner C, Geiger S, Kurts C, et al. Transfer of MHC-class-I molecules among liver sinusoidal cells facilitates hepatic immune surveillance. *J Hepatol.* (2014) 61:600–8. doi: 10.1016/j.jhep.2014.04.028
40. Kruse N, Neumann K, Schrage A, Derkow K, Schott E, Erben U, et al. Priming of CD4+ T cells by liver sinusoidal endothelial cells induces CD25low forkhead box protein 3-regulatory T cells suppressing autoimmune hepatitis. *Hepatology.* (2009) 50:1904–13. doi: 10.1002/hep.23191
41. Klugewitz K, Blumenthal-Barby F, Schrage A, Knolle PA, Hamann A, Crispe IN. Immunomodulatory effects of the liver: deletion of activated CD4+ effector cells and suppression of IFN-gamma-producing cells after intravenous protein immunization. *J Immunol.* (2002) 169:2407–13. doi: 10.4049/jimmunol.169.5.2407
42. Tokita D, Shishida M, Ohdan H, Onoe T, Hara H, Tanaka Y, et al. Liver sinusoidal endothelial cells that endocytose allogeneic cells suppress T cells with indirect allospecificity. *J Immunol.* (2006) 177:3615–24. doi: 10.4049/jimmunol.177.6.3615
43. Schurich A, Berg M, Stabenow D, Böttcher J, Kern M, Schild HJ, et al. Dynamic regulation of CD8 T cell tolerance induction by liver sinusoidal endothelial cells. *J Immunol.* (2010) 184:4107–14. doi: 10.4049/jimmunol.0902580
44. Diehl L, Schurich A, Grochtmann R, Hegenbarth S, Chen L, Knolle PA. Tolerogenic maturation of liver sinusoidal endothelial cells promotes B7-homolog 1-dependent CD8+ T cell tolerance. *Hepatology.* (2007) 47:296–305. doi: 10.1002/hep.21965
45. Yang Z, Li Q, Wang X, Jiang X, Zhao D, Lin X, et al. C-type lectin receptor LSECtin-mediated apoptotic cell clearance by macrophages directs intestinal repair in experimental colitis. *Proc Natl Acad Sci USA.* (2018) 115:11054–9. doi: 10.1073/pnas.1804094115
46. Tang L, Yang J, Liu W, Tang X, Chen J, Zhao D, et al. Liver sinusoidal endothelial cell lectin, LSECtin, negatively regulates hepatic T-cell immune response. *Gastroenterology.* (2009) 137:1498–508.e1-5. doi: 10.1053/j.gastro.2009.07.051
47. Bilzer M, Roggel F, Gerbes AL. Role of Kupffer cells in host defense and liver disease. *Liver Int.* (2006) 26:1175–86. doi: 10.1111/j.1478-3231.2006.01342.x
48. Jenne CN, Kubes P. Immune surveillance by the liver. *Nat Immunol.* (2013) 14:996–1006. doi: 10.1038/ni.2691
49. Thomson AW, Knolle PA. Antigen-presenting cell function in the tolerogenic liver environment. *Nat Rev Immunol.* (2010) 10:753–66. doi: 10.1038/nri2858
50. Bissell DM, Wang SS, Jarnagin WR, Roll FJ. Cell-specific expression of transforming growth factor-beta in rat liver. Evidence for autocrine regulation of hepatocyte proliferation. *J Clin Invest.* (1995) 96:447–55. doi: 10.1172/JCI118055
51. Knolle PA, Uhrig A, Protzer U, Trippler M, Duchmann R, Meyer zum Büschenfelde KH, et al. Interleukin-10 expression is autoregulated at the transcriptional level in human and murine Kupffer cells. *Hepatology.* (1998) 27:93–9. doi: 10.1002/hep.510270116
52. You Q, Cheng L, Kedl RM, Ju C. Mechanism of T cell tolerance induction by murine hepatic Kupffer cells. *Hepatology.* (2008) 48:978–90. doi: 10.1002/hep.22395
53. Roland CR, Walp L, Stack RM, Flye MW. Outcome of Kupffer cell antigen presentation to a cloned murine Th1 lymphocyte depends on the inducibility of nitric oxide synthase by IFN-gamma. *J Immunol.* (1994) 153:5453–64.
54. Li T, Zhu JY, Wang FS, Leng XS. Down-Regulation of donor Kupffer cell B7 expression reduced recipient lymphocyte activation and secretion of interleukin-2 *in vitro. Transpl Proc.* (2015) 47:2985–90. doi: 10.1016/j.transproceed.2015.10.038
55. Heymann F, Peusquens J, Ludwig-Portugall I, Kohlhepp M, Ergen C, Niemietz P, et al. Liver inflammation abrogates immunological tolerance induced by Kupffer cells. *Hepatology.* (2015) 62:279–91. doi: 10.1002/hep.27793
56. Breous E, Somanathan S, Vandenberghe LH, Wilson JM. Hepatic regulatory T cells and Kupffer cells are crucial mediators of systemic T cell tolerance to antigens targeting murine liver. *Hepatology.* (2009) 50:612–21. doi: 10.1002/hep.23043
57. Kamei T, Callery MP, Flye MW. Kupffer cell blockade prevents induction of portal venous tolerance in rat cardiac allograft transplantation. *J Surg Res.* (1990) 48:393–6. doi: 10.1016/0022-4804(90)90001-I
58. Sato K, Yabuki K, Haba T, Maekawa T. Role of Kupffer cells in the induction of tolerance after liver transplantation. *J Surg Res.* (1996) 63:433–8. doi: 10.1006/jsre.1996.0288
59. Callery MP, Kamei T, Flye MW. Kupffer cell blockade inhibits induction of tolerance by the portal venous route. *Transplantation.* (1989) 47:1092–4. doi: 10.1097/00007890-198906000-00041
60. Houssin D, Bellon B, Brunaud MD, Gugenheim J, Settaf A, Meriggi F, et al. Interactions between liver allografts and lymphocytotoxic alloantibodies in inbred rats. *Hepatology.* (1986) 6:994–8. doi: 10.1002/hep.1840060531
61. Gugenheim J, Amorosa L, Gigou M, Fabiani B, Rouger P, Gane P, et al. Specific absorption of lymphocytotoxic alloantibodies by the liver in inbred rats. *Transplantation.* (1990) 50:309–13. doi: 10.1097/00007890-199008000-00027
62. Chen Y, Liu Z, Liang S, Luan X, Long F, Chen J, et al. Role of Kupffer cells in the induction of tolerance of orthotopic liver transplantation in rats. *Liver Transpl.* (2008) 14:823–36. doi: 10.1002/lt.21450
63. Morita M, Joyce D, Miller C, Fung JJ, Lu L, Qian S. Rejection triggers liver transplant tolerance: involvement of mesenchyme-mediated immune control mechanisms in mice. *Hepatology.* (2015) 62:915–31. doi: 10.1002/hep.27909
64. Beattie L, Sawtell A, Mann J, Frame TCM, Teal B, de Labastida Rivera F, et al. Bone marrow-derived and resident liver macrophages display unique transcriptomic signatures but similar biological functions. *J Hepatol.* (2016) 65:758–68. doi: 10.1016/j.jhep.2016.05.037
65. Ramachandran P, Pellicoro A, Vernon MA, Boulter L, Aucott RL, Ali A, et al. Differential Ly-6C expression identifies the recruited macrophage

phenotype, which orchestrates the regression of murine liver fibrosis. *Proc Natl Acad Sci USA.* (2012) 109:E3186–95. doi: 10.1073/pnas.1119964109
66. Banchereau J, Steinman RM. Dendritic cells and the control of immunity. *Nature.* (1998) 392:245–52. doi: 10.1038/32588
67. Steinman RM, Hawiger D, Nussenzweig MC. Tolerogenic dendritic cells. *Annu Rev Immunol.* (2003) 21:685–711. doi: 10.1146/annurev.immunol.21.120601.141040
68. Merad M, Sathe P, Helft J, Miller J, Mortha A. The dendritic cell lineage: ontogeny and function of dendritic cells and their subsets in the steady state and the inflamed setting. *Ann Rev Immunol.* (2013) 31:563–604. doi: 10.1146/annurev-immunol-020711-074950
69. Haniffa M, Collin M, Ginhoux F. Ontogeny and functional specialization of dendritic cells in human and mouse. *Adv Immunol.* (2013) 120:1–49. doi: 10.1016/B978-0-12-417028-5.00001-6
70. Steptoe RJ, Patel RK, Subbotin VM, Thomson AW. Comparative analysis of dendritic cell density and total number in commonly transplanted organs: morphometric estimation in normal mice. *Transpl Immunol.* (2000) 8:49–56. doi: 10.1016/S0966-3274(00)00010-1
71. Creus AD, Abe M, Lau AH, Hackstein H, Raimondi G, Thomson AW. Low TLR4 expression by liver dendritic cells correlates with reduced capacity to activate allogeneic T cells in response to endotoxin. *J Immunol.* (2005) 174:2037–45. doi: 10.4049/jimmunol.174.4.2037
72. Biswas SK, Lopez-Collazo E. Endotoxin tolerance: new mechanisms, molecules and clinical significance. *Trends Immunol.* (2009) 30:475–87. doi: 10.1016/j.it.2009.07.009
73. Pillarisetty VG, Shah AB, Miller G, Bleier JI, DeMatteo RP. Liver dendritic cells are less immunogenic than spleen dendritic cells because of differences in subtype composition. *J Immunol.* (2004) 172:1009–17. doi: 10.4049/jimmunol.172.2.1009
74. Bertolino P, McCaughan GW, Bowen DG. Role of primary intrahepatic T-cell activation in the "liver tolerance effect." *Immunol Cell Biol.* (2002). 80:84–92. doi: 10.1046/j.0818-9641.2001.01048.x
75. Thomson AW, Drakes ML, Zahorchak AF, O'Connell PJ, Steptoe RJ, Qian S, et al. Hepatic dendritic cells: immunobiology and role in liver transplantation. *J Leukoc Biol.* (1999) 66:322–30. doi: 10.1002/jlb.66.2.322
76. O'Connell PJ, Morelli AE, Logar AJ, Thomson AW. Phenotypic and functional characterization of mouse hepatic CD8 alpha$^+$ lymphoid-related dendritic cells. *J Immunol.* (2000) 165:795–803. doi: 10.4049/jimmunol.165.2.795
77. Chen Y, Jiang G, Yang HR, Gu X, Wang L, Hsieh CC, et al. Distinct response of liver myeloid dendritic cells to endotoxin is mediated by IL-27. *J Hepatol.* (2009) 51:510–9. doi: 10.1016/j.jhep.2009.04.026
78. Abe M, Tokita D, Raimondi G, Thomson AW. Endotoxin modulates the capacity of CpG-activated liver myeloid DC to direct Th1-type responses. *Eur J Immunol.* (2006) 36:2483–93. doi: 10.1002/eji.200535767
79. Khanna A, Morelli AE, Zhong C, Takayama T, Lu L, Thomson AW. Effects of liver-derived dendritic cell progenitors on Th1- and Th2-like cytokine responses *in vitro* and *in vivo*. *J Immunol.* (2000) 164:1346–54. doi: 10.4049/jimmunol.164.3.1346
80. Bamboat ZM, Stableford JA, Plitas G, Burt BM, Nguyen HM, Welles AP, et al. Human liver dendritic cells promote T cell hyporesponsiveness. *J Immunol.* (2009) 182:1901–11. doi: 10.4049/jimmunol.0803404
81. Moseman EA, Liang X, Dawson AJ, Panoskaltsis-Mortari A, Krieg AM, Liu YJ, et al. Human plasmacytoid dendritic cells activated by CpG oligodeoxynucleotides induce the generation of CD4$^+$CD25$^+$ regulatory T cells. *J Immunol.* (2004) 173:4433–42. doi: 10.4049/jimmunol.173.7.4433
82. Matta BM, Raimondi G, Rosborough BR, Sumpter TL, Thomson AW. IL-27 production and STAT3-dependent upregulation of B7-H1 mediate immune regulatory functions of liver plasmacytoid dendritic cells. *J Immunol.* (2012) 188:5227–37. doi: 10.4049/jimmunol.1103382
83. Ito T, Yang M, Wang YH, Lande R, Gregorio J, Perng OA, et al. Plasmacytoid dendritic cells prime IL-10-producing T regulatory cells by inducible costimulator ligand. *J Exp Med.* (2007) 204:105–15. doi: 10.1084/jem.20061660
84. Siu JHY, Surendrakumar V, Richards JA, Pettigrew GJ. T cell allorecognition pathways in solid organ transplantation. *Front Immunol.* (2018) 9:2548. doi: 10.3389/fimmu.2018.02548
85. Lin CM, Gill RG. Direct and indirect allograft recognition: pathways dictating graft rejection mechanisms. *Curr Opin Organ Transplant.* (2016) 21:40–4. doi: 10.1097/MOT.0000000000000263
86. Yokota S, Yoshida O, Ono Y, Geller DA, Thomson AW. Liver transplantation in the mouse: insights into liver immunobiology, tissue injury, and allograft tolerance. *Liver Transpl.* (2016) 22:536–46. doi: 10.1002/lt.24394
87. Li W, Lu L, Wang Z, Wang L, Fung JJ, Thomson AW, et al. Il-12 antagonism enhances apoptotic death of T cells within hepatic allografts from Flt3 ligand-treated donors and promotes graft acceptance. *J Immunol.* (2001) 166:5619–28. doi: 10.4049/jimmunol.166.9.5619
88. Steptoe RJ, Fu F, Li W, Drakes ML, Lu L, Demetris AJ, et al. Augmentation of dendritic cells in murine organ donors by Flt3 ligand alters the balance between transplant tolerance and immunity. *J Immunol.* (1997) 159:5483–91.
89. Yoshida O, Kimura S, Dou L, Matta BM, Yokota S, Ross MA, et al. DAP12 deficiency in liver allografts results in enhanced donor DC migration, augmented effector T cell responses and abrogation of transplant tolerance. *Am J Transplant.* (2014) 14:1791–805. doi: 10.1111/ajt.12757
90. Marino J, Babiker-Mohamed MH, Crosby-Bertorini P, Paster JT, LeGuern C, Germana S, et al. Donor exosomes rather than passenger leukocytes initiate alloreactive T cell responses after transplantation. *Sci Immunol.* (2016) 1:aaf8759. doi: 10.1126/sciimmunol.aaf8759
91. Liu Q, Rojas-Canales DM, Divito SJ, Shufesky WJ, Stolz DB, Erdos G, et al. Donor dendritic cell-derived exosomes promote allograft-targeting immune response. *J Clin Invest.* (2016) 126:2805–20. doi: 10.1172/JCI84577
92. Harshyne LA, Watkins SC, Gambotto A, Barratt-Boyes SM. Dendritic cells acquire antigens from live cells for cross-presentation to CTL. *J Immunol.* (2001) 166:3717–23. doi: 10.4049/jimmunol.166.6.3717
93. Game DS, Rogers NJ, Lechler RI. Acquisition of HLA-DR and costimulatory molecules by T cells from allogeneic antigen presenting cells. *Am J Transplant.* (2005) 5:1614–25. doi: 10.1111/j.1600-6143.2005.00916.x
94. Russo V, Zhou D, Sartirana C, Rovere P, Villa A, Rossini S, et al. Acquisition of intact allogeneic human leukocyte antigen molecules by human dendritic cells. *Blood.* (2000) 95:3473–7. doi: 10.1182/blood.V95.11.3473.011k06_3473_3477
95. Ono Y, Perez-Gutierrez A, Nakao T, Dai H, Camirand G, Yoshida O, et al. Graft-infiltrating PD-L1 high cross-dressed dendritic cells regulate anti-donor T cell responses in mouse liver transplant tolerance. *Hepatology.* (2017) 67:1499–515. doi: 10.1097/01.tp.0000520343.32573.7c
96. Naranjo-Gómez M, Raïch-Regué D, Oñate C, Grau López L, Ramo Tello C, Pujol-Borrell R, et al. Comparative study of clinical grade human tolerogenic dendritic cells. *J Transl Med.* (2011) 9:89. doi: 10.1186/1479-5876-9-89
97. Penna G, Adorini L. 1 alpha,25-dihydroxyvitamin D3 inhibits differentiation, maturation, activation, and survival of dendritic cells leading to impaired alloreactive T cell activation. *J Immunol.* (2000). 164:2405–11. doi: 10.4049/jimmunol.164.5.2405
98. Turnquist HR, Raimondi G, Zahorchak AF, Fischer RT, Wang Z, Thomson AW. Rapamycin-conditioned dendritic cells are poor stimulators of allogeneic CD4$^+$ T cells, but enrich for antigen-specific Foxp3$^+$ T regulatory cells and promote organ transplant tolerance. *J Immunol.* (2007) 178:7018–31. doi: 10.4049/jimmunol.178.11.7018
99. Ochando J, Ordikhani F, Jordan S, Boros P, Thomson AW. Tolerogenic dendritic cells in organ transplantation. *Transpl Int.* (2019) 33:113–27. doi: 10.1111/tri.13504
100. Rosen SJ, Harris PE, Hardy MA. State of the art: role of the dendritic cell in induction of allograft tolerance. *Transplantation.* (2018) 102:1603–13. doi: 10.1097/TP.0000000000002239
101. Thomson AW, Ezzelarab MB. Regulatory dendritic cells: profiling, targeting, and therapeutic application. *Curr Opin Organ Transplant.* (2018) 23:538–45. doi: 10.1097/MOT.0000000000000565
102. Thomson AW, Metes DM, Ezzelarab MB, Raïch-Regué D. Regulatory dendritic cells for human organ transplantation. *Transpl Rev.* (2019) 33:130–6. doi: 10.1016/j.trre.2019.05.001
103. Reynaert H, Thompson MG, Thomas T, Geerts A. Hepatic stellate cells: role in microcirculation and pathophysiology of portal hypertension. *Gut.* (2002) 50:571–81. doi: 10.1136/gut.50.4.571
104. Tsuchida T, Friedman SL. Mechanisms of hepatic stellate cell activation. *Nat Rev Gastroenterol Hepatol.* (2017) 14:397–411. doi: 10.1038/nrgastro.2017.38
105. Venturi C, Reding R, Quinones JA, Sokal E, Rahier J, Bueno J, et al. Relevance of activated hepatic stellate cells in predicting the development of pediatric liver allograft fibrosis. *Liver Transpl.* (2016) 22:822–9. doi: 10.1002/lt.24412
106. Charles R, Chou H-S, Wang L, Fung JJ, Lu L, Qian S. Human hepatic stellate cells inhibit T-cell response through B7-H1 pathway. *Transplantation.* (2013) 96:17–24. doi: 10.1097/TP.0b013e318294caae

107. Chinnadurai R, Grakoui A. B7-H4 mediates inhibition of T cell responses by activated murine hepatic stellate cells. *Hepatology.* (2010) 52:2177–85. doi: 10.1002/hep.23953
108. Yu M-C, Chen C-H, Liang X, Wang L, Gandhi CR, Fung JJ, et al. Inhibition of T-cell responses by hepatic stellate cells via B7-H1-mediated T-cell apoptosis in mice. *Hepatology.* (2004) 40:1312–21. doi: 10.1002/hep.20488
109. Schildberg FA, Wojtalla A, Siegmund SV, Endl E, Diehl L, Abdullah Z, et al. Murine hepatic stellate cells veto CD8 T cell activation by a CD54-dependent mechanism. *Hepatology.* (2011) 54:262–72. doi: 10.1002/hep.24352
110. Jiang Z, Chen Y, Feng X, Jiang J, Chen T, Xie H, et al. Hepatic stellate cells promote immunotolerance following orthotopic liver transplantation in rats via induction of T cell apoptosis and regulation of Th2/Th3-like cell cytokine production. *Exp Ther Med.* (2013) 5:165–9. doi: 10.3892/etm.2012.801
111. Sumpter TL, Dangi A, Matta BM, Huang C, Stolz DB, Vodovotz Y, et al. Hepatic stellate cells undermine the allostimulatory function of liver myeloid dendritic cells via STAT3-dependent induction of IDO. *J Immunol.* (2012) 189:3848–58. doi: 10.4049/jimmunol.1200819
112. Yang HR, Hsieh CC, Wang L, Fung JJ, Lu L, Qian S. A critical role of TRAIL expressed on cotransplanted hepatic stellate cells in prevention of islet allograft rejection. *Microsurgery.* (2010) 30:332–7. doi: 10.1002/micr.20697
113. Chen CH, Kuo LM, Chang Y, Wu W, Goldbach C, Ross MA, et al. *In vivo* immune modulatory activity of hepatic stellate cells in mice. *Hepatology.* (2006) 44:1171–81. doi: 10.1002/hep.21379
114. Chou HS, Hsieh CC, Yang HR, Wang L, Arakawa Y, Brown K, et al. Hepatic stellate cells regulate immune response by way of induction of myeloid suppressor cells in mice. *Hepatology.* (2011) 53:1007–19. doi: 10.1002/hep.24162
115. Höchst B, Schildberg FA, Sauerborn P, Gäbel YA, Gevensleben H, Goltz D, et al. Activated human hepatic stellate cells induce myeloid derived suppressor cells from peripheral blood monocytes in a CD44-dependent fashion. *J Hepatol.* (2013) 59:528–35. doi: 10.1016/j.jhep.2013.04.033
116. Dunham RM, Thapa M, Velazquez VM, Elrod EJ, Denning TL, Pulendran B, et al. Hepatic stellate cells preferentially induce $Foxp3^+$ regulatory T cells by production of retinoic acid. *J Immunol.* (2013) 190:2009–16. doi: 10.4049/jimmunol.1201937
117. Dangi A, Sumpter TL, Kimura S, Stolz DB, Murase N, Raimondi G, et al. Selective expansion of allogeneic regulatory T cells by hepatic stellate cells: role of endotoxin and implications for allograft tolerance. *J Immunol.* (2012) 188:3667–77. doi: 10.4049/jimmunol.1102460
118. Kumar S, Wang J, Thomson AW, Gandhi CR. Hepatic stellate cells increase the immunosuppressive function of natural $Foxp3^+$ regulatory T cells via IDO-induced AhR activation. *J Leukoc Biol.* (2017) 101:429–38. doi: 10.1189/jlb.2A0516-239R
119. Jiang G, Yang H-R, Wang L, Wildey GM, Fung J, Qian S, et al. Hepatic stellate cells preferentially expand allogeneic $CD4^+$ $CD25^+$ $FoxP3^+$ regulatory T cells in an IL-2-dependent manner. *Transplantation.* (2008) 86:1492–502. doi: 10.1097/TP.0b013e31818bfd13
120. Tay SS, Lu B, Sierro F, Benseler V, McGuffog CM, Bishop GA, et al. Differential migration of passenger leukocytes and rapid deletion of naive alloreactive CD8 T cells after mouse liver transplantation. *Liver Transpl.* (2013) 19:1224–35. doi: 10.1002/lt.23720
121. Klugewitz K, Adams DH, Emoto M, Eulenburg K, Hamann A. The composition of intrahepatic lymphocytes: shaped by selective recruitment? *Trends Immunol.* (2004) 25:590–4. doi: 10.1016/j.it.2004.09.006
122. Mikulak J, Bruni E, Oriolo F, Di Vito C, Mavilio D. Hepatic natural killer cells: organ-specific sentinels of liver immune homeostasis and physiopathology. *Front Immunol.* (2019) 10:946. doi: 10.3389/fimmu.2019.00946
123. Zheng M, Sun H, Tian Z. Natural killer cells in liver diseases. *Front Med.* (2018) 12:269–79. doi: 10.1007/s11684-018-0621-4
124. Ruggeri L, Mancusi A, Capanni M, Martelli MF, Velardi A. Exploitation of alloreactive NK cells in adoptive immunotherapy of cancer. *Curr Opin Immunol.* (2005) 17:211–7. doi: 10.1016/j.coi.2005.01.007
125. Lanier LL. NK cell recognition. *Annu Rev Immunol.* (2005) 23:225–74. doi: 10.1146/annurev.immunol.23.021704.115526
126. Harmon C, Sanchez-Fueyo A, O'Farrelly C, Houlihan DD. Natural killer cells and liver transplantation: orchestrators of rejection or tolerance? *Am J Transplant.* (2016) 16:751–7. doi: 10.1111/ajt.13565
127. Moroso V, Metselaar HJ, Mancham S, Tilanus HW, Eissens D, van der Meer A, et al. Liver grafts contain a unique subset of natural killer cells that are transferred into the recipient after liver transplantation. *Liver Transpl.* (2010) 16:895–908. doi: 10.1002/lt.22080
128. Cuff AO, Robertson FP, Stegmann KA, Pallett LJ, Maini MK, Davidson BR, et al. Eomeshi NK cells in human liver are long-lived and do not recirculate but can be replenished from the circulation. *J Immunol.* (2016) 197:4283–91. doi: 10.4049/jimmunol.1601424
129. Cerboni C, Zingoni A, Cippitelli M, Piccoli M, Frati L, Santoni A. Antigen-activated human T lymphocytes express cell-surface NKG2D ligands via an ATM/ATR-dependent mechanism and become susceptible to autologous NK- cell lysis. *Blood.* (2007) 110:606–15. doi: 10.1182/blood-2006-10-052720
130. Cooper MA, Fehniger TA, Fuchs A, Colonna M, Caligiuri MA. NK cell and DC interactions. *Trends Immunol.* (2004) 25:47–52. doi: 10.1016/j.it.2003.10.012
131. Yu JD, Long TZ, Li GL, Lv LH, Lin HM, Huang YH, et al. Donor liver natural killer cells alleviate liver allograft acute rejection in rats. *HBPD INT.* (2011) 10:386–92. doi: 10.1016/S1499-3872(11)60065-9
132. Lassen MG, Lukens JR, Dolina JS, Brown MG, Hahn YS. Intrahepatic IL-10 maintains $NKG2A^+Ly49^-$ Liver NK cells in a functionally hyporesponsive state. *J Immunol.* (2010) 184:2693–701. doi: 10.4049/jimmunol.0901362
133. Jamil KM, Hydes TJ, Cheent KS, Cassidy SA, Traherne JA, Jayaraman J, et al. STAT4-associated natural killer cell tolerance following liver transplantation. *Gut.* (2017) 66:352–61. doi: 10.1136/gutjnl-2015-309395
134. Garrod KR, Liu FC, Forrest LE, Parker I, Kang SM, Cahalan MD. NK cell patrolling and elimination of donor-derived dendritic cells favor indirect alloreactivity. *J Immunol.* (2010) 184:2329–36. doi: 10.4049/jimmunol.0902748
135. Rulifson IC, Szot GL, Palmer E, Bluestone JA. Inability to induce tolerance through direct antigen presentation. *Am J Transplant.* (2002) 2:510–9. doi: 10.1034/j.1600-6143.2002.20604.x
136. Yu G, Xu X, Vu MD, Kilpatrick ED, Li XC. NK cells promote transplant tolerance by killing donor antigen-presenting cells. *J Exp Med.* (2006) 203:1851–8. doi: 10.1084/jem.20060603
137. Laffont S, Seillet C, Ortaldo J, Coudert JD, Guéry JC. Natural killer cells recruited into lymph nodes inhibit alloreactive T-cell activation through perforin-mediated killing of donor allogeneic dendritic cells. *Blood.* (2008) 112:661–71. doi: 10.1182/blood-2007-10-120089
138. Li L, Wozniak LJ, Rodder S, Heish S, Talisetti A, Wang Q, et al. A common peripheral blood gene set for diagnosis of operational tolerance in pediatric and adult liver transplantation. *Am J Transplant.* (2012) 12:1218–28. doi: 10.1111/j.1600-6143.2011.03928.x
139. Sarwal MM. Fingerprints of transplant tolerance suggest opportunities for immunosuppression minimization. *Clin Biochem.* (2016) 49:404–10. doi: 10.1016/j.clinbiochem.2016.01.007
140. Margalit M, Ilan Y. Induction of immune tolerance: a role for natural killer T lymphocytes? *Liver Int.* (2005) 25:501–4. doi: 10.1111/j.1478-3231.2005.01147.x
141. Morita M, Fujino M, Li XK, Kimura H, Nakayama T, Taniguchi M, et al. Spontaneous tolerance involving natural killer T cells after hepatic grafting in mice. *Transpl Immunol.* (2007) 18:142–5. doi: 10.1016/j.trim.2007.05.015
142. Mackay CR, Marston WL, Dudler L. Naive and memory T cells show distinct pathways of lymphocyte recirculation. *J Exp Med.* (1990) 171:801–17. doi: 10.1084/jem.171.3.801
143. Bertolino P, Bowen DG, McCaughan GW, Fazekas de St. Groth B. Antigen-specific primary activation of $CD8^+$ T cells within the liver. *J Immunol.* (2001) 166:5430–8. doi: 10.4049/jimmunol.166.9.5430
144. Lohse A, Knolle P, Bilo K, Uhrig A, Waldmann C, Ibe M, et al. Antigen-presenting function and B7 expression of murine sinusoidal endothelial cells and kupffer cells. *Gastroenterology.* (1996) 110:1175–81. doi: 10.1053/gast.1996.v110.pm8613007
145. Mühlbauer M, Fleck M, Schütz C, Weiss T, Froh M, Blank C, et al. PD-L1 is induced in hepatocytes by viral infection and by interferon-α and -γ and mediates T cell apoptosis. *J Hepatol.* (2006) 45:520–8. doi: 10.1016/j.jhep.2006.05.007
146. Maier H, Isogawa M, Freeman GJ, Chisari FV. PD-1: PD-L1 interactions contribute to the functional suppression of virus-specific $CD8^+$ T lymphocytes in the liver. *J Immunol.* (2007) 178:2714–20. doi: 10.4049/jimmunol.178.5.2714
147. De Bleser PJ, Niki T, Rogiers V, Geerts A. Transforming growth factor-β gene expression in normal and fibrotic rat liver. *J Hepatol.* (1997) 26:886–93. doi: 10.1016/S0168-8278(97)80257-7
148. Carambia A, Freund B, Schwinge D, Heine M, Laschtowitz A,

Huber S, et al. TGF-β-dependent induction of $CD4^+CD25^+Foxp3^+$ Tregs by liver sinusoidal endothelial cells. *J Hepatol.* (2014) 61:594–9. doi: 10.1016/j.jhep.2014.04.027
149. Crispe IN. Liver antigen-presenting cells. *J Hepatol.* (2011) 54:357–65. doi: 10.1016/j.jhep.2010.10.005
150. Horst AK, Neumann K, Diehl L, Tiegs G. Modulation of liver tolerance by conventional and nonconventional antigen-presenting cells and regulatory immune cells. *Cell Mol Immunol.* (2016) 13:277–92. doi: 10.1038/cmi.2015.112
151. Mehrfeld C, Zenner S, Kornek M, Lukacs-Kornek V. The contribution of non-professional antigen-presenting cells to immunity and tolerance in the liver. *Front Immunol.* (2018) 9:635. doi: 10.3389/fimmu.2018.00635
152. Crispe IN, Dao T, Klugewitz K, Mehal WZ, Metz DP. The liver as a site of T-cell apoptosis: graveyard, or killing field? *Immunol Rev.* (2000) 174:47–62. doi: 10.1034/j.1600-0528.2002.017412.x
153. Huang L, Soldevila G, Leeker M, Flavell R, Crispe IN. The liver eliminates T cells undergoing antigen-triggered apoptosis *in vivo*. *Immunity.* (1994) 1:741–9. doi: 10.1016/S1074-7613(94)80016-2
154. Mehal WZ, Juedes AE, Crispe IN. Selective retention of activated $CD8^+$ T cells by the normal liver. *J Immunol.* (1999) 163:3202–10.
155. Benseler V, Warren A, Vo M, Holz LE, Tay SS, Couteur DGL, et al. Hepatocyte entry leads to degradation of autoreactive CD8 T cells. *Proc Natl Acad Sci USA.* (2011) 108:16735–40. doi: 10.1073/pnas.1112251108
156. Qian S, Lu L, Fu F, Li Y, Li W, Starzl TE, et al. Apoptosis within spontaneously accepted mouse liver allografts: evidence for deletion of cytotoxic T cells and implications for tolerance induction. *J Immunol.* (1997) 158:4654–61.
157. Thai NL, Li Y, Fu F, Qian S, Demetris AJ, Duquesnoy RJ, et al. Interleukin-2 and interleukin-12 mediate distinct effector mechanisms of liver allograft rejection. *Liver Transpl Surg.* (1997) 3:118–29. doi: 10.1002/lt.500030204
158. Clouston AD, Jonsson JR, Balderson GA, Fawcett J, Lynch SV, Kelso A, et al. Lymphocyte apoptosis and cell replacement in human liver allografts. *Transplantation.* (2002) 73:1828–34. doi: 10.1097/00007890-200206150-00022
159. McLane LM, Abdel-Hakeem MS, Wherry EJ. CD8 T cell exhaustion during chronic viral infection and cancer. *Annu Rev Immunol.* (2019) 37:457–95. doi: 10.1146/annurev-immunol-041015-055318
160. Wherry EJ, Kurachi M. Molecular and cellular insights into T cell exhaustion. *Nat Rev Immunol.* (2015) 15:486–99. doi: 10.1038/nri3862
161. Hashimoto M, Kamphorst AO, Im SJ, Kissick HT, Pillai RN, Ramalingam SS, et al. CD8 T cell exhaustion in chronic infection and cancer: opportunities for interventions. *Annu Rev Med.* (2018) 69:301–18. doi: 10.1146/annurev-med-012017-043208
162. Mueller SN, Ahmed R. High antigen levels are the cause of T cell exhaustion during chronic viral infection. *Proc Natl Acad Sci USA.* (2009) 106:8623–8. doi: 10.1073/pnas.0809818106
163. Han S, Asoyan A, Rabenstein H, Nakano N, Obst R. Role of antigen persistence and dose for $CD4^+$ T-cell exhaustion and recovery. *Proc Natl Acad Sci USA.* (2010) 107:20453–8. doi: 10.1073/pnas.1008437107
164. Zuniga EI, Harker JA. T cell exhaustion due to persistent antigen: quantity not quality? *Eur J Immunol.* (2012) 42:2285–9. doi: 10.1002/eji.201242852
165. Steger U, Denecke C, Sawitzki B, Karim M, Jones ND, Wood KJ. Exhaustive differentiation of alloreactive $CD8^+$ T cells: critical for determination of graft acceptance or rejection. *Transplantation.* (2008) 85:1339–47. doi: 10.1097/TP.0b013e31816dd64a
166. Netea MG, Balkwill F, Chonchol M, Cominelli F, Donath MY, Giamarellos-Bourboulis EJ, et al. A guiding map for inflammation. *Nat Immunol.* (2017) 18:826–31. doi: 10.1038/ni.3790
167. Zhou L, Chong MMW, Littman DR. Plasticity of $CD4^+$ T cell lineage differentiation. *Immunity.* (2009) 30:646–55. doi: 10.1016/j.immuni.2009.05.001
168. Besançon A, Baas M, Goncalves T, Valette F, Waldmann H, Chatenoud L, et al. The induction and maintenance of transplant tolerance engages both regulatory and anergic $CD4^+$ T cells. *Front Immunol.* (2017) 8:218. doi: 10.3389/fimmu.2017.00218
169. Burrell BE, Nakayama Y, Xu J, Brinkman CC, Bromberg JS. Treg induction, migration, and function in transplantation. *J Immunol.* (2012) 189:4705–11. doi: 10.4049/jimmunol.1202027
170. Romano M, Fanelli G, Albany CJ, Giganti G, Lombardi G. Past, present, and future of regulatory T cell therapy in transplantation and autoimmunity. *Front Immunol.* (2019) 10:43. doi: 10.3389/fimmu.2019.00043
171. Li W, Kuhr CS, Zheng XX, Carper K, Thomson AW, Reyes JD, et al. New insights into mechanisms of spontaneous liver transplant tolerance: the role of Foxp3-expressing $CD25^+CD4^+$ regulatory T cells. *Am J Transplant.* (2008) 8:1639–51. doi: 10.1111/j.1600-6143.2008.02300.x
172. Jiang X, Morita M, Sugioka A, Harada M, Kojo S, Wakao H, et al. The importance of $CD25^+$ $CD4^+$ regulatory T cells in mouse hepatic allograft tolerance. *Liver Transpl.* (2006) 12:1112–8. doi: 10.1002/lt.20787
173. Davies HS, Pollard SG, Calne RY. Soluble HLA antigens in the circulation of liver graft recipients. *Transplantation.* (1989) 47:524–7. doi: 10.1097/00007890-198903000-00025
174. Schwartz RH. Costimulation of T lymphocytes: the role of CD28, CTLA-4, and B7/BB1 in interleukin-2 production and immunotherapy. *Cell.* (1992) 71:1065–8. doi: 10.1016/S0092-8674(05)80055-8
175. Sumimoto R, Kamada N. Specific suppression of allograft rejection by soluble class I antigen and complexes with monoclonal antibody. *Transplantation.* (1990) 50:678–82. doi: 10.1097/00007890-199010000-00029
176. Geissler EK, Korzun WJ, Graeb C. Secreted donor-MHC class I antigen prolongs liver allograft survival and inhibits recipient anti-donor cytotoxic T lymphocyte responses. *Transplantation.* (1997) 64:782–6. doi: 10.1097/00007890-199709150-00024
177. Geissler EK, Graeb C, Tange S, Guba M, Jauch KW, Scherer MN. Effective use of donor MHC class I gene therapy in organ transplantation: prevention of antibody-mediated hyperacute heart allograft rejection in highly sensitized rat recipients. *Hum Gene Ther.* (2000) 11:459–69. doi: 10.1089/10430340050015923
178. Graeb C, Justl M, Scherer MN, Andrassy J, Frank E, Zuelke C, et al. Use of an adenoviral vector to express soluble donor-major histocompatibility complex molecules capable of suppressing the immune response in rat transplant recipients. *Hum Immunol.* (2002) 63:844–52. doi: 10.1016/S0198-8859(02)00460-3
179. Qian S, Fu F, Li Y, Lu L, Rao AS, Starzl TE, et al. Impact of donor MHC class I or class II antigen deficiency on first- and second-set rejection of mouse heart or liver allografts. *Immunology.* (1996) 88:124–9. doi: 10.1046/j.1365-2567.1996.d01-633.x
180. Spencer SC, Fabre JW. Water-soluble form of RT1.A class I MHC molecules in the kidney and liver of the rat. *Immunogenetics.* (1987) 25:91–8. doi: 10.1007/BF00364273
181. Hausmann R, Zavazava N, Steinmann J, Müller-Ruchholtz W. Interaction of papain-digested HLA class I molecules with human alloreactive cytotoxic T lymphocytes (CTL). *Clin Exp Immunol.* (1993) 91:183–8. doi: 10.1111/j.1365-2249.1993.tb03376.x
182. Gansuvd B, Hagihara M, Munkhbat B, Kanai N, Morita N, Munkhtuvshin N, et al. Inhibition of Epstein-Barr virus (EBV)-specific $CD8^+$ cytotoxic T lymphocyte (CTL) activity by soluble HLA class I *in vitro*. *Clin Exp Immunol.* (2000) 119:107–14. doi: 10.1046/j.1365-2249.2000.01092.x
183. Behrens D, Lange K, Fried A, Yoo-Ott KA, Richter K, Fändrich F, et al. Donor-derived soluble MHC antigens plus low-dose cyclosporine induce transplantation unresponsiveness independent of the thymus by down-regulating T cell-mediated alloresponses in a rat transplantation model. *Transplantation.* (2001) 72:1974–82. doi: 10.1097/00007890-200112270-00018
184. Semiletova NV, Shen XD, Feldman DM, Busuttil RW, Kupiec-Weglinski JW, Ghobrial RM. Donor MHC class I peptides in conjunction with self-epitopes induce donor-specific tolerance in a dose-dependent manner but unable to abrogate chronic rejection. *Transplant Proc.* (2005) 37:1937–9. doi: 10.1016/j.transproceed.2005.02.114
185. Doenecke A, Frank E, Scherer MN, Schlitt HJ, Geissler EK. Prolongation of heart allograft survival after long-term expression of soluble MHC class I antigens and vIL-10 in the liver by AAV-plasmid-mediated gene transfer. *Langenbecks Arch Surg.* (2008) 393:343–8. doi: 10.1007/s00423-008-0298-2
186. Porto JD, Johansen TE, Catipović B, Parfiit DJ, Tuveson D, Gether U, et al. A soluble divalent class I major histocompatibility complex molecule inhibits alloreactive T cells at nanomolar concentrations. *Proc Natl Acad Sci USA.* (1993) 90:6671–5. doi: 10.1073/pnas.90.14.6671
187. O'Herrin SM, Slansky JE, Tang Q, Markiewicz MA, Gajewski TF, Pardoll DM, et al. Antigen-Specific blockade of t cells *in vivo* using dimeric mhc peptide. *J Immunol.* (2001) 167:2555–60. doi: 10.4049/jimmunol.167.5.2555
188. Fried A, Berg M, Sharma B, Bonde S, Zavazava N. Recombinant dimeric MHC antigens protect cardiac allografts from rejection and visualize alloreactive T cells. *J Leukocyte Biol.* (2005)

78:595–604. doi: 10.1189/jlb.0205078

189. Schlitt HJ, Kanehiro H, Raddatz G, Steinhoff G, Richter N, Nashan B, et al. Persistence of donor lymphocytes in liver allograft recipients. *Transplantation.* (1993) 56:1001–7. doi: 10.1097/00007890-199310000-00042
190. Starzl TE, Demetris AJ, Trucco M, Murase N, Ricordi C, Ildstad S, et al. Cell migration and chimerism after whole-organ transplantation: the basis of graft acceptance. *Hepatology.* (1993) 17:1127–52. doi: 10.1002/hep.1840170629
191. Starzl TE, Demetris AJ, Trucco M, Ramos H, Zeevi A, Rudert WA, et al. Systemic chimerism in human female recipients of male livers. *Lancet.* (1992) 340:876–7. doi: 10.1016/0140-6736(92)93286-V
192. Hammond EJ, Ng RL, Stanley MA, Munro AJ. Prolonged survival of cultured keratinocyte allografts in the nonimmunosuppressed mouse. *Transplantation.* (1987) 44:106–12. doi: 10.1097/00007890-198707000-00022
193. Stone JP, Critchley WR, Major T, Rajan G, Risnes I, Scott H, et al. Altered immunogenicity of donor lungs via removal of passenger leukocytes using *ex vivo* lung perfusion. *Am J Transplant.* (2016) 16:33–43. doi: 10.1111/ajt.13446
194. Brown K, Nowocin AK, Meader L, Edwards LA, Smith RA, Wong W. Immunotoxin against a donor mhc class ii molecule induces indefinite survival of murine kidney allografts. *Am J Transplant.* (2016) 16:1129–38. doi: 10.1111/ajt.13584
195. Bishop GA, Sun J, DeCruz DJ, Rokahr KL, Sedgwick JD, Sheil AG, et al. Tolerance to rat liver allografts. III. Donor cell migration and tolerance-associated cytokine production in peripheral lymphoid tissues. *J Immunol.* (1996) 156:4925–31.
196. Sun J, McCaughan GW, Gallagher ND, Sheil AG, Bishop GA. Deletion of spontaneous rat liver allograft acceptance by donor irradiation. *Transplantation.* (1995) 60:233–6. doi: 10.1097/00007890-199508000-00004
197. Shimizu Y, Goto S, Lord R, Vari F, Edwards-Smith C, Chiba S, et al. Restoration of tolerance to rat hepatic allografts by spleen-derived passenger leukocytes. *Transpl Int.* (1996) 9:593–5. doi: 10.1111/j.1432-2277.1996.tb00920.x
198. Sun J, Sheil AG, Wang C, Wang L, Rokahr K, Sharland A, et al. Tolerance to rat liver allografts: IV. Acceptance depends on the quantity of donor tissue and on donor leukocytes. *Transplantation.* (1996) 62:1725–30. doi: 10.1097/00007890-199612270-00005
199. Sharland A, Yan Y, Wang C, Bowen DG, Sun J, Sheil AG, et al. Evidence that apoptosis of activated T cells occurs in spontaneous tolerance of liver allografts and is blocked by manipulations which break tolerance. *Transplantation.* (1999) 68:1736–45. doi: 10.1097/00007890-199912150-00018
200. Devlin J, Doherty D, Thomson L, Wong T, Donaldson P, Portmann B, et al. Defining the outcome of immunosuppression withdrawal after liver transplantation. *Hepatology.* (1998) 27:926–33. doi: 10.1002/hep.510270406
201. Girlanda R, Rela M, Williams R, O'Grady JG, Heaton ND. Long-term outcome of immunosuppression withdrawal after liver transplantation. *Transplant Proc.* (2005) 37:1708–9. doi: 10.1016/j.transproceed.2005.03.070
202. Wood K, Sachs DH. Chimerism and transplantation tolerance: cause and effect. *Immunol Today.* (1996) 17:584–7. doi: 10.1016/S0167-5699(96)10069-4
203. Zanella G, Reif AE, Buenviaje OL, Asakuma R, Deterling RAJ. On prolonged survival of massive skin allografts in mice. *Transplantation.* (1968) 6:885–94. doi: 10.1097/00007890-196811000-00003
204. Lappé MA, Graff RG, Snell GD. The importance of target size in the destruction of skin grafts with non-H-2 incompatibility. *Transplantation.* (1969) 7:372–7. doi: 10.1097/00007890-196905000-00006
205. Wang C, Sheil AGR, Sun J. Outcome of different models of multiorgan transplantation in rats. *Microsurgery.* (1999) 19:318–23. doi: 10.1002/(SICI)1098-2752-1999-19:7<318::AID-MICR5>3.0.CO;2-P
206. Dirsch O, Li J, He Q, Ji Y, Gu YL, Dahmen U. Induction of rejection after small-for-size liver transplantation: size matters. *J Invest Surg.* (2008) 21:288–98. doi: 10.1080/08941930802216823
207. Yang ZF, Ho DWY, Chu ACY, Wang YQ, Fan ST. Linking inflammation to acute rejection in small-for-size liver allografts: the potential role of early macrophage activation. *Am J Transplant.* (2004) 4:196–209. doi: 10.1046/j.1600-6143.2003.00313.x
208. Shiraishi M, Csete ME, Yasunaga C, Drazan KE, Jurim O, Cramer DV, et al. Regeneration-induced accelerated rejection in reduced-size liver grafts. *Transplantation.* (1994) 57:336–40. doi: 10.1097/00007890-199402150-00004
209. Bishop GA, Sun J, Sheil AG, McCaughan GW. High-dose/activation-associated tolerance: a mechanism for allograft tolerance. *Transplantation.* (1997) 64:1377–82. doi: 10.1097/00007890-199711270-00001
210. Fong TL, Bunnapradist S, Jordan SC, Selby RR, Cho YW. Analysis of the united network for organ sharing database comparing renal allografts and patient survival in combined liver-kidney transplantation with the contralateral allografts in kidney alone or kidney-pancreas transplantation. *Transplantation.* (2003) 76:348–53. doi: 10.1097/01.TP.0000071204.03720.BB
211. He C, Schenk S, Zhang Q, Valujskikh A, Bayer J, Fairchild RL, et al. Effects of T cell frequency and graft size on transplant outcome in mice. *J Immunol.* (2004) 172:240–7. doi: 10.4049/jimmunol.172.1.240
212. Ganbold A, Andersen S, Tay SS, Cunningham E, Ilie V, Krishnan S, et al. Expression of common gamma chain signalling cytokines and their receptors distinguishes rejection from tolerance in a rat organ transplant model. *Transplant Immunol.* (2012) 27:89–94. doi: 10.1016/j.trim.2012.08.001
213. Tay SS, Wong YC, McDonald DM, Wood NAW, Roediger B, Sierro F, et al. Antigen expression level threshold tunes the fate of CD8 T cells during primary hepatic immune responses. *Proc Natl Acad Sci USA.* (2014) 111:E2540–9. doi: 10.1073/pnas.1406674111

5

Clinical and Basic Research Progress on Treg-Induced Immune Tolerance in Liver Transplantation

Xuhao Ni[1,2,3,4]*, Qi Wang*[1,2,3,4]*, Jian Gu*[1,2,3,4] *and Ling Lu*[1,2,3,4*]

[1]Jiangsu Cancer Hospital, Jiangsu Institute of Cancer Research, Nanjing Medical University Affiliated Cancer Hospital, Nanjing, China, [2] Hepatobiliary Center, The First Affiliated Hospital of Nanjing Medical University, Nanjing, China, [3] Research Unit of Liver Transplantation and Transplant Immunology, Chinese Academy of Medical Sciences, Nanjing, China, [4] Key Laboratory of Liver Transplantation, Chinese Academy of Medical Sciences, NHC Key Laboratory of Living Donor Liver Transplantation, Nanjing, China

***Correspondence:**
Ling Lu
lvling@njmu.edu.cn

Rejection after organ transplantation is a cause of graft failure. Effectively reducing rejection and inducing tolerance is a challenge in the field of transplantation immunology. The liver, as an immunologically privileged organ, has high rates of spontaneous and operational tolerance after transplantation, allowing it to maintain its normal function for long periods. Although modern immunosuppression regimens have serious toxicity and side effects, it is very risky to discontinue immunosuppression regimens blindly. A more effective treatment to induce immune tolerance is the most sought-after goal in transplant medicine. Tregs have been shown to play a pivotal role in the regulation of immune balance, and infusion of Tregs can also effectively prevent rejection and cure autoimmune diseases without significant side effects. Given the immune characteristics of the liver, the correct use of Tregs can more effectively induce the occurrence of operational tolerance for liver transplants than for other organ transplants. This review mainly summarizes the latest research advances regarding the characteristics of the hepatic immune microenvironment, operational tolerance, Treg generation *in vitro*, and the application of Tregs in liver transplantation. It is hoped that this review will provide a deeper understanding of Tregs as the most effective treatment to induce and maintain operational tolerance after liver transplantation.

Keywords: clinical trial, Foxp3, operational tolerance, regulatory T cell, liver transplantation

INTRODUCTION

Liver transplantation is effective for end-stage liver disease and acute liver failure, even when used as the sole treatment (1). Over the past few decades, surgical techniques for liver transplantation have matured. Modern immunosuppression regimens have greatly reduced the early mortality of transplant patients. However, diseases caused by the side effects of those regimens also reduce long-term quality of life and increase long-term mortality for recipients, who risk adverse effects such as renal insufficiency and renal failure, cholangitis and bile duct stones caused by biliary tract injury, and tumours caused by immunodeficiency (2). Therefore, exploring more effective and less toxic treatments to induce immune tolerance has become the chief scientific concern in transplantation.

Immune tolerance refers to a specific non-responsive state that the immune system exhibits when exposed to antigenic substances (3). The study of immune tolerance induction has achieved promising results in animal experiments; for example, allografts could maintain good graft function without the use of immunosuppression regimens. For decades, a small number of transplant recipients have shown no signs of rejection and good graft function with long-term discontinuation of immunosuppressants, a phenomenon known as spontaneous operational tolerance (4). In the 1990s, the University of Pittsburgh in the United States found that approximately 20% of liver transplant patients could safely stop all immunosuppressant therapy after the transplant had been in place for many years (5). However, organ damage or failure caused by the side effects of immunosuppressants often occurred early postoperatively and was irreversible. Hence, how to induce early operational tolerance of transplantation through intervention measures is an important research topic at present.

Tregs are a subgroup of immune cells with strong regulatory functions that play an important role in maintaining immune homeostasis and inducing immune tolerance (6). In 1995, Sakaguchi et al. discovered and defined it as a $CD4^{+}CD25^{+}$ T cell subset originating from the thymus (7). But $Foxp3^{+}$ T cells were called Tregs when the key transcription factor Foxp3 was discovered in 2003 (8). Current research has clarified that Tregs regulate immune balance mainly by means of direct cell contact and indirect secretion of cytokines (9). Tregs are related to the occurrence of spontaneous immune tolerance after transplantation, and there is a high quantity of Tregs in these patients (10). In recent years, multiple centres have applied *in vitro*-induced Tregs to the induction of early or late tolerance in patients with liver transplantation, and some progress has been achieved (11). This review will systematically summarize the latest research progress and look forward to future research directions.

THE IMMUNOLOGIC CHARACTERISTICS OF LIVER

The liver was defined as a non-immune organ in the past and is mainly responsible for the functions of material metabolism, nutrient storage and decomposition of toxic substances. Transformed into continuous understanding of the characteristics of liver tissue, we know that it is also an extremely complex immune organ, with functions such as secreting acute phase proteins, complement components, cytokines and chemokines, and contains a variety of resident immune cells with self-renewal capabilities (11, 12). The liver has been stimulated by a large number of external antigens for a long time because it receives blood from the entire digestive tract, but the liver maintains its autoimmune balance through an extremely complex regulatory network. The recipient immune system is mainly composed of resident immune cells from donors and circulating immune cells from recipients after transplantation. However, the liver, unlike other solid organs, is more likely to coexist with the donor's immune cell to form immune tolerance, which is inseparable from the internal environment unique to the liver. An explanation may be the presence of chimerism, which is developed by lymphocytes and dendritic cells from donors migrating to the lymph nodes and thymus of recipients, releasing soluble MHC molecules, deleting colonies and exhausting alloreactive T-cells (13). In addition, the portal vein and hepatic artery converge in the hepatic sinus, which results in hypoperfusion pressure, slow blood flow, and a hypoxic state in the sinusoidal area. This provides a favourable place for adaptive immune cells and innate immune cells to contact and respond to each other.

The liver has its own unique innate immune system and plays a key role in the development of immune tolerance after liver transplantation, including liver-derived dendritic cells, Kupffer cells, sinusoidal endothelial cells, natural killer cells, and natural killer T cells (14). A large number of studies have shown that the maturity of dendritic cells in the liver is much lower than that of peripheral lymphoid organs (15–20). Immature dendritic cells display lower expression of MHC-II, costimulatory signalling molecules and IL-12p70 and high expression of IL-10, IL-27 and TGF-β (21–23). Therefore, it is conducive to the expansion of Tregs and the maintenance of their functions but inhibits T cell activation (17, 24–26). Chen et al. recently confirmed that immature dendritic cells overexpressing IL-10 and Fasl display lower expression of MHC-II, CD80 and CD86, which could effectively induce early immune tolerance after liver transplantation in rats (27). Experimental results from our centre showed that galectin-1 induces peripheral monocytes to differentiate into immature dendritic cells, promotes their expression of IL-27 and TGF-β, induces differentiation and expansion of Tregs, and effectively induces immune tolerance after liver transplantation in rats (28). The above conclusions favourably determine the important role of immature liver dendritic cells in the induction of immune tolerance after liver transplantation. Kupffer cells, as the main resident macrophages in the liver, play a critical role in the inflammatory response caused by ischaemia-reperfusion in liver transplantation (29, 30). However, studies have also found that Kupffer cells can induce Tregs to proliferate and secrete IL-10 through direct contact with Tregs while inhibiting T cell activation by secreting PGE2 and 15d-PGJ2 (31–34). Sinusoidal endothelial cells, as the main components of liver non-parenchymal cells, can induce T cell apoptosis by inducing the expression of PD-L1 and inhibiting T cell secretion of IL-2, thereby inducing immune tolerance (35, 36). Meanwhile, studies have shown that hepatic sinusoidal endothelial cells can induce $CD4^{+}$ T cells to differentiate into $CD4^{+}CD25^{low}Foxp3^{-}$specific T cell subsets with inhibitory activity (37). NK cells have been demonstrated to play dual roles in liver immunity (38). NK cells have been clarified to inhibit dendritic cell activation and promote hepatic tolerance by secreting TGF-β and IL-10, which further induce the expansion of Tregs (39). The above research conclusions suggest that in addition to directly affecting T cells, liver innate immunity can simultaneously induce the differentiation and proliferation of suppressive T cell subsets, especially Tregs.

TREGS DEVELOPMENTS AND FOXP3 REGULATION

Over the past 20 years, the biological characteristics and immune regulation mechanisms of Tregs have been widely studied. Tregs are classified as thymus-derived Tregs (tTregs) and peripheral-derived Tregs (pTregs) according to the different sites where Tregs differentiate (40, 41). However, tTregs and pTregs are not only different in the place of differentiation but also in the manner of differentiation. tTregs are mainly induced by autoantigens in the thymus, and CD4 single-positive cells express Foxp3 under moderate autoantigen and IL-2 signal stimulation *via* TCR (42, 43). pTregs are mainly induced by foreign antigens, and peripheral $CD4^+$ naïve T cells express Foxp3 under the stimulation of bacterial or food antigens and differentiate into pTregs (44, 45). Studies have also confirmed that TCR is essential for the activation, maturation, and functions of Tregs (46, 47). TCR signal activation plays a key role in the differentiation and activation of Tregs and pTregs. Sidwell et al. found that the transcription factor Bach2 inhibits signal transduction downstream of TCR and affects Treg activation. ChIP-seq and ATAC-seq revealed that Bach2 antagonizes TCR-induced IRF4 and DNA binding activity and restricts chromatin accessibility (48). Using single-cell RNA sequencing, Zemmour et al. analysed the variation in TCR expression profiles between Tregs and $CD4^+Foxp3^-$T cells (49). However, there are no reports about alloantigen-reactive Tregs in patients with liver transplantation. Single-cell analysis can provide a deeper understanding of the specificity of TCRs and related transcription factors or key factors and, in combination with ChIP-seq and ATAC-seq, further analyse specific mechanisms. In addition to TCR signalling, TGF-β and IL-2 signalling also play an important role in Treg development, whether in the thymus or in the periphery. Our previous results showed that TGF-β signalling plays a pivotal role in iTreg (induced in cell culture) induction, which mainly depends on downstream SMAD2/3 activation (50). A recent study reported that 5-aza-dC efficiently generates Foxp3+ iTreg TCR-stimulated $CD4^+Foxp3^-$ T cells in the absence of exogenous TGF-β and IL-2, and they further discovered that the function of 5-aza-dC on Treg generation is critically dependent on TGF-βR and IL-2R signalling (51). Although those studies provided us with a deep understanding of the molecular mechanisms underlying the process of Foxp3 induction, we need to look for more drugs or molecules to assist TGF-β and IL-2 in inducing stable iTregs.

The maintenance of the phenotype and function of Tregs depended on the stable expression of Foxp3 and the function of Foxp3 protein. In 2017, we systematically summarized the important regulatory molecular mechanisms affecting Foxp3 at the level of transcription, translation, and post-translational modification (52). The execution of these suppressive functions requires the proper regulation of Foxp3 genes within Treg cells. Many transcription factors can bind to the promoter regions of its gene, such as NAFT, RUNX1, and IRF4 (53–55). Previous data have shown that atRA increases histone acetylation on the Foxp3 gene promoter and CpG demethylation in the region of the Foxp3 locus (56, 57). Our recent research found that YAP upregulates activin receptor expression through binding to TEAD, thereby promoting the activation of the TGF-β/SMAD2/3 signalling pathway, stabilizing and increasing Foxp3 expression and Treg function (58). At the same time, we confirmed for the first time that Foxp3 is regulated by K63-type polyubiquitination. When TRAF6 is defective in Tregs, K63-type polyubiquitination of Foxp3 is significantly inhibited, and its nuclear distribution is significantly abnormal (59). The post-translational modification of Foxp3 has been gradually valued. In addition to ubiquitination, Foxp3 lysine acetylation is also important. Dahiya et al. found that HDAC10 regulates Foxp3 protein stability and transcriptional activity, and HDAC10 deficiency leads to a significant decline in Treg immunosuppressive function (60). Xiao et al. recently found that EZH2 inhibits Foxp3 transcription by downregulating RUNX1 and upregulating SMAD7 expression, further clarifying that methylation modification plays an important role in the regulation of Foxp3 transcription (61). Many studies have deeply determined the molecular mechanism of Foxp3 and other important factors regulating the function of Tregs (62–64). However, the recognition of alloantigen-reactive Tregs is still almost completely unknown. We need to establish an effective system to analyse the regulatory characteristics of alloantigen-reactive Tregs so that we can better and more effectively induce and maintain them and induce stable and durable immune tolerance.

TREGS AND OPERATIONAL TOLERANCE

Operational tolerance is different from what we usually call immune tolerance. This means that the allograft does not suffer a rejection reaction and maintains good graft function and normal histology. Because of the unique histological and immune microenvironment characteristics of the liver, it is more prone to spontaneous operational tolerance than other solid and non-solid organs. At first, Starzl found that some patients who discontinued immunosuppressive drugs due to serious side effects did not develop rejection and form natural tolerance (65). Subsequently, Mazariegos recruited 95 liver transplant recipients who had taken immunosuppressive drugs for a long time after operation and had stable liver function to perform withdrawal experiments and found that spontaneous operational tolerance occurred in approximately 20% of recipients (66). The results of clinical withdrawal experiments from multiple centres in the world also confirmed the above conclusions (67–74). The overall incidence of spontaneous operational tolerance in liver transplant recipients remains unknown. Considering that blind withdrawal early can lead to more serious consequences, how to induce early operational tolerance in liver transplant recipients is a major scientific issue in the transplant world today.

Tregs induce immune tolerance through a variety of pathways, including direct and indirect pathways. For example, Tregs interact with B cells, T cells and DCs and inhibit their activation and proliferation by expressing PD-1, CTLA-4, CD39 and LAG-3. It can also secrete the anti-inflammatory cytokines IL-10, IL-25 and TGF-β to inhibit T cell activation, releasing perforin and granzyme to promote target cell apoptosis and competing with T cells for binding to IL-2 by expressing CD25 (75, 76). Th17 cells produce IL-17A, IL-21 and IL-22, which have been shown to promote immunopathology and autoinflammatory diseases (77). Many studies have shown that Tregs suppress Th 17 cell proliferation and control its response (78). Early studies found that the occurrence of acute rejection after liver transplantation was inversely related to the number of peripheral circulating Tregs and the ratio of Tregs/Th17 cells (79–82). Li et al. used a CD25 antibody (250 μg/d, IP) to treat a mouse transplantation model and found that it reduced the proportion of CD4+CD25+ Treg/CD3+ T cells and significantly reduced the incidence of spontaneous tolerance in transplanted mice (83). A clinical trial of withdrawal of recipients who took immunosuppressive drugs after liver transplantation with stable liver function for more than 2 years found that the level of Foxp3 mRNA in peripheral blood of recipients who did not have rejection after withdrawal was increased a rate of 3.5 times each time and continued to increase until the drug was completely withdrawn, but the recipients who experienced a rejection after drug withdrawal could not see this phenomenon (74). Recent studies have used flow cytometry to detect the ratio of Tregs/Th17 in the peripheral blood of patients with rejection within 2 weeks to 1 month after living donor liver transplantation and found that the occurrence of early rejection is directly related to the low number of Tregs (80). Therefore, we can easily predict that Treg immunotherapy may be the most effective way to induce operational tolerance in the early stage.

EX VIVO REGULATORY T CELLS GENERATION

Since Tregs only account for 5-10% of peripheral blood CD4+ T cells, to obtain a sufficient number of Tregs, we need to expand Tregs *in vitro*. Currently, there are two methods expanding Tregs *in vitro* for clinical applications that are certified by GMP (84). Considering the timeliness of magnetic bead sorting, GMP stipulated that two-step magnetic bead sorting (CliniMACS) is used to obtain human peripheral blood CD4+ CD25+ Tre (85). Treg expansion *in vitro* is mainly divided into polyclonal Treg expansion and alloantigen-reactive Treg expansion. Polyclonal Tregs are expanded by using CD3 and CD28 antibody-coated magnetic beads and IL-2 recombinant protein (86, 87). However, this expansion method inevitably led to the loss of Foxp3 and changed the Treg phenotype, and the effector T cells also expanded and mixed in the presence of IL-2. We and other laboratories added rapamycin and all-trans retinoic acid to effectively maintain Foxp3 expression and inhibit effector T cell expansion (57, 88). Due to the poor specificity of polyclonal Treg antigens, we are now focusing more on alloantigen-reactive Treg expansion. Alloantigen-reactive Tregs can be expanded by using donor antigen-presenting cells, such as dendritic cells, B cells, and peripheral blood mononuclear cells (89). Putnam et al. used CD40L-activated allogeneic B cells for the first time to stimulate and select alloantigen-reactive Tregs and then performed 200-4000 times in 16 days with magnetic beads coated with CD3 and CD28 antibodies and IL-2 recombinant protein (90). Our centre designed a method inducing alloantigen-reactive Tregs and is applying for Republic of South Africa Patents (International Application NO: PCT/CN2018/075730). The invention adopts rapamycin combined with TGF-β cells to induce human T cells into alloantigen-reactive Tregs with immunosuppressive function *in vitro* by the action of DC cells from donors. Podestà et al. used PBMCs to establish an allogeneic mixed lymphocyte system, applied this system to expand alloantigen-reactive Tregs, and added ceprizumab, a CD2 monoclonal antibody. They found that ceprizumab can greatly reduce the proportion of CD4+ and CD8+ effector and memory T cells and at the same time selectively promote alloantigen-reactive Treg expansion (91). This study suggests that we can modify polyclonal Tregs and alloantigen-reactive Tregs *in vitro* based on the biological characteristics of Tregs and the regulatory mechanism of Foxp3 stability so that they have stronger expansion ability and stability.

THE APPLICATION OF TREGS IN LIVER TRANSPLANTATION

As of January 2020, there are very few clinical trials reporting that Tregs successfully induced operational tolerance in patients with liver transplant in the early stage, almost all of which are in phase I/II clinical trials. Ex vivo expanded polyclonal regulatory T-cell therapy is being utilized in the ThRIL trial at King's College Hospital, UK [clinicaltrials.gov NCT02166177]. The DeLTA and ARTEMIS trials at University of California, San Francisco, USA, are using donor-alloantigen-reactive regulatory T cells (darTregs) [NCT02188719] NCT02474199. A preliminary study from Japan showed that Tregs can safely and effectively induce operational tolerance in the early stage of recipients after living liver transplantation. Treg-enriched allogeneic lymphocytes were obtained by co-culturing recipient spleen lymphocytes and irradiated donor lymphocytes in the presence of CD80 and CD86 antibodies, which were reinfused (23.30 + 14.38×106/kg) on the 13th day after living-donor liver transplantation. Dug withdrawal gradually started after 6 months and completed withdrawal until 18 months. Ten patients were included in this study, and no severe side effects occurred after cell therapy. All patients had normal liver function and liver histology. Seven patients achieved operational tolerance. Three of seven patients resumed taking low-dose immunosuppressive drugs due to autoimmune liver disease. However, this study has no long-term data or follow-up (92). This study suggests that

TABLE 1 | The clinical trial for tregs in liver transplantation.

Status	Study Title	Conditions	Trial ID
Active, not recruiting	Safety Study of Using Regulatory T Cells Induce Liver Transplantation Tolerance	Chronic Rejection of Liver Transplant	NCT01624077
Recruiting	Liver Transplantation With Tregs at MGH	Liver Transplantation	NCT03577431
Active, not recruiting	Efficacy of Low Dose, SubQ Interleukin-2 (IL-2) to Expand Endogenous Regulatory T-Cells in Liver Transplant Recipients	Liver Transplantation	NCT02739412
Completed	Donor Alloantigen Reactive Tregs (darTregs) for Calcineurin Inhibitor (CNI) Reduction	Liver Transplant Recipient, Living Donor (of the Respective Liver Transplant Recipient)	NCT02474199
Completed	Safety and Efficacy Study of Regulatory T Cell Therapy in Liver Transplant Patients	End-stage Liver Disease	NCT01678937

Tregs induce operational tolerance to be safe and effective (**Table 1**).

FUTURE DIRECTIONS

Along with the application of Tregs in inducing operational tolerance after solid organ transplantation and non-solid organ transplantation (93–95), it has been clearly confirmed that Tregs can effectively induce and maintain operational tolerance early without significant side effects. However, although the biological characteristics of Tregs and the molecular regulatory mechanisms of Foxp3 are understood in depth, little is known about the heterogeneity of alloantigen-reactive Tregs in different organs. In the future, it is necessary to further characterize the phenotypic and functional differences in alloantigen-reactive Tregs between different organs *via* modern omics analysis. With that knowledge, we could effectively modify Tregs during *in vitro* expansion to obtain Tregs with stronger suppressive activity and stability and generate common Car-Tregs with antigen-specific properties. For Car-Tregs, it is important to determine and verify the best target for engineered Treg cells, as well as consider whether the target molecule on these cells could be a soluble antigen instead of a surface molecule.

The mass production process of Treg cells is still not perfect, mainly due to the limitations of reagents and equipment. Combining MACS with FACS may further improve this process. The low proliferation rate of Treg cells *in vitro* is in stark contrast to their highly proliferative state *in vivo*. Suitable media, growth factors and stimulants for Treg cells have not been developed. In addition, current Treg cell manufacturing processes are expensive and labour intensive. Maximizing automation not only reduces costs but also improves repeatability and standardization.

Meanwhile, because there is still no effective way to evaluate the outcome of Treg infusion *in vivo*, we need to compare the differences in Treg heterogeneous subgroups *in vivo* before and after Treg therapy and to clarify the phenotypic and functional differences. A better understanding of how Treg cells maintain tissue integrity during homeostasis and in autoimmunity and organ transplantation, whether (and how) Treg cells change their identity in autoimmunity and whether Treg cells from patients with autoimmune disease are intrinsically defective and thus unsuitable for therapeutic use will also be critical to establish a Treg immunotherapy evaluation system that can guide the withdrawal process. In addition to Tregs alone, we need to explore the efficacy of Tregs combined with other immune cell therapies, such as MSCs, DCs or others. In the next few years, as clinical experimental data from other centres are reported, we will achieve a deeper understanding of the efficacy, safety, and side effects of Treg therapy in liver transplantation. However, we still need to establish a safe, effective and unified system to facilitate the implementation of Treg.

AUTHOR CONTRIBUTIONS

XN, QW and JG participated in manuscript writing and editing. LL contributed to manuscript editing. All authors contributed to the article and approved the submitted version.

REFERENCES

1. Bodzin AS, Baker TB. Liver Transplantation Today: Where We are Now and Where We are Going. *Liver Transpl* (2018) 24(10):1470–5. doi: 10.1002/lt.25320
2. Mukherjee S, Mukherjee U. A Comprehensive Review of Immunosuppression Used for Liver Transplantation. *J Transplant* (2009) 2009p:701464. doi: 10.1155/2009/701464
3. Stolp J, Zaitsu M, Wood KJ. Immune Tolerance and Rejection in Organ Transplantation. *Methods Mol Biol* (2019) 1899:159–80. doi: 10.1007/978-1-4939-8938-6_12
4. Salisbury EM, Game DS, Lechler RI. Transplantation Tolerance. *Pediatr Nephrol* (2014) 29(12):2263–72. doi: 10.1007/s00467-013-2659-5
5. Sanchez-Fueyo A. Hot-Topic Debate on Tolerance: Immunosuppression Withdrawal. *Liver Transpl* (2011) 17(Suppl 3):S69–73. doi: 10.1002/lt.22421
6. Sakaguchi S. Regulatory T Cells: History and Perspective. *Methods Mol Biol* (2011) 707:3–17. doi: 10.1007/978-1-61737-979-6_1
7. Sakaguchi S. Regulatory T Cells: Key Controllers of Immunologic Self-Tolerance. *Cell* (2000) 101(5):455–8. doi: 10.1016/S0092-8674(00)80856-9
8. Hori S, Nomura T, Sakaguchi S. Control of Regulatory T Cell Development by the Transcription Factor Foxp3. *Science* (2003) 299(5609):1057–61. doi: 10.1126/science.1079490
9. Schmidt A, Oberle N, Krammer PH. Molecular Mechanisms of Treg-Mediated T Cell Suppression. *Front Immunol* (2012) 3:51. doi: 10.3389/fimmu.2012.00051
10. Romano M, Tung SL, Smyth LA, Lombardi G. Treg Therapy in Transplantation: A General Overview. *Transpl Int* (2017) 30(8):745–53. doi: 10.1111/tri.12909
11. Crispe IN. The Liver as a Lymphoid Organ. *Annu Rev Immunol* (2009) 27:147–63. doi: 10.1146/annurev.immunol.021908.132629
12. Nemeth E, Baird AW, O'Farrelly C. Microanatomy of the Liver Immune System. *Semin Immunopathol* (2009) 31(3):333–43. doi: 10.1007/s00281-009-0173-4
13. Mineo D, Ricordi C. Chimerism and Liver Transplant Tolerance. *J Hepatol* (2008) 49(3):478–80. doi: 10.1016/j.jhep.2008.06.021
14. Huang H, Lu Y, Zhou T, Gu G, Xia Q. Innate Immune Cells in Immune Tolerance After Liver Transplantation. *Front Immunol* (2018) 9:2401. doi:

10.3389/fimmu.2018.02401

15. Svensson M, Maroof A, Ato M, Kaye PM. Stromal Cells Direct Local Differentiation of Regulatory Dendritic Cells. *Immunity* (2004) 21(6):805–16. doi: 10.1016/j.immuni.2004.10.012
16. Wakkach A, Fournier N, Brun V, Breittmayer JP, Cottrez F, Groux H. Characterization of Dendritic Cells That Induce Tolerance and T Regulatory 1 Cell Differentiation in Vivo. *Immunity* (2003) 18(5):605–17. doi: 10.1016/S1074-7613(03)00113-4
17. Pillarisetty VG, Shah AB, Miller G, Bleier JI, DeMatteo RP. Liver Dendritic Cells are Less Immunogenic Than Spleen Dendritic Cells Because of Differences in Subtype Composition. *J Immunol* (2004) 172(2):1009–17. doi: 10.4049/jimmunol.172.2.1009
18. De Creus A, Abe M, Lau AH, Hackstein H, Raimondi G, Thomson AW. Low TLR4 Expression by Liver Dendritic Cells Correlates With Reduced Capacity to Activate Allogeneic T Cells in Response to Endotoxin. *J Immunol* (2005) 174(4):2037–45. doi: 10.4049/jimmunol.174.4.2037
19. Kingham TP, Chaudhry UI, Plitas G, Katz SC, Raab J, DeMatteo RP. Murine Liver Plasmacytoid Dendritic Cells Become Potent Immunostimulatory Cells After Flt-3 Ligand Expansion. *Hepatology* (2007) 45(2):445–54. doi: 10.1002/hep.21457
20. Tokita D, Sumpter TL, Raimondi G, Zahorchak AF, Wang Z, Nakao A, et al. Poor Allostimulatory Function of Liver Plasmacytoid DC is Associated With Pro-Apoptotic Activity, Dependent on Regulatory T Cells. *J Hepatol* (2008) 49 (6):1008–18. doi: 10.1016/j.jhep.2008.07.028
21. He W, Chen L, Zheng L, Luo L, Gao L. Prolonged Survival Effects Induced by Immature Dendritic Cells and Regulatory T Cells in a Rat Liver Transplantation Model. *Mol Immunol* (2016) 79:92–7. doi: 10.1016/j.molimm.2016.10.004
22. Chen Y, Jiang G, Yang HR, Gu X, Wang L, Hsieh CC, et al. Distinct Response of Liver Myeloid Dendritic Cells to Endotoxin is Mediated by IL-27. *J Hepatol* (2009) 51(3):510–9. doi: 10.1016/j.jhep.2009.04.026
23. Nakamoto N, Ebinuma H, Kanai T, Chu PS, Ono Y, Mikami Y, et al. CCR9+ Macrophages are Required for Acute Liver Inflammation in Mouse Models of Hepatitis. *Gastroenterology* (2012) 142(2):366–76. doi: 10.1053/j.gastro.2011.10.039
24. Rastellini C, Lu L, Ricordi C, Starzl TE, Rao AS, Thomson AW. Granulocyte/Macrophage Colony-Stimulating Factor-Stimulated Hepatic Dendritic Cell Progenitors Prolong Pancreatic Islet Allograft Survival. *Transplantation* (1995) 60(11):1366–70.
25. Mascanfroni ID, Yeste A, Vieira SM, Burns EJ, Patel B, Sloma I, et al. IL-27 Acts on Dcs to Suppress the T Cell Response and Autoimmunity by Inducing Expression of the Immunoregulatory Molecule CD39. *Nat Immunol* (2013) 14 (10):1054–63. doi: 10.1038/ni.2695
26. Matta BM, Raimondi G, Rosborough BR, Sumpter TL, Thomson AW. IL-27 Production and STAT3-Dependent Upregulation of B7-H1 Mediate Immune Regulatory Functions of Liver Plasmacytoid Dendritic Cells. *J Immunol* (2012) 188(11):5227–37. doi: 10.4049/jimmunol.1103382
27. Chen L, Zhang L, Zhu Z, He W, Gao L, Zhang W, et al. Effects of IL-10- and Fasl-Overexpressing Dendritic Cells on Liver Transplantation Tolerance in a Heterotopic Liver Transplantation Rat Model. *Immunol Cell Biol* (2019) 97 (8):714–25. doi: 10.1111/imcb.12252
28. Lu H, Dai X, Li X, Sun Y, Gao Y, Zhang C. Gal-1 Regulates Dendritic Cells-Induced Treg/Th17 Balance Though NF-Kappab/Relb-IL-27 Pathway. *Ann Transl Med* (2019) 7(22):628. doi: 10.21037/atm.2019.11.02
29. Karimi MH, Geramizadeh B, Malek-Hosseini SA. Tolerance Induction in Liver. *Int J Organ Transplant Med* (2015) 6(2):45–54.
30. Knolle PA, Uhrig A, Protzer U, Trippler M, Duchmann R, Meyer zum Buschenfelde KH, et al. Interleukin-10 Expression is Autoregulated At the Transcriptional Level in Human and Murine Kupffer Cells. *Hepatology* (1998) 27(1):93–9. doi: 10.1002/hep.510270116
31. Breous E, Somanathan S, Vandenberghe LH, Wilson JM. Hepatic Regulatory T Cells and Kupffer Cells are Crucial Mediators of Systemic T Cell Tolerance to Antigens Targeting Murine Liver. *Hepatology* (2009) 50(2):612–21. doi: 10.1002/hep.23043
32. Wiegard C, Frenzel C, Herkel J, Kallen KJ, Schmitt E, Lohse AW. Murine Liver Antigen Presenting Cells Control Suppressor Activity of CD4+CD25+ Regulatory T Cells. *Hepatology* (2005) 42(1):193–9. doi: 10.1002/hep.20756
33. You Q, Cheng L, Kedl RM, Ju C. Mechanism of T Cell Tolerance Induction by Murine Hepatic Kupffer Cells. *Hepatology* (2008) 48(3):978–90. doi: 10.1002/hep.22395
34. Thorgersen EB, Barratt-Due A, Haugaa H, Harboe M, Pischke SE, Nilsson PH, et al. The Role of Complement in Liver Injury, Regeneration, and Transplantation. *Hepatology* (2019) 70(2):725–36. doi: 10.1002/hep.30508
35. Schurich A, Berg M, Stabenow D, Bottcher J, Kern M, Schild HJ, et al. Dynamic Regulation of CD8 T Cell Tolerance Induction by Liver Sinusoidal Endothelial Cells. *J Immunol* (2010) 184(8):4107–14. doi: 10.4049/jimmunol.0902580
36. Robinson KA, Orent W, Madsen JC, Benichou G. Maintaining T Cell Tolerance of Alloantigens: Lessons From Animal Studies. *Am J Transplant* (2018) 18(8):1843–56. doi: 10.1111/ajt.14984
37. Kruse N, Neumann K, Schrage A, Derkow K, Schott E, Erben U, et al. Priming of CD4+ T Cells by Liver Sinusoidal Endothelial Cells Induces CD25low Forkhead Box Protein 3- Regulatory T Cells Suppressing Autoimmune Hepatitis. *Hepatology* (2009) 50(6):1904–13. doi: 10.1002/hep.23191
38. Tian Z, Chen Y, Gao B. Natural Killer Cells in Liver Disease. *Hepatology* (2013) 57(4):1654–62. doi: 10.1002/hep.26115
39. Mikulak J, Bruni E, Oriolo F, Di Vito C, Mavilio D. Hepatic Natural Killer Cells: Organ-Specific Sentinels of Liver Immune Homeostasis and Physiopathology. *Front Immunol* (2019) 10:946. doi: 10.3389/fimmu.2019.00946
40. Singer A, Adoro S, Park JH. Lineage Fate and Intense Debate: Myths, Models and Mechanisms of CD4- Versus CD8-Lineage Choice. *Nat Rev Immunol* (2008) 8(10):788–801. doi: 10.1038/nri2416
41. Kretschmer K, Apostolou I, Hawiger D, Khazaie K, Nussenzweig MC, von Boehmer H. Inducing and Expanding Regulatory T Cell Populations by Foreign Antigen. *Nat Immunol* (2005) 6(12):1219–27. doi: 10.1038/ni1265
42. Famili F, Wiekmeijer AS, Staal FJ. The Development of T Cells From Stem Cells in Mice and Humans. *Future Sci OA* (2017) 3(3):FSO186. doi: 10.4155/fsoa-2016-0095
43. Tanoue T, Atarashi K, Honda K. Development and Maintenance of Intestinal Regulatory T Cells. *Nat Rev Immunol* (2016) 16(5):295–309. doi: 10.1038/nri.2016.36
44. Luu M, Steinhoff U, Visekruna A. Functional Heterogeneity of Gut-Resident Regulatory T Cells. *Clin Transl Immunol* (2017) 6(9):e156. doi: 10.1038/cti.2017.39
45. Shevach EM, Thornton AM. Ttregs, Ptregs, and Itregs: Similarities and Differences. *Immunol Rev* (2014) 259(1):88–102. doi: 10.1111/imr.12160
46. Levine AG, Arvey A, Jin W, Rudensky AY. Continuous Requirement for the TCR in Regulatory T Cell Function. *Nat Immunol* (2014) 15(11):1070–8. doi: 10.1038/ni.3004
47. Vahl JC, Drees C, Heger K, Heink S, Fischer JC, Nedjic J, et al. Continuous T Cell Receptor Signals Maintain a Functional Regulatory T Cell Pool. *Immunity* (2014) 41(5):722–36. doi: 10.1016/j.immuni.2014.10.012
48. Sidwell T, Liao Y, Garnham AL, Vasanthakumar A, Gloury R, Blume J, et al. Attenuation of TCR-Induced Transcription by Bach2 Controls Regulatory T Cell Differentiation and Homeostasis. *Nat Commun* (2020) 11(1):252. doi: 10.1038/s41467-019-14112-2
49. Zemmour D, Zilionis R, Kiner E, Klein AM, Mathis D, Benoist C. Single-Cell Gene Expression Reveals a Landscape of Regulatory T Cell Phenotypes Shaped by the TCR. *Nat Immunol* (2018) 19(3):291–301. doi: 10.1038/s41590-018-0051-0
50. Lu L, Wang J, Zhang F, Chai Y, Brand D, Wang X, et al. Role of SMAD and Non-SMAD Signals in the Development of Th17 and Regulatory T Cells. *J Immunol* (2010) 184(8):4295–306. doi: 10.4049/jimmunol.0903418
51. Freudenberg K, Lindner N, Dohnke S, Garbe AI, Schallenberg S, Kretschmer K. Critical Role of TGF-Beta and IL-2 Receptor Signaling in Foxp3 Induction by an Inhibitor of DNA Methylation. *Front Immunol* (2018) 9:125. doi: 10.3389/fimmu.2018.00125
52. Lu L, Barbi J, Pan F. The Regulation of Immune Tolerance by FOXP3. *Nat Rev Immunol* (2017) 17(11):703–17. doi: 10.1038/nri.2017.75
53. Wu Y, Borde M, Heissmeyer V, Feuerer M, Lapan AD, Stroud JC, et al. FOXP3 Controls Regulatory T Cell Function Through Cooperation With NFAT. *Cell* (2006) 126(2):375–87. doi: 10.1016/j.cell.2006.05.042
54. Ono M, Yaguchi H, Ohkura N, Kitabayashi I, Nagamura Y, Nomura T, et al. Foxp3 Controls Regulatory T-Cell Function by Interacting With AML1/Runx1. *Nature* (2007) 446(7136):685–9. doi: 10.1038/nature05673
55. Zheng Y, Chaudhry A, Kas A, deRoos P, Kim JM, Chu TT, et al. Regulatory T-Cell Suppressor Program Co-Opts Transcription Factor IRF4 to Control T(H) 2 Responses. *Nature* (2009) 458(7236):351–6. doi: 10.1038/nature07674
56. Lu L, Ma J, Li Z, Lan Q, Chen M, Liu Y, et al. All-Trans Retinoic Acid Promotes TGF-Beta-Induced Tregs Via Histone Modification But Not DNA Demethylation on Foxp3 Gene Locus. *PLoS One* (2011) 6(9):e24590. doi: 10.1371/journal.pone.0024590

57. Lu L, Lan Q, Li Z, Zhou X, Gu J, Li Q, et al. Critical Role of All-Trans Retinoic Acid in Stabilizing Human Natural Regulatory T Cells Under Inflammatory Conditions. *Proc Natl Acad Sci U S A* (2014) 111(33):E3432–40. doi: 10.1073/pnas.1408780111
58. Ni X, Tao J, Barbi J, Chen Q, Park BV, Li Z, et al. YAP is Essential for Treg-Mediated Suppression of Antitumor Immunity. *Cancer Discov* (2018) 8 (8):1026–43. doi: 10.1158/2159-8290.CD-17-1124
59. Ni X, Kou W, Gu J, Wei P, Wu X, Peng H, et al. TRAF6 Directs FOXP3 Localization and Facilitates Regulatory T-Cell Function Through K63-Linked Ubiquitination. *EMBO J* (2019) 38(9):e99766. doi: 10.15252/embj.201899766
60. Dahiya S, Beier UH, Wang L, Han R, Jiao J, Akimova T, et al. HDAC10 Deletion Promotes Foxp3(+) T-Regulatory Cell Function. *Sci Rep* (2020) 10 (1):424. doi: 10.1038/s41598-019-57294-x
61. Xiao XY, Li YT, Jiang X, Ji X, Lu X, Yang B, et al. EZH2 Deficiency Attenuates Treg Differentiation in Rheumatoid Arthritis. *J Autoimmun* (2020) 108:102404. doi: 10.1016/j.jaut.2020.102404
62. Andersen L, Gulich AF, Alteneder M, Preglej T, Orola MJ, Dhele N, et al. The Transcription Factor MAZR/PATZ1 Regulates the Development of FOXP3 (+) Regulatory T Cells. *Cell Rep* (2019) 29(13):4447–59.e6. doi: 10.1016/j.celrep.2019.11.089
63. Xiong Y, Wang L, Di Giorgio E, Akimova T, Beier UH, Han R, et al. Inhibiting the Coregulator Corest Impairs Foxp3+ Treg Function and Promotes Antitumor Immunity. *J Clin Invest* (2020) 130(4):1830–42. doi: 10.1172/JCI131375
64. Qiu R, Zhou L, Ma Y, Zhou L, Liang T, Shi L, et al. Regulatory T Cell Plasticity and Stability and Autoimmune Diseases. *Clin Rev Allergy Immunol* (2020) 58 (1):52–70. doi: 10.1007/s12016-018-8721-0
65. Starzl TE. Cell Migration and Chimerism–a Unifying Concept in Transplantation–With Particular Reference to HLA Matching and Tolerance Induction. *Transplant Proc* (1993) 25(1 Pt 1):8–12.
66. Mazariegos GV, Reyes J, Marino IR, Demetris AJ, Flynn B, Irish W, et al. Weaning of Immunosuppression in Liver Transplant Recipients. *Transplantation* (1997) 63(2):243–9. doi: 10.1097/00007890-199701270-00012
67. Devlin J, Doherty D, Thomson L, Wong T, Donaldson P, Portmann B, et al. Defining the Outcome of Immunosuppression Withdrawal After Liver Transplantation. *Hepatology* (1998) 27(4):926–33. doi: 10.1002/hep.510270406
68. Girlanda R, Rela M, Williams R, O'Grady JG, Heaton ND. Long-Term Outcome of Immunosuppression Withdrawal After Liver Transplantation. *Transplant Proc* (2005) 37(4):1708–9. doi: 10.1016/j.transproceed.2005.03.070
69. Takatsuki M, Uemoto S, Inomata Y, Sakamoto S, Hayashi M, Ueda M, et al. Analysis of Alloreactivity and Intragraft Cytokine Profiles in Living Donor Liver Transplant Recipients With Graft Acceptance. *Transpl Immunol* (2001) 8(4):279–86. doi: 10.1016/S0966-3274(01)00027-2
70. Eason JD, Cohen AJ, Nair S, Alcantera T, Loss GE. Tolerance: is It Worth the Risk? *Transplantation* (2005) 79(9):1157–9. doi: 10.1097/01.TP.0000162084.46555.10
71. Tryphonopoulos P, Tzakis AG, Weppler D, Garcia-Morales R, Kato T, Madariaga JR, et al. The Role of Donor Bone Marrow Infusions in Withdrawal of Immunosuppression in Adult Liver Allotransplantation. *Am J Transplant* (2005) 5(3):608–13. doi: 10.1111/j.1600-6143.2004.00743.x
72. Tisone G, Orlando G, Cardillo A, Palmieri G, Manzia TM, Baiocchi L, et al. Complete Weaning Off Immunosuppression in HCV Liver Transplant Recipients is Feasible and Favourably Impacts on the Progression of Disease Recurrence. *J Hepatol* (2006) 44(4):702–9. doi: 10.1016/j.jhep.2005.11.047
73. Assy N, Adams PC, Myers P, Simon V, Minuk GY, Wall W, et al. Randomized Controlled Trial of Total Immunosuppression Withdrawal in Liver Transplant Recipients: Role of Ursodeoxycholic Acid. *Transplantation* (2007) 83(12):1571–6. doi: 10.1097/01.tp.0000266678.32250.76
74. Pons JA, Revilla-Nuin B, Baroja-Mazo A, Ramirez P, Martinez-Alarcon L, Sanchez-Bueno F, et al. Foxp3 in Peripheral Blood is Associated With Operational Tolerance in Liver Transplant Patients During Immuno suppression Withdrawal. *Transplantation* (2008) 86(10):1370–8. doi: 10.1097/TP.0b013e318188d3e6
75. Vignali DA, Collison LW, Workman CJ. How Regulatory T Cells Work. *Nat Rev Immunol* (2008) 8(7):523–32. doi: 10.1038/nri2343
76. Sojka DK, Huang YH, Fowell DJ. Mechanisms of Regulatory T-Cell Suppression - a Diverse Arsenal for a Moving Target. *Immunology* (2008) 124(1):13–22. doi: 10.1111/j.1365-2567.2008.02813.x
77. Wu X, Tian J, Wang S. Insight Into Non-Pathogenic Th17 Cells in Autoimmune Diseases. *Front Immunol* (2018) 9:1112. doi: 10.3389/fimmu.2018.01112
78. Lee GR. The Balance of Th17 Versus Treg Cells in Autoimmunity. *Int J Mol Sci* (2018) 19(3):730. doi: 10.3390/ijms19030730
79. Demirkiran A, Kok A, Kwekkeboom J, Kusters JG, Metselaar HJ, Tilanus HW, et al. Low Circulating Regulatory T-Cell Levels After Acute Rejection in Liver Transplantation. *Liver Transpl* (2006) 12(2):277–84. doi: 10.1002/lt.20612
80. He Q, Fan H, Li JQ, Qi HZ. Decreased Circulating CD4+CD25highFoxp3+ T Cells During Acute Rejection in Liver Transplant Patients. *Transplant Proc* (2011) 43(5):1696–700. doi: 10.1016/j.transproceed.2011.03.084
81. Zhou Y, Yang X, Zhang H, Jiang J. The Roles of T Helper Type 17/ Regulatory T Cells in Acute Rejection After Liver Transplantation in Rats. *Transplantation* (2015) 99(6):1126–31. doi: 10.1097/TP.0000000000000666
82. Editors PO. Retraction: The Ratio of Circulating Regulatory T Cells (Tregs)/ Th17 Cells is Associated With Acute Allograft Rejection in Liver Transplantation. *PLoS One* (2019) 14(9):e0222348. doi: 10.1371/journal.pone.0222348
83. Li W, Carper K, Liang Y, Zheng XX, Kuhr CS, Reyes JD, et al. Anti-CD25 Mab Administration Prevents Spontaneous Liver Transplant Tolerance. *Transplant Proc* (2006) 38(10):3207–8. doi: 10.1016/j.transproceed.2006.10.094
84. MacDonald KN, Piret JM, Levings MK. Methods to Manufacture Regulatory T Cells for Cell Therapy. *Clin Exp Immunol* (2019) 197(1):52–63. doi: 10.1111/cei.13297
85. Di Ianni M, Del Papa B, Zei T, Iacucci Ostini R, Cecchini D, Cantelmi MG, et al. T Regulatory Cell Separation for Clinical Application. *Transfus Apher Sci* (2012) 47(2):213–6. doi: 10.1016/j.transci.2012.06.007
86. Levings MK, Sangregorio R, Roncarolo MG. Human Cd25(+)Cd4(+) T Regulatory Cells Suppress Naive and Memory T Cell Proliferation and Can Be Expanded in Vitro Without Loss of Function. *J Exp Med* (2001) 193 (11):1295–302. doi: 10.1084/jem.193.11.1295
87. Hoffmann P, Eder R, Kunz-Schughart LA, Andreesen R, Edinger M. Large-Scale in Vitro Expansion of Polyclonal Human CD4(+)CD25high Regulatory T Cells. *Blood* (2004) 104(3):895–903. doi: 10.1182/blood-2004-01-0086
88. Safinia N, Vaikunthanathan T, Fraser H, Thirkell S, Lowe K, Blackmore L, et al. Successful Expansion of Functional and Stable Regulatory T Cells for Immunotherapy in Liver Transplantation. *Oncotarget* (2016) 7(7):7563–77. doi: 10.18632/oncotarget.6927
89. Tang Q, Bluestone JA. Regulatory T-Cell Therapy in Transplantation: Moving to the Clinic. *Cold Spring Harb Perspect Med* (2013) 3(11):a015552. doi: 10.1101/cshperspect.a015552
90. Putnam AL, Safinia N, Medvec A, Laszkowska M, Wray M, Mintz MA, et al. Clinical Grade Manufacturing of Human Alloantigen-Reactive Regulatory T Cells for Use in Transplantation. *Am J Transplant* (2013) 13(11):3010–20. doi: 10.1111/ajt.12433
91. Podesta MA, Binder C, Sellberg F, DeWolf S, Shonts B, Ho SH, et al. Siplizumab Selectively Depletes Effector Memory T Cells and Promotes a Relative Expansion of Alloreactive Regulatory T Cells in Vitro. *Am J Transplant* (2020) 20(1):88–100. doi: 10.1111/ajt.15533
92. Todo S, Yamashita K, Goto R, Zaitsu M, Nagatsu A, Oura T, et al. A Pilot Study of Operational Tolerance With a Regulatory T-Cell-Based Cell Therapy in Living Donor Liver Transplantation. *Hepatology* (2016) 64(2):632–43. doi: 10.1002/hep.28459
93. Massart A, Ghisdal L, Abramowicz M, Abramowicz D. Operational Tolerance in Kidney Transplantation and Associated Biomarkers. *Clin Exp Immunol* (2017) 189(2):138–57. doi: 10.1111/cei.12981
94. Romano M, Fanelli G, Albany CJ, Giganti G, Lombardi G. Past, Present, and Future of Regulatory T Cell Therapy in Transplantation and Autoimmunity. *Front Immunol* (2019) 10:43. doi: 10.3389/fimmu.2019.00043
95. Mancusi A, Piccinelli S, Velardi A, Pierini A. CD4(+)FOXP3(+) Regulatory T Cell Therapies in HLA Haploidentical Hematopoietic Transplantation. *Front Immunol* (2019) 10:2901. doi: 10.3389/fimmu.2019.02901

6

Immune Tolerance Induction Using Cell-Based Strategies in Liver Transplantation: Clinical Perspectives

Pusen Wang [1†], Zhongyi Jiang [1†], Chunguang Wang [1], Xueni Liu [1], Hao Li [1], Dingyin Xu [2] and Lin Zhong [1*]*

[1] Department of General Surgery, Shanghai General Hospital, Shanghai Jiao Tong University School of Medicine, Shanghai, China, [2] Department of Hepatobiliary Surgery, Ruian People's Hospital, Ruian, China

***Correspondence:**
Dingyin Xu
xudy2004@sina.com
Lin Zhong
zhongl_3284@hotmail.com*

† These authors have contributed equally to this work

Liver transplantation (LT) has become the best chance and a routine practice for patients with end-stage liver disease and small hepatocellular carcinoma. However, life-long immunosuppressive regimens could lead to many post-LT complications, including cancer recurrence, infections, dysmetabolic syndrome, and renal injury. Impeccable management of immunosuppressive regimens is indispensable to ensure the best long-term prognosis for LT recipients. This is challenging for these patients, who probably have a post-LT graft survival of more than 10 or even 20 years. Approximately 20% of patients after LT could develop spontaneous operational tolerance. They could maintain normal graft function and histology without any immunosuppressive regimens. Operational tolerance after transplantation has been an attractive and ultimate goal in transplant immunology. The liver, as an immunoregulatory organ, generates an immune hyporesponsive microenvironment under physiological conditions. In this regard, LT recipients may be ideal candidates for studies focusing on operative tolerance. Cell-based strategies are one of the most promising methods for immune tolerance induction, including chimerism induced by hematopoietic stem cells and adoptive transfer of regulatory T cells, regulatory dendritic cells, regulatory macrophages, regulatory B cells, and mesenchymal stromal cells. The safety and the efficacy of many cell products have been evaluated by prospective clinical trials. In this review, we will summarize the latest perspectives on the clinical application of cell-based strategies in LT and will address a number of concerns and future directions regarding these cell products.

Keywords: immune tolerance, liver transplantation, hematopoietic stem cells, regulatory cells, mesenchymal stromal cells

INTRODUCTION

Liver transplantation (LT) has become the best chance for patients with end-stage liver disease and small hepatocellular carcinoma with chronic liver disease since it was first performed in 1963 (1, 2). With the development of new immunosuppressive regimens and the improvement of surgical techniques, LT has become a routine practice and is increasingly conducted around the world. However, most recipients need open-ended and even lifelong immunosuppression to achieve ideal long-term outcomes. This open-ended immunosuppressive therapy can result in many post-LT complications, such as cancer recurrence, dysmetabolic syndrome, infections, and renal injury. Interestingly, some LT recipients who are taken off immunosuppression for different reasons accidently develop immune tolerance. Among highly selected LT recipients, some of them could discontinue all immunosuppression for more than 1 year while maintaining a stable allograft status, which is defined as "operational tolerance" (3, 4). For these reasons, tolerance of LT has been an attractive and ultimate goal in transplant immunology. Approximately 20% of recipients could become completely tolerant without any immunosuppressant drugs after LT (5–7), whereas such "operational tolerance" is reported only anecdotally in recipients of other organs (8).

The liver has been generally recognized as an immunoregulatory organ (9, 10). It consists in parenchymal and innate immune cells, including hepatocytes and cholangiocytes, liver sinusoidal endothelial cells, hepatic stellate cells, Kupffer cells, stromal cells, liver-derived dendritic cells, natural killer (NK) cells, natural killer T (NKT) cells, and so on (11). The complex interactions between these cells and immune cells contribute to the induction of immune tolerance in the liver (12). The liver receives blood from both the portal vein and the hepatic artery. In the portal vein, the liver confronts various antigens from digested food and the gut microbiome under physiological conditions (13). The immune reaction is tightly controlled and regulated, generating liver-protective immunity while these antigens pass through sinusoids. The responsible mechanisms are associated with various elements, including immature and non-professional antigen-presenting cells, exhausted lymphocytes, transforming growth factor β (TGFβ), and interleukin (IL)-10 in the cytokine milieu, and high proportions of regulatory cells (14). Compared to that in other solid organ transplantations, the incidence of chronic rejection in LT is lower (15). With this background, LT recipients may be ideal candidates for clinical trials studying operative tolerance. A reproducible strategy to induce stable transplant tolerance may achieve success first in LT.

Substantial progress has been made toward immune tolerance induction and in the study of relevant mechanisms in animal models. However, the translation of these strategies into clinical transplantation remains challenging. In addition to novel immunomodulatory drugs such as belatacept, the most promising strategy is cell-based therapy. A variety of cell products were tested to induce tolerance in preclinical experiments, but only a small part of them were evaluated in clinical studies, including induction of chimerism by hematopoietic stem cells and adoptive transfer of regulatory cells and mesenchymal stromal cells. There are many advantages of cell-based strategies, such as low toxicity and long-term efficacy. In addition, a cell-based strategy is expected to control many kinds of inflammatory cells and generate donor antigen-specific tolerance (16). In this review, we mainly focus on cell-based strategies of tolerance induction in LT by clarifying the translational potential of these strategies.

HEMATOPOIETIC STEM CELLS FOR TOLERANCE INDUCTION

Since the first successful application of mixed chimerism in tolerance induction in human kidney transplantation in 2008 (17), mixed chimerism induced by donor hematopoietic stem cell (HSC) infusion remains one of the most effective treatments for tolerance induction. Chimerism can be defined as tissues from two genetically distinct organisms coexisting in one organism (18). Mixed chimerism, in which both donor and recipient HSCs coexist, leads to donor-specific transplantation tolerance and retains immunocompetence for primary immune responses (19–22). Additionally, mixed chimerism can be induced through a non-myeloablative conditioning protocol, which represents a lower risk and severity of graft-vs.-host disease (GVHD) than the fully allogeneic chimerism induced by myeloablative conditioning.

In LT, the application of hematopoietic chimerism to achieve graft tolerance has been studied by various groups. The St. Mary's Hospital group reported that full donor chimerism induced by HSC transplantation could maintain stable allograft tolerance without immunosuppressants. Two patients were immunosuppressant-free with normal liver function for 6 and 7 years (**Table 1**) (23). Donckier et al. reported two pilot studies in which donor stem cell infusion under non-myeloablative conditioning was used to induce tolerance in living donor liver transplantation (LDLT). Both patients, who were treated with pretransplant conditioning using cyclophosphamide and anti-thymocyte globulin (ATG), discontinued immunosuppressive therapies 90 and 28 days after transplantation without subsequent rejection episodes (**Table 1**) (24). In the other study, three prospectively enrolled patients were treated with post-transplant conditioning using high doses of ATG and donor $CD34^+$ stem cell infusion (5.3–10 × 10^6 cells/kg) (**Figure 1**; **Table 1**). Two of the three recipients successfully discontinued immunosuppression early without subsequent graft deterioration. Of note is that both patients developed acute rejection during follow-up (25). These results are promising. However, among the four immunosuppression-free patients, Donckier et al. reported relatively short follow-ups from 270 days to 561 days. In another study conducted by the University of Miami group, unprocessed donor bone marrow cell infusion without conditioning therapy was investigated for tolerance induction (**Figure 1**; **Table 1**). A total of 104 patients of at least 3 years post-transplantation were enrolled, among which 45 patients received donor bone marrow cell infusions (5.94 ± 0.4 × 10^8 cells/kg) during the early post-operative period and 59 patients did not. Immunosuppressive therapies were tapered slowly over 3 years after their enrollment. Twenty patients, 10 from each group, were immunosuppression-free during follow-up without a significant difference (26). These data indicate that chimerism-based strategies can produce long-term tolerance, but conditioning therapy seems indispensable. In the application of mixed chimerism for tolerance induction in LT, any risk of acute or chronic GVHD should be avoided. Although many studies reported less frequent incidences of

TABLE 1 | Clinical studies/trials of cell-based strategies for tolerance induction in LT.

Cell type	Sample size/stage	Cell dose (total)	Reference/trial ID
HSC			
Allogeneic, HSC transplantation	2 cases		23
Purified donor CD34$^+$ stem cells	2 cases	3.3–5.7 × 10^6 cells/kg	24
Purified donor CD34+ stem cells	3 cases	5.3–10 × 10^6 cells/kg	25
Donor bone marrow cells	104 cases	5.94 ± 0.4 × 10^8 cells/kg	26
Autologous, HSC transplantation	Phase II		NCT02549586
Treg			
Autologous, donor alloantigen-specific specific Treg	Phase I	0.34–6.37× 10^6 cells/kg	46, UMIN-000015789
Autologous, polyclonal Treg	Phase I/II	0.5–4.5 × 10^6 cells/kg	47, NCT02166177
Autologous, donor alloantigen-specific specific Treg	Phase I	1 × 10^6 cells/kg	NCT01624077
Autologous, donor alloantigen-specific specific Treg	Phase I/II	1–2.5 × 10^6 cells/kg	NCT03577431
Autologous, donor alloantigen-specific specific Treg	Phase I	25–960 × 10^6 cells/kg	NCT02188719
Autologous, donor alloantigen-specific specific Treg	Phase I/II	300–500 × 10^6 cells/kg	NCT02474199
DCreg			
Donor DCreg (infusion at 7 days before LT)	Phase I/II	2.5–10 × 10^6 cells/kg	NCT03164265
Donor DCreg (infusion at 7 days prior to IS weaning)	Phase I/II		NCT04208919
MSC			
Third-party BM-derived MSC	Phase I	1.9–2.7× 10^6 cells/kg	91, NCT01429038
Third-party BM-derived MSC	Phase I	1–2 × 10^6 cells/kg	NCT02260375
Allogeneic, MSC	Phase I/II	6 × 10^6 cells/kg	NCT02706132
Umbilical cord derived MSC	Phase I	3 × 10^6 cells/kg	NCT01690247
Donor BM-derived MSC (pediatric LT)	Phase I	2 × 10^6 cells/kg	NCT02957552

LT, liver transplantation; HSC, hematopoietic stem cell; Treg, regulatory T cell; DCreg, regulatory DC cell; IS, immunosuppression; MSC, mesenchymal stromal cell; BM, bone marrow.

GVHD using non-myeloablative conditioning regimen (27), there is still a risk of GVHD with durable mixed chimerism (28, 29). Therefore, modifications of the conditioning protocol and maybe delayed HSC infusion might be important next steps for chimerism-induced tolerance in LT.

In addition to donor HSC infusion, autologous hematopoietic stem cell transplantation (HSCT) has also been studied for tolerance induction. Autologous HSCT may reset the deregulated immune system into a tolerant status by regenerating new autotolerant T and B cells and increasing immune regulatory mechanisms (30–32). The therapeutic efficacy of autologous HSCT for various autoimmune diseases has been reported by clinical trials, such as trials in systemic and multiple sclerosis (33–35), Crohn's disease (36), and scleroderma (37). In LT, there is an ongoing clinical trial evaluating the ability of autologous HSCT to induce tolerance (NCT02549586) (**Figure 1**; **Table 1**). The researchers plan to recruit 10 liver transplant recipients. The purified HSCs will be infused following a chemotherapy- and ATG-based conditioning regimen. The immunosuppressive drugs will be withdrawn at 6 months post-HSCT.

REGULATORY T CELLS FOR TOLERANCE INDUCTION

Regulatory T cells (Tregs), commonly distinguished into natural Tregs (nTregs) and inducible Tregs (iTregs) (38), are a population of CD4+ cells that constitutively express the Forkhead box P3 (Foxp3) transcription factor. In 2001, human Tregs were initially identified as CD4+CD25+ T cells (39), which comprise 5–10% of total peripheral CD4+ T cells (40). Over the past two decades, Tregs have been studied and are known to be responsible for maintaining immune homeostasis and tolerance (41, 42). The adoptive transfer of Tregs has been successful and proven effective in murine (43, 44) and non-human primate transplantation models (45).

In the LT setting, tolerance induction by Treg infusion has been reported in two clinical trials to date (46, 47). Researchers from Hokkaido University reported a pilot study of tolerance induction with Treg-based cell therapy in living donor LT in 2016 (46). In this study, donor-antigen-specific iTregs were obtained *ex vivo* by coculturing recipient lymphocytes with irradiated donor cells and anti-CD80/CD86 mAbs for 2 weeks. At day 13 after LT, the expanded cells were administered to the recipients at a mean dose of 3.39 × 10^6/kg CD4$^+$CD25$^+$Foxp3$^+$ cells (**Figure 1**; **Table 1**). This dose is much lower than the dose of nTregs for transplant cell therapy since donor-antigen-specific iTregs are considered to be more potent than nTregs (48, 49). The infusion caused no significant adverse events. After infusion, the immunosuppressive agent weaning program was initiated at 6 months post-LT and completely discontinued at 18 months. Among the 10 consecutively enrolled patients, seven completely stopped their immunosuppressive regimen for 16–33 months with normal graft function and histology.

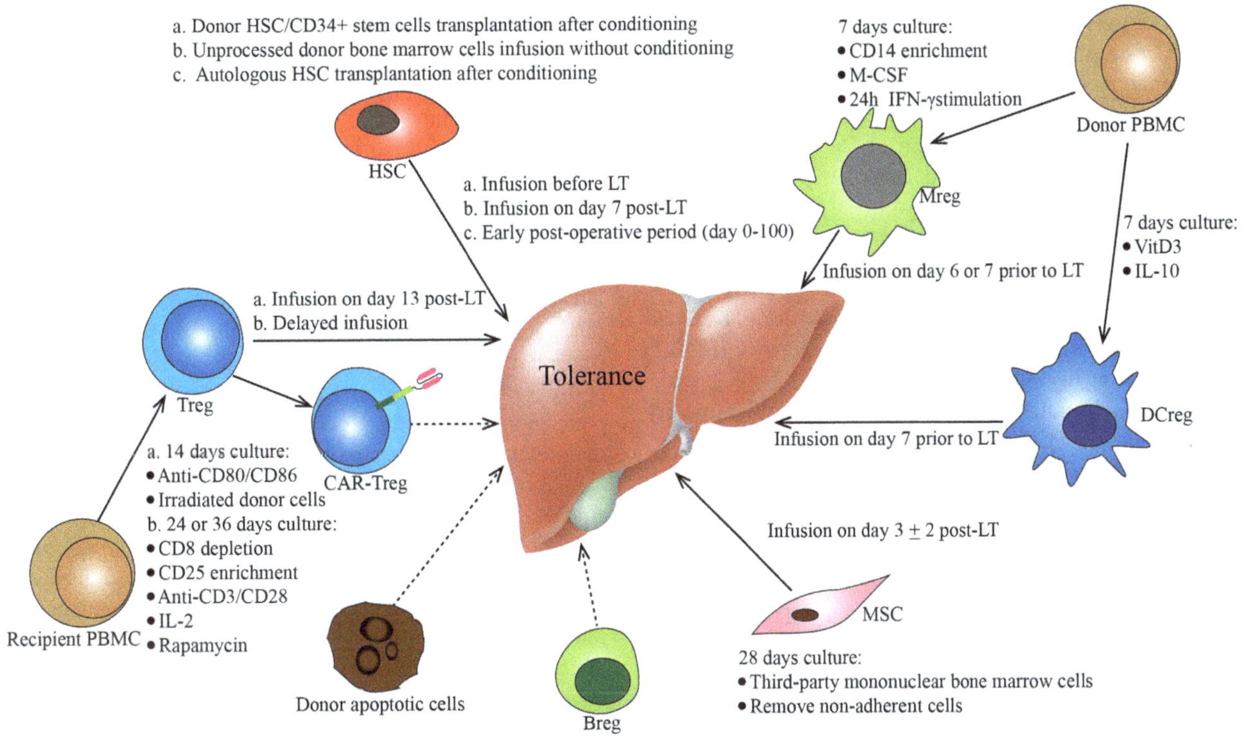

FIGURE 1 | Protocols of various cell-based strategies for tolerance induction in liver transplantation. This figure summarizes the different cell-based therapies described in the manuscript. Cell types, culture conditions, dosages (i.e., cell number), and administration conditions are mentioned for each cell-based therapy. Breg, regulatory B cells; CAR, chimeric antigen receptor; DCreg, regulatory dendritic cells; HSC, hematopoietic stem cells; MSC, mesenchymal stroma cells; PBMC, peripheral blood mononuclear cells; Treg, regulatory CD4+ T cells.

The other three recipients who had autoimmune liver diseases developed acute cellular rejection and resumed reduced doses of immunotherapy. This is the first study of successful operational tolerance induction using the adoptive transfer of Tregs in LT.

More recently, the King's College London group published the results of their phase I clinical trial, ThRIL, evaluating the safety and the efficacy profile of Treg therapy in LT recipients (47). In this trial, patients with an autoimmune disease were excluded. Tregs isolated from the recipients were expanded under polyclonal conditions *ex vivo* using anti-CD3/CD28 beads, IL-2, and rapamycin for 24 or 36 days. Three patients awaiting LT were enrolled and received an infusion of 1×10^6 Tregs/kg 83–110 days post-transplant, while the other six patients were recruited 6–12 months post-transplant and received an infusion of 4.5×10^6 Tregs/kg 112–151 days after enrollment (**Figure 1**; **Table 1**). Of note is that one of the patients who received an infusion of 4.5×10^6 Tregs developed a fever of >39°C associated with rigors, which was classified as a dose-limiting toxicity. In general, this autologous non-specific Treg transfer was considered to be safe and exerted potentially beneficial donor-specific immunosuppressive effects.

Treg-induced immune regulation is the best-studied and core mechanism of tolerance. Both preliminary clinical studies demonstrated the safety and the efficacy of Treg strategies in human LT, which has great potential for future clinical translation. Many other registered phase I/II clinical trials assessing the safety and the efficacy of Treg infusion are in progress (NCT01624077, NCT03577431, NCT02188719, and NCT02474199) (**Table 1**). However, multicenter studies with large sample sizes need to be conducted, and future studies should focus on the protocol of Treg infusion, such as cell dosage, timing/frequency of infusion, optimal immunosuppressive regimen, and its late complications. Additionally, some other approaches to generate antigen-specific Tregs can be promising in LT, such as chimeric antigen receptor (CAR) transduction (50). It was shown that the adoptive transfer of Tregs engineered with a CAR which targets HLA-A2 can suppress skin allograft rejection in humanized mouse models (51, 52). Therefore, these modified cells may have a great potential in LT.

REGULATORY DENDRITIC CELLS FOR TOLERANCE INDUCTION

Dendritic cells (DCs) were first identified by Steinman and Cohn in 1973 (53, 54) and have proved potent antigen-presenting cells linking the innate and the adaptive immune responses (55). Over the following years, based on their morphological features, ontogenies, locations, and functions, various DC subsets have been identified, including conventional DCs (cDCs), plasmacytoid DCs (pDCs), Langerhans cells (LCs), and inflammatory DCs (56, 57). It has been reported that DCs can be either immunogenic or tolerogenic in different states (58, 59). Of note is that the ablation of DCs could break the self-tolerance of $CD4^+$ T cells and result in spontaneous fatal autoimmunity (60).

Tolerogenic DCs or regulatory DCs (DCregs) are characterized by a low expression of MHC gene products (MHC class I and II) and co-stimulatory molecules (CD80 and CD86) and a high expression of co-inhibitory ligands (PD-L1) and death-inducing ligands (FasL). In terms of functions, DCregs are resistant to maturation, able to produce anti-inflammatory cytokines (IL-10 and TGFβ), and impair T cell proliferation.

In LT, tolerance induction by DCregs is ongoing as phase I/II clinical trials conducted by the University of Pittsburgh group (61). Actually, the safety, the tolerability, and the feasibility of autologous DCreg infusion have been confirmed by various clinical studies in autoimmune disorders, such as rheumatoid arthritis (62, 63), type 1 diabetes (64), and Crohn's disease (65). In a preclinical non-human primate renal transplant model, it has been demonstrated that a single pretransplant DCreg infusion can prolong MHC-mismatched renal allograft survival (66–68). In an ongoing trial (NCT03164265), according to preclinical experience, DCregs are generated from monocytes of prospective living donors in the presence of VitD3 and IL-10. Then, the expanded cells are infused at a dose of 2.5–10 × 10^6/kg (54) into the respective recipients 7 days before transplantation (**Figure 1**; **Table 1**). Weaning and withdrawal of the immunosuppressive drugs begin at 12 and 18 months post-transplantation, respectively.

More recently, the University of Pittsburgh group registered another clinical trial evaluating the delayed infusion of DCreg for tolerance induction in LDLT (NCT04208919) (**Table 1**). In this clinical trial, recipients who are between 1 and 3 years after transplantation will be enrolled. Those enrolled patients will receive a single infusion of donor-derived DCreg. At 1 week after that, immunosuppression weaning will be initiated slowly. Since preclinical experience to date has proven that DCreg infusion is safe, the results of their clinical trials are awaited with great interest.

REGULATORY MACROPHAGES FOR TOLERANCE INDUCTION

Macrophages are immune cells of hematopoietic origin that provide crucial innate immune defense and have tissue-specific functions in the regulation and the maintenance of organ homeostasis (69). Various macrophage subsets with distinct functions have been identified, including classically activated macrophages (M1 macrophages), alternatively activated macrophages (M2 macrophages), regulatory macrophages (Mregs), tumor-associated macrophages, and myeloid-derived suppressor cells (70–73).

Human Mregs reflect a unique state of macrophage differentiation, distinguished from macrophages in other activation states by their particular mode of derivation, robust phenotype, and potent T cell-suppressing function (74). According to the protocol from University Hospital Regensburg (74, 75), Mregs could be generated from $CD14^+$ blood monocytes in the presence of M-CSF and a further 24-h stimulation with IFN-γ after 7 days of culture. In terms of cell surface phenotype, these cells are homogeneously $CD14^{-/low}HLA\text{-}DR^+CD80^{-/low}CD86^+CD16^-TLR2^-CD163^{-/low}$ (75). In this pilot study, these cells were administered 1 week prior to transplantation to two living-donor renal transplant recipients at doses of 7.1 × 10^6 and 8 × 10^6 cells/kg (75) (**Figure 1**). Both patients were weaned to low-dose tacrolimus monotherapy and maintained normal graft function. Of note is that the infused cells were ^{111}In-labeled, which is different from that of other studies. The tracking results showed that the donor-derived Mregs remained viable for more than 30 days and migrated from the pulmonary vasculature *via* the blood to the liver, spleen, and bone marrow. The clinical trial of Mreg treatment for renal transplantation was registered as the One study, in which donor-derived Mregs (2.5–7.5 × 10^6 cells/kg) were infused 6–7 days before transplantation into recipients of a living donor renal transplant (NCT02085629). However, in LT, there is no registered clinical trial about Mregs to date.

MESENCHYMAL STROMAL CELLS FOR TOLERANCE INDUCTION

Mesenchymal stromal cells (MSCs) are plastic-adherent non-hematopoietic multipotent cells that are able to differentiate into osteoblasts, adipocytes, and chondroblasts under standard *in vitro* differentiating conditions (76). In terms of cell surface phenotype as measured by flow cytometry, these cells express CD105, CD73, and CD90 and lack expression (<2% positive) of CD45, CD34, CD14, or CD11b, CD79a or CD19, and HLA class II (76, 77). Bone marrow was first and most commonly used to isolate MSCs for clinical applications since 2004 (78). Over the last few years, other sources of MSCs have been found and proposed for clinical use, including adipose tissue (79), dental tissues (80), placenta (81), umbilical cord tissue (82), and cord blood (83). MSC-induced immunosuppression targets both the innate (84) and the adaptive immune systems (85). A variety of studies documented the potent immunosuppressive capacity of MSCs *in vitro* and *in vivo* (86–88). The immunoregulatory effect of MSCs is dose dependent and seems independent of MHC (89). The effects of autologous MSC infusion have been evaluated in kidney transplantation in a randomized controlled trial with a large sample size (90). In this study, MSC infusion resulted in a lower incidence of acute rejection, a lower risk of opportunistic infection, and better renal function at 1 year.

In LT, MSC therapy has been evaluated in a phase I–II clinical study (91). In this study, MSCs were generated by isolating mononuclear BM cells with Ficoll and expanding them in a 4 week culture. Third-party unrelated MSCs were infused at a dose of 1.5–3 × 10^6/kg on post-transplantation day 3 ± 2 in 10 patients (**Figure 1**; **Table 1**). Compared with 10 control liver transplant recipients, patients who received MSC infusion did not have an impairment of organ functions or an increased rate of opportunistic infection or malignancies. Weaning and withdrawal of the immunosuppressive drugs were attempted from month 6 to 12 post-transplantation. Among nine MSC recipients, tacrolimus and mycophenolate mofetil withdrawal were successfully achieved in only one patient, while the other eight patients failed due to either graft rejection or a significant increase in transaminases.

The very fast tapering of immunosuppressive drugs within 3 months might explain the failure of tolerance induction using MSCs in this study (91, 92). MSC-induced immunoregulation might be disrupted by very fast drug discontinuation, which could promote effector T cell activation (92). In addition, lack of induction therapy, insufficient MSC dosage, timing of infusion, infusion routes, and different sources might also account for the failure. As far as we know, MSC infusion for tolerance induction in LT is being studied by various other registered clinical trials (NCT02260375, NCT02706132, NCT01690247, and NCT02957552) (**Table 1**), including that using donor-derived MSC and that using umbilical-cord-derived MSC. Indeed these variables should be studied in future studies to achieve better results.

REGULATORY B CELLS FOR TOLERANCE INDUCTION

Regulatory B cells (Bregs) are immunosuppressive cells that support immunological tolerance (93, 94). Bregs express immune-regulatory cytokines, including IL-10, TGF-β, and IL-35, through which Bregs can suppress the differentiation of various pro-inflammatory lymphocytes (93, 94).

The role of Bregs in transplant tolerance has been studied mostly in rodents using heart (95, 96) and islet (97, 98) graft models. Stable immune tolerance to solid organ and islet cell grafts can be induced using antibodies directed at CD45RB, and this tolerance is dependent on Bregs (95, 97, 98). Furthermore, graft rejection in B cell-deficient mice after islet transplantation could be reversed to tolerance by the adoptive transfer of B cells from tolerant mice (97). The mechanisms of Breg-induced tolerance remain unclear, and research is still active. Breg-dependent islet transplant tolerance also requires the functions of natural killer cells and Tregs (98). Although promising, many questions remain unsolved in Breg-based strategies, such as the method of *ex vivo* culture and the expansion and the ability of tolerance induction in large animals. The field of Breg-induced tolerance is very immature and has a long way to go before translation into clinical LT.

APOPTOTIC CELLS FOR TOLERANCE INDUCTION

Apoptosis is a genetically programmed cell death mechanism occurring during the elimination of unwanted or dangerous cells. Apoptotic cells exhibit immunomodulatory properties through various mechanisms, including inhibiting pathogenic T or B cell responses and inducing pro-tolerogenic/regulatory cells (99). In addition to those specific cell populations, apoptotic cell-based therapy is another promising strategy for tolerance induction in transplantation. In many animal studies, apoptotic cells, mainly apoptotic splenocytes in transplantation setting, favor the engraftment of liver (100, 101), cardiac (102, 103), islet (104), and hematopoietic (105) allografts.

In LT, tolerance induction using apoptotic cells was studied in rats by two groups. Researchers from Zhejiang University reported that donor apoptotic cells can promote liver graft acceptance using a rat LT model (106). In this study, apoptotic splenic lymphocytes induced by ultraviolet-C (UVC) irradiation at a dosage of 5 × 10^7 cells/rat were infused intravenously at 7 days before LT. In terms of mechanism, they found increased peripheral blood Tregs in rats treated with UVC-irradiated lymphocytes. In another study performed by the Zhejiang University group, they showed that the combination of tolerogenic DCs and apoptotic lymphocytes alleviates rejection after LT (100). The other group, Zhejiang Cancer Hospital group, also reported that preinfusion of apoptotic lymphocytes can induce immune tolerance in a rat LT model (101). The apoptotic cells used in this study were obtained from donor peripheral blood. Lymphocytes irradiated by X-ray from an electron linear accelerator at an absorbed dose of 2.0 Gy were infused intravenously at a dosage of 5 × 10^7 cells/rat 7 days before operation. However, there are no clinical studies or studies using nonhuman primate transplantation models considering the immunoregulatory role of apoptotic cells in LT. This can be an important next step in the field.

CONCERNS

There are many concerns for cell-based therapies. First, for allogenic/autologous HSC infusion, intense myeloablative or non-myeloablative conditioning therapy may not be tolerated by patients with end-stage liver disease. Of note is that, in the absence of conditioning therapy, donor HSC infusion may show no significant effect in LT (26). Various non-myeloablative conditioning regimens of reduced intensity are now being studied, revised, and improved to induce tolerance with less toxicity (27, 107–109). Second, protocols of these regulatory cell-based therapies are not clearly established. The optimal dose of regulatory cells could be highly important for those strategies using non-donor-specific therapies. Overdose may result in original disease recurrence, infection, and other immunosuppression-related complications. In addition, there is no current consensus regarding the method and the timing of administration. The potential influence of different protocols needs to be observed in a study with long follow-up. Third, the purity of *in vitro*-expanded cells represents another significant concern. After stimulation, culture, and expansion, cell products without classical confirmed markers cannot be purified. There are subpopulations in these cell products that have different functions, such as resting and activated Tregs, highly suppressive

Tregs, and non-Treg FoxP3$^+$ cells (110–113). Additionally, Tregs can acquire the expression of transcription factors associated with effector T cell programs (called Th-like Tregs), which is called Treg cell plasticity (114). These Th-like Tregs can be pro-inflammatory rather than suppressive, which play an opposite role in tolerance induction. Fourth, the stability of infused cells has not been determined. Except for one study (75), none of the studies thus far have used cell products that were radioactively labeled. Without genetic or radioactive labels, *in vivo* homing and the stability of infused cells are difficult to detect. Fifth, at least for now, another drawback of cell-based therapy is the cost. Basic researches, clinical trials, and products of these cell-based therapies are very costly. Last but not least, the selection of patients is one of the top issues. Allogenic/autologous HSC infusion may not be conducted in patients with end-stage organ disease considering the toxicity of recipient conditioning (115, 116). Regulatory cells may play a detrimental role in patients with hepatitis B infection (117, 118), hepatitis C infection (119, 120), or hepatocellular carcinoma (121, 122). Pilot studies or phase I/II clinical trials with small sample sizes are unable to uncover all potential risks. It is vital to conduct high-quality studies with large sample sizes to assess the safety and the efficacy of these cellular strategies in tolerance induction.

SUMMARY AND OUTLOOK

Undoubtedly, cell-based strategies have a great potential in tolerance induction in transplantation. In particular, LT provides a great opportunity to achieve this goal because of an immunoregulatory microenvironment in the liver. Compared to immunosuppressant drugs, cell products can generate donor-specific tolerance with low toxicity and long-term efficacy. Theoretically, they could maintain normal graft function without immunosuppression and keep the protective properties of the immune system intact. Various cell products using different infusion protocols are being evaluated in clinical studies (**Figure 1**). These preliminary clinical studies have demonstrated a promising breakthrough in tolerance induction using cell-based therapies, including HSCs, Tregs, Mregs, DCregs, and MSCs. Breg-induced tolerance has mostly been studied in animal models, and the field is still in its infancy. The clinical studies or trials exploring the safety and the efficacy of cell-based strategies for tolerance induction in LT are listed in **Table 1**. Many excellent translational results may show up in the next few years. However, various problems with these strategies remain challenging. These strategies are not equally effective in each patient, suggesting that diverse mechanisms of immune tolerance exist among different individuals. Identifying useful biomarkers of immune tolerance that could guide the gradual tapering of immunosuppression after cell-based therapies is necessary. In addition, the heterogeneity of immunological status and health state between patients makes tolerance induction difficult with a universal protocol. The combination of cell products and other therapies as well as individualized treatment might provide ideal results. However, more high-quality clinical studies focusing on these strategies need to be performed for practical translation from bench to bedside.

AUTHOR CONTRIBUTIONS

PW and ZJ wrote this manuscript and prepared the table and the figure. LZ and DX devised and supervised this project. CW, XL, and HL assisted in the literature search and manuscript editing. All authors contributed to the article and approved the submitted version.

REFERENCES

1. Starzl TE, Marchioro TL, Vonkaulla KN, Hermann G, Brittain RS, Waddell RW. Homotransplantation of the liver in humans. *Surg Gynecol Obstet.* (1963) 117:659–76.
2. Starzl TE. The long reach of liver transplantation. *Nat Med.* (2012) 18:1489–92. doi: 10.1038/nm.2927
3. Benitez C, Londono MC, Miquel R, Manzia TM, Abraldes JG, Lozano JJ, et al. Prospective multicenter clinical trial of immunosuppressive drug withdrawal in stable adult liver transplant recipients. *Hepatology.* (2013) 58:1824–35. doi: 10.1002/hep.26426
4. Feng S, Ekong UD, Lobritto SJ, Demetris AJ, Roberts JP, Rosenthal P, et al. Complete immunosuppression withdrawal and subsequent allograft function among pediatric recipients of parental living donor liver transplants. *JAMA.* (2012) 307:283–93. doi: 10.1001/jama.2012014
5. Adams DH, Sanchez-Fueyo A, Samuel D. From immunosuppression to tolerance. *J Hepatol.* (2015) 62(Suppl. 1):S170–85. doi: 10.1016/j.jhep.2015.02.042
6. Crispe IN, Giannandrea M, Klein I, John B, Sampson B, Wuensch S. Cellular and molecular mechanisms of liver tolerance. *Immunol Rev.* (2006) 213:101–18. doi: 10.1111/j.1600-065X.2006.00435.x
7. Feng S. Spontaneous and induced tolerance for liver transplant recipients. *Curr Opin Organ Transplant.* (2016) 21:53–8. doi: 10.1097/MOT.0000000000000268
8. Taner T. Liver transplantation: rejection and tolerance. *Liver Transpl.* (2017) 23:S85–8. doi: 10.1002/lt.24840
9. Demetris AJ, Bellamy CO, Gandhi CR, Prost S, Nakanuma Y, Stolz BD. Functional immune anatomy of the liver-as an allograft. *Am J Transplant.* (2016) 16:1653–80. doi: 10.1111/ajt.13749
10. Tiegs G, Lohse WA. Immune tolerance: what is unique about the liver. *J Autoimmun.* (2010) 34:1–6. doi: 10.1016/j.jaut.2009.08.008
11. Huang H, Lu Y, Zhou T, Gu G, Xia Q. Innate immune cells in immune tolerance after liver transplantation. *Front Immunol.* (2018) 9:2401. doi: 10.3389/fimmu.2018.02401
12. Zheng M, Tian Z. Liver-mediated adaptive immune tolerance. *Front Immunol.* (2019) 10:2525. doi: 10.3389/fimmu.2019.02525
13. Chaudhry S, Emond J, Griesemer A. Immune cell trafficking to the liver. *Transplantation.* (2019) 103:1323–37. doi: 10.1097/TP.0000000000002690
14. Feng S, Bucuvalas J. Tolerance after liver transplantation: where are we? *Liver Transpl.* (2017) 23:1601–14. doi: 10.1002/lt.24845
15. Wu SL, Pan EC. Tolerance and chimerism and allogeneic bone marrow/stem cell transplantation in liver transplantation. *World J Gastroenterol.* (2013) 19:5981–7. doi: 10.3748/wjg.v19.i36.5981
16. Ten Brinke A, Martinez-Llordella M, Cools N, Hilkens CMU, van Ham SM, Sawitzki B, et al. Ways forward for tolerance-inducing cellular therapies- an AFACTT perspective. *Front Immunol.* (2019) 10:181. doi: 10.3389/fimmu.2019.00181
17. Kawai T, Cosimi AB, Spitzer TR, Tolkoff-Rubin N, Suthanthiran M, Saidman SL, et al. HLA-mismatched renal transplantation without maintenance immunosuppression. *N Engl J Med.* (2008) 358:353–61. doi: 10.1056/NEJMoa071074
18. Wu S, Xu H, Ravindra K, Ildstad TS. Composite tissue allotransplantation: past, present and future-the history and expanding applications of CTA as a new frontier in transplantation. *Transplant Proc.* (2009) 41:463–5. doi: 10.1016/j.transproceed.2009.01.027
19. Ildstad ST, Sachs HD. Reconstitution with syngeneic plus allogeneic or xenogeneic bone marrow leads to specific acceptance of allografts or xenografts. *Nature.* (1984) 307:168–70. doi: 10.1038/307168a0

20. Ruedi E, Sykes M, Ildstad ST, Chester CH, Althage A, Hengartner H, et al. Antiviral T cell competence and restriction specificity of mixed allogeneic (P1 + P2—-P1) irradiation chimeras. *Cell Immunol.* (1989) 121:185–95. doi: 10.1016/0008-8749(89)90016-6
21. Mache CJ, Schwinger W, Spendel S, Zach O, Regauer S, Ring E. Skin transplantation to monitor clinical donor-related tolerance in mixed hematopoietic chimerism. *Pediatr Transplant.* (2006) 10:128–31. doi: 10.1111/j.1399-3046.2005.00412.x
22. Trivedi HL, Vanikar AV, Modi PR, Shah VR, Vakil JM, Trivedi VB, et al. Allogeneic hematopoietic stem-cell transplantation, mixed chimerism, and tolerance in living related donor renal allograft recipients. *Transplant Proc.* (2005) 37:737–42. doi: 10.1016/j.transproceed.2005.01.028
23. Kim SY, Kim DW, Choi JY, Kim DG, Min WS, Lee JW, et al. Full donor chimerism using stem-cell transplantation for tolerance induction in the human leukocyte antigen-matched liver transplant setting. *Transplantation.* (2009) 88:601–3. doi: 10.1097/TP.0b013e3181b164d5
24. Donckier V, Troisi R, Toungouz M, Colle I, Van Vlierberghe H, Jacquy C, et al. Donor stem cell infusion after non-myeloablative conditioning for tolerance induction to HLA mismatched adult living-donor liver graft. *Transpl Immunol.* (2004) 13:139–46. doi: 10.1016/j.trim.2004.05.004
25. Donckier V, Troisi R, Le Moine A, Toungouz M, Ricciardi S, Colle I, et al. Early immunosuppression withdrawal after living donor liver transplantation and donor stem cell infusion. *Liver Transpl.* (2006) 12:1523–8. doi: 10.1002/lt.20872
26. Tryphonopoulos P, Tzakis AG, Weppler D, Garcia-Morales R, Kato T, Madariaga JR, et al. The role of donor bone marrow infusions in withdrawal of immunosuppression in adult liver allotransplantation. *Am J Transplant.* (2005) 5:608–13. doi: 10.1111/j.1600-6143.2004.00743.x
27. Sasaki H, Oura T, Spitzer TR, Chen YB, Madsen JC, Allan J, et al. Preclinical and clinical studies for transplant tolerance via the mixed chimerism approach. *Hum Immunol.* (2018) 79:258–65. doi: 10.1016/j.humimm.2017.11.008
28. Peggs KS, Thomson K, Hart DP, Geary J, Morris EC, Yong K, et al. Dose-escalated donor lymphocyte infusions following reduced intensity transplantation: toxicity, chimerism, disease responses. *Blood.* (2004) 103:1548–56. doi: 10.1182/blood-2003-05-1513
29. Perruche S, Marandin A, Kleinclauss F, Angonin R, Fresnay S, Baron MH, et al. Association of mixed hematopoietic chimerism with elevated circulating autoantibodies and chronic graft-versus-host disease occurrence. *Transplantation.* (2006) 81:573–82. doi: 10.1097/01.tp.0000183878.53367.77
30. Swart JF, Delemarre EM, van Wijk F, Boelens JJ, Kuball J, van Laar JM, et al. Haematopoietic stem cell transplantation for autoimmune diseases. *Nat Rev Rheumatol.* (2017) 13:244–56. doi: 10.1038/nrrheum.2017.7
31. Muraro PA, Martin R, Mancardi GL, Nicholas R, Sormani MP, Saccardi R. Autologous haematopoietic stem cell transplantation for treatment of multiple sclerosis. *Nat Rev Neurol.* (2017) 13:391–405. doi: 10.1038/nrneurol.2017.81
32. Muraro PA, Robins H, Malhotra S, Howell M, Phippard D, Desmarais C, et al. T cell repertoire following autologous stem cell transplantation for multiple sclerosis. *J Clin Invest.* (2014) 124:1168–72. doi: 10.1172/JCI71691
33. Burt RK, Oliveira MC, Shah SJ, Moraes DA, Simoes B, Gheorghiade M, et al. Cardiac involvement and treatment-related mortality after non-myeloablative haemopoietic stem-cell transplantation with unselected autologous peripheral blood for patients with systemic sclerosis: a retrospective analysis. *Lancet.* (2013) 381:1116–24. doi: 10.1016/S0140-6736(12)62114-X
34. Mancardi GL, Sormani MP, Gualandi F, Saiz A, Carreras E, Merelli E, et al. Autologous hematopoietic stem cell transplantation in multiple sclerosis: a phase II trial. *Neurology.* (2015) 84:981–8. doi: 10.1212/WNL.0000000000001329
35. Muraro PA, Pasquini M, Atkins HL, Bowen JD, Farge D, Fassas A, et al. Multiple sclerosis-autologous hematopoietic stem cell transplantation long-term outcomes study: long-term outcomes after autologous hematopoietic stem cell transplantation for multiple sclerosis. *JAMA Neurol.* (2017) 74:459–69. doi: 10.1001/jamaneurol.2016.5867
36. Pineton de Chambrun G, Pariente B, Seksik P, Altwegg R, Vuitton L, Stefasnescu C, et al. Adalimumab for patients with Crohn's disease complicated by intra-abdominal abscess: a multicentre, prospective, observational cohort study. *J Crohns Colitis.* (2019) 13(Suppl. 1):S616. doi: 10.1093/ecco-jcc/jjz045
37. Sullivan KM, Goldmuntz EA, Keyes-Elstein L, McSweeney PA, Pinckney A, Welch B, et al. Myeloablative autologous stem-cell transplantation for severe scleroderma. *N Engl J Med.* (2018) 378:35–47. doi: 10.1056/NEJMoa1703327
38. Yadav M, Louvet C, Davini D, Gardner JM, Martinez-Llordella M, Bailey-Bucktrout S, et al. Neuropilin-1 distinguishes natural and inducible regulatory T cells among regulatory T cell subsets *in vivo*. *J Exp Med.* (2012) 209:1713–22, S1–19. doi: 10.1084/jem.20120822
39. Dieckmann D, Plottner H, Berchtold S, Berger T, Schuler G. *Ex vivo* isolation and characterization of $CD4^+CD25^+$ T cells with regulatory properties from human blood. *J Exp Med.* (2001) 193:1303–10. doi: 10.1084/jem.193.11.1303
40. Wang YM, Ghali J, Zhang GY, Hu M, Wang Y, Sawyer A, et al. Development and function of $Foxp3^+$ regulatory T cells. *Nephrology.* (2016) 21:81–5. doi: 10.1111/nep.12652
41. Sakaguchi S, Miyara M, Costantino CM, Hafler AD. FOXP3+ regulatory T cells in the human immune system. *Nat Rev Immunol.* (2010) 10:490–500. doi: 10.1038/nri2785
42. Sakaguchi S. Regulatory T cells: key controllers of immunologic self-tolerance. *Cell.* (2000) 101:455–8. doi: 10.1016/S0092-8674(00)80856-9
43. Chandrasekharan D, Issa F, Wood JK. Achieving operational tolerance in transplantation: how can lessons from the clinic inform research directions? *Transpl Int.* (2013) 26:576–89. doi: 10.1111/tri.12081
44. van der Net JB, Bushell A, Wood KJ, Harden NP. Regulatory T cells: first steps of clinical application in solid organ transplantation. *Transpl Int.* (2016) 29:3–11. doi: 10.1111/tri.12608
45. Ezzelarab MB, Zhang H, Guo H, Lu L, Zahorchak AF, Wiseman RW, et al. Regulatory T cell infusion can enhance memory T cell and alloantibody responses in lymphodepleted nonhuman primate heart allograft recipients. *Am J Transplant.* (2016) 16:1999–2015. doi: 10.1111/ajt.13685
46. Todo S, Yamashita K, Goto R, Zaitsu M, Nagatsu A, Oura T, et al. A pilot study of operational tolerance with a regulatory T-cell-based cell therapy in living donor liver transplantation. *Hepatology.* (2016) 64:632–43. doi: 10.1002/hep.28459
47. Sanchez-Fueyo A, Whitehouse G, Grageda N, Cramp ME, Lim TY, Romano M, et al. Applicability, safety and biological activity of regulatory T cell therapy in liver transplantation. *Am J Transplant.* (2019) 20:1125–36. doi: 10.1111/ajt.15700
48. Tang Q, Bluestone AJ. Regulatory T-cell therapy in transplantation: moving to the clinic. *Cold Spring Harb Perspect Med.* (2013) 3:a015552. doi: 10.1101/cshperspect.a015552
49. Sagoo P, Ali N, Garg G, Nestle FO, Lechler RI, Lombardi G. Human regulatory T cells with alloantigen specificity are more potent inhibitors of alloimmune skin graft damage than polyclonal regulatory T cells. *Sci Transl Med.* (2011) 3:83ra42. doi: 10.1126/scitranslmed.3002076
50. Raffin C, Vo LT, Bluestone AJ. Treg cell-based therapies: challenges and perspectives. *Nat Rev Immunol.* (2020) 20:158–72. doi: 10.1038/s41577-019-0232-6
51. Noyan F, Zimmermann K, Hardtke-Wolenski M, Knoefel A, Schulde E, Geffers R, et al. Prevention of allograft rejection by use of regulatory T cells with an MHC-specific chimeric antigen receptor. *Am J Transplant.* (2017) 17:917–30. doi: 10.1111/ajt.14175
52. Boardman DA, Philippeos C, Fruhwirth GO, Ibrahim MA, Hannen RF, Cooper D, et al. Expression of a chimeric antigen receptor specific for donor HLA class I enhances the potency of human regulatory T cells in preventing human skin transplant rejection. *Am J Transplant.* (2017) 17:931–43. doi: 10.1111/ajt.14185
53. Steinman RM, Cohn AZ. Identification of a novel cell type in peripheral lymphoid organs of mice. I. Morphology, quantitation, tissue distribution. *J Exp Med.* (1973) 137:1142–62. doi: 10.1084/jem.137.5.1142
54. Steinman RM, Cohn AZ. Identification of a novel cell type in peripheral lymphoid organs of mice. II. Functional properties *in vitro*. *J Exp Med.* (1974) 139:380–97. doi: 10.1084/jem.139.2.380
55. Mellman I. Dendritic cells: master regulators of the immune response. *Cancer Immunol Res.* (2013) 1:145–9. doi: 10.1158/2326-6066.CIR-13-0102
56. Naik SH, Sathe P, Park HY, Metcalf D, Proietto AI, Dakic A, et al. Development of plasmacytoid and conventional dendritic cell subtypes from single precursor cells derived *in vitro* and *in vivo*. *Nat Immunol.* (2007) 8:1217–26. doi: 10.1038/ni1522
57. Balan S, Saxena M, Bhardwaj N. Dendritic cell subsets and locations. *Int Rev Cell Mol Biol.* (2019) 348:1–68. doi: 10.1016/bs.ircmb.2019.07.004
58. Vander Lugt B, Riddell J, Khan AA, Hackney JA, Lesch J, DeVoss

J, et al. Transcriptional determinants of tolerogenic and immunogenic states during dendritic cell maturation. *J Cell Biol.* (2017) 216:779–92. doi: 10.1083/jcb.201512012
59. Steinman RM, Hawiger D, Nussenzweig CM. Tolerogenic dendritic cells. *Annu Rev Immunol.* (2003) 21:685–711. doi: 10.1146/annurev.immunol.21.120601.141040
60. Ohnmacht C, Pullner A, King SB, Drexler I, Meier S, Brocker T, et al. Constitutive ablation of dendritic cells breaks self-tolerance of CD4 T cells and results in spontaneous fatal autoimmunity. *J Exp Med.* (2009) 206:549–59. doi: 10.1084/jem.20082394
61. Thomson AW, Humar A, Lakkis FG, Metes MD. Regulatory dendritic cells for promotion of liver transplant operational tolerance: rationale for a clinical trial and accompanying mechanistic studies. *Hum Immunol.* (2018) 79:314–21. doi: 10.1016/j.humimm.2017.10.017
62. Benham H, Nel HJ, Law SC, Mehdi AM, Street S, Ramnoruth N, et al. Citrullinated peptide dendritic cell immunotherapy in HLA risk genotype-positive rheumatoid arthritis patients. *Sci Transl Med.* (2015) 7:290ra87. doi: 10.1126/scitranslmed.aaa9301
63. Bell GM, Anderson AE, Diboll J, Reece R, Eltherington O, Harry RA, et al. Autologous tolerogenic dendritic cells for rheumatoid and inflammatory arthritis. *Ann Rheum Dis.* (2017) 76:227–34. doi: 10.1136/annrheumdis-2015-208456
64. Giannoukakis N, Phillips B, Finegold D, Harnaha J, Trucco M. Phase I (safety) study of autologous tolerogenic dendritic cells in type 1 diabetic patients. *Diabetes Care.* (2011) 34:2026–32. doi: 10.2337/dc11-0472
65. Jauregui-Amezaga A, Cabezon R, Ramirez-Morros A, Espana C, Rimola J, Bru C, et al. Intraperitoneal administration of autologous tolerogenic dendritic cells for refractory Crohn's disease: a phase I study. *J Crohns Colitis.* (2015) 9:1071–8. doi: 10.1093/ecco-jcc/jjv144
66. Ezzelarab MB, Zahorchak AF, Lu L, Morelli AE, Chalasani G, Demetris AJ, et al. Regulatory dendritic cell infusion prolongs kidney allograft survival in nonhuman primates. *Am J Transplant.* (2013) 13:1989–2005. doi: 10.1111/ajt.12310
67. Ezzelarab MB, Raich-Regue D, Lu L, Zahorchak AF, Perez-Gutierrez A, Humar A, et al. Renal allograft survival in nonhuman primates infused with donor antigen-pulsed autologous regulatory dendritic cells. *Am J Transplant.* (2017) 17:1476–89. doi: 10.1111/ajt.14182
68. Ezzelarab MB, Lu L, Guo H, Zahorchak AF, Shufesky WF, Cooper DK, et al. Eomesodermin(lo) CTLA4(hi) alloreactive CD8+ memory T cells are associated with prolonged renal transplant survival induced by regulatory dendritic cell infusion in CTLA4 immunoglobulin-treated nonhuman primates. *Transplantation.* (2016) 100:91–102. doi: 10.1097/TP.0000000000000871
69. Lavin Y, Mortha A, Rahman A, Merad M. Regulation of macrophage development and function in peripheral tissues. *Nat Rev Immunol.* (2015) 15:731–44. doi: 10.1038/nri3920
70. Martinez FO, Sica A, Mantovani A, Locati M. Macrophage activation and polarization. *Front Biosci.* (2008) 13:453–61. doi: 10.2741/2692
71. Mantovani A, Sica A, Sozzani S, Allavena P, Vecchi A, Locati M. The chemokine system in diverse forms of macrophage activation and polarization. *Trends Immunol.* (2004) 25:677–86. doi: 10.1016/j.it.2004.09.015
72. Murray PJ, Allen JE, Biswas SK, Fisher EA, Gilroy DW, Goerdt S, et al. Macrophage activation and polarization: nomenclature and experimental guidelines. *Immunity.* (2014) 41:14–20. doi: 10.1016/j.immuni.2014.06.008
73. Murray PJ, Wynn AT. Protective and pathogenic functions of macrophage subsets. *Nat Rev Immunol.* (2011) 11:723–37. doi: 10.1038/nri3073
74. Hutchinson JA, Riquelme P, Geissler EK, Fandrich F. Human regulatory macrophages. *Methods Mol Biol.* (2011) 677:181–92. doi: 10.1007/978-1-60761-869-0_13
75. Hutchinson JA, Riquelme P, Sawitzki B, Tomiuk S, Miqueu P, Zuhayra M, et al. Cutting edge: immunological consequences and trafficking of human regulatory macrophages administered to renal transplant recipients. *J Immunol.* (2011) 187:2072–8. doi: 10.4049/jimmunol.1100762
76. Dominici M, Le Blanc K, Mueller I, Slaper-Cortenbach I, Marini F, Krause D, et al. Minimal criteria for defining multipotent mesenchymal stromal cells. The international society for cellular therapy position statement. *Cytotherapy.* (2006) 8:315–7. doi: 10.1080/14653240600855905
77. Friedenstein AJ, Piatetzky S II, Petrakova KV. Osteogenesis in transplants of bone marrow cells. *J Embryol Exp Morphol.* (1966) 16:381–90.
78. Le Blanc K, Rasmusson I, Sundberg B, Gotherstrom C, Hassan M, Uzunel M, et al. Treatment of severe acute graft-versus-host disease with third party haploidentical mesenchymal stem cells. *Lancet.* (2004) 363:1439–41. doi: 10.1016/S0140-6736(04)16104-7
79. Orbay H, Tobita M, Mizuno H. Mesenchymal stem cells isolated from adipose and other tissues: basic biological properties and clinical applications. *Stem Cells Int.* (2012) 2012:461718. doi: 10.1155/2012/461718
80. La Noce M, Paino F, Spina A, Naddeo P, Montella R, Desiderio V, et al. Dental pulp stem cells: state of the art and suggestions for a true translation of research into therapy. *J Dent.* (2014) 42:761–8. doi: 10.1016/j.jdent.2014.02.018
81. In 't Anker PS, Scherjon SA, Kleijburg-van der Keur C, de Groot-Swings GM, Claas FH, Fibbe WE, et al. Isolation of mesenchymal stem cells of fetal or maternal origin from human placenta. *Stem Cells.* (2004) 22:1338–45. doi: 10.1634/stemcells.2004-0058
82. Sarugaser R, Lickorish D, Baksh D, Hosseini MM, Davies EJ. Human umbilical cord perivascular (HUCPV) cells: a source of mesenchymal progenitors. *Stem Cells.* (2005) 23:220–9. doi: 10.1634/stemcells.2004-0166
83. Flynn A, Barry F, O'Brien T. UC blood-derived mesenchymal stromal cells: an overview. *Cytotherapy.* (2007) 9:717–26. doi: 10.1080/14653240701584578
84. Le Blanc K, Mougiakakos D. Multipotent mesenchymal stromal cells and the innate immune system. *Nat Rev Immunol.* (2012) 12:383–96. doi: 10.1038/nri3209
85. Beyth S, Borovsky Z, Mevorach D, Liebergall M, Gazit Z, Aslan H, et al. Human mesenchymal stem cells alter antigen-presenting cell maturation and induce T-cell unresponsiveness. *Blood.* (2005) 105:2214–9. doi: 10.1182/blood-2004-07-2921
86. Barry FP, Murphy JM, English K, Mahon PB. Immunogenicity of adult mesenchymal stem cells: lessons from the fetal allograft. *Stem Cells Dev.* (2005) 14:252–65. doi: 10.1089/scd.2005.14.252
87. Lazarus HM, Koc ON, Devine SM, Curtin P, Maziarz RT, Holland HK, et al. Cotransplantation of HLA-identical sibling culture-expanded mesenchymal stem cells and hematopoietic stem cells in hematologic malignancy patients. *Biol Blood Marrow Transplant.* (2005) 11:389–98. doi: 10.1016/j.bbmt.2005.02.001
88. Di Nicola M, Carlo-Stella C, Magni M, Milanesi M, Longoni PD, Matteucci P, et al. Human bone marrow stromal cells suppress T-lymphocyte proliferation induced by cellular or nonspecific mitogenic stimuli. *Blood.* (2002) 99:3838–43. doi: 10.1182/blood.V99.10.3838
89. Le Blanc K, Tammik L, Sundberg B, Haynesworth SE, Ringden O. Mesenchymal stem cells inhibit and stimulate mixed lymphocyte cultures and mitogenic responses independently of the major histocompatibility complex. *Scand J Immunol.* (2003) 57:11–20. doi: 10.1046/j.1365-3083.2003.01176.x
90. Tan J, Wu W, Xu X, Liao L, Zheng F, Messinger S, et al. Induction therapy with autologous mesenchymal stem cells in living-related kidney transplants: a randomized controlled trial. *JAMA.* (2012) 307:1169–77. doi: 10.1001/jama.2012.316
91. Detry O, Vandermeulen M, Delbouille MH, Somja J, Bletard N, Briquet A, et al. Infusion of mesenchymal stromal cells after deceased liver transplantation: a phase I-II, open-label, clinical study. *J Hepatol.* (2017) 67:47–55. doi: 10.1016/j.jhep.2017.03.001
92. Casiraghi F, Perico N, Remuzzi G. Mesenchymal stromal cells for tolerance induction in organ transplantation. *Hum Immunol.* (2018) 79:304–13. doi: 10.1016/j.humimm.2017.12.008
93. Rosser EC, Mauri C. Regulatory B cells: origin, phenotype, and function. *Immunity.* (2015) 42:607–12. doi: 10.1016/j.immuni.2015.04.005
94. Mauri C, Bosma A. Immune regulatory function of B cells. *Annu Rev Immunol.* (2012) 30:221–41. doi: 10.1146/annurev-immunol-020711-074934
95. Deng S, Moore DJ, Huang X, Lian MM, Mohiuddin M, Velededeoglu E, et al. Cutting edge: transplant tolerance induced by anti-CD45RB requires B lymphocytes. *J Immunol.* (2007) 178:6028–32. doi: 10.4049/jimmunol.178.10.6028
96. Huang X, Moore DJ, Mohiuddin M, Lian MM, Kim JI, Sonawane S, et al. Inhibition of ICAM-1/LFA-1 interactions prevents B-cell-dependent anti-CD45RB-induced transplantation tolerance. *Transplantation.* (2008) 85:675–80. doi: 10.1097/TP.0b013e3181663422
97. Lee KM, Kim JI, Stott R, Soohoo J, O'Connor MR, Yeh H, et al. Anti-CD45RB/anti-TIM-1-induced tolerance requires regulatory B cells. *Am J Transplant.* (2012) 12:2072–8. doi: 10.1111/j.1600-6143.2012.04055.x

98. Schuetz C, Lee KM, Scott R, Kojima L, Washburn L, Liu L, et al. Regulatory B cell-dependent islet transplant tolerance is also natural killer cell dependent. *Am J Transplant.* (2017) 17:1656–62. doi: 10.1111/ajt.14265
99. Saas P, Daguindau E, Perruche S. Concise review: apoptotic cell-based therapies-rationale, preclinical results and future clinical developments. *Stem Cells.* (2016) 34:1464–73. doi: 10.1002/stem.2361
100. Peng Y, Ye Y, Jia J, He Y, Yang Z, Zhu X, et al. Galectin-1-induced tolerogenic dendritic cells combined with apoptotic lymphocytes prolong liver allograft survival. *Int Immunopharmacol.* (2018) 65:470–82. doi: 10.1016/j.intimp.2018.10.019
101. Feng JF, Chen F, Liu H, Liu J. Induction of immune tolerance by pre-infusion of apoptotic lymphocytes derived from peripheral blood of donor rats before liver transplantation. *Minerva Chir.* (2013) 68:183–9.
102. Sun E, Gao Y, Chen J, Roberts AI, Wang X, Chen Z, et al. Allograft tolerance induced by donor apoptotic lymphocytes requires phagocytosis in the recipient. *Cell Death Differ.* (2004) 11:1258–64. doi: 10.1038/sj.cdd.4401500
103. Wang Z, Larregina AT, Shufesky WJ, Perone MJ, Montecalvo A, Zahorchak AF, et al. Use of the inhibitory effect of apoptotic cells on dendritic cells for graft survival via T-cell deletion and regulatory T cells. *Am J Transplant.* (2006) 6:1297–311. doi: 10.1111/j.1600-6143.2006.01308.x
104. Mougel F, Bonnefoy F, Kury-Paulin S, Borot S, Perruche S, Kantelip B, et al. Intravenous infusion of donor apoptotic leukocytes before transplantation delays allogeneic islet graft rejection through regulatory T cells. *Diabetes Metab.* (2012) 38:531–7. doi: 10.1016/j.diabet.2012.08.008
105. Bittencourt MC, Perruche S, Contassot E, Fresnay S, Baron MH, Angonin R, et al. Intravenous injection of apoptotic leukocytes enhances bone marrow engraftment across major histocompatibility barriers. *Blood.* (2001) 98:224–30. doi: 10.1182/blood.V98.1.224
106. Cheng J, Zhou L, Qin YS, Wang Y, Xie HY, Feng XW, et al. Donor apoptotic lymphocyte transfusion-induced liver allograft tolerance by up-regulation of $CD4^{+}CD25^{+}$ regulatory T cells in peripheral blood. *Transplant Proc.* (2009) 41:3893–7. doi: 10.1016/j.transproceed.2009.05.033
107. Kawai T, Poncelet A, Sachs DH, Mauiyyedi S, Boskovic S, Wee SL, et al. Long-term outcome and alloantibody production in a non-myeloablative regimen for induction of renal allograft tolerance. *Transplantation.* (1999) 68:1767–75. doi: 10.1097/00007890-199912150-00022
108. Leventhal JR, Mathew JM, Salomon DR, Kurian SM, Friedewald JJ, Gallon L, et al. Nonchimeric HLA-identical renal transplant tolerance: regulatory immunophenotypic/genomic biomarkers. *Am J Transplant.* (2016) 16:221–34. doi: 10.1111/ajt.13416
109. Scandling JD, Busque S, Shizuru JA, Lowsky R, Hoppe R, Dejbakhsh-Jones S, et al. Chimerism, graft survival, and withdrawal of immunosuppressive drugs in HLA matched and mismatched patients after living donor kidney and hematopoietic cell transplantation. *Am J Transplant.* (2015) 15:695–704. doi: 10.1111/ajt.13091
110. Miyara M, Chader D, Sage E, Sugiyama D, Nishikawa H, Bouvry D, et al. Sialyl lewis x (CD15s) identifies highly differentiated and most suppressive FOXP3high regulatory T cells in humans. *Proc Natl Acad Sci USA.* (2015) 112:7225–30. doi: 10.1073/pnas.1508224112
111. Joller N, Lozano E, Burkett PR, Patel B, Xiao S, Zhu C, et al. Treg cells expressing the coinhibitory molecule TIGIT selectively inhibit proinflammatory Th1 and Th17 cell responses. *Immunity.* (2014) 40:569–81. doi: 10.1016/j.immuni.2014.02.012
112. Miyara M, Yoshioka Y, Kitoh A, Shima T, Wing K, Niwa A, et al. Functional delineation and differentiation dynamics of human CD4+ T cells expressing the FoxP3 transcription factor. *Immunity.* (2009) 30:899–911. doi: 10.1016/j.immuni.2009.03.019
113. Kurtulus S, Sakuishi K, Ngiow SF, Joller N, Tan DJ, Teng MW, et al. TIGIT predominantly regulates the immune response via regulatory T cells. *J Clin Invest.* (2015) 125:4053–62. doi: 10.1172/JCI81187
114. Shi H, Chi H. Metabolic control of treg cell stability, plasticity, tissue-specific heterogeneity. *Front Immunol.* (2019) 10:2716. doi: 10.3389/fimmu.2019.02716
115. Fehr T, Sykes M. Clinical experience with mixed chimerism to induce transplantation tolerance. *Transpl Int.* (2008) 21:1118–35. doi: 10.1111/j.1432-2277.2008.00783.x
116. Mazariegos GV. Immunosuppression withdrawal after liver transplantation: what are the next steps? *Transplantation.* (2011) 91:697–9. doi: 10.1097/TP.0b013e31820c85a3
117. Liu C, Xu L, Xia C, Long Y, Liu C, Lu S, et al. Increased proportion of functional subpopulations in circulating regulatory T cells in patients with chronic hepatitis B. *Hepatol Res.* (2019) 50:439–52. doi: 10.1111/hepr.13472
118. Pal S, Nandi M, Dey D, Chakraborty BC, Shil A, Ghosh S, et al. Myeloid-derived suppressor cells induce regulatory T cells in chronically HBV infected patients with high levels of hepatitis B surface antigen and persist after antiviral therapy. *Aliment Pharmacol Ther.* (2019) 49:1346–59. doi: 10.1111/apt.15226
119. Carpentier A, Conti F, Stenard F, Aoudjehane L, Miroux C, Podevin P, et al. Increased expression of regulatory Tr1 cells in recurrent hepatitis C after liver transplantation. *Am J Transplant.* (2009) 9:2102–12. doi: 10.1111/j.1600-6143.2009.02743.x
120. Utsumi M, Takaki A, Umeda Y, Koike K, Napier SC, Watanabe N, et al. Frequency of regulatory T-cell and hepatitis C viral antigen-specific immune response in recurrent hepatitis C after liver transplantation. *Transpl Immunol.* (2014) 31:33–41. doi: 10.1016/j.trim.2014.05.006
121. Lan YT, Fan XP, Fan YC, Zhao J, Wang K. Change in the Treg/Th17 cell imbalance in hepatocellular carcinoma patients and its clinical value. *Medicine (Baltimore).* (2017) 96:e7704. doi: 10.1097/MD.0000000000007704
122. Langhans B, Nischalke HD, Kramer B, Dold L, Lutz P, Mohr R, et al. Role of regulatory T cells and checkpoint inhibition in hepatocellular carcinoma. *Cancer Immunol Immunother.* (2019) 68:2055–66. doi: 10.1007/s00262-019-02427-4

7

The Human Immune Response to Cadaveric and Living Donor Liver Allografts

Angus Hann[1,2†], *Daniel-Clement Osei-Bordom*[2†], *Desley A. H. Neil*[2,3], *Vincenzo Ronca*[2], *Suz Warner*[2,4] *and M. Thamara P. R. Perera*[1,4*]

[1] The Liver Unit, Queen Elizabeth Hospital Birmingham, Birmingham, United Kingdom, [2] Institute of Immunology and Immunotherapy, University of Birmingham, Birmingham, United Kingdom, [3] Department of Cellular Pathology, University Hospitals Birmingham NHS Foundation Trust, Birmingham, United Kingdom, [4] The Liver Unit, Birmingham Children's Hospital, Birmingham, United Kingdom

***Correspondence:**
M. Thamara P. R. Perera
thamara.perera@uhb.nhs.uk

† These authors have contributed equally to this work

The liver is an important contributor to the human immune system and it plays a pivotal role in the creation of both immunoreactive and tolerogenic conditions. Liver transplantation provides the best chance of survival for both children and adults with liver failure or cancer. With current demand exceeding the number of transplantable livers from donors following brain death, improved knowledge, technical advances and the desire to prevent avoidable deaths has led to the transplantation of organs from living, ABO incompatible (ABOi), cardiac death donors and machine based organ preservation with acceptable results. The liver graft is the most well-tolerated, from an immunological perspective, of all solid organ transplants. Evidence suggests successful cessation of immunosuppression is possible in ~20–40% of liver transplant recipients without immune mediated graft injury, a state known as "operational tolerance." An immunosuppression free future following liver transplantation is an ambitious but perhaps not unachievable goal. The initial immune response following transplantation is a sterile inflammatory process mediated by the innate system and the mechanisms relate to the preservation-reperfusion process. The severity of this injury is influenced by graft factors and can have significant consequences. There are minimal experimental studies that delineate the differences in the adaptive immune response to the various forms of liver allograft. Apart from ABOi transplants, antibody mediated hyperacute rejection is rare following liver transplant. T-cell mediated rejection is common following liver transplantation and its incidence does not differ between living or deceased donor grafts. Transplantation in the first year of life results in a higher rate of operational tolerance, possibly due to a bias toward Th2 cytokines (IL4, IL10) during this period. This review further describes the current understanding of the immunological response toward liver allografts and highlight the areas of this topic yet to be fully understood.

Keywords: liver, transplant, immunity, tolerance, rejection, cadaveric, living donor

INTRODUCTION

At present, orthotopic liver transplantation (OLT) is the only effective treatment option for many conditions (1). Unfortunately the demand for organs exceeds the supply, each year in the United Kingdom ~15% of patients awaiting a liver transplant either die or are delisted due to disease progression (2). Improvements in surgical technique, graft preservation techniques, perioperative care and immunosuppression has resulted in better short term graft function and patient survival (1). The detrimental effects of long term immunosuppression in regards to malignancies, metabolic disturbances, cardiovascular disease, renal failure and opportunistic infections are well-recognized (3, 4). These contribute significantly to the longer term morbidity and mortality in transplant patients (5, 6). The withdrawal of immunosuppression would eliminate these complications and is therefore highly desirable (7). The term "operational tolerance" implies a state of stable graft function following cessation of immunosuppressive medications and without evidence of rejection or graft injury (6). Operational tolerance is known to occur spontaneously following OLT more frequently than any other solid organ transplant (8). Immunosuppression withdrawal trials suggest that the rate of spontaneous operational tolerance may be as high as 40% in adults and 60% in pediatric patients post OLT (4, 9). Research focused on detecting biomarkers that identify patients who have a higher probability of developing operational tolerance are ongoing, as this would allow an expedited withdrawal of immunosuppression (10). However, a major aim in the field of transplantation is the development of tolerance inducing therapies. Therapeutic administration of interleukin-2 (IL-2), Regulatory T cells (Tregs), and dendritic cells (DC) are all being investigated, some of which are in phase II clinical trials. Further advancement in this area requires a detailed understanding of the immunophysiology of the liver and the interaction with the systemic immune system.

The allograft implanted during OLT can be from either a living or deceased donor. Procurement of a deceased individuals organs can occur following brain death (DBD) or cardiac death (DCD) and the organ can be split between two recipients depending on the volume of parenchyma required. Deceased donors are scarce in many countries and implanting organs from different ABO blood groups may be the only option to save a recipient's life, this is known as ABO incompatible (ABOi) liver transplantation. Early reports of ABOi OLT utilizing conventional immunosuppressive regimes and deceased donors yielded significantly inferior results (11). However, the introduction of modern therapies such as rituximab, a chimeric monoclonal antibody against the protein CD20 on B lymphocytes, has enabled living donor ABOi OLT to be common practice in many countries with equivalent results to conventional living donation (11). Liver transplantation for pediatric patients is more challenging due to lack of size matched donors. Pediatric patients most commonly receive a segmental graft that could be from a split, reduced size or living donor liver transplant (12). It is likely that variations in both the graft types and indications for OLT influence the immune response elicited. Understanding these in detail will allow further refinement of immunosuppressive regimes and tolerance inducing therapies.

METHODS

Relevant existing publications for this narrative review were identified by searching the Pubmed, EMBASE and Medline databases. The search was limited to the English language, but no other filters were utilized. The following terms were utilized (in a variety of combinations); *liver, transplant, immune response, innate, acquired, cell, antibody, rejection, ischaemia reperfusion, cadaveric, living donor, ABO incompatible, pediatric, pediatric.* Any additional publications relevant to this review were then identified by manually searching article reference lists.

IMMUNE FUNCTION OF THE LIVER

The liver is one of the two organs in human body with a dual blood supply, deriving blood from both arterial and portal venous blood. Therefore, it is exposed to both systemic and enterically derived pathogens (13). Portal venous blood delivers essential gut derived nutrients to the liver, however it also contains a significant volume of foreign antigens (13). Once a pathogen breaches our first defensive barrier, the intestinal epithelium, it will travel to the liver and therefore this organ is essential in the defense against harmful pathogens (14). However, unrestrained immune activation against non-pathogenic foreign antigens would have a detrimental result. The liver has a unique "tolerogenic" property which prevents this occurring. A large population of immune cells reside in the liver including macrophages (Kupffer cells), lymphocytes and dendritic cells. In addition, both the hepatic stellate cells (HSCs) and hepatocytes have immune functionality. Under certain inflammatory conditions, hepatocytes can express MHC II molecules and along with HSCs have been shown to interact with lymphocytes (13). The immune surveillance and pathogen clearance within the liver occurs predominantly at the hepatic sinusoids (14).

Systemic infection has a significant effect on the liver. Sepsis is known to induce changes in gene and protein expression and this alteration in hepatocellular function is known as the acute phase response. This response is triggered by IL-6 and IL-1 from monocytes and stimulates hepatocytes to release numerous acute phase proteins (APPs) (14). A number of these proteins then proceed to augment the systemic immune system by opsonising, further cellular activation or via direct action of complement (14). APPs have a further role in the abrogation of the immune response to prevent tissue injury from an over response (15). It has been shown that APPs such as serum amyloid A and Cxcl1/KC result in the mobilization of myeloid derived suppressor cells (MDSCs) which suppress inflammation and T cell responses in particular (15). Bacteraemia is reported to be ten times more common in patients with cirrhosis and it is associated with a fourfold increase in mortality in comparison to those without cirrhosis (14, 16). An imbalance of both the defense mechanisms and counterregulatory responses are likely contributory to the susceptibility of these patients to life threatening sepsis.

The liver is also a target of multiple autoimmune diseases. Autoimmune liver disease (AILD) is comprised of autoimmune hepatitis (AIH), primary biliary cirrhosis (PBC), and primary sclerosing cholangitis (PSC). AIH results from a T cell mediated insult on autoantigens and causes a chronic hepatitis with an interface and lobular hepatitic component, however the portal/interface component usually predominate (17). A subset of T-cells, known as Tregs ($CD4^{pos}$, $CD25^{high}$, $CD127^{LOW}$, $FoxP3^{pos}$), are key components of the immunosuppressive arm of the immune system, suppressing effector cell activity and restoring immune homeostasis. Multiple immunosuppressive mechanisms have been attributed to Tregs such as the secretion of anti-inflammatory cytokines and inhibitor molecules (e.g., CTLA4), depletion of crucial growth factors, disruption of effector cell metabolism by promoting the accumulation of adenosine nucleosides, consuming scarce amino acids and also by direct cytotoxic killing of effector cells (18). The number and function of Tregs are reduced in AIH, giving rise to the theory of unchecked or un-inhibited effector cell activity perpetuating the inflammatory cascade. AILD and liver allograft rejection both rely on leukocyte recruitment to the liver, and subsequent migration from the vasculature into the tissue. In most tissues, migration across the vascular endothelium occurs at post capillary venules (19). However, a study utilizing intravital microscopy demonstrated that in 80% of leukocytes adhere to the endothelium in the hepatic sinusoids and this is where the majority of leukocyte extravasation occurs in the liver (19, 20). Shear stress in the sinusoids in low and therefore the "rolling" process described for leukocyte extravasation is not required (19). Recruitment and adhesion of leukocytes is enhanced by hepatic sinusoidal endothelium expressing peptide molecules vascular adhesion protein 1 (VAP-1), VCAM-1, ICAM-1, CD44 (19). The recruitment of lymphocytes (in particular Th2) to the liver is enhanced by VAP-1. An additional molecule known as the common lymphatic endothelial and vascular endothelial receptor 1 has been demonstrated to recruit Tregs to the liver and promote transendothelial migration (19, 21). These recruitment mechanisms used by the liver are preserved after transplantation (19). The grafts endothelial cells are the first donor cells to encounter recipient leukocytes and their activation is likely an early event that leads to immune cell migration into the graft (22).

A hepatic allograft has immunoprotective benefits. The frequency of renal allograft TCMR is significantly lower in combined liver-kidney recipients in comparison to kidney alone recipients (23). In addition, less frequent and severe episodes of renal allograft rejection have been demonstrated when kidney transplants occurred in patients with previous liver transplants (24) Similar immunoprotective benefits were less pronounced when renal transplants followed heart and lung transplantation (24). Suggested mechanisms of protection are immune exhaustion due to high antigen burden, chimerism, and T cell deletion within the liver (23, 24). Chimerism refers to the presence of donor cells within the recipient's circulation and occurs due to cell migration from the graft (23, 25). Hematopoietic and T cells from the liver allograft migrate into the recipients circulation and if donor cells comprise more than 1% of the tissue it is referred to as macrochimerism, if they comprise <1% it is known as microchimerism (23). The persistence of chimerism has been associated with less rejection and is postulated to have a role in tolerance induction (25). T-cell deletion is suggested to occur within the liver due to direct contact with parenchymal cells (23). It has been suggested by Abrol et al. that the tolerance inducing effect of the liver in combined liver-kidney transplantation is due to a cell type from within the donor liver migrating to the other transplanted organ and inducing immune regulatory effects (23).

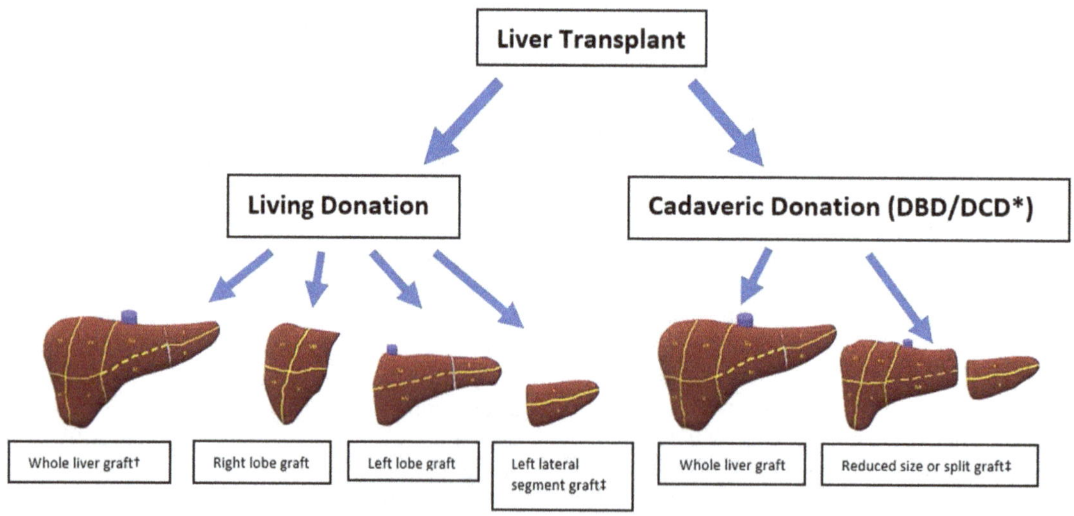

FIGURE 1 | Different types of liver allografts. * DCD grafts not split. † Living donation of whole liver only possible with domino transplantation. ‡ Either of these grafts is suitable for an auxiliary transplant.

THE DIFFERENT TYPES OF LIVER TRANSPLANT ALLOGRAFTS

The first liver transplant recipient to survive more than 24 h following the procedure was a 19-month-old infant who received a whole liver graft obtained from a 18-month-old brain dead donor (26). This pivotal procedure was performed by Thomas Starzl and his team in 1967 and subsequently numerous different types of liver grafts have been utilized by transplant clinicians. The main initial distinction between grafts is whether they were obtained from a deceased or living donor (**Figure 1**).

A liver obtained from a deceased individual is known as a deceased donor graft and depending on the terminal event, these donors can be considered to have experienced brain death (DBD) or circulatory death (DCD). The universal definition of brain death is "The irreversible loss of the capacity for consciousness, combined with irreversible loss of the capacity to breathe and therefore irreversible cessation of the integrative function of the brainstem" and strict neurological criteria need to be satisfied to make this diagnosis (27). DBD donors therefore have spontaneous cardiovascular activity providing organ perfusion and are receiving mechanical ventilation, both of which are maintained until cold perfusate is administered to the graft. DCD donors are individuals who do not meet the strict brain death criteria but are receiving life sustaining treatment that is deemed to provide no overall benefit. In this scenario the organ support is withdrawn, and death is determined by the standard cardiorespiratory criteria. Therefore, DCD donation involves a period of circulatory arrest with resultant ischaemia prior to cold perfusion of the graft. This is known as the donor warm ischaemic time (dWIT). The modified Maastricht criteria (**Table 1**) is used to sub classify the DCD donors based on the time of expected dWIT, and safety of organs used in transplantation (28). Deceased donor grafts can be implanted as whole or split grafts. Splitting of a cadaveric graft in most instances would provide an extended right lobe graft to an adult and a left lateral section to a pediatric recipient. Due to supply not meeting demand, the use of grafts from cadaveric donors with suboptimal features are known as extended criteria donors (ECD) (29). These include advanced donor age, graft steatosis and a DCD donor which are all features associated with poorer transplant outcomes (29).

Living donor liver transplantation (LDLT) occurs when a live individual undergoes a partial hepatectomy and donates this portion of their liver. The type of hepatectomy will depend on the volume of parenchyma the recipient requires. The donor can be either biologically related or biologically unrelated. All living donor grafts will be partial grafts, the only exception to this would be when "Domino" transplantation occurs. A "Domino" transplant occurs when recipient A undergoes a total hepatectomy and this explanted liver is transplanted into recipient B, recipient A can survive as they receive a separate cadaveric or living donor graft (30). This strategy is possible when recipient A suffers from one of several hereditary metabolic diseases as these livers are otherwise normal. Familial Amyloid Polyneuropathy is the most common reason for domino liver transplantation (30). An auxiliary liver transplantation is another type of graft in which either a remnant or the entire native liver is left within the recipient (31). Auxillary transplantation is most commonly used in the setting of acute liver failure as a "therapeutic bridge" until the native liver regenerates (31).

TABLE 1 | Modified Maastricht criteria for donation following cardiac death.

	Sub-category	Description
Category I—Found dead (Uncontrolled)	IA	Unexpected cardiac arrest out of hospital without attempted resuscitation
	IB	Unexpected cardiac arrest in hospital without attempted resuscitation
Category II—Witnessed cardiac arrest (Uncontrolled)	IIA	Unexpected cardiac arrest out of hospital with unsuccessful resuscitation
	IIB	Unexpected cardiac arrest in hospital with unsuccessful resuscitation
Category III—Withdrawal of life support (Controlled)		Expected, planned cardiac arrest after withdrawal of care
Category IV—Cardiac arrest whilst brain dead (Uncontrolled, controlled)		Sudden cardiac arrest following brain death but prior to planned organ recovery

Categories used to classify donation following cardiac death (22).

POST REPERFUSION SYNDROME AND PRESERVATION-REPERFUSION INJURY

An intense inflammatory response occurs immediately post OLT due to multiple factors including surgical stress, tissue trauma, preservation-reperfusion injury (PRI), blood loss and alloantigen recognition. Traditionally the liver grafts are preserved *ex-situ* in cold storage, thus without perfusion or oxygen delivery. These preservation conditions minimize oxidative phosphorylation and reduce metabolic activity to ~10% of the normal rate, the energy of which is mainly derived by anaerobic metabolism (32). In addition to ischaemia, hypothermic preservation conditions have a deleterious effects on the cell organelles, cytoskeletons and membranes (33). Re-establishment of blood flow results in the release of reactive oxygen species (ROS) from the mitochondria which in turn cause the release of proinflammatory cytokines from Kupffer cells (34, 35). This predominantly innate immune response is known as PRI and is also characterized by liver sinusoidal endothelial cell (LSEC) dysfunction (35). Intraoperative cardiovascular instability can occur immediately following re-establishment of blood flow due to a large efflux of metabolic substrates from the damaged liver, this entity is known as postreperfusion syndrome (PRS) (36). Release of cytokines (Tumor necrosis factor-α, IL-1, Interferon-γ, tumor necrosis factor-β) results in the accumulation of neutrophils (35). Previous literature has suggested that the immunogenicity of the graft is increased with PRI due to interactions between the innate and adaptive immune system (37). Enhanced T-cell priming is thought to result from this interaction and contribute to both acute and chronic rejection (37). Advanced donor age, graft steatosis and prolonged cold ischaemic time are associated with more severe PRI manifestations (38). PRI has physiological consequences and is considered the main cause of primary non function (PNF) and delayed graft function (DGF) (34, 39). In livers with severe PRI, ~40% will manifest PNF (40). **Figure 2** further demonstrates how the different events in the transplant process relate to the immune response.

The human immune system is commonly divided into innate and adaptive components with separate effector cells and activation pathways. However, evidence suggests third division of the immune system referred to as "innate-like" exists and is comprised of both B and T lymphocyte subsets (41). A characteristic of these cells is a rapid and robust response to antigens with limited memory capabilities (41). Natural Killer T cells (NKT) are one type of innate-like cell that is present in the liver sinusoids and has been implicated in the transplant PRI process (42). NKT cells are subclassified into type I and type II based on the expression of invariant TCR-α and minimal TCR-β (Type 1) in comparison to diverse TCR-α and TCR-β (type II) (42). In a murine experimental model of PRI, type I NKT cells were found to induce injury and with an increased intracellular expression and secretion of IFN-γ. Type II NKT were shown to be protective against PRI and the proposed mechanism was that they inhibit the pro-inflammatory effects of type I NKT cells (43).

LIVER ALLOGRAFT REJECTION

Acute T-cell mediated rejection (TCMR) is the most common immune mediated complication following liver transplantation (44). Less frequent immune complications are recurrence of an AILD, plasma cell rich rejection, antibody mediated rejection (AMR) and unresolved TCMR/AMR progressing to chronic rejection. Allorecognition of transplanted tissue is known to occur via three pathways; direct, indirect and semi-direct (45). The direct pathway involves the recipients T-cells recognizing the donor MHC molecules on donor antigen presenting cells (APCs). The indirect pathway occurs when the donor antigen is processed by recipient APCs and recipient MHC molecules expressed. The semi direct pathway involves cell exchange either via exosomes or the process of trogocytosis, which is the active transfer of plasma membrane fragments from an antigen presenting cell to a lymphocyte via cell conjugation (45, 46). The semi-direct pathway is yet to be completely understood but it is believed to involve the transfer of complete MHC-peptide complexes from donor APCs to recipient APCs. This results in a recipient APC displaying both a self and donor MHC molecule, both with an attached donor antigen. This brings both the direct and indirect pathway together onto a single APC and allows additional interaction between the two CD-4 or CD-8 T-cells that bind with each MHC:peptide complex, therefore forming a 3 cell model (45). All pathways lead to increased secretion of IL-2 and other inflammatory cytokines

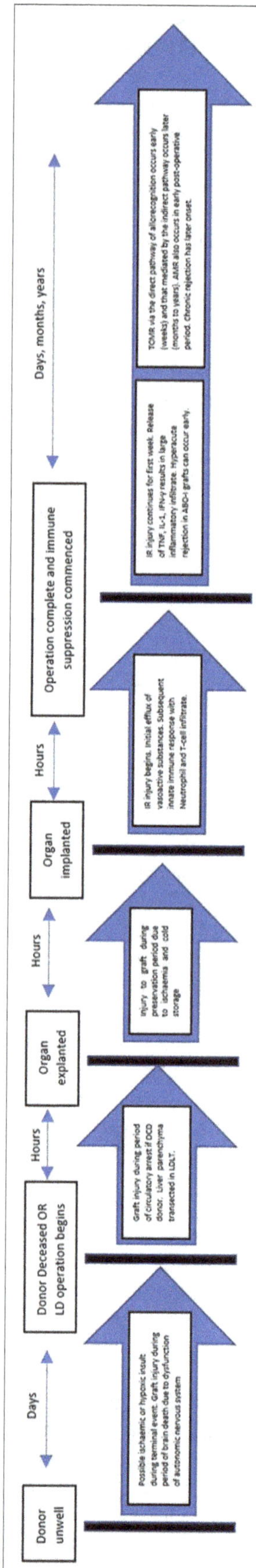

FIGURE 2 | Pathway of a graft from donor to recipient. The journey of a liver allograft from donor to recipient. LDLT, Living donor liver transplantationl; IR: Ischaemia reperfusion; TCMR, T-cell mediated rejection, AMR, Antibody mediated rejection.

which induce T-cell proliferation. The initial alloreactive T cell response is driven by the direct pathway with the indirect pathway assuming the main role as time progresses (8, 45).

The diagnosis of graft rejection is made via liver biopsy and graded in severity via the Banff criteria (47, 48). In addition to criteria for typical TCMR and chronic rejection, the 2016 update of the Banff working group recognized what had previously been termed *de novo* autoimmune hepatitis as a form of plasma cell rich rejection and added criteria for the diagnosis of acute and chronic AMR (48). Modern immunosuppressive agents have resulted in a reduction of early acute rejection from 60 to 33.5% (49, 50). This finding concurs with other authors that reported TCMR to occur most commonly in the early post-transplant period (47). Early TCMR is a result of the direct alloantigen presentation pathway and is characterized by pleomorphic portal inflammation, bile duct injury and the lack of necro-inflammatory interface activity (48). The indirect alloantigen presentation pathway is thought to result in the late TCMR and has predominantly mononuclear portal inflammatory change, less subendothelial inflammation than early TCMR but more interface and necro-inflammatory perivenular activity (48, 51). Early TCMR generally responds to treatment and graft loss as a result is reported to be <1% (52). Late TCMR is less responsive and a preceding episode of moderate-severe early TCMR has been identified as a risk factor, however Jadloweic et al. reported more than half of the patients who experience late TCMR had no history of early TCMR (49). The implications of late TCMR are more sinister with a higher rate of graft loss due to chronic rejection or cholestasis (49). Chronic rejection occurs relatively rarely with a reported rate of 3–5% following liver transplant (53). Chronic rejection is defined as 50% bile duct loss and/or a foam cell arteriopathy, it typically occurs early following non-responsive acute rejection, and is increasingly recognized to have an antibody mediated component (48, 53).

Acute AMR causes graft dysfunction due to donor specific antibody (DSA) interaction to antigens on the graft. DSAs may be pre-existing (preformed) or develop post-transplant in response to foreign antigen (*de novo* antibodies). DSAs may be against HLA antigens, which are the most readily detected by current assays, or non-HLA antigens such as anti-glutathione S transferase (GSTT-1) and anti-angiotensine 2 receptor (54, 55). The development of anti GSTT-1 antibodies has been demonstrated to occur in recipients who are negative for the GSTT-1 gene but receive a graft from a GSTT-1 positive donor (55). These anti-GSTT1 antibodies have been shown to be pathogenic and are implicated in periportal inflammation, fibrosis and the loss of bile ducts (55). The understanding of AMR is evolving, it is also believed to often occur concurrently with ACR. The liver exhibits strong ABO and MHC I antigen expression on all liver cells in normal circumstances, however the MHC I expression on hepatocytes is weaker (56). Liver allografts in comparison to kidneys are highly resistant to HLA alloantibodies and numerous mechanisms are proposed to explain this phenomenon (57). Secretion of soluble HLA class 1 molecules which form immune complexes with alloantibodies and then subsequently undergo clearance by Kupffer cells is one such mechanism (57). Davies et al. demonstrated that the liver graft also continues to deliver HLA class I antigens into the recipients serum for the lifetime of the graft, thus generating called DSAs (58). Resistance to AMR is also enhanced by the fenestrated endothelium of the sinusoidal network as occlusion by activated immune complexes does not result in the same degree of ischaemia as other transplanted organs (23). The main clinical manifestations are graft dysfunction, transaminitis, and thrombocytopenia (48). The histological changes that occur are oedema, endothelial cell swelling, leukocyte sludging or margination and vascular deposition of tissue complement component 4d (C4d) (48). The catastrophic Vasculitis and intravascular thrombosis associated with hyperacute rejection of renal allografts is exceedingly rare following liver transplant (44, 59). Approximately 13% of liver transplant recipients have persisting DSA positivity and the most commonly found is the anti-HLA class II DSAs (60, 61). Del bello et al. found in a cohort type study that 5 of out the 21 subjects with *de novo* DSA formation experienced acute AMR and the average liver fibrosis score was higher in this subjects with DSAs (60). This latter finding is similar to previous authors who have associated DSA positivity with progressive fibrosis, graft loss and poorer patient survival (48, 61). Anastomotic biliary strictures have also been associated with the presence of anti-HLA class II DSAs in patients who have undergone ABO compatible transplantation (62). Rationale for this observation is that biliary structures receive their entire blood supply from the peri-biliary capillary plexus and therefore is not protected from occlusion by immune complexes in the same manner as the hepatic sinusoids (23). Establishing the histopathological evidence for the entity of chronic AMR is frequently challenging due to confounding factors (48). The Banff working group has established criteria for probable and possible chronic AMR. The histology findings associated with chronic AMR are low levels of portal, periportal, perivenular lymphoplasmacytic inflammation and interface necro-inflammatory activity with non-inflammatory fibrosis (48).

THE IMMUNE RESPONSE TO CADAVERIC GRAFTS

During the initial decades of OLT, only cadaveric grafts from DBD donors were utilized. DCD programs emerged to expand the organ donor pool and consequently reduce waitlist mortality (63). At present, nearly a third of organ donations in the UK occur following DCD and the proportion of liver transplants utilizing DCD organs increased from 6.3% in 2005 to 26.3% in 2010 (64, 65). The inferior outcomes of DCD liver grafts was their higher rate of of PNF, non-anastomotic biliary complications, graft loss and poorer overall survival (65). However, the complication profile has changed over time with increased experience. Ischaemic injury occurs to the biliary epithelium during the dWIT making these grafts more susceptible to ischaemic cholangiopathy (65). It has been demonstrated that DCD grafts experience a more severe PRI with greater elevation of alanine transaminase (AST) and cell death (66). This may result in the devastating consequence of primary non-function (67). Despite DBD donation avoiding a period of circulatory arrest and subsequent warm ischaemia, significant detrimental changes are already thought to have occurred within the graft as a result of brain death. The physiological changes that take place during brain death have been described as an "autonomic storm" with initial intense parasympathetic response followed by short lived sympathetic activation (68). The decline in sympathetic activity is accompanied by myocardial depression and at all stages of this process the liver is subjected to an ischaemic type injury (68). In addition, there is widespread activation of inflammatory mediators irrespective of any hemodynamic instability (69).

An experimental animal study utilizing a rat model investigated the differing proinflammatory (TLR4, HMGB1, IL-1β, IL-6, TNF-α, MCP-1, E-selectin, and P selectin) cytoprotective (HO-1, VEGF, Hif-1α) and injury gene (P21, Bax, Bcl-2) expression associated with DCD and DBD grafts, utilizing a living donor liver as a reference (70). Directly after organ retrieval, DBD grafts demonstrated a down regulation of TLR4 but an upregulation of IL-6 (326-fold), IL-1β (15-fold), TNF-α (22- fold), P-selectin (41.7-fold), and E-selectin (12.9-fold) in comparison to LD grafts (70). The DCD livers only demonstrated an increase in HMGB1 directly after retrieval, in comparison to the living donor group. In addition, HO-1 expression increased to a larger extent in the DBD (12-fold) than the DCD (5.6-fold) livers in comparison to the living donor liver. As indicated by gene expression, the DBD and DCD grafts responded differently a period of cold ischaemia. After 12 h of cold ischaemia, the DBD livers inflammatory gene expression did not change significantly from immediately post retrieval. However, DCD Livers demonstrated a 4-fold increase in IL-6, 30-fold increase in MCP-1 and 4-fold increase in E-selectin in comparison to living donor grafts (70). The pro-apoptotic gene Bcl-2 increased significantly (4.6-fold) in the DCD livers in comparison to both DBD and liver donor livers. DBD livers showed a further 17-fold increase in HO-1 gene expression after a period of cold ischaemia in comparison to the living donor grafts. These findings demonstrate a pronounced inflammatory process is occurring in the liver at the time of retrieval in DBD livers, likely as a result of the physiological and inflammatory changes that occur during brain death. It was proposed that not enough time had elapsed following the short but significant period of warm ischaemia in the DCD livers to see a significant increase in inflammatory and apoptotic genes at the time of retrieval.

A recent cohort study that compared DCD and DBD grafts demonstrated equivalent outcomes in regards to primary non-function, acute cellular rejection, need for retransplantation and patient survival at 3 years (71). Pitarch Martinez et al. (71) demonstrated an acute cellular rejection rate of 20% in DCD and 16.4% in DBD grafts that was not statistically significant ($P = 0.685$) (71). However, in this cohort the DCD grafts needed to meet strict criteria (Maastricht III, WiT <30 min, Donor age ≤65) and their recipients had lower MELD scores. Doyle et al. performed a similar cohort type study and had similar findings with the rate of rejection being 24.5 and 26.5% in the DCD and DBD group, respectively ($P = 0.84$), the early rejection rate (≤30 days) was identical (72). A case matched study by Pine et al. comparing DBD to DCD grafts also demonstrated a similar rate of both acute and chronic rejection however primary non-function was higher in the DCD group (2/39 vs. 0/39) (73). PRI is thought to be increased in DCD grafts and this has been demonstrated by a greater elevation in early post-operative transaminases (74). Despite innate immunity being the main driver of PRI, it has been suggested that this is positively correlated with subsequent graft rejection (75). Mechanisms for this include trafficking of DCs into the graft and enhanced T cell priming (37). The results of the aforementioned clinical studies have not demonstrated this effect.

A study by Xystrakis et al. investigated the frequency and function of T-cell subsets in liver perfusate fluid obtained from DBD, DCD and living donors. The perfusate fluid was obtained from the graft at the end of the cold storage period and was analyzed by flow cytometry, cell sorting and culture (76). The frequency of memory and naïve T-cell subsets in the perfusate did not differ between all graft types but the frequency of $CD69^+$ CD8 T-cells was significantly higher in the perfusate from DBD grafts (76). In addition, the proportion of IL-2 and IFN-γ produced by CD8 T-cells was higher in DBD grafts. These authors concluded that the process of brain death is associated with the release of non-specific inflammatory mediators (76). Jaseem et al. compared immunohistochemical findings of preimplantation liver biopsies from living and deceased (DBD) donor grafts (77). Significantly higher levels of $CD3^+$ lymphocytes and Kuppfer cells were found in the DBD grafts. In addition, the adhesion molecule ICAM-1 was found to be expressed at higher levels in the DBD grafts (77). A higher percentage of $CD3^+$ lymphocytes in the preimplantation biopsy was associated with subsequent acute rejection in the DBD graft recipients (77). These authors concluded that the process of brain death resulted in a significant increase in inflammatory cell recruitment and migration into the liver allograft in comparison to living donor grafts. However, clinical outcomes of the recipients did not differ (77).

The literature describing humoral responses in ABO compatible DCD grafts is sparse. Levitsky et al. (78) compared the differences of both preformed and *de-novo* DSAs in living donor with deceased donor recipients, however the results for DCD and DBD subgroups were not published (78). This study did not demonstrate a difference in either preformed or *de-novo* DSA formation in either graft group. The presence of DSAs, either preformed or *de-novo*, did not affect patient survival in either graft group but did affect the graft survival (78). The deceased donor recipients with *de-novo* DSAs had higher rates of graft failure ($P = 0.005$) (56). Coexisting TCMR or recurrent viral hepatitis is thought to increase the DSA mediated damage as inflammation within the liver increases MHC I expression and induces MHC II expression. As previously mentioned, DSAs can be directed at either of these MHC molecules. Inlet and mononuclear septal venulitis have been suggested as the cause of the interface hepatitis that occurs with the presence of *de novo* DSA formation (56).

THE IMMUNE RESPONSE TO LIVING DONOR GRAFTS

The lack of suitable deceased donor livers for transplantation and the associated waitlist mortality has prompted the development of living donor liver transplantation (LDLT). The first successful LDLT was performed in Australia in 1989, a female adult donated her left lobe and it was implanted into her to 17-month-old son who suffered from biliary atresia (79). Following this pivotal event, LDLT has been performed around the world and at present one third of pediatric liver transplants involve a living donor (80). Particular political, cultural and religious beliefs in Asian countries have resulted in very low rates of deceased donors but the highest rates of LDLT (81, 82). Initially, LDLT procedures were limited to adult-pediatric with left lateral segment grafts (81). Significant progress has occurred and at present adult-adult LDLT with right lobe grafts are now being performed (81). LDLT is technically challenging as the graft must have an adequate volume of parenchyma, portal and arterial inflow, venous outflow and biliary drainage. The transplantation of a substantially smaller hepatic allograft in LDLT puts the recipient at the additional risk of small-for-size-syndrome (SFSS) (82). Other additional risks inherent with LDLT are the surgical risks posed to the donor (83). Inference based on the experience from living donor kidney transplantation would suggest that LDLT would have superior immunological outcomes, however this is yet to be conclusively demonstrated (84).

In the United states, adult-to-adult LDLT is increasing in frequency with a 82% graft survival at 1 year and a 10 years overall survival post-transplant that exceeded deceased donor transplantation (70 vs. 64%) (83). Avoidance of a graft exposed to the physiological perturbations of brain death and minimal cold ischaemic time are both thought to reduce the initial inflammatory response and subsequent immune activation. In addition, there may be HLA matching between genetically related donors and recipients (84). The evidence regarding the immunological benefits of adult-to adult LDLT is conflicting at present. Shaked et al. demonstrated in their retrospective review a similar rate of biopsy proven acute cellular rejection, more recurrent episodes and more frequent graft loss as a result in LDLT in comparison to deceased donor transplants (84). Subsequent to this, Levitsky et al. demonstrated that the incidence of acute cellular rejection was significantly lower in LDLT patients who received a graft from a biologically related donor in comparison to a non-biologically related and deceased donors (85). Another pertinent finding from this study relating to all liver transplant recipients was that an episode of biopsy proven cellular rejection significantly increased the patients risk of subsequent graft loss and death. The humoral immune response following LDLT has also been investigated by Levitsky et al. (78) and these authors found no difference in preformed or *de novo* donor specific antibody formation in LDLT in comparison to cadaveric graft recipients (DSA) (78). It was demonstrated however that *de novo* DSA positivity was associated with higher graft failure in both LDLT and cadaveric graft recipients and this relationship was proportional to the quantity of DSA present.

Experimental data indicates that inflammatory cell and cytokine concentrations are significantly lower in living donor grafts prior to retrieval, reperfusion and post reperfusion in comparison to brain death donors (68). Liver biopsies taken at various timepoints during the retrieval and transplant procedure by Weiss et al. (68) demonstrated that the mRNA concentration of CD3 and CD25 to be significantly lower in LDLT grafts in comparison to those from DBD donors. These authors concluded that although the presence of immune cells and cytokines increase as the LDLT procedure progresses, the level of immune activation is far less intense than that in transplants with DBD grafts (68). Interestingly, the LDLT recipients in this study had significantly lower transaminases in the post-operative period compared with DBD recipients which signifies a milder PRI. These authors also demonstrated a lower incidence of biopsy proven rejection in the 24 months post-transplant for LDLT in comparison to DBD graft recipients (38 vs. 28%, $P = 0.04$) (68). De Jonge et al. performed biopsies on both cadaveric and living donor grafts prior to retrieval (PRE), following cold perfusion (COLD) and post reperfusion in the recipient (POST) (86). Gene expression was analyzed and there was an upregulation of inflammatory genes between the PRE and POST biopsy in the cadaveric grafts, these included genes for IL-8 and ICAM-1. In the living donor grafts there was also an upregulation of genes for SOCS3, Hepatocyte growth factor (HGF) and NFκB1 from the PRE to the POST reperfusion sample and these are all associated with regeneration (86). The parenchymal transection during living donor procurement may be the initiating stimulus for this. There was also upregulation of MHC II genes in the living donor grafts and it was suggested that smaller grafts are associated with increased alloreactivity (86).

ABO INCOMPATIBLE GRAFTS

Transplanting organs across the ABO blood groups has for a long time been associated with poor outcomes due to increased graft loss and worse patient survival (87). The blood antigens are expressed on hepatic vasculature, biliary epithelium and hepatocytes and all are a target for AMR. Despite knowledge of these reactions and the inferior results, a compatible graft may not be available and an emergency situation may necessitate ABO incompatible transplant to prevent certain death (88). Since its initial inception, numerous immune modulating strategies and therapies have been implemented and a recent meta-analyses found no difference in patient survival following an ABO incompatible in comparison to an ABO compatible transplant (89, 90).

Acute AMR is a feared consequence of ABO-I liver transplantation and can often lead to loss of the graft. Numerous interventions have been attempted to mitigate the risk of AMR and these include; preoperative plasmapheresis, splenectomy, local infusions, mycophenolate mofetil, and rituximab (91) Several studies have failed to demonstrate a correlation between preoperative ABO antibody titer and AMR (92). It has been the implementation of rituximab, an anti CD20 monoclonal antibody that has yielded the greatest improvement in outcomes

(92–94). Commonly used AMR prophylaxis regimes include a single dose of Rituximab 2–3 weeks prior to transplantation (92, 94). Plasmapheresis aims to reduce the ABO antibody titer and is commonly performed both prior to transplantation and post operatively, however the antibody titer level targeted with this modality varies between institution (92). Undertaking a splenectomy on the recipient at the time of transplantation initially gained acceptance as this organ is the site of antibody production and harbors a large amount of B cells and plasma cells (92). However, studies have failed to demonstrate a benefit from this procedure, especially following the introduction of rituximab (92, 93).

Acute AMR in the ABO incompatible graft can result in graft failure via two types of injuries; liver necrosis in the first 1–2 post-operative weeks or diffuse intra-hepatic bile duct injury in the subsequent 2–3 months (92). These injuries are thought to occur because the hepatic vascular endothelium and biliary epithelium exhibit ABO antigens and therefore are sites for antibody-antigen binding with subsequent complement activation, cytokine production, cell migration and thrombus formation (93). The biliary damage manifests as diffuse biliary strictures and can result directly from the antibody-antigen reaction or secondary to ischaemia from intrahepatic arterial thrombosis (ischaemic cholangiopathy) (94). Song et al. compared outcomes in a cohort of patients that underwent either ABO compatible LDLT or ABO incompatible LDLT following the introduction of Rituximab in the desensitization protocol (94). The difference in patient survival, biopsy proven TCMR and post-operative LFTs were not significant. Biliary strictures were more common in the ABO incompatible group (20.7 vs. 14.2%, $p = 0.038$) with non-anastomotic biliary strictures occurring in 12 (8.5%) of the ABO incompatible recipients. Interestingly, all 12 underwent liver biopsy and only one case had histopathological evidence of AMR. No recipient of an ABO compatible graft developed a non-anastomotic biliary stricture (94).

IMMUNE RESPONSE IN THE PEDIATRIC PATIENT

The outcomes of pediatric liver transplantation have improved significantly over the last several decades and a 2012 study demonstrated a 1 and 10 years survival of 95 and 88%, respectively (95, 96). The indications for transplantation differs in the pediatric population with the most common indication in the US being biliary atresia (95, 97). In contrast to adults, transplantation for viral hepatitis and malignant tumors are a rare occurrence. Approximately 8% of liver transplants each year in the US are performed on children with an equal portion receiving either a whole or split graft (98). A large Canadian transplant center reported LDLT to comprise 46% of all pediatric LT. The same authors reported that the LDLT grafts comprised the left lateral section, left and right lobe in 82.8%, 3.7% and 13.4% respectively between 2000 and 2015 (99). Operational tolerance, post-transplant lymphoproliferative disorder (PTLD) and graft fibrosis occur more commonly in this patient population.

An individual's immune system needs to rapidly adapt as it makes the transition from intra-uterine life to the antigen rich outside world (100). Initially there is a heavy reliance on innate mechanisms, with maturation of the immune system gradually occurring as we progress through childhood. Acute cellular rejection is a common occurrence in this population with reported incidence of up to 60% (95). In a retrospective cohort study of 46 children who received a split graft from a living relative, 44 episodes of ACR occurred over 10 years of follow up with 35 of these in the first 6 weeks post op (101). It is believed that younger children (<1 year of age) are more likely to become immunologically tolerant of their graft, but the mechanism is yet defined (102, 103). Byun et al. compared outcomes of pediatric recipients that underwent OLT at <12 months of age with those older than 12 months and found the rate of ACR to be similar (30.2 and 33.0%, $P = 0.848$) in each group (104). This differs from a previous study utilizing the SPLIT database which demonstrated the rate of ACR in those <12 months was significantly less than in older pediatric recipients (0.20 vs. 0.44 episodes per patient-year, $P = 0.001$) (105). A large retrospective cohort study by Talisetti et al. assessed numerous factors and their relationship with operational tolerance (106). A recipient age of <12 months was the only variable significantly associated with a higher rate of developing operational tolerance (106). It has been demonstrated that in early infancy the Th2 cytokines (IL4, IL10) predominate over the Th1 cytokines (IL-2, IFN-γ) and this may contribute to graft acceptance in this age group (107). This is supported by the fact that pediatric patients that experienced TCMR had a higher proportion of Th1 cytokines (107).

Post-operative frequency of TREGs and IL-4 are higher in pediatric recipients who receive a LD graft in comparison to a deceased donor graft cadaveric (108). Favorable immunological outcomes would be expected as TREGs and IL-4 are both associated with immunotolerance, however the clinical evidence is less clear. In the retrospective cohort study published be Kehar et al. compared TCMR rates between pediatric LD and deceased donor recipients. The 1, 3 and 5 years TCMR rejection free survival was 64.4%, 61.1%, and 61.1% for LD and 55%, 44.4%, and 43.4% for cadaveric graft recipients respectively, however this difference was not statistically significant ($P = 0.08$) (99). Alonso et al. found that the incidence of rejection was the same in pediatric cadaveric graft compared to LD recipients (78 vs. 74%) but there was a higher rate of steroid resistant rejection in the cadaveric graft group (43 vs. 13%, $P \leq 0.01$). Kehar et al. found no difference in rejection rates between pediatric patients that received a graft from a genetically related compared with unrelated donor ($P = 0.4$) (99).

IMPLICATIONS FOR CLINICAL PRACTICE

There is variation in both the standard post-operative immunosuppression and rejection treatment regimens utilized by transplant centers around the world. The immunosuppressant drug most commonly used long term is the calcineurin inhibitor, tacrolimus, based on evidence of improved efficacy (109, 110).

There does not appear to be clinical evidence that altering standard immunosuppressive regimes based on the type of graft is beneficial, the only exception to this would be the implementation of pre-operative Rituximab infusions for ABO-I transplants. Pediatric patients that are transplanted at <12 months of age appear to have a more immunotolerant profile. This should be considered when planning transplantation for their native liver disease as it may optimize graft survival and minimize morbidity from immunosuppression. The inflammatory insult on the hepatic allograft that occurs during the period of brain death is undeniable. Administration of corticosteroids to the donor prior to organ retrieval has been investigated in a randomized controlled trial but provided no benefit (111). Further research is needed in this area as it may improve outcomes and result in the increased utilization of grafts. The desire to minimize graft injury during the preservation period has led to the development of machine perfusion strategies such as hypothermic (HMP) and normothermic machine perfusion (NMP). A recent randomized controlled trial of NMP demonstrated increased organ utilization and a reduction in preservation-reperfusion injury, as evidenced by a significant reduction in post-operative LFTs (112). Administration of anti-inflammatory and immune mediating therapies directly to the hepatic allograft via the machine perfusion circuit is a growing area of research interest (113).

Tolerance inducing therapies are showing promising results in clinical studies. In a landmark pilot study, Todo et al. showed that a single post-operative infusion of TREG cells allowed accelerated withdrawal of immunosuppression at 6 months post LDLT and 70% of these individuals achieved operational tolerance (114). The patients that experienced rejection in this pilot study were transplanted for AILD, suggesting that these individuals may require additional strategies (114). This study utilized recipient TREG cells that were co-cultured with irradiated donor leukocytes obtained several weeks before transplantation, an opportunity that does not exist in the deceased donor transplantation setting. The participants also underwent splenectomy at the time of transplantation. Sanchez-Fueyo et al. recently published results of a phase 1 clinical trial investigating the safety, applicability and biological activity of treg administration post cadveric liver transplantation (115). The treg cells in this study are autologous and not exposed to donor antigens during the culture process Subjects in this study received a doses of either 0.5–1 or 3–4.5 million tregs/kg. Nine subjects were enrolled and only a single subject who received the higher dose experienced a transfusion reaction (115). The frequency of tregs in the peripheral blood of subjects who received the higher dose remained elevated for 1 month and this likely reflected the infused tregs as the subpopulation that increased was similar to the infused cells (115). Although it did not reach statistical significance, donor specific hyporesponsiveness in the group that received the larger dose of tregs was observed (115). Tregs exert their suppressive effects on multiple different immune cells via both direct and indirect mechanisms (116). Direct mechanisms include IL-10, IL-35, TGF-β, secretion which results in apoptotic cell death of target effector cells. Depletion of extracellular ATP and IL-2 via the expression of CD39/CD73 and CD25, respectively, are examples of the indirect mechanisms (117). Other tolerance inducing therapies currently under investigation include Dendritic Cells, IL-2 and regulatory macrophages. Their rationale and current place in clinical transplantation are outlined elsewhere (118, 119).

CONCLUSION

The field of liver transplantation has advanced significantly since the 1960's. Progress has been made in organ preservation, post-operative care, immunosuppression and optimal utility of different grafts to ensure those in need get the best possible access to this lifesaving procedure. Grafts previously not possible such as ABOi LDLT are now commonplace in many centers with acceptable results. Based on existing literature, a similar immune response is elicited to the majority of grafts following implantation, comprising an initial innate inflammatory response due to preservation-reperfusion mechanisms followed by a predominantly cell mediated response. However, contribution from the innate-like and humoral components of the immune system to PRI and graft rejection are becoming increasingly recognized. Grafts from brain dead donors appear to have a higher inflammatory cell infiltrate and cytokine concentration at retrieval than DCD or living donor grafts, however clinical differences in rejection as a result are not evident. It is likely that both cell and antibody mediated injury results in the morbidity associated with chronic rejection. Acute TCMR is common following OLT but undergoing transplant in the first year of life seems protective. Hyperacute graft rejection of the liver is exceedingly rare. Strong clinical evidence that a DBD, DCD or LDLT graft is associated with a lower rate of TCMR is not apparent. Research into tolerance inducing therapies has shown promising results and the results of larger, phase II trial are eagerly awaited.

AUTHOR'S NOTE

AH was employed by the University Hospital Birmingham NHS Trust as a clinical research fellow.

AUTHOR CONTRIBUTIONS

AH and D-CO-B performed the literature search and constructed the manuscript. DN, VR, SW, and MP reviewed and contributed to the manuscript. All authors contributed to the article and approved the submitted version.

REFERENCES

1. Jadlowiec CC, Taner T. Liver transplantation: current status and challenges *World J Gastroenterol.* (2016) 22:4438–45. doi: 10.3748/wjg.v22.i18.4438
2. Neuberger J. Liver transplantation in the United Kingdom. *Liver Transpl.* (2016) 22:1129–35. doi: 10.1002/lt.24462
3. Euvrard S, Kanitakis J, Claudy A. Skin cancers after organ transplantation. *N Engl J Med.* (2003) 348:1681–91. doi: 10.1056/NEJMra022137

4. Benitez C, Londono MC, Miquel R, Manzia TM, Abraldes JG, Lozano JJ, et al. Prospective multicenter clinical trial of immunosuppressive drug withdrawal in stable adult liver transplant recipients. *Hepatology.* (2013) 58:1824–35. doi: 10.1002/hep.26426
5. Ojo AO, Held PJ, Port FK, Wolfe RA, Leichtman AB, Young EW, et al. Chronic renal failure after transplantation of a nonrenal organ. *N Engl J Med.* (2003) 349:931–40. doi: 10.1056/NEJMoa021744
6. Whitehouse GP, Hope A, Sanchez-Fueyo A. Regulatory T-cell therapy in liver transplantation. *Transpl Int.* (2017) 30:776–84. doi: 10.1111/tri.12998
7. Orlando G, Manzia T, Baiocchi L, Sanchez-Fueyo A, Angelico M, Tisone G. The Tor vergata weaning off immunosuppression protocol in stable HCV liver transplant patients: the updated follow up at 78 months. *Transpl Immunol.* (2008) 20:43–7. doi: 10.1016/j.trim.2008.08.007
8. Taner T. Liver transplantation: rejection and tolerance. *Liver Transpl.* (2017) 23(S1):S85–S8. doi: 10.1002/lt.24840
9. Feng S, Ekong UD, Lobritto SJ, Demetris AJ, Roberts JP, Rosenthal P, et al. Complete immunosuppression withdrawal and subsequent allograft function among pediatric recipients of parental living donor liver transplants. *JAMA.* (2012) 307:283–93. doi: 10.1001/jama.2011.2014
10. Baroja-Mazo A, Revilla-Nuin B, Parrilla P, Martinez-Alarcon L, Ramirez P, Pons JA. Tolerance in liver transplantation: biomarkers and clinical relevance. *World J Gastroenterol.* (2016) 22:7676–91. doi: 10.3748/wjg.v22.i34.7676
11. Dahlgren US, Bennet W. ABO-Incompatible liver transplantation - a review of the historical background and results. *Int Rev Immunol.* (2019) 38:118–28. doi: 10.1080/08830185.2019.1601720
12. Perera MT, Gozzini S, Mayer D, Sharif K, Bennett J, Muiesan P, et al. Safe use of segmental liver grafts from donors after cardiac death (DCD) in children with acute liver failure. *Transpl Int.* (2009) 22:757–60. doi: 10.1111/j.1432-2277.2009.00886.x
13. Jenne CN, Kubes P. Immune surveillance by the liver. *Nat Immunol.* (2013) 14:996–1006. doi: 10.1038/ni.2691
14. Strnad P, Tacke F, Koch A, Trautwein C. Liver - guardian, modifier and target of sepsis. *Nat Rev Gastroenterol Hepatol.* (2017) 14:55–66. doi: 10.1038/nrgastro.2016.168
15. Sander LE, Sackett SD, Dierssen U, Beraza N, Linke RP, Muller M, et al. Hepatic acute-phase proteins control innate immune responses during infection by promoting myeloid-derived suppressor cell function. *J Exp Med.* (2010) 207:1453–64. doi: 10.1084/jem.20091474
16. Bartoletti M, Giannella M, Caraceni P, Domenicali M, Ambretti S, Tedeschi S, et al. Epidemiology and outcomes of bloodstream infection in patients with cirrhosis. *J Hepatol.* (2014) 61:51–8. doi: 10.1016/j.jhep.2014.03.021
17. Liberal R, Krawitt EL, Vierling JM, Manns MP, Mieli-Vergani G, Vergani D. Cutting edge issues in autoimmune hepatitis. *J Autoimmunity.* (2016) 75:6–19. doi: 10.1016/j.jaut.2016.07.005
18. Lu L, Barbi J, Pan F. The regulation of immune tolerance by FOXP3. *Nat Rev Immunol.* (2017) 17:703–17. doi: 10.1038/nri.2017.75
19. Shetty S, Adams DH, Hubscher SG. Post-transplant liver biopsy and the immune response: lessons for the clinician. *Expert Rev Clin Immunol.* (2012) 8:645–61. doi: 10.1586/eci.12.65
20. Wong J, Johnston B, Lee SS, Bullard DC, Smith CW, Beaudet AL, et al. A minimal role for selectins in the recruitment of leukocytes into the inflamed liver microvasculature. *J Clin Invest.* (1997) 99:2782–90. doi: 10.1172/JCI119468
21. Shetty S, Weston CJ, Oo YH, Westerlund N, Stamataki Z, Youster J, et al. Common lymphatic endothelial and vascular endothelial receptor-1 mediates the transmigration of regulatory T cells across human hepatic sinusoidal endothelium. *J Immunol.* (2011) 186:4147–55. doi: 10.4049/jimmunol.1002961
22. Briscoe DM, Alexander SI, Lichtman AH. Interactions between T lymphocytes and endothelial cells in allograft rejection. *Curr Opin Immunol.* (1998) 10:525–31. doi: 10.1016/S0952-7915(98)80218-5
23. Abrol N, Jadlowiec CC, Taner T. Revisiting the liver's role in transplant alloimmunity. *World J Gastroenterol.* (2019) 25:3123–35. doi: 10.3748/wjg.v25.i25.3123
24. Schachtner T, Stein M, Reinke P. Kidney transplant recipients after nonrenal solid organ transplantation show low alloreactivity but an increased risk of infection. *Transpl Int.* (2016) 29:1296–306. doi: 10.1111/tri.12856
25. Bettens F, Tiercy JM, Campanile N, Giostra E, Majno P, Rubbia L, et al. Microchimerism after liver transplantation: absence of rejection without abrogation of anti-donor cytotoxic T-lymphocyte-mediated alloreactivity. *Liver Transpl.* (2005) 11:290–7. doi: 10.1002/lt.20360
26. Starzl TE, Groth CG, Brettschneider L, Penn I, Fulginiti VA, Moon JB, et al. Orthotopic homotransplantation of the human liver. *Ann Surgery.* (1968) 168:392–415. doi: 10.1097/00000658-196809000-00009
27. McGee A, Gardiner D. Differences in the definition of brain death and their legal impact on intensive care practice. *Anaesthesia.* (2019) 74:569–72. doi: 10.1111/anae.14568
28. Thuong M, Ruiz A, Evrard P, Kuiper M, Boffa C, Akhtar MZ, et al. New classification of donation after circulatory death donors definitions and terminology. *Transpl Int.* (2016) 29:749–59. doi: 10.1111/tri.12776
29. Vodkin I, Kuo A. Extended criteria donors in liver transplantation. *Clin Liver Dis.* (2017) 21:289–301. doi: 10.1016/j.cld.2016.12.004
30. Kitchens WH. Domino liver transplantation: indications, techniques, and outcomes. *Transpl Rev (Orlando, Fla).* (2011) 25:167–77. doi: 10.1016/j.trre.2011.04.002
31. Rela M, Kaliamoorthy I, Reddy MS. Current status of auxiliary partial orthotopic liver transplantation for acute liver failure. *Liver Transpl.* (2016) 22:1265–74. doi: 10.1002/lt.24509
32. Bellini MI, Yiu J, Nozdrin M, Papalois V. The effect of preservation temperature on liver, kidney, and pancreas tissue ATP in animal and preclinical human models. *J Clin Med.* (2019) 8:1421. doi: 10.3390/jcm8091421
33. Fondevila C, Busuttil RW, Kupiec-Weglinski JW. Hepatic ischemia/reperfusion injury–a fresh look. *Exp Mol Pathol.* (2003) 74:86–93. doi: 10.1016/S0014-4800(03)00008-X
34. Boteon YL, Afford SC. Machine perfusion of the liver: which is the best technique to mitigate ischaemia-reperfusion injury? *World J Transpl.* (2019) 9:14–20. doi: 10.5500/wjt.v9.i1.14
35. Peralta C, Jimenez-Castro MB, Gracia-Sancho J. Hepatic ischemia and reperfusion injury: effects on the liver sinusoidal milieu. *J Hepatol.* (2013) 59:1094–106. doi: 10.1016/j.jhep.2013.06.017
36. Jayant K, Reccia I, Shapiro AMJ. Normothermic ex-vivo liver perfusion: where do we stand and where to reach? *Expert Rev Gastroenterol Hepatol.* (2018) 12:1045–58. doi: 10.1080/17474124.2018.1505499
37. Martins PN, Chandraker A, Tullius SG. Modifying graft immunogenicity and immune response prior to transplantation: potential clinical applications of donor and graft treatment. *Transpl Int.* (2006) 19:351–9. doi: 10.1111/j.1432-2277.2006.00301.x
38. Dar WA, Sullivan E, Bynon JS, Eltzschig H, Ju C. Ischaemia reperfusion injury in liver transplantation: cellular and molecular mechanisms. *Liver Int.* (2019) 39:788–801. doi: 10.1111/liv.14091
39. Zhai Y, Petrowsky H, Hong JC, Busuttil RW, Kupiec-Weglinski JW. Ischaemia-reperfusion injury in liver transplantation–from bench to bedside. *Nat Rev Gastroenterol Hepatol.* (2013) 10:79–89. doi: 10.1038/nrgastro.2012.225
40. Martins PN, Chang S, Mahadevapa B, Martins AB, Sheiner P. Liver grafts from selected older donors do not have significantly more ischaemia reperfusion injury. *HPB (Oxword).* (2011) 13:212–20. doi: 10.1111/j.1477-2574.2010.00275.x
41. Van Kaer L, Postoak JL, Wang C, Yang G, Wu L. Innate, innate-like and adaptive lymphocytes in the pathogenesis of MS and EAE. *Cell Mol Immunol.* (2019) 16:531–9. doi: 10.1038/s41423-019-0221-5
42. Ware R, Kumar V. Complexity and function of natural killer T cells with potential application to hepatic transplant survival. *Liver Transpl.* (2017) 23:1589–92. doi: 10.1002/lt.24950
43. Arrenberg P, Maricic I, Kumar V. Sulfatide-mediated activation of type II natural killer T cells prevents hepatic ischemic reperfusion injury in mice. *Gastroenterology.* (2011) 140:646–55. doi: 10.1053/j.gastro.2010.10.003
44. Choudhary NS, Saigal S, Bansal RK, Saraf N, Gautam D, Soin AS. Acute and chronic rejection after liver transplantation: what a clinician needs to know. *J Clin Exp Hepatol.* (2017) 7:358–66. doi: 10.1016/j.jceh.2017.10.003
45. Gokmen MR, Lombardi G, Lechler RI. The importance of the indirect pathway of allorecognition in clinical transplantation. *Curr Opin Immunol.* (2008) 20:568–74. doi: 10.1016/j.coi.2008.06.009
46. Joly E, Hudrisier D. What is trogocytosis and what is its purpose? *Nat Immunol.* (2003) 4:815. doi: 10.1038/ni0903-815
47. Demetris AJ, Batts KP, Dhillon AP, Ferrell L, Fung J, Geller SA, et al. Banff schema for grading liver allograft rejection: an international consensus document. *Hepatology.* (1997) 25:658–63. doi: 10.1002/hep.510250328

48. Demetris AJ, Bellamy C, Hubscher SG, O'Leary J, Randhawa PS, Feng S, et al. (2016). Comprehensive update of the banff working group on liver allograft pathology: introduction of antibody-mediated rejection. *Am J Transpl.* (2016) 16:2816–35. doi: 10.1111/ajt.13909
49. Jadlowiec CC, Morgan PE, Nehra AK, Hathcock MA, Kremers WK, Heimbach JK, et al. Not all cellular rejections are the same: differences in early and late hepatic allograft rejection. *Liver Transpl.* (2019) 25:425–35. doi: 10.1002/lt.25411
50. Klintmalm GB, Nery JR, Husberg BS, Gonwa TA, Tillery GW. Rejection in liver transplantation. *Hepatology.* (1989) 10:978–85. doi: 10.1002/hep.1840100615
51. Demetris AJ, Adeyi O, Bellamy CO, Clouston A, Charlotte F, Czaja A, et al. Liver biopsy interpretation for causes of late liver allograft dysfunction. *Hepatology.* (2006) 44:489–501. doi: 10.1002/hep.21280
52. Demetris AJ, Ruppert K, Dvorchik I, Jain A, Minervini M, Nalesnik MA, et al. Real-time monitoring of acute liver-allograft rejection using the banff schema. *Transplantation.* (2002) 74:1290–6. doi: 10.1097/00007890-200211150-00016
53. Demetris A, Adams D, Bellamy C, Blakolmer K, Clouston A, Dhillon AP, et al. Update of the international banff schema for liver allograft rejection: working recommendations for the histopathologic staging and reporting of chronic rejection. An international panel. *Hepatology.* (2000) 31:792–9. doi: 10.1002/hep.510310337
54. Wozniak LJ, Venick RS. Donor-specific antibodies following liver and intestinal transplantation: clinical significance, pathogenesis and recommendations. *Int Rev Immunol.* (2019) 38:106–17. doi: 10.1080/08830185.2019.1630404
55. Aguilera I, Sousa JM, Nunez-Roldan A. Clinical relevance of GSTT1 mismatch in solid organ and hematopoietic stem cell transplantation. *Hum Immunol.* (2013) 74:1470–3. doi: 10.1016/j.humimm.2013.06.004
56. Demetris AJ, Bellamy CO, Gandhi CR, Prost S, Nakanuma Y, Stolz DB. Functional immune anatomy of the liver-as an allograft. *Am J Transpl.* (2016) 16:1653–80. doi: 10.1111/ajt.13749
57. O'Leary JG, Michelle Shiller S, Bellamy C, Nalesnik MA, Kaneku H, Jennings LW, et al. Acute liver allograft antibody-mediated rejection: an inter-institutional study of significant histopathological features. *Liver Transpl.* (2014) 20:1244–55. doi: 10.1002/lt.23948
58. Davies HS, Pollard SG, Calne RY. Soluble HLA antigens in the circulation of liver graft recipients. *Transplantation.* (1989) 47:524–7. doi: 10.1097/00007890-198903000-00025
59. Zhang R. Donor-specific antibodies in kidney transplant recipients. *Clin J Am Soc Nephrol CJASN.* (2018) 13:182–92. doi: 10.2215/CJN.00700117
60. Del Bello A, Congy-Jolivet N, Muscari F, Lavayssiere L, Esposito L, Cardeau-Desangles I, et al. Prevalence, incidence and risk factors for donor-specific anti-HLA antibodies in maintenance liver transplant patients. *Am J Transpl.* (2014) 14:867–75. doi: 10.1111/ajt.12651
61. Kaneku H, O'Leary JG, Banuelos N, Jennings LW, Susskind BM, Klintmalm GB, et al. *De novo* donor-specific HLA antibodies decrease patient and graft survival in liver transplant recipients. *Am J Transpl.* (2013) 13:1541–8. doi: 10.1111/ajt.12212
62. Iacob S, Cicinnati VR, Dechene A, Lindemann M, Heinemann FM, Rebmann V, et al. Genetic, immunological and clinical risk factors for biliary strictures following liver transplantation. *Liver Int.* (2012) 32:1253–61. doi: 10.1111/j.1478-3231.2012.02810.x
63. Schlegel A, Kalisvaart M, Scalera I, Laing RW, Mergental H, Mirza DF, et al. The UK DCD risk score: a new proposal to define futility in donation-after-circulatory-death liver transplantation. *J Hepatol.* (2018) 68:456–64. doi: 10.1016/j.jhep.2017.10.034
64. Neuberger J. An update on liver transplantation: a critical review. *J Autoimmunity.* (2016) 66:51–9. doi: 10.1016/j.jaut.2015.08.021
65. Callaghan CJ, Charman SC, Muiesan P, Powell JJ, Gimson AE, van der Meulen JH. Outcomes of transplantation of livers from donation after circulatory death donors in the UK: a cohort study. *BMJ Open.* (2013) 3:e003287. doi: 10.1136/bmjopen-2013-003287
66. Xu J, Sayed BA, Casas-Ferreira AM, Srinivasan P, Heaton N, Rela M, et al. The impact of ischemia/reperfusion injury on liver allografts from deceased after cardiac death versus deceased after brain death donors. *PLoS ONE.* (2016) 11:e0148815. doi: 10.1371/journal.pone.0148815
67. Taner T, Heimbach JK. Somethig wicked this way comes. *Hepatology.* (2020) 71:1119–21. doi: 10.1002/hep.31015
68. Weiss S, Kotsch K, Francuski M, Reutzel-Selke A, Mantouvalou L, Klemz R, et al. Brain death activates donor organs and is associated with a worse I/R injury after liver transplantation. *Am J Transpl.* (2007) 7:1584–93. doi: 10.1111/j.1600-6143.2007.01799.x
69. van Der Hoeven JA, Ter Horst GJ, Molema G, de Vos P, Girbes AR, Postema F, et al. Effects of brain death and hemodynamic status on function and immunologic activation of the potential donor liver in the rat. *Ann Surgery.* (2000) 232:804–13. doi: 10.1097/00000658-200012000-00009
70. Saat TC, Susa D, Kok NF, van den Engel S, Roest HP, van der Laan LJ, et al. Inflammatory genes in rat livers from cardiac- and brain death donors. *J Surg Res.* (2015) 198:217–27. doi: 10.1016/j.jss.2015.04.057
71. Pitarch Martinez M, Sanchez Perez B, Leon Diaz FJ, Fernandez Aguilar JL, Perez Daga JA, Montiel Casado MC, et al. Donation after cardiac death in liver transplantation: an additional source of organs with similar results to donation after brain death. *Transpl Proc.* (2019) 51:4–8. doi: 10.1016/j.transproceed.2018.02.208
72. Doyle MB, Collins K, Vachharajani N, Lowell JA, Shenoy S, Nalbantoglu I, et al. Outcomes using grafts from donors after cardiac death. *J Am College Surg.* (2015) 221:142–52. doi: 10.1016/j.jamcollsurg.2015.03.053
73. Pine JK, Aldouri A, Young AL, Davies MH, Attia M, Toogood GJ, et al. Liver transplantation following donation after cardiac death: an analysis using matched pairs. *Liver Transpl.* (2009) 15:1072–82. doi: 10.1002/lt.21853
74. Meurisse N, Vanden Bussche S, Jochmans I, Francois J, Desschans B, Laleman W, et al. Outcomes of liver transplantations using donations after circulatory death: a single-center experience. *Transpl Proc.* (2012) 44:2868–73. doi: 10.1016/j.transproceed.2012.09.077
75. Oliveira THC, Marques PE, Proost P, Teixeira MMM. Neutrophils: a cornerstone of liver ischemia and reperfusion injury. *Lab Invest J Tech Methods Pathol.* (2018) 98:51–62. doi: 10.1038/labinvest.2017.90
76. Xystrakis E, Yuksel M, Lin F, Huang X, Pop OT, Quaglia A, et al. Impact of donation mode on the proportion and function of t lymphocytes in the liver. *PLoS ONE.* (2015) 10:e0139791. doi: 10.1371/journal.pone.0139791
77. Jassem W, Koo DD, Cerundolo L, Rela M, Heaton ND, Fuggle SV. Leukocyte infiltration and inflammatory antigen expression in cadaveric and living-donor livers before transplant. *Transplantation.* (2003) 75:2001–7. doi: 10.1097/01.TP.0000061605.30685.03
78. Levitsky J, Kaneku H, Jie C, Walsh RC, Abecassis M, Tambur AR. Donor-Specific HLA antibodies in living versus deceased donor liver transplant recipients. *Am J Transpl.* (2016) 16:2437–44. doi: 10.1111/ajt.13757
79. Strong RW, Lynch SV, Ong TH, Matsunami H, Koido Y, Balderson GA. Successful liver transplantation from a living donor to her son. *N Engl J Med.* (1990) 322:1505–7. doi: 10.1056/NEJM199005243222106
80. Hackl C, Schmidt KM, Susal C, Dohler B, Zidek M, Schlitt HJ. Split liver transplantation: current developments. *World J Gastroenterol.* (2018) 24:5312–21. doi: 10.3748/wjg.v24.i47.5312
81. Chen CL, Kabiling CS, Concejero AM. Why does living donor liver transplantation flourish in Asia? *Nat Rev Gastroenterol Hepatol.* (2013) 10:746–51. doi: 10.1038/nrgastro.2013.194
82. Tulla KA, Jeon H. Living donor liver transplantation: technical innovations. *Gastroenterol Clin North Am.* (2018) 47:253–65. doi: 10.1016/j.gtc.2018.01.001
83. Abu-Gazala S, Olthoff KM. Status of adult living donor liver transplantation in the united states: results from the adult-to-adult living donor liver transplantation cohort study. *Gastroenterol Clin North Am.* (2018) 47:297–311. doi: 10.1016/j.gtc.2018.01.004
84. Shaked A, Ghobrial RM, Merion RM, Shearon TH, Emond JC, Fair JH, et al. Incidence and severity of acute cellular rejection in recipients undergoing adult living donor or deceased donor liver transplantation. *Am J Transpl.* (2009) 9:301–8. doi: 10.1111/j.1600-6143.2008.02487.x
85. Levitsky J, Goldberg D, Smith AR, Mansfield SA, Gillespie BW, Merion RM, et al. Acute rejection increases risk of graft failure and death in recent liver transplant recipients. *Clin Gastroenterol Hepatol.* (2017) 15:584–93.e2. doi: 10.1016/j.cgh.2016.07.035
86. de Jonge J, Kurian S, Shaked A, Reddy KR, Hancock W, Salomon DR, et al. Unique early gene expression patterns in human adult-to-adult living donor liver grafts compared to deceased donor grafts. *Am J Transpl.* (2009) 9:758–72. doi: 10.1111/j.1600-6143.2009.02557.x
87. Gordon RD, Iwatsuki S, Esquivel CO, Todo S, Makowka L, Tzakis A, et al. Experience with primary liver transplantation across ABO blood groups. *Transpl Proc.* (1987) 19:4575–9.

88. Goss MB, Rana A. ABO-incompatible liver transplantation: is it a viable option with modern innovation? *Clin Liver Dis.* (2017) 10:124–9. doi: 10.1002/cld.673
89. Yadav DK, Hua YF, Bai X, Lou J, Que R, Gao S, et al. ABO-incompatible adult living donor liver transplantation in the era of rituximab: a systematic review and meta-analysis. *Gastroenterol Res Pract.* (2019) 2019:8589402. doi: 10.1155/2019/8589402
90. Lee EC, Kim SH, Park SJ. Outcomes after liver transplantation in accordance with ABO compatibility: a systematic review and meta-analysis. *World J Gastroenterol.* (2017) 23:6516–33. doi: 10.3748/wjg.v23.i35.6516
91. Raut V, Uemoto S. Management of ABO-incompatible living-donor liver transplantation: past and present trends. *Surg Today.* (2011) 41:317–22. doi: 10.1007/s00595-010-4437-3
92. Oh J, Kim JM. Immunologic strategies and outcomes in ABO-incompatible living donor liver transplantation. *Clin Mol Hepatol.* (2019) 26:1–6. doi: 10.3350/cmh.2019.0023
93. Kim JM, Kwon CH, Joh JW, Kang ES, Park JB, Lee JH, et al. ABO-incompatible living donor liver transplantation is suitable in patients without ABO-matched donor. *J Hepatol.* (2013) 59:1215–22. doi: 10.1016/j.jhep.2013.07.035
94. Song GW, Lee SG, Hwang S, Kim KH, Ahn CS, Moon DB, et al. Biliary stricture is the only concern in ABO-incompatible adult living donor liver transplantation in the rituximab era. *J Hepatol.* (2014) 61:575–82. doi: 10.1016/j.jhep.2014.04.039
95. Cuenca AG, Kim HB, Vakili K. Pediatric liver transplantation. *Semin Pediatr Surg.* (2017) 26:217–23. doi: 10.1053/j.sempedsurg.2017.07.014
96. Ng VL, Alonso EM, Bucuvalas JC, Cohen G, Limbers CA, Varni JW, et al. Health status of children alive 10 years after pediatric liver transplantation performed in the US and Canada: report of the studies of pediatric liver transplantation experience. *J Pediatr.* (2012) 160:820–6.e3. doi: 10.1016/j.jpeds.2011.10.038
97. Branford WV. Acute epigastric pain and blood amylase activity. *Southern Med Surg.* (1948) 110:41–4.
98. Rawal N, Yazigi N. Pediatric liver transplantation. *Pediatr Clin North Am.* (2017) 64:677–84. doi: 10.1016/j.pcl.2017.02.003
99. Kehar M, Parekh RS, Stunguris J, De Angelis M, Van Roestel K, Ghanekar A, et al. Superior outcomes and reduced wait times in pediatric recipients of living donor liver transplantation. *Transpl Direct.* (2019) 5:e430. doi: 10.1097/TXD.0000000000000865
100. Levy O. Innate immunity of the newborn: basic mechanisms and clinical correlates. *Nat Rev Immunol.* (2007) 7:379–90. doi: 10.1038/nri2075
101. Dattani N, Baker A, Quaglia A, Melendez HV, Rela M, Heaton N. Clinical and histological outcomes following living-related liver transplantation in children. *Clin Res Hepatol Gastroenterol.* (2014) 38:164–71. doi: 10.1016/j.clinre.2013.10.009
102. Seyfert-Margolis V, Feng S. Tolerance: is it achievable in pediatric solid organ transplantation? *Pediatr Clin North Am.* (2010) 57:523–38. doi: 10.1016/j.pcl.2010.01.015
103. Sanchez-Fueyo A. Hot-topic debate on tolerance: immunosuppression withdrawal. *Liver Transpl.* (2011) 17(Suppl. 3):S69–73. doi: 10.1002/lt.22421
104. Byun J, Yi NJ, Lee JM, Suh SW, Yoo T, Choi Y, et al. Long term outcomes of pediatric liver transplantation according to age. *J Korean Med Sci.* (2014) 29:320–7. doi: 10.3346/jkms.2014.29.3.320
105. Shepherd RW, Turmelle Y, Nadler M, Lowell JA, Narkewicz MR, McDiarmid SV, et al. Risk factors for rejection and infection in pediatric liver transplantation. *Am J Transpl.* (2008) 8:396–403. doi: 10.1111/j.1600-6143.2007.02068.x
106. Talisetti A, Hurwitz M, Sarwal M, Berquist W, Castillo R, Bass D, et al. Analysis of clinical variables associated with tolerance in pediatric liver transplant recipients. *Pediat Transpl.* (2010) 14:976–9. doi: 10.1111/j.1399-3046.2010.01360.x
107. Ganschow R, Broering DC, Nolkemper D, Albani J, Kemper MJ, Rogiers X, et al. Th2 cytokine profile in infants predisposes to improved graft acceptance after liver transplantation. *Transplantation.* (2001) 72:929–34. doi: 10.1097/00007890-200109150-00031
108. Briem-Richter A, Leuschner A, Haag F, Grabhorn E, Ganschow R. Cytokine concentrations and regulatory T cells in living donor and deceased donor liver transplant recipients. *Pediatr Transpl.* (2013) 17:185–90. doi: 10.1111/petr.12044
109. Muduma G, Saunders R, Odeyemi I, Pollock RF. Systematic review and meta-analysis of tacrolimus versus ciclosporin as primary immunosuppression after liver transplant. *PLoS ONE.* (2016) 11:e0160421. doi: 10.1371/journal.pone.0160421
110. Haddad E, McAlister V, Renouf E, Malthaner R, Kjaer MS, Gluud LL. Cyclosporin versus tacrolimus for liver transplanted patients. *Cochrane Database Syst Rev.* (2006) 2006:CD005161. doi: 10.1002/14651858.CD005161.pub2
111. Amatschek S, Wilflingseder J, Pones M, Kainz A, Bodingbauer M, Mühlbacher F, et al. The effect of steroid pretreatment of deceased organ donors on liver allograft function: a blinded randomized placebo-controlled trial. *J Hepatol.* (2012) 56:1305–9. doi: 10.1016/j.jhep.2012.01.020
112. Nasralla D, Coussios CC, Mergental H, Akhtar MZ, Butler AJ, Ceresa CDL, et al. A randomized trial of normothermic preservation in liver transplantation. *Nature.* (2018) 557:50–6. doi: 10.1038/s41586-018-0047-9
113. Dengu F, Abbas SH, Ebeling G, Nasralla D. Normothermic machine perfusion (NMP) of the liver as a platform for therapeutic interventions during ex-vivo liver preservation: a review. *J Clin Med.* (2020) 9:1046. doi: 10.3390/jcm9041046
114. Todo S, Yamashita K, Goto R, Zaitsu M, Nagatsu A, Oura T, et al. A pilot study of operational tolerance with a regulatory T-cell-based cell therapy in living donor liver transplantation. *Hepatology.* (2016) 64:632–43. doi: 10.1002/hep.28459
115. Sánchez-Fueyo A, Whitehouse G, Grageda N, Cramp ME, Lim TY, Romano M, et al. Applicability, safety, and biological activity of regulatory T cell therapy in liver transplantation. *Am J Transplant.* (2020) 20:1125–36. doi: 10.1111/ajt.15700
116. Romano M, Fanelli G, Albany CJ, Giganti G, Lombardi G. Past, present, and future of regulatory T cell therapy in transplantation and autoimmunity. *Front Immunol.* (2019) 10:43. doi: 10.3389/fimmu.2019.00043
117. Castoldi L, De Rai P, Zerbi A, Frulloni L, Uomo G, Gabbrielli A, et al. Long term outcome of acute pancreatitis in Italy: results of a multicentre study. *Digest Liver Dis.* (2013) 45:827–32. doi: 10.1016/j.dld.2013.03.012
118. Thomson AW, Humar A, Lakkis FG, Metes DM. Regulatory dendritic cells for promotion of liver transplant operational tolerance: rationale for a clinical trial and accompanying mechanistic studies. *Hum Immunol.* (2018) 79:314–21. doi: 10.1016/j.humimm.2017.10.017
119. Whitehouse G, Gray E, Mastoridis S, Merritt E, Kodela E, Yang JHM, et al. IL-2 therapy restores regulatory T-cell dysfunction induced by calcineurin inhibitors. *Proc Natl Acad Sci USA.* (2017) 114:7083–8. doi: 10.1073/pnas.1620835114

8

Organ Restoration with Normothermic Machine Perfusion and Immune Reaction

Alessandro Parente[1†], *Daniel-Clement Osei-Bordom*[1,2,3†], *Vincenzo Ronca*[1,2,4], *M. Thamara P. R. Perera*[1] and *Darius Mirza*[1,2*]

[1] Liver Unit, Queen Elizabeth Hospital, University Hospitals Birmingham NHS Foundation Trust, Birmingham, United Kingdom, [2] Centre for Liver and Gastrointestinal Research, Institute of Immunology and Immunotherapy, University of Birmingham, Birmingham, United Kingdom, [3] National Institute for Health Research Birmingham Liver Biomedical Research Centre, University Hospitals Birmingham National Health Service Foundation Trust, Birmingham, United Kingdom, [4] Division of Gastroenterology and Centre for Autoimmune Liver Diseases, Department of Medicine and Surgery, University of Milan Bicocca, Milan, Italy

***Correspondence:**
Darius Mirza
darius.mirza@uhb.nhs.uk

† Joint first authors

Liver transplantation is the only recognized effective treatment for end-stage liver disease. However, organ shortages have become the main challenge for patients and physicians within the transplant community. Waiting list mortality remains an issue with around 10% of patients dying whilst waiting for an available organ. The post-transplantation period is also associated with an adverse complication rate for these specific cohorts of high-risk patients, particularly regarding patient and graft survival. Ischaemia reperfusion injury (IRI) has been highlighted as the mechanism of injury that increases parenchymal damage, which eventually lead to significant graft dysfunction and other poor outcome indicators. The consequences of IRI in clinical practice such as reperfusion syndrome, primary non-function of graft, allograft dysfunction, ischaemic biliary damage and early biliary complications can be life-threatening. IRI dictates the development of a significant inflammatory response that drives the pathway to eventual cell death. The main mechanisms of IRI are mitochondrial damage due to low oxygen tension within the hepatic micro-environment and severe adenosine triphosphate (ATP) depletion during the ischaemic period. After the restoration of normal blood flow, this damage is further enhanced by reoxygenation as the mitochondria respond to reperfusion by releasing reactive oxygen species (ROS), which in turn activate Kupffer cells within the hepatic micro-environment, leading to a pro-inflammatory response and eventual parenchymal cell apoptosis and associated tissue degradation. Machine perfusion (MP) is one emergent strategy considered to be one of the most important advances in organ preservation, restoration and transplantation. Indeed, MP has the potential to rescue frequently discarded organs and has been shown to limit the extent of IRI, leading to suppression of the deleterious pro-inflammatory response. This immunomodulation reduces the prevalence of allograft rejection, the use of immunosuppression therapy and minimizes post-transplant complications. This review aims to update the current knowledge of MP with a focus on normothermic machine liver perfusion (NMLP) and its potential role in immune response pathways.

Keywords: normothermic machine liver perfusion, immune activation, hepatic microenvironment, graft survival, liver transplantation

INTRODUCTION

Liver transplantation (LT) is the only effective and definitive therapy for end stage liver disease. However, the increasing disparity between the number of organ donors and the number of wait-listed patients has become a constant challenge for the transplant community worldwide, with an overall waiting list mortality between 15 and 20% in the UK (1).

Based on these concerns, sub-optimal grafts, which are those from "Extended Criteria Donors" (ECDs), have been used for LT to ameliorate the difference between organ demand and availability. There are limited guidelines on the use of these grafts from ECDs, hence the numerous clinical trials being carried out to review the viability and functionality they may possess. ECDs are considered to be: (1) older aged (≥60 years old) brain death donors (DBD), (2) donors (aged 50–59 years old) with underlying medical co-morbidities(two of either stroke, hypertension, or serum creatinine >1.5 mg/dL), (3) donors with high-grade steatosis, and (4) cardiac death donors (DCD) or donors whose liver is subjected to prolonged cold ischaemia time (CIT). Historically, transplanted grafts from ECDs had poorer graft outcomes including primary non-function (PNF), early allograft dysfunction (EAD) and ischaemic cholangiopathy (2). MP protocols from clinical trials such as Dual Hypothermic Oxygenated Perfusion of DCD Liver Grafts (DHOPE) and Consortium on Organ Preservation in Europe (COPE) project have developed diverse methods to manipulate the immune response and restore marginal organs to a state where they are deemed transplantable. In this setting, the overall donor pool could be expanded, which could lighten the burden on the transplantation list and reduce waitlist mortality. This review will look at normothermic machine perfusion (NMP) and its effect on the immune reaction upon on the graft during the transplantation phase.

THE RATIONALE OF ORGAN PRESERVATION BY MACHINE PERFUSION

Static cold storage (SCS) has been the standard preservation method for liver grafts pre-transplantation. The basis of this preservation technique is inducing hypothermic conditions to reduce cellular activity, theoretically reducing the consumption of mitochondrial ATP substrate stores, increasing anaerobic metabolism and leading to an increase in lactate production within the parenchymal cells. Despite the fact that the liver microenvironment is ordinarily hypoxic, a further hypoxic insult is detrimental to hepatocytes. At low temperatures cells sustain a basal activity that, in a hypoxic environment, induces ATP depletion and lactic acid accumulation. Decreasing levels of ATP induce cellular lysis via the loss of the normal electrolyte cell membrane gradients, which triggers the activation of proteolytic enzymes (3). Mitochondrial damage develops due to lack of available metabolic substrates namely oxygen and ATP. This is the metabolic pathway and underlying cause of ischaemia reperfusion injury (IRI) (4). The period of oxygen deprivation, and then the restoration of normal oxygenated blood flow to the liver propagates the IRI cascade. After reperfusion the mitochondria react by releasing all the toxins generated and accumulated during the ischaemic period, which encompasses the time from donor graft vessel clamp time to cold ischaemia time. These toxins include the reactive oxygen species (ROS) which activate pro-inflammatory cascades and, eventually, cell apoptotic pathways (5–7).

Within the liver allograft, the oxygen deprivation that provokes the release of damage associated molecular patterns (DAMPs), such as HMGB-1, which promote the inflammatory response by activating Antigen Presenting Cells (APCs), like dendritic and resident immune cell subsets, Kupffer cells. However, ECD livers have a lower tolerance of hypoxia, leading to a more severe IRI and more serious clinical consequences, such as reperfusion syndrome, allograft dysfunction, ischaemic biliary damage and early biliary complications. There is currently an array of new preservation methods with varied perfusate fluid types and machine perfusion methods in normothermic machine perfusion. Nonetheless, hypothermic machine perfusion (HMP) and subnormothermic machine perfusion (SNMP) play a dynamic role in mediating the immune response in a number of visceral organ transplantations including the kidneys, liver, pancreas, intestine, heart and lung (8).

Machine perfusion (MP) has been key in preserving Donors after Circulatory Death (DCD) allografts. MP has shown promise in utilizing DCD kidneys for transplantation, with the MP-preserved renal allografts performing better when compared with simple cold storage (9–11). Taylor et al. highlighted the significance of this result, with the aim to widen the renal donor pool without fear of transplanting a graft susceptible to numerous post-operative complications and adverse long-term outcomes. There are some complications that occur more frequently in the early post-transplant phase in the MP DCD kidney group, including significantly higher incidences of early delayed graft function and primary non-function cases when compared with matched MP DBD donor grafts. However, on evaluation of long-term outcomes, renal function in the MP DCD kidney group recovers within 5–6 months post-transplantation, and both DCD and DBD donor kidneys have equal serum creatinine levels at this timepoint (12). Studies including Weissenbacher et al. have demonstrated that prolonged perfusion whilst recirculating urine in with the perfusate in order to maintain the composition of the perfusate fluid has beneficial effects on the graft and ensures stability of the perfusate (13).

Abbreviations: CIT, Cold Ischemia Time; DAMPs, Damage Associated Molecular Patterns; DBD, Donation after Brain Death; DCD, Donation after Cardiac Death; DHOPE, Dual Hypothermic Oxygenated Perfusion; EAD, Early Allograft Dysfunction; ECD, Extended Criteria Donors; HMP- Hypothermic Machine Perfusion; HOPE- Hypothermic Oxygenated Perfusion; IFN, Interferon; IFOT, Ischaemia Free Organ Transplantation; IL, Interleukin; IRI, Ischaemic Reperfusion Injury; LT, Liver Transplantation; MAPCs, Multipotent Adult Progenitor Cells; MP, Machine Perfusion; NLR, Nucleotide-binding Oligomerization Domain (NOD)-like receptors; NMLP, Normothermic Machine Liver Perfusion; PAMPS, Pathogen-Associated Molecular Patterns; PNF, Primary Non-Function; PRR, Pathogen Recognition Receptor; RIG-I, Retinoic acid-Inducible Gene-I-like receptors; ROS, Reactive Oxygen Species; SNMP, Subnormothermic Machine Perfusion; TLR, Toll Like Receptors; TNF, Tumor Necrosis Factor; WIT, Warm Ischaemia Time.

NMP in liver (NMLP) and renal grafts reduce peak creatinine, improve graft survival, and allow organ recovery after periods of cold ischaemia. The energy requirements that the graft demands whilst being on NMP means that there is a requirement for an oxygen carrier, oxygen, and nutrient supplementation within the perfusion circuit to support physiological metabolic rates. By doing so research groups have reduced the effect of reperfusion tissue injury and subsequent graft dysfunction (14). Hypothermic Machine Perfusion (HMP) has clearly been shown to be advantageous in the preservation of both DBD and DCD allografts of the liver, kidneys, and pancreas. HMP in renal allografts lowers the incidence of poor clinical parameters in sub-optimal grafts post-renal transplantation (15, 16). HMP use has increased due to decreased Delayed Graft Function (DGF) occurrence for ECD, DCD, and DBD donor kidneys (17). With ECD, DCD, and DBD grafts, HMP allows an extensive review and assessment of the renal organ prior to transplantation, according to the "Predictive Score Model for Delayed Graft Function Based on Hypothermic Machine Perfusion Variables in Kidney Transplantation (18)."

There are similar studies of hypothermic machine perfusion of the pancreases, that demonstrated reduced graft oedema and reduced islet and acinar damage (19, 20). One study using 20 human pancreases in a hypothermic pulsatile perfusion of marginal human pancreas-duodenum organs for 24 h showed that this strategy was feasible with no deleterious parenchymal effect (21). Further observations highlighted that the ideal parameters for hypothermic continuous perfusion of pancreases has been difficult to ascertain. Branchereau et al. demonstrated that whilst using a hypothermic oxygenated continuous circuit at 25 mmHg for 24 h, none of the pancreas grafts used in the study showed signs of, or produced markers of, cellular injury, oedema, or necrosis. The tissue level of adenosine triphosphate (ATP) is a long-established marker of graft viability and functionality and is universal for all solid organ transplants (22). ATP is also a marker of the viability of machine-perfusion treated grafts (23). The Branchereau study highlighted that the tissue-biopsies of the pancreases in the HMP-group had a higher concentration of ATP levels when compared to the control group (21, 24). The maintenance of low pulsatile perfusion pressures in turn prevents endothelial damage and increased vasculature thrombosis (24, 25). We see that the low pressures and the pulsatile action may activate endothelial protective genes, including Kruppel-like factor 2, which is overexpressed by the endothelium during perfusion and has an antithrombotic action and promotes effective local microcirculation (26).

Huang et al. (27) used sub-normothermic machine liver perfusion (SNMLP) in whole and split liver NMLP. The study highlighted that ATP generation during perfusion is a potential viability marker that may be predictive of allograft function after transplantation. The ATP:ADP and ATP:AMP ratios increased similarly between split lobes and whole grafts within the first 2 h and decreased slightly by the 3rd hour among both the whole liver and split liver groups in this study. The increase of the energy ratios is an important marker for good graft function. No significant differences were seen when comparing left and right lobes for the energy ratios during the split machine perfusion model. This highlights the potential in the split technique, as we can hypothesize that both lobes will behave metabolically and physiologically in the same way (28). In essence, if each lobe has good function, we are therefore able to further increase the donor pool by utilizing what previously was one suboptimal liver allograft into two viable transplantable allografts (27, 29, 30).

With improving viability of grafts on MP, research groups often seek to use quantitative analysis of DAMPs (HMGB-1, cfDNA, etc.) and PAMPs (Pathogen-Associated Molecular Patterns) in tissue and perfusate as markers of graft restoration and the dampening of intraparenchymal immune reactions highlighted in various SNMP and HMP studies, such as the Huang and Porte groups, respectively. For extended perfusion and to improve graft function in most visceral allografts using HMP, the circuit requires oxygenation. Transforming the HMP into a hypothermic oxygenated perfusion further attenuates the immune reaction in liver donor grafts during extended MP restoration (31). Dual hypothermic oxygenated machine perfusion (DHOPE), a new clinical preservation technique developed by the Porte group, attempts to preserve donor liver grafts of poorer quality for longer periods of time (24 h). This facilitates transplantation by expanding the donor pool to include both marginal and sub-marginal human and porcine livers. The study highlighted that extended end-ischaemic DHOPE enabled successful preservation of porcine and discarded human liver grafts for up to 24 h (with required perfusion temperatures to be remain between 8 and 10°C) (31). Specific markers and cytokines were measured to compare and quantify hepatocellular injury and the production of deleterious pro-inflammatory cytokines. Alanine aminotransferase (ALT), HMGB 1, and cell-free DNA (cfDNA) (32) are markers used to detect and quantify nuclear subcellular injury and cell damage with necrosis. Tumor necrosis factor alpha (TNF-α) and Interleukin 6 (IL-6) were markers of initiation and development of a proinflammatory response (33), whilst malondialdehyde (MDA) was used to detect lipid peroxidation seen in oxidative stress. MDA was found in the perfusate and the liver parenchyma during tissue sampling in this study (34). DHOPE also quantified intracellular ATP as a marker of the energy status and viability of the grafts pre- and post-DHOPE (35).

ALT, HMGB-1, and cfDNA were not elevated by extended DHOPE preservation in the perfusate for the livers after re-warming. There were no histological necrotic changes in the DHOPE group. Levels of MDA were not increased in liver biopsies at the end of DHOPE ($p = 0125$) or at the end of reperfusion ($p = 0.604$) when compared to the control static cold storage group. Perfusate levels of HMGB-1, cfDNA, TNF-α, and IL-6 remained low in both livers during the entire period of DHOPE. The reduction in pro-inflammatory cytokines downregulates chemokine and chemoattractant production, which in turn dampens the immune reaction in the DHOPE livers. Von Willebrand factor (vWF), a marker of endothelial injury of the vasculature, was also not increased. vWF, DAMPs and PAMPs are present in endothelial injury and endothelial activation (26). Endothelial activation within inflamed allograft vessels allows the binding of vWF followed by platelets. This then promotes the opening of endothelial junctions and facilitates leucocyte transmigration to the site of liver injury and inflammation, leading to immunothrombosis and potential allograft demise. DAMPs generated are recognized by pathogen recognition receptors (PRRs), such as Toll-like receptors (TLRs) and cytoplasmic Nod-like receptors (NLRs), which drive an immune response.

The immune cells such as mast cells, macrophages, dendritic cells, innate lymphoid cells, and basophils recruited to site of inflammation and injury by chemokines express PRRs on their surface, sensing and binding with PAMPs and DAMPs. PRR activation leads to the production of proinflammatory cytokines including TNF-α, IL-1, vasoactive amines (e.g., histamine and serotonin), nitric oxide (NO), reactive oxygen species (ROS), neuropeptides, and arachidonic acid metabolites (e.g., prostaglandins and leukotrienes). This cascade of pro-inflammatory cytokine production induces damage and inflammation leading to the disruption of the integrity of macro- and micro- endothelial barriers.

NMP and HMP diminish the progression of endothelial damage and generation of DAMPs that drive a pro-inflammatory immune reaction. Tietjen et al. (36) have shown that with the use of *ex vivo* machine perfusion there are windows of opportunity to deliver therapeutics to the organ directly. The group targeted endothelial cells as their primary targets for reducing ischaemic-reperfusion injury (IRI) in renal allografts during NMP. Therapeutics have been developed to target endothelial cell injury and improve long-term outcomes. The group used nanoparticles (NP) to serve as a delivery mechanism of key medications, using surface conjugation of an anti-CD31 antibody (also known as anti-platelet endothelial cell adhesion molecule-1 (PECAM-1) antibody) to enhance targeting of NPs to graft endothelial cells of human kidneys undergoing NMP.

Similar studies have also used NMP to deliver therapeutics to reduce the immune response driven by IRI. Thompson et al. used multi-potent adult progenitor cells (MAPCs) to minimize IRI (37). MAPC-treated kidneys demonstrated improved physiological parameters when compared to the control group. Parameters including improved urine output $p = 0.009$), reduced expression of novel injury biomarker, Neutrophil gelatinase-associated lipocalin, (NGAL) ($p = 0.012$), and improved microvascular perfusion and down regulation of pro-inflammatory cytokines. Laing et al. utilized NMLP to deliver MAPCs, demonstrating that these MAPCs can be delivered to the liver prior to host immune cell involvement and with maintenance of continuous perfusion. The study showed trans-endothelial migration of MAPCs into vasculature and parenchymal endothelium. Whilst in the endothelium, MAPCs secreted soluble factors that would have anti-inflammatory and immunomodulatory benefits in a human model of liver transplantation (38).

NORMOTHERMIC MACHINE PERFUSION

Early NMLP studies (39, 40) describe how perfusing the graft at a physiological temperature has been revived and is at the forefront of "bench to bedside" practice in transplantation. In contrast to Simple cold storage (SCS) is a process by which the preservation solution is infused into the organ and then stored statically at hypothermic temperatures; the principles of NMLP is to maintain physiological conditions by supplementation of key metabolic substrates during perfusion of the organ. This is obtained with inflow of human blood or an oxygen-carrying blood substitute at 37°C, which simulates physiological conditions. In this environment, cell metabolism is maintained thanks to normal oxygen tensions within the perfusate, preventing ischaemic changes and providing the substrate for ATP production. In this setting, feasibility and safety were demonstrated and IRI and its consequences were shown to be reduced (41–43).

The main features and potential appeal of NMLP is to offer the possibility for assessing graft viability, for graft reconditioning and for improving high-risk potential liver allografts (44). This ability has been crucial, as many potentially transplantable livers might otherwise be discarded if deemed suboptimal without the means to recondition and improving the graft function prior to assessing the grafts' function in simulated physiological conditions.

There are four NMLP devices that are available: the OrganOx metra® (OrganOx Ltd., Oxford, UK), the Liver Assist (Organ Assist®, Groningen, the Netherlands), the Cleveland circuit (Cleveland Clinic, Cleveland, Ohio, US) and the OCS™ Liver System (Transmedics, Andover, Massachusetts, US). The mechanism of action is the same with four common main components: an oxygenator, a blood reservoir, a pump that can be single or double for hepatic artery and portal vein inflow and a heat exchanger.

Early human application of NMLP in the UK was documented by the Birmingham Machine Perfusion Group (45–47). The group compared outcomes of NMLP of DBDs and DCDs liver allografts to a matched control SCS group: the first 20 patients were transplanted with NMP primed grafts and described adequate outcomes (48). No grafts in either arm of the trial had primary non-function as a complication. Three patients' grafts (15%), had early allograft dysfunction (EAD) in the NMLP group compared to nine patients (23%) in the control SCS group. Median intensive care unit and hospital stays were comparable between the NMLP and SCS groups. Four DBD-NMLP patients in the trial developed anastomotic biliary strictures, which were treated with stenting. Patient survival at 1 year in the NMLP group was 95%, with 1 death at 9 months accounted for by an alcohol abuse relapse (46).

Bral et al. reported preliminary single-center North American experience using the OrganOx metra® device with nine liver grafts, which were matched with SCS grafts (49). There was no statistically significant difference in peak AST levels in the first 7 days in NMLP and SCS preserved grafts ($p = 0.52$), and there was no statistically difference in bilirubin levels during the first 7 days between the groups ($p = 0.35$). There was also no statistically significant difference in graft survival at 30 days in an intention-to-treat analysis ($p = 0.25$). Intensive care and hospital stays were higher in the NMLP group. This preliminary experience demonstrates feasibility as well as the potential technical risks of NMLP and highlights a need for larger, randomized studies with long-term follow up to assess functionality of NMP in the clinical setting (50).

Nasralla et al. published the result of a large multinational, open-label, two-arm, parallel randomized controlled trial on NMLP versus SCS (50). The trial randomized 334 livers, allocating 164 to SCS and 170 to NMLP using the NMLP OrganOx metra® device. Eventually, 101 SCS and 121 NMLP were successfully transplanted. They reported that peak AST levels during the first 7 days after LT were reduced by 49.4% in the NMLP group compared to SCS when adjusted by center and donor type (geometric mean ratio 0.506, 95% confidence interval 0.388–0.659; $P < 0.001$). There was one case of PNF in the NMLP group, whereas no cases of PNF were reported in the SCS group. EAD rates were available in 216 recipients: the odds of developing EAD in the NMLP arm (12 out of 119) were 74% lower than the SCS arm (29 out of 97; odds ratio 0.263, 95% confidence interval 0.126–0.550; $P < 0.001$). The median bilirubin level in the first week after surgery was lower in NMLP recipients (2.25 mg dl^{-1}, 95% confidence interval 1.23–4.28) than in the SCS group (2.87 mg dl^{-1}, 95% confidence interval 1.52–5.00; $P = 0.029$). There was no difference in median intensive care unit stay ($P = 0.339$) as well as hospital stay ($P = 0.926$) or the need for renal replacement therapy in the first postoperative week ($P = 0.621$) between the two groups. Graft survival at 1 year in the NMLP group was 0.950 (95% confidence interval 0.893–0.977), compared with the SCS 0.960 (95% confidence interval 0.897–0.985) ($P = 0.695$) (50).

The COPE (Consortium on Organ Preservation in Europe) project (51, 52) demonstrated significant reductions in peak AST and EAD rates in NMLP livers. However, it was stated that a larger trial with a longer follow-up period is mandatory to establish and assess whether there is a major difference in graft or patient survival.

Ghinolfi et al. reported the results of 20 livers from donors 70 years old or older randomized with SCS, thus 10 livers were perfused with NMLP Organ Assist® (53). The results showed no PNF in either group. There were two cases of EAD in NMLP and 1 case in SCS. No differences were observed in either a post-operative transaminitis or bilirubin peak in the first 7 post-operative days. In the NMLP arm of the trial, one graft was lost due to hepatic artery thrombosis, but no other vascular complications were observed in any other trial patients. In the SCS group, one patient died due to sepsis. Furthermore, the researchers performed biopsies and demonstrated that there was histological evidence of reduced IRI, demonstrated by a significant decrease in mitochondrial volume density and intracellular lipid droplets at the end of transplantation in the NMLP group vs. the SCS group ($P < 0.001$). All these reports are summarized in **Table 1**.

NORMOTHERMIC MACHINE PERFUSION FOR ORGAN PRESERVATION

As the demand for livers for transplantation grows worldwide, maximizing graft utilization is paramount. In this setting, NMLP allows groups to assess the liver viability and to chronologically evaluate the quality of at-risk grafts requiring restoration. Evidence shows that NMLP could play a role in reconditioning and restoring organs such as DCD or steatotic livers to optimize potentially transplantable liver allografts. The latter are considered to be grafts from ECDs, especially with the biopsy-proven macrosteatosis lipid concentration at 30–40%. In fact, macrosteatotic livers have been shown to have the poorest graft outcomes in terms of PNF and graft dysfunction, and consequently many of them are declined. The reason for this poor function seems to be excessive cytoplasmic fatty acids, which enhance lipoperoxidation, thus releasing more free radicals and reactive oxygen species (54). This induces disruption of cells, releasing PAMPs and DAMPs and therefore triggering the activation of TLRs (specifically TLR2 and TLR4), RIG-I-like receptors and NOD-like receptors, which all drive a pro-inflammatory response (55).

In experimental models, NMLP has been associated with reduction of triglyceride content as well as increased bile and urea production, and this process is enhanced with the

TABLE 1 | Outcomes of Normothermic machine perfusion (NMP).

References	Study Type	NMP device	Donor type	N° graft NMP vs. SCS	Graft Survival at 180/365 days NMP vs. SCS	Patient Survival at 180/365 days NMP vs. SCS	Median AST peak 7 days
Ravikumar et al. (46)	Observational	OrganOx metra®	DBD + DCD	20 vs. 39	180 days: 100% vs. 97.5%	180 days: 100% vs. 97.5%	417 vs. 902
Perera et al. (45)	Observational	OrganOx metra®	DCD	1 vs. 0	365 days: 100%	365 days: 100%	NA
Mergental et al. (47)	Observational	OrganOx metra®	DBD+DCD	5 vs. 0	180 days: 100%	NA	NA
Bral et al. (49)	Nonrandomized pilot study	OrganOx metra®	DBD+DCD	10 vs. 30	180 days: 80% vs. 100%	180 days: 89% vs. 100%	1,252 vs. 839
Nasralla et al. (50)	RCT	OrganOx metra®	DBD+DCD	121 vs. 101	365 days: 95% vs. 96%	365 days: 94.9 vs. 95.8%	167.5 vs. 318.5
Ghinolfi et al. (53)	RCT	Liver Assist®	DBD	10 vs. 10	180 days: 90% vs. 90%	180 days: 100% vs. 90%	709 vs. 574

RCT, randomized controlled trial; DBD, donor brain death; DCD, donor cardiac death; SCS, static cold storage; AST, aspartate aminotransferase.

implementation of liver defatting protocols (56). NMLP alone in human steatotic livers did not demonstrate encouraging results; a Liu et al. study reported that after 24 h of NMLP there was no reduction in tissue steatosis (57, 58). Pharmacological-induced defatting feasibility trials have shown some promise in widening the donor pool. Nagrath et al. reported that after 48 h of NMLP, administering a defatting cocktail produced a 35% reduction in the intracellular lipid content within the livers for this model (59, 60). Other studies of pharmacologically induced defatting agents during NMLP used 10 mmol of L-carnitine added to the perfusate in order to improve mitochondrial oxidation of fatty acids, obtaining a 10% reduction in macrosteatosis (61).

Boteon et al. allocated ten discarded steatotic livers into two NMLP groups: the treatment group had the perfusate supplemented with a defatting cocktail, whereas the control group was without supplementation. The defatting cocktail reduced tissue triglycerides by 38% and macro-vesicular steatosis by 40% over 6 h. Moreover, grafts in the defatting group displayed augmented and improved metabolic functional parameters such as urea production ($P = 0.03$), lower release of alanine aminotransferase ($P = 0.049$), and higher bile production ($P = 0.008$) with a higher bile pH ($P = 0.03$). Furthermore, the treatment reduced expression of key markers of IRI as well as activation of immune cells (CD14- found in neutrophils and macrophages; CD11b- found in NK cells and macrophages) and reduced the release of pro-inflammatory cytokines in the perfusate, particularly TNF-α and IL-1β (62).

NMLP has proven to maximize organ utilization and offer the opportunity for organ reconditioning and rehabilitation by circumventing the mechanisms of IRI and their deleterious consequences to the allograft. Further, the defatting of human grafts opens the possibility of treating declined steatotic livers and enhancing their utilization rate. Defatting trials have shown improvements in hepatic microcirculation, downregulation of Kupffer cells, and reduced release of inflammatory mediators during reperfusion, resulting in a reduction in subsequent reperfusion tissue injury. Although these findings are promising, rigorous research with clear long-term outcome data is required before it can be considered a widely accepted clinical option (63).

IMMUNE RESPONSE AND NMLP

NMLP significantly improves post LT outcomes with a reduction of the IRI in CIT. NMLP therefore enhances ATP restoration by decreasing the anaerobic metabolism of cells, leading to less accumulation of metabolites such as lactate, which affect the acid-base balance within the hepatic microenvironment and often enhance proteolytic enzymatic activity and liver tissue degradation (64). Jassem et al. detailed results regarding the immune response after NMLP (65). The study matched 12 DBD grafts perfused with NMLP and 27 DBD grafts preserved with SCS. At the end NMLP or SCS, they performed serial biopsies pre- and post-reperfusion for both histological and transcriptomic analysis of the perfusate and parenchyma from the livers in the study. Intrahepatic lymphocytes were extracted were recognized to be representative of liver-resident lymphocytes (66). The group found that in the SCS group there was a higher level of gene expression of immune-related genes, in particular pro-inflammatory cytokines, and also increased expression of genes involved in humoral immunity, platelet activity and neutrophil chemotaxis, when compared to the NMLP group. Moreover, several genes linked to the stress response and cell apoptosis, such as thrombomodulin (THBD) and IFN-γ, were up-regulated in the SCS cohort but not in the NMLP livers in the post-reperfusion phase of the study. The study assessed the effect of NMLP on the differentiation of T helper cells: Th1 (IL-2, IL-17, IFN-γ), Th2 (IL-4) as well as on Treg (IL-10 and TGF-β) cytokine production by intrahepatic CD4+. CD8+ T cells have also shown to secrete cytokines which effect T cells differentiation. NMLP grafts had significantly lower amounts of CD4+ T cells producing IL-4 ($p < 0.05$), IL-2 ($p < 0.001$), IFN-γ ($p < 0.05$), and IL-17 ($p < 0.0001$). There were no significant differences found in the production of the anti-inflammatory, regulatory cytokines IL-10 or Transforming Growth Factor-Beta (TGF-β). NMLP significantly decreased the proportions of CD8+ T cells subsets producing IFN-γ ($p < 0.001$), while slight reductions in IL-17 were also observed. There were no changes in IL-2 production by CD8+ T cells after NMLP. Studies have identified that within the perfusate and liver tissue samples in both NMP and SCS there is a significant increase in regulatory T helper cells and regulatory cytokines implementing immune tolerance in liver grafts (65, 67). We also see a statistically significant abundance of intrahepatic Tregs in NMP when compared to SCS (4.36% ± 3.27 vs. 1.9% ± 1.8, $p = 0.0156$), and in conjunction with the presence of IL-2 this promotes an expansion and proliferation of the Treg subset. In regards to the clinical parameters of long-term functionality and survival of graft measured in the study, the peak AST and peak INR in the first 7 post-operative days were significantly lower in the NMLP group compared with the SCS group ($p < 0.01$ and $p = 0.07$, respectively), thus suggesting that the NMLP group had grafts with a greater functionality and survival probability than the SCS group (65).

Intrahepatic lymphocyte populations have been identified as being integral in initiating the innate and adaptive immune responses. Certain lymphocytes subsets have a varied prevalence in the NMP and SCS. $CD3^{-}CD19^{+}$ B cells, $CD3^{+}CD4^{+}$ T cells and $CD3^{+}CD56^{+}$ Natural Killer (NK) T (NKT)-like cells were statistically similar in the liver tissue and perfusate of both populations in both NMP and SCS (68). Intrahepatic NK cells are contributors in acute and chronic allograft rejection and are a key cell subset in amplifying the inflammatory process. NK cells were more prevalent in tissue and perfusate from the SCS samples when compared to NMP samples. NMP livers showed a significant up-regulation of genes involved in immune-trafficking compared to SCS in both pre-reperfusion and post-reperfusion stages. In biopsies collected pre- and post-reperfusion, the Jassem et al. study demonstrated significantly lower quantities of apoptotic and necrotic cells in NMLP compared to SCS, as well as reduced quantities of neutrophil clusters within the parenchyma when NMLP livers were compared with SCS livers in both pre- and post-reperfusion stages. The group concluded that NMLP minimizes inflammation and cell death, and promotes liver restoration and regeneration (65).

THE FUTURE OF ORGAN PRESERVATION

Sub-normothermic machine liver perfusion (SNMLP) has become a prominent technique in preserving livers at lower temperatures on the perfusion circuit. A research group stored the human liver graft at −4°C with the supercooling method followed by sub-normothermic machine perfusion. This technique could extend up to 27 h of *ex vivo* preservation of the liver, without altering the viability of the organ. In super-cooling livers, the parenchyma can withstand the stress of simulated transplantation by *ex vivo* normothermic reperfusion with blood (69). The results have shown some promising clinical outcomes (70, 71).

Other studies like Eshmuminov et al. have attempted to increase the length of time for reconditioning on NMP and have demonstrated graft viability on animal models perfused for 7 days without the need for additional blood products or perfusate exchange (72). This novel approach was conducted using ten human livers declined for transplantation. After 7 days of perfusion, 6 out of 10 human livers showed preserved function as indicated by bile production, synthesis of coagulation factors, maintained cellular energy (ATP) and an intact liver structure (72).

The boundaries of NMLP have attempted to be pushed to meet the demands of transplantation as well as improving outcomes of these marginal livers used. The proof of concept study developed by Wu et al. raises the possibility of an ischaemia-free organ transplantation (IFOT). In essence, by removing the total element of IRI by preventing it whilst continually maintaining the blood supply for the organ at a physiological temperature throughout the procurement period until implantation, we may be able to eliminate the threat of graft dysfunction secondary to IRI. The group maintained NMLP during procurement and preservation until implantation and the recipient experienced no post-reperfusion syndrome. Initial investigations including liver function tests as well as histological analysis demonstrated a low injury to hepatocytes and vascular and biliary epithelium during preservation and post-transplantation. Moreover, they stated that the inflammatory cytokine levels were much lower in IFOT than those in conventional procedures (73).

Undoubtedly, there is an impending influx of innovative technologies will open new horizons for organ preservation and restoration and in return reduce mortality on transplant waiting lists. Despite clinical trials in the field being in their infancy, the results so far have been very encouraging with promising graft and patient outcomes. However, with few medical governing bodies embracing and introducing machine perfusion preservation for transplantable organs into their guidelines, further work in the form of multi-center randomized controlled trials with a focus on long-term outcome data is required in order to establish best clinical practice for liver preservation and restoration.

AUTHOR CONTRIBUTIONS

AP and D-CO-B conducted the literature research and co-wrote the paper. VR was aided in the writing of the immunological aspects of the paper as well as performed integral editing of parts of the review. MP and DM supervised and edited the overall review up to submission. All authors contributed to the article and approved the submitted version.

REFERENCES

1. Neuberger J. Liver transplantation in the United Kingdom. *Liver Transplant.* (2016) 22:1129–35. doi: 10.1002/lt.24462
2. Jiménez-Romero C, Caso Maestro O, Cambra Molero F, Justo Alonso I, Alegre Torrado C, Manrique Municio A, et al. Using old liver grafts for liver transplantation: Where are the limits? *World J. Gastroenterol.* (2014) 20:10691–702. doi: 10.3748/wjg.v20.i31.10691
3. Kalogeris T, Baines CP, Krenz M, Korthuis RJ. Cell biology of ischemia/reperfusion injury. *Int Rev Cell Mol Biol.* (2012) 298:229–317. doi: 10.1016/B978-0-12-394309-5.00006-7
4. Soares ROS, Losada DM, Jordani MC, Évora P, Castro-E-Silva O. Ischemia/reperfusion injury revisited: An overview of the latest pharmacological strategies. *Int J Mol Sci.* (2019) 20:5034. doi: 10.3390/ijms20205034
5. Jaeschke H, Molecular mechanisms of hepatic ischemia-reperfusion injury and preconditioning. *Am J Physiol Gastrointest Liver Physiol.* (2003) 284:G15–G26. doi: 10.1152/ajpgi.00342.2002
6. Clavien PA, Harvey PR, Strasberg SM. Preservation_and_reperfusion_injuries_in_liver.1.pdf. *Transplantation*(1992) 53:957–78. doi: 10.1097/00007890-199205000-00001
7. Zhai Y, Petrowsky H, Hong JC, Busuttil RW, Kupiec-Weglinski JW. Ischaemia-reperfusion injury in liver transplantation-from bench to bedside. *Nat Rev Gastroenterol Hepatol.* (2013) 10:79–89. *doi: 10.1038/nrgastro.2012.225*
8. Soo E, Marsh C, Steiner R, Stocks L, McKay DB. Optimizing organs for transplantation; advancements in perfusion and preservation methods. *Transplant. Rev.* (2020) 34:100514. doi: 10.1016/j.trre.2019.100514
9. Giwa S, Lewis JK, Alvarez L, Langer R, Roth AE, Church GM. The promise of organ and tissue preservation to transform medicine HHS Public Access Author manuscript. *Nat Biotechnol.* (2017) 35:30–542. doi: 10.1038/nbt.3889
10. Taylor MJ, Baicu C. Organs : the clinical perspective. *Cell.* (2011) 60:1–38. doi: 10.1016/j.cryobiol.2009.10.006
11. Baicu SC, Taylor MJ, Brockbank KGM. The role of preservation solution on acid-base regulation during machine perfusion of kidneys. *Clin Transplant.* (2006) 20:113–21. doi: 10.1111/j.1399-0012.2005.00451.x
12. Patel SVB, Sener A, Bhattacharjee RN, Luke PPW. Machine preservation of donor kidneys in transplantation. *Transl Androl Urol.* (2019) 8:118–25. doi: 10.21037/tau.2019.03.06
13. Weissenbacher A, Lo Faro L, Boubriak O, Soares MF, Roberts IS, Hunter JP, et al. Twenty-four-hour normothermic perfusion of discarded human kidneys with urine recirculation. *Am J Transplant.* (2019) 19:178–192. doi: 10.1111/ajt.14932
14. Kasimsetty SG, Hawkes A, Barekatain K, Soo E, Welch AK, McKay DB. TLR2 and NODs1 and 2 cooperate in inflammatory responses associated with renal ischemia reperfusion injury. *Transpl Immunol.* (2020) 58:101260. doi: 10.1016/j.trim.2019.101260
15. Summers DM, Watson CJE, Pettigrew GJ, Johnson RJ, Collett D, Neuberger JM, et al. Kidney donation after circulatory death (DCD): state of the art. *Kidney Int.* (2015) 88:241–9. doi: 10.1038/ki.2015.88
16. Rijkse E, IJzermans JN, Minnee RC. Machine perfusion in abdominal organ transplantation: Current use in the Netherlands. *World J. Transplant.* (2020) 10:15–28. doi: 10.5500/wjt.v10.i1.15
17. Umberto M. The marginal kidney donor. *Curr Opin Organ Transpl.* (2014) 19:372–80. doi: 10.1097/MOT.0000000000000081
18. Ding CG, Li Y, Tian XH, Hu XJ, Tian PX, Ding XM, et al. Predictive score model for delayed graft function based on hypothermic machine perfusion variables in kidney transplantation. *Chin Med J. (Engl).* (2018) 131:2651–7. doi: 10.4103/0366-6999.245278
19. Hamaoui K, Papalois V. Machine perfusion and the pancreas: will it increase the donor pool? *Curr Diab Rep.* (2019) 19:56. doi: 10.1007/s11892-019-1165-y

20. Leemkuil M, Lier G, Engelse MA, Ploeg RJ, De Koning EJP, T'Hart NA,et al. Hypothermic oxygenated machine perfusion of the human donor pancreas. *Transplant Direct.* (2018) 4:1-8. doi: 10.1097/TXD.0000000000000829
21. Branchereau J, Renaudin K, Kervella D, Bernadet S, Karam G, Blancho G. Hypothermic pulsatile perfusion of human pancreas: preliminary technical feasibility study based on histology. *Cryobiology.* (2018) 85:56–62. doi: 10.1016/j.cryobiol.2018.10.002
22. Bellini MI, Yiu J, Nozdrin M, Papalois V. The effect of preservation temperature on liver, kidney, and pancreas tissue ATP in animal and preclinical human models. *J Clin Med.* (2019) 8:1421. doi: 10.3390/jcm8091421
23. Resch T, Cardini B, Oberhuber R, Weissenbacher A, Dumfarth J, Krapf C, et al. Transplanting marginal organs in the era of modern machine perfusion and advanced organ monitoring. *Front. Immunol.* (2020) 11:631. doi: 10.3389/fimmu.2020.00631
24. Branchereau J, Hunter J, Friend P, and Ploeg R. Pancreas preservation: clinical practice and future developments. *Curr. Opin. Organ Transplant.* (2020) 25:329–35. doi: 10.1097/MOT.0000000000000784
25. Tortajada P, Pittau G, Ciacio O, Schwarz L, Fernandez de sevilla E, Durbach A, et al. Pancreas preservation by pulsatile hypothermic machine perfusion. *Hpb.* (2018) 20:S825. doi: 10.1016/j.hpb.2018.06.2479
26. Hamaoui K. *Machine Perfusion for Assessing and optimizing Kidney and Pancreas Allografts*, Doctoral thesis (PhD), London: Imperial College London. (2016).
27. Huang V, Karimian N, Detelich D, Raigani S, Geerts S, Beijert I, et al. Split-liver ex situ machine perfusion: a novel technique for studying organ preservation and therapeutic interventions. *J. Clin. Med.* (2020) 9:269. doi: 10.3390/jcm9010269
28. She WH, Chok KSH, Fung JYY, Chan ACY, Lo CM. Outcomes of right-lobe and left-lobe living-donor liver transplantations using small-for-size grafts. *World J Gastroenterol.* (2017) 23:4270–7. doi: 10.3748/wjg.v23.i23.4270
29. Spada M, Angelico R, Grimaldi C, Francalanci P, Saffioti MC, Rigamonti A, et al. The new horizon of split liver transplantation: ex situ liver splitting during hypothermic oxygenated machine perfusion. *Liver Transpl.* (2020) 2. doi: 10.1002/lt.25843
30. Takahashi H. Machine perfusion preservation for porcine split liver graft. *Transplantation.* (2018) 102:2018. doi: 10.1097/01.tp.0000543067.37529.d9
31. Brüggenwirth IMA, van Leeuwen OB, de Vries Y, Bodewes SB, Adelmeijer J, Wiersema-Buist J. Extended hypothermic oxygenated machine perfusion enables ex situ preservation of porcine livers for up to 24 hours. *JHEP Rep.* (2020) 2:100092. doi: 10.1016/j.jhepr.2020.100092
32. Krenzien F, Katou S, Papa A, Sinn B, Benzing C, Feldbrügge L, et al. Increased cell-free DNA plasma concentration following liver transplantation is linked to portal hepatitis and inferior survival. *J. Clin. Med.* (2020) 9:1543. doi: 10.3390/jcm9051543
33. Liu A, Fang H, Dirsch O, Jin H, Dahmen U. Oxidation of hmgb1 causes attenuation of its pro-inflammatory activity and occurs during liver ischemia and reperfusion. *PLoS ONE.* (2012) 7:e35379. doi: 10.1371/journal.pone.0035379
34. Van Rijn R, Van Den Berg AP, Erdmann JI, Heaton N, Van Hoek B, De Jonge J, et al. Study protocol for a multicenter randomized controlled trial to compare the efficacy of end-ischemic dual hypothermic oxygenated machine perfusion with static cold storage in preventing non-anastomotic biliary strictures after transplantation of liver gra. *BMC Gastroenterol.* (2019) 19:1–12. doi: 10.1186/s12876-019-0956-6
35. De Vries Y, Berendsen TA, Fujiyoshi M, Van Den Berg AP, Blokzijl H, De Boer MT, et al. Transplantation of high-risk donor livers after resuscitation and viability assessment using a combined protocol of oxygenated hypothermic, rewarming and normothermic machine perfusion: study protocol for a prospective, single-arm study (DHOPE-COR-NMP tri. *BMJ Open.* (2019) 9:1–8. doi: 10.1136/bmjopen-2018-028596
36. Tietjen GT, Hosgood SA, DiRito J, Cui J, Deep D, Song E, et al. Nanoparticle targeting to the endothelium during normothermic machine perfusion of human kidneys. *Sci Transl Med.* (2017) 9. doi: 10.1126/scitranslmed.aam6764
37. Thompson ER, Bates L, Ibrahim IK, Sewpaul A, Stenberg B, McNeill A, et al. Novel delivery of cellular therapy to reduce ischemia reperfusion injury in kidney transplantation. *Am J Transplant.* (2020) 1–13. doi: 10.1111/ajt.16100
38. Laing RW, Stubblefield S, Wallace L, Roobrouck VD, Bhogal RH, Schlegel A, et al. The delivery of multipotent adult progenitor cells to extended criteria human donor livers using normothermic machine perfusion. *Front. Immunol.* (2020) 11:1–18. doi: 10.3389/fimmu.2020.01226
39. Akateh C, Beal EW, Whitson BA, Black SM. Normothermic ex-vivo liver perfusion and the clinical implications for liver transplantation. *J Clin Transl Hepatol.* (2018) 6:1–7. doi: 10.14218/JCTH.2017.00048
40. Starzl TE, Groth CG, Brettschneider L, Moon JB, Fulginiti VA, Cotton EK, et al. Extended survival in 3 cases of orthotopic homotransplantation of the human liver. *Surgery.* (1968) 63:549–63. doi: 10.1097/00007890-196810000-00022
41. Schön MR, Kollmar O, Wolf S, Schrem H, Matthes M, Akkoc N, et al. Liver transplantation after organ preservation with normothermic extracorporeal perfusion. *Ann Surg.* (2001) 233:114–23. doi: 10.1097/00000658-200101000-00017
42. Brockmann J, Reddy S, Coussios C, Pigott D, Guirriero D, Hughes D. Normothermic perfusion: a new paradigm for organ preservation. *Ann Surg.* (2009) 250:1–6. doi: 10.1097/SLA.0b013e3181a63c10
43. Guibert EE, Petrenko AY, Balaban CL, Somov AY, Rodriguez JV, Fuller BJ. Organ preservation: current concepts and new strategies for the next decade. *Transfus Med Hemotherapy.* (2011) 38:125–42. doi: 10.1159/000327033
44. Mergental H, Stephenson BTF, Laing RW, Kirkham AJ, Neil DAH, Wallace LL, et al. Development of clinical criteria for functional assessment to predict primary nonfunction of high-risk livers using normothermic machine perfusion. *Liver Transplant.* (2018) 24:1453–69. doi: 10.1002/lt.25291
45. Perera T, Mergental H, Stephenson B, Roll GR, Cilliers H, Liang R, et al. First human liver transplantation using a marginal allograft resuscitated by normothermic machine perfusion. *Liver Transplant.* (2016) 22:120–4. doi: 10.1002/lt.24369
46. Ravikumar R, Jassem W, Mergental H, Heaton N, Mirza D, Perera MT, et al. Liver transplantation after ex vivo normothermic machine preservation: a phase 1 (first-in-man) clinical trial. *Am J Transplant.* (2016) 16:1779–87. doi: 10.1111/ajt.13708
47. Mergental H, Perera MTPR, Laing RW, Muiesan P, Isaac JR, Smith A, Mirza DF. Transplantation of declined liver allografts following normothermic ex-situ evaluation. *Am J Transplant.* (2016) 16:3235–45. doi: 10.1111/ajt.13875
48. Laing RW, Mergental H, Yap C, Kirkham A, Whilku M, Barton D, et al. Viability testing and transplantation of marginal livers (VITTAL) using normothermic machine perfusion: study protocol for an open-label, non-randomised, prospective, single-arm trial. *BMJ Open.* (2017) 7:e017733. doi: 10.1136/bmjopen-2017-017733.
49. Bral M, Gala-Lopez B, Bigam D, Kneteman N, Malcolm A, Livingstone S, et al. Preliminary single-center canadian experience of human normothermic ex vivo liver perfusion: results of a clinical trial. *Am J Transplant.* (2017) 17:1071–80. doi: 10.1111/ajt.14049
50. Nasralla D, Coussios CC, Mergental H, Akhtar MZ, Butler AJ, Ceresa CDL, et al. A randomized trial of normothermic preservation in liver transplantation. *Nature.* (2018) 557:50–6. doi: 10.1038/s41586-018-0047-9
51. von Horn C, Baba HA, Hannaert P, Hauet T, Leuvenink H, Paul A, et al. Controlled oxygenated rewarming up to normothermia for pretransplant reconditioning of liver grafts. *Clin Transplant.* (2017) 31:1–7. doi: 10.1111/ctr.13101
52. von Horn C, Hannaert P, Hauet T, Leuvenink H, Paul A, Minor T. Cold flush after dynamic liver preservation protects against ischemic changes upon reperfusion – an experimental study. *Transpl Int.* (2019) 32:218–24. doi: 10.1111/tri.13354
53. Ghinolfi D, Rreka E, De Tata V, Franzini M, Pezzati D, Fierabracci V, et al. Pilot, open, randomized, prospective trial for normothermic machine perfusion evaluation in liver transplantation from older donors. *Liver Transplant.* (2019) 25:436–49. doi: 10.1002/lt.25362
54. George J, Pera N, Phung N, Leclercq I, Hou JY, Farrell G. Lipid peroxidation, stellate cell activation and hepatic fibrogenesis in a rat model of chronic steatohepatitis. *J Hepatol.* (2003) 39:756–64. doi: 10.1016/S0168-8278(03)00376-3
55. Teramoto, K, Bowers, JL, Kruskal, JB, Clouse M. Hepatic microcirculatory changes after reperfusion in fatty and normal liver transplantation in the rat. *Transplantation.* (1993) 56:1076–82. doi: 10.1097/00007890-199311000-00005
56. Jamieson RW, Zilvetti M, Roy D, Hughes D, Morovat A, Coussios CC, et al. Hepatic steatosis and normothermic perfusion-preliminary experiments in a porcine model. *Transplantation.* (2011) 92:289–95. doi: 10.1097/TP.0b013e318223d817

57. Liu, Q, Berendsen T, Izamis M, Uygun B, Yarmush ML, Uygun K. Perfusion defatting at subnormothermic temperatures in steatotic rat livers. *Transplant Proc.* (2013) 45:3209–13. doi: 10.1016/j.transproceed.2013.05.005
58. Liu Q, Nassar A, Buccini L, Iuppa G, Soliman B, Pezzati D, et al. Lipid metabolism and functional assessment of discarded human livers with steatosis undergoing 24 hours of normothermic machine perfusion. *Liver Transplant.* (2018) 24:233–45. doi: 10.1002/lt.24972
59. Nagrath D, Xu H, Tanimura Y, Zuo R, Berthiaume F, Avila M, et al. Metabolic preconditioning of donor organs: defatting fatty livers by normothermic perfusion *ex vivo*. *Metab Eng.* (2009) 11:274–83. doi: 10.1016/j.ymben.2009.05.005
60. Yarmush G, Santos L, Yarmush J, Koundinyan S, Saleem M, Nativ NI, et al. Metabolic flux distribution during defatting of steatotic human hepatoma (HepG2) cells. *Metabolites.* (2016) 6:1. doi: 10.3390/metabo60 10001
61. Banan B, Watson R, Xu M, Lin Y, Chapman W. Development of a normothermic extracorporeal liver perfusion system toward improving viability and function of human extended criteria donor livers. *Liver Transplant.* (2016) 22:979–93. doi: 10.1002/lt.24451
62. Boteon YL, Attard J, Boteon APCS, Wallace L, Reynolds G, Hubscher S. Manipulation of lipid metabolism during normothermic machine perfusion: effect of defatting therapies on donor liver functional recovery. *Liver Transplant.* (2019) 25:1007–22. doi: 10.1002/lt. 25439
63. Boteon YL, Boteon APCS, Attard J, Mergental H, Mirza DF, Bhogal RH, et al. *Ex situ* machine perfusion as a tool to recondition steatotic donor livers: troublesome features of fatty livers and the role of defatting therapies. A systematic review. *Am J Transplant.* (2018) 18:2384–99. doi: 10.1111/ajt.14992
64. Ceresa CDL, Nasralla D, Coussios CC, Friend PJ. The case for normothermic machine perfusion in liver transplantation. *Liver Transplant.* (2018) 24:269–75. doi: 10.1002/lt.25000
65. Jassem W, Xystrakis E, Ghnewa YG, Yuksel M, Pop O, Martinez-Llordella M, et al. Normothermic machine perfusion (NMP) inhibits proinflammatory responses in the liver and promotes regeneration. *Hepatology.* (2019) 70:682–95. doi: 10.1002/hep.30475
66. Xystrakis E, Yuksel M, Lin F, Huang X, Pop OT, Quaglia A, et al. Impact of donation mode on the proportion and function of T lymphocytes in the liver. *PLoS ONE.* (2015) 10:1–16. doi: 10.1371/journal.pone.0139791
67. Ravaioli M, De Pace V, Angeletti A, Comai G, Vasuri F, Baldassarre M, et al. Hypothermic oxygenated new machine perfusion system in liver and kidney transplantation of extended criteria donors:first italian clinical trial. *Sci. Rep.* (2020) 10:1–11. doi: 10.1038/s41598-020-62979-9
68. Fahrner R, Dondorf F, Ardelt M, Settmacher U, Rauchfuss F. Role of NK, NKT cells and macrophages in liver transplantation. *World J Gastroenterol.* (2016) 22:6135–44. doi: 10.3748/wjg.v22.i27.6135
69. de Vries RJ, Tessier SN, Banik PD, Nagpal S, Cronin SEJ, Ozer S, et al. Supercooling extends preservation time of human livers. *Nat Biotechnol.* (2019) 37:1131–6. doi: 10.1038/s41587-019-0223-y
70. Bruinsma BG, Berendsen TA, Izamis ML, Yeh H, Yarmush ML, Uygun K. Supercooling preservation and transplantation of the rat liver. *Nat Protoc.* (2015) 10:484–94. doi: 10.1038/nprot.2015.011
71. Berendsen TA, Bruinsma BG, Puts CF, Saeidi N, Usta OB, Uygun BE. Supercooling enables long-term transplantation survival following 4 days of liver preservation. *Nat Med.* (2014) 20:790–3. doi: 10.1038/nm.3588
72. Eshmuminov D, Becker D, Bautista Borrego L, Hefti M, Schuler MJ, Hagedorn C, et al. An integrated perfusion machine preserves injured human livers for 1 week. *Nat Biotechnol.* (2020) 38:189–98. doi: 10.1038/s41587-019-0374-x
73. He X, Guo Z, Zhao Q, Ju W, Wang D, Wu L, et al. The first case of ischemia-free organ transplantation in humans: a proof of concept. *Am J Transplant.* (2018) 18:737–44. doi: 10.1111/ajt.14583

9

Antigen-Specific Immunotherapy for Treatment of Autoimmune Liver Diseases

*Naomi Richardson, Sky T. H. Ng and David C. Wraith**

Institute of Immunology and Immunotherapy, College of Medical and Dental Sciences, University of Birmingham, Birmingham, United Kingdom

***Correspondence:**
David C. Wraith
d.wraith@bham.ac.uk

The liver is a critical organ in controlling immune tolerance. In particular, it is now clear that targeting antigens for presentation by antigen presenting cells in the liver can induce immune tolerance to either autoantigens from the liver itself or tissues outside of the liver. Here we review immune mechanisms active within the liver that contribute both to the control of infectious diseases and tolerance to self-antigens. Despite its extraordinary capacity for tolerance induction, the liver remains a target organ for autoimmune diseases. In this review, we compare and contrast known autoimmune diseases of the liver. Currently patients tend to receive strong immunosuppressive treatments and, in many cases, these treatments are associated with deleterious side effects, including a significantly higher risk of infection and associated health complications. We propose that, in future, antigen-specific immunotherapies are adopted for treatment of liver autoimmune diseases in order to avoid such adverse effects. We describe various therapeutic approaches that either are in or close to the clinic, highlight their mechanism of action and assess their suitability for treatment of autoimmune liver diseases.

Keywords: immunoregulation, liver, autoimmune disease, immunotherapy, T-cell

IMMUNOLOGY OF THE LIVER, AN OVERVIEW

The liver is a complex immune-rich organ with a propensity toward tolerance, central to its role in blood filtration and toxin removal. This characteristic is most striking in cases of successful liver transplantation in which patients can be safely weaned off immunosuppression and in multi-organ transplants where transplanting liver alongside other organs including lung and heart prevents multi-organ rejection (1–4).

As the liver receives both arterial blood and blood from the gut via the portal vein, it is regularly exposed to both dietary and microbial antigens, which could establish excessive and prolonged inflammation, tissue damage and fibrosis if unregulated. Therefore, diverse populations of immune cells, stromal cells and hepatocytes work in synergy to resolve localized inflammation and avoid unnecessary immune responses to innocuous stimuli (5, 6). The liver microenvironment is well-adapted to maintain homeostasis due to its unique populations of antigen-presenting cells (APC) with tolerogenic characteristics, feedback mechanisms to control inflammation, high density of innate immune cells and richness of suppressive soluble mediators (summarized in **Figure 1** and **Table 1**).

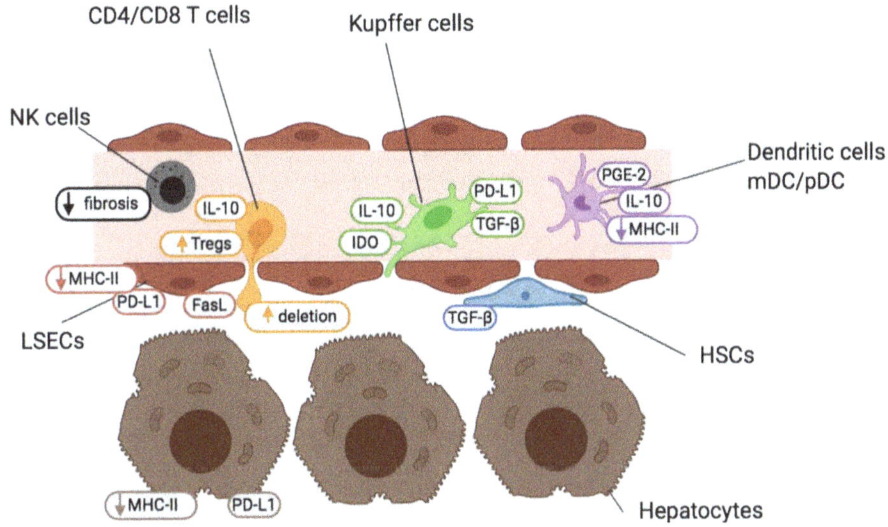

FIGURE 1 | Cells of the liver sinusoid environment and their functions help maintain a state of homeostatic tolerance in the liver. Non-parenchymal resident liver cells including Kupffer cells (green), hepatic stellate cells (HSCs; blue), liver sinusoidal endothelial cells (LSECs; red) and dendritic cells (myeloid mDC and plasmacytoid pDC; purple) are situated within, or in close proximity to, liver sinusoids forming an early detection system to identify pathogens and maintain barrier function. They contribute to the maintenance of a high anti-inflammatory TGF-β and IL-10 cytokine milieu under steady-state conditions and in the face of common bacterial and food antigens to which the liver is continuously exposed. The liver also contains high numbers of innate-like immune cells such as NK cells (gray), and δT cells (not shown). NK cells act as pro-inflammatory agents, and promote the recruitment of effector immune cells, but are also key regulators of fibrosis. Both non-parenchymal antigen-presenting cells and hepatocytes (brown) offer a reduced antigen-presentation capacity and lower levels of costimulation than other antigen-presenting cells elsewhere in the body. This helps promote an environment of low T cell (orange) activation under normal conditions and maintain a state of "active" tolerance, whereby if required, inflammation and T cell activation is readily engaged.

For example, cells of the hepatic sinusoids are continuously exposed to Gram-negative bacterial endotoxin e.g., lipopolysaccharide (LPS), which is detectable in portal vein blood but not systemic circulation (32). These cells when engaging with LPS via Toll-like receptor 4 (TLR4) are adapted to have an increased activating threshold to avoid hyper-active signaling and to better remove LPS from the blood stream (33).

Innate Immune Cells in the Liver

The liver is enriched for innate immune cells which help trigger strong activating signals for inflammation in situations where tolerance is unsuitable, e.g., pathogen infection. Around 50% of liver resident lymphocytes are NK cells (**Figure 1**, gray), notably higher than in most tissues (34). Similarly, numbers of unconventional T cells, NK-T and γδT cells, are increased in the liver to recognize lipid antigens and bacterial pathogens, respectively (35, 36). Activated NK and NKT cells produce significant amounts of cytokines, including strongly inflammatory TNF-α and GM-CSF in response to viral and bacterial pathogens, to shift the balance from tolerance to inflammation. Activated liver NK cells produce IFN-γ and exert cytotoxicity due to TRAIL receptor binding and in response to IL-18 released by Kupffer cells (7, 8). Intriguingly, cytotoxic NKs also contribute to prevention of fibrosis by IFN-γ dependent arrest and apoptosis of hepatic stellate cells (HSCs) as well as directly killing activated HSC (37, 38). The role of γδT cells in the liver is currently less well-defined, but they are known to accumulate in both human fibrotic liver and experimental liver injury models and are producers of IL-17 (39, 40).

Antigen-Presentation in the Liver

The liver is home to a wide range of APC with a tolerogenic bias, including liver sinusoidal endothelial cells (LSECs; **Figure 1**, red), resident myeloid and plasmacytoid dendritic cells (mDCs and pDCs; **Figure 1**, purple), Kupffer cells (KCs; **Figure 1**, green) and hepatic stellate cells (HSCs; **Figure 1**, blue). Antigen-presentation and costimulatory capacity of resting APC in the liver is generally low, contributing to the liver's state of active tolerance.

Dendritic Cells

Mouse and human liver resident DCs are tolerogenic under steady-state conditions, as they display a more immature phenotype with significantly lower expression of MHC Class II and CD80/CD86 than DCs found elsewhere (9). When activated by TLR4 ligands, liver DCs produce substantial amounts of anti-inflammatory prostaglandin E2 (PGE2) (11) and IL-10 whereas blood DCs produce almost exclusively inflammatory cytokines. Therefore, liver DCs are less capable to provide sufficiently strong signals required to activate T cells. Instead, DC-T cell interactions generate more CD25+FoxP3+ Tregs and IL-4 producing Th2 cells by an IL-10 dependent mechanism (9). IL-10 also downregulates the expression of CCR7 on circulating DCs preventing their re-circulation to secondary lymphoid tissue (13).

TABLE 1 | Summary of tolerogenic functions exerted by non-parenchymal liver cells and hepatocytes and their physiological effects.

Cell type	Mechanisms	Effects	References
NK	Become cytotoxic in response to IL-18 and TRAIL receptor ligation	Direct and indirect killing of activated HSCs	(7, 8)
DCs (myeloid and plasmacytoid)	Expression of low MHC-II and costimulatory molecules CD80/CD86 and CD40, low secretion of IL-12	Poor T cell priming - induction of anergy or deletion of antigen-specific T cells. Poor differentiation of naïve CD4+ T cells to Th1 effector cells	(9, 10)
	Secretion of IL-10	Bias toward generation of CD25+FoxP3+ Tregs and Th2 cells Reduced production of pro-inflammatory cytokines TNF-α, IL-6 and ROS by monocytes	(9)
	Production of PGE-2	Inhibition of T cell proliferation and induces apoptosis, induction of regulatory dendritic cells	(11)
	Expression of PD-L1	Inhibition of T cell activation and induction of apoptosis of activated T cells	(12)
Tregs	Production of IL-10	Downregulation of CCR7 on liver DCs preventing their recirculation to secondary lymphoid tissues	(13)
LSECs	Production of PGE2 and IL-10	Inhibition of T cell proliferation, decreased pro-inflammatory cytokine production, increased Treg generation	(14, 15)
	Cross-presentation of antigen to CD8+ T cells	CD8+ T cells are rendered unresponsive, preferential deletion when PD-1/PD-L1 engaged	(16, 17)
	Expression of PD-L1	Inhibition of T cell activation and induction of apoptosis of activated T cells	(18)
	Expression of FasL	Allospecific T cells crossing LSEC barrier undergo apoptosis	(19)
	Expression of low MHC-II and costimulatory molecules CD80/CD86 and CD40	Poor T cell priming - naïve CD4 do not effectively differentiate to Th1 effector cells. Th1 and Th17 cells lose effector potency in contact with LSECs	(18)
Kupffer cells	Production of IDO, PGE2, TGF-β and IL-10	Reduced production of pro-inflammatory cytokines TNF-α, IL-6, increased Treg generation	(20)
	Low expression of MHC-II, CD80, CD86, and CD40	Poor direct T cell priming - naïve CD4 do not effectively differentiate to effector cells	(21)
	Production of prostaglandins	Inhibit dendritic cells priming of T cells, reduced Th1 and Th17 output	(21, 22)
	Scavengers of antigen at steady-state	Induce/maintain T cell tolerance to antigen by expansion of IL-10 producing Tregs and arrest of CD4+ Tconv	(22)
HSCs	Expression of PD-L1 and TRAIL when activated	Inhibition of T cell activation and induction of TRAIL-mediated apoptosis	(23, 24)
	Production of TGF-β and retinoic acid	Increased Treg differentiation	(25, 26)
Hepatocytes	MHC-II expression with very low expression of costimulatory molecules	Poor T cell priming - induction of anergy or deletion of antigen-specific T cells	(27, 28)
	Expression of PD-L1	Inhibition of T cell activation and induction of apoptosis of activated T cells	(29, 30)
	Activation of Notch signaling pathway on Th1	Diverts Th1 CD4+ T cells to synthesize IL-10	(31)

Liver Sinusoidal Endothelial Cells

LSECs express both MHC-I and MHC–II, and are as capable at antigen-uptake as DCs (41). They can, therefore, prime CD4+ T cells and cross-present antigen to CD8+ T cells, a function which is modulated by liver IL-10 (14). In both cases, the interaction between LSEC and T cell is biased toward tolerance. Naïve CD4 T cells primed by LSECs do not receive high costimulation, or an IL-12 stimulus from neighboring tolerogenic DCs and, therefore, do not effectively differentiate to Th1 effector cells (42–44). Th1 and Th17 cells when in contact with tolerogenic LSECs are unable to produce high levels of IFN-γ and IL-17, respectively (18). LSECs constitutive expression of PDL-1 when cross-presenting antigen to CD8+ T cells renders these T cells unresponsive and establishes a PDL-1 dependent antigen-specific T cell tolerance in the liver (16, 17). Futhermore, as T cells transmigrate across the LSEC barrier to enter the liver parenchyma, the LSECs are able to detect allospecificity and induce T cell death both directly and indirectly via the Fas/FasL pathway (19, 45).

Kupffer Cells

KCs are liver-resident, immobile macrophages located within the sinusoidal lumen. They are hugely abundant, constituting 80% of the body's entire macrophage population and around 35% of non-parenchymal cells within the liver (5). KCs have been found to be essential mediators of homeostatic tolerance in the liver. KCs express significantly lower levels of MHC-II and costimulatory molecules compared to dendritic cells, meaning that they are incapable of sufficiently priming T cells on their own. Notably, they can block dendritic cell priming of antigen-specific T cells in a prostaglandin-dependent manner *in vitro* (21). Under steady-state conditions, KCs survey the sinusoids for dead cell debris, pathogens and particulates to phagocytose and this surveillance role can both establish tolerance or rapid response to pathogen depending on the physiological context. KCs phagocytose and present non-pathogen derived antigenic particulate matter and generate a skew in liver CD4+ T cells toward non-responsiveness (22). Heymann et al. shed light on the efficacy of KCs to induce tolerance by tracking OVA-loaded liposomes using intra-vital microscopy. KCs were the primary cell type within the liver to internalize labeled particulates and promoted the expansion of CD25+FoxP3+ OVA-specific Tregs *in vivo*. Both KC depletion and liver inflammation prevented tolerance induction (22).

Their essential sentinel role is further highlighted in mouse models lacking in KCs, where mice are fatally unable to clear a range of bacterial infections (46–48). When encountering pathogen, KCs rapidly release pro-inflammatory cytokines TNF-α, IL-6, and IL-1, promoting the recruitment of granulocytes and neutrophils to clear pathogens (46, 49). Following initial pro-inflammatory function, KCs then express the suppressive mediator IDO and release PGE-2, IL-10, and TGF-β to quench localized inflammation (21, 42, 50).

Targeting KCs to induce antigen-specific tolerance is a promising avenue when considering immunotherapeutic particle delivery for treatment of autoimmune diseases, but would require administration in contexts without liver inflammation. It may therefore not be the most appropriate method for addressing liver autoimmune diseases without prior immune suppressive treatment.

Hepatic Stellate Cells

HSCs can also act as APCs and present antigens via MHC-I, MHC-II and CD1d (51). They are powerful producers of TGF-β and retinoic acid within the liver, helping to maintain a generalized immunosuppressive milieu at homeostasis and promoting Treg differentiation and residence within the liver (25, 26). However, when HSCs become activated in the presence of pathogens or strong inflammatory signals, they rapidly metabolize stored Vitamin A and differentiate into myofibroblasts, secreting extra-cellular matrix proteins. Therefore, HSC are key drivers of hepatic fibrosis and associated deterioratio to cirrhosis (52).

Hepatocytes

Hepatocytes themselves possess tolerogenic properties, as they are MHC-II expressing in the absence or very low expression of costimulatory molecules (27, 28). In mice, hepatocytes in inflammatory conditions can activate a Notch and IFN-γ dependent pathway to divert Th1 CD4+ T cells to synthesize IL-10 (31). PD-L1 is also inducible in hepatocytes by viral infection and by type 1 and type II interferons, mediating apoptosis of activated T cells (29).

At present, it is unclear exactly which of these tolerance-promoting mechanisms fail in the pathogenesis of autoimmune liver diseases, and at which time in disease progression. The consequence of these homeostatic mechanisms failing, however, can be devastating for liver function, impairing tissue regeneration and causing fibrosis. In the case of autoimmune liver diseases, immunological targeting of liver self-antigens catalyzes a system of inflammation and chronic liver disease. It will be important to understand which mechanisms break down in the process of developing autoimmune liver disease, in order to best intervene with tolerance promoting treatments.

AUTOIMMUNE LIVER DISEASE

Autoimmune liver disease (AILD) can be divided into 3 distinct clinical diseases, autoimmune hepatitis (AIH), primary biliary cholangitis (PBC) and primary sclerosing cholangitis (PSC). They are distinguished by the molecular and cellular targets of immune pathology alongside the location of observed liver damage (**Figure 2**). Biliary dominant PBC and PSC affect cholangiocytes lining bile ducts. PBC destroys small, interlobular bile ducts while PSC targets larger bile ducts and is characterized by inflammatory fibrosis in the intrahepatic and extrahepatic biliary tree (53, 54). In AIH, the target is hepatocytes themselves, leading to interface hepatitis and significant lymphocyte infiltration primarily around the portal tracts (55). All 3 diseases will develop to severe liver fibrosis without medical intervention.

DISEASE CHARACTERISTICS AND EPIDEMIOLOGY

AIH is a chronic progressive liver-disease that mainly affects women (70–80% cases) and can be diagnosed in adults and children of any age or ethnicity (56). As symptoms and biochemical indicators are widely heterogenous between patients, the International Autoimmune Hepatitis Group (IAIHG) developed a scoring system based on specific criteria to improve early diagnosis (57, 58). Early diagnosis is imperative as cirrhosis is already present at diagnosis of a third of AIH patients and liver cirrhosis is the primary risk factor associated with development of hepatocellular carcinoma (56). AIH is a rare disease affecting between 16 and 20 cases per 100,000 (59–62) but appears to be increasing in prevalence. A long-term Danish study observed an almost 2-fold increase in the annual incidence rate of AIH between 1994 and 2012 (63).

PBC affects around 35/100,000 individuals, and is most common in women (9:1 female: male) and those over 50 years old (64). Reports have also indicated increasing prevalence of PBC over time (65). In around 10% of PBC patients, there will be overlap disease with features of AIH (66).

PSC is lowest in prevalence, and most commonly found in Northern Europe with 5.5–8.5 patients per 100,000 individuals in the UK, which has increased by about 50% since 1991 (67, 68). Unlike AIH and PBC, PSC is more common in men than in women (3:1) and although disease can occur at any age it has a peak incidence around 40 (69).

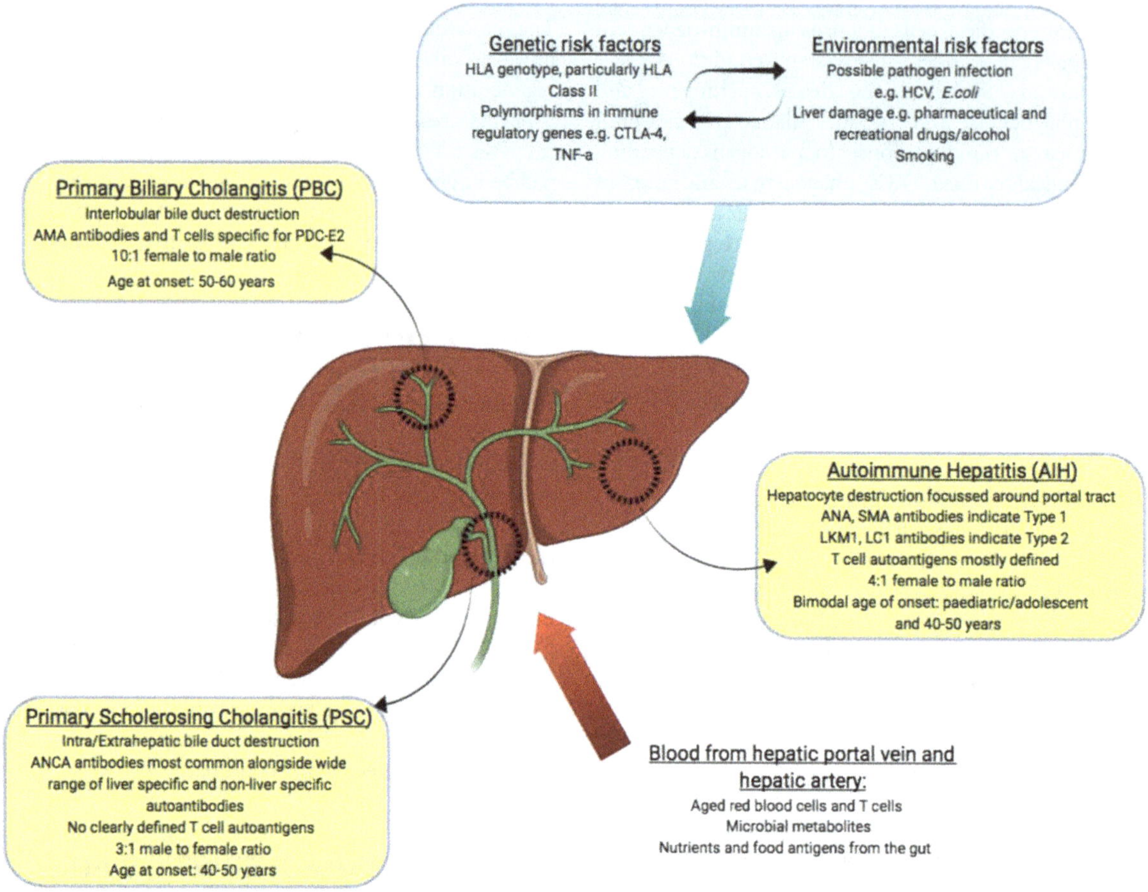

FIGURE 2 | Summary of autoimmune liver diseases: tissues affected, and key features of disease (yellow boxes). Blood borne factors which challenge the maintenance of immune tolerance are listed as inputs (red arrow). Genetic, environmental and lifestyle factors which could affect the maintenance of tolerance are listed as inputs (blue box and arrow).

GENETIC ASSOCIATIONS

There is evidence for genetic factors playing a role in pathogenesis of all 3 AILD disease classes, with both major histocompatibility complex HLA genes and non-HLA genes showing disease associations (70). Exactly how HLA confers increased disease risk is unknown, but is presumed to be related to how antigens are presented and recognized by the immune system.

AIH-1 usually presenting in middle age has been linked to HLA-DRB1*0301 and HLA-DRB1*0401 with co-expression of these risk alleles indicating a double-dose effect (71–73). AIH-2 affects around 10% of AIH patients, exhibits a more aggressive phenotype and has been related to the presence of HLA-DRB1*07 and DRB1*03 in cohorts in the UK and Brazil (74). AIH-2 is most commonly diagnosed in childhood and has even been recorded in infants, suggesting a potentially different etiology to AIH1 (75). Around 20% of AIH patients suffer concomitant autoimmune diseases, most commonly thyroiditis (also HLA-DR3), inflammatory bowel disease (IBD), Type 1 diabetes (also HLA-DR4/HLA-DR3) and Addisons disease (HLA-DR4) (76).

PBC susceptibility is highly associated with HLA-DRB1*08 in Europe and North America (77). In contrast HLA-DRB1*11 and HLA-DRB1*13 were found to be protective toward PBC (78).

PSC is generally associated with HLA-DRB1*0301 in Norwegian and British patients (79). In patients with both PSC and inflammatory bowel disease, PSC is also associated with HLA-DRB1*13 but only with individuals with IBD (80).

GWAS studies have also identified association between specific polymorphisms within regulatory genes and AIH, PBC, PSC development. Notably for AIH and PBC but not for PSC, these include CTLA-4 and TNF-α genes (81–86) which are identified in similar studies of wide ranging autoimmune disorders (87, 88). TNF-α is located in the HLA-DR/DP locus; therefore, its appearance in GWAS studies of autoimmune diseases is unsurprising. However, at present it is unclear whether its influence is merely by association via linkage disequilibrium, or whether its function and downstream signaling actively contributes to the strong correlation of certain HLA haplotypes to autoimmunity. A further interesting correlation between TNF-α and CTLA-4 noted that single nucleotide polymorphism (SNP) rs1800629 of the TNF-α gene, leading to increased

TNF-α production, amplified the CTLA4 SNP risk associated with rs231725, and that the combination of both SNPs was significantly more common in PBC patients compared to healthy controls (84). Studies in PBC have also identified common variant in IL-12 and IL-12R which indicate a role for aberrant IL-12 signaling in disease pathogenesis (89).

The specific triggers that lead to development of AILD are as yet poorly understood, due to the complex nature of genetic and environmental (drug and foreign pathogen) influences. It is thought that environmental stressors on a background of genetic predisposition in the form of HLA haplotypes and general tolerogenic "fitness" (Tregs and feedback loops) could help establish chronic autoimmune liver injury. AILD patients commonly present other autoimmune diseases, suggesting that immune dysregulation is not isolated to the liver in these cases.

AUTOANTIGENS AND AUTOANTIBODIES

Characteristic of all autoimmune diseases, AIH and PBC have autoantibodies present in patient's circulation. In both diseases, there are a some well-defined autoantibodies that are used to diagnose patients; however, the autoantigens that these antibodies are specific for is less well-defined. In contrast, PSC patients do not possess defined liver-specific autoantibodies. The strongest biomarker associated with PSC is elevated serum alkaline phosphatase levels, indicative of cholestasis (69, 90). PSC is usually diagnosed by MRI imaging of the biliary tree to identify cholestasis and/or strictures (69, 91, 92). Up to 80% of PSC patients also present with inflammatory bowel disease (IBD), indicating a general gastrointestinal inflammatory phenotype (93). Taken alongside the fact that PSC is more common in men and has less strong HLA associations, the lack of known autoantibodies calls into question whether the disease is strictly autoimmune, or whether it is autoinflammatory in nature (94).

Suspected AIH patients are scored according to International AIH Group published criteria to determine a diagnosis of AIH (57, 58). For clinical and research purposes, patients are grouped into AIH-1 or AIH-2 by the presence of different autoantibody profiles to liver antigens. The definitive clinical distinction between AIH subtypes is challenging, and age-matched patients usually follow similar trajectories and treatment protocols regardless of patient autoantibody profiles (95).

The vast majority (≈75%) of AIH-1 patients are positive for anti-nuclear antibodies (ANA) and/or anti-smooth muscle antibodies (SMA) (62, 63). However, these autoantibodies are not limited to AIH-1 patients and the autoantigens responsible are not well-defined (96, 97). ANA can react to histones, ribonucleoproteins ds-DNA and chromatin (98). SMA also have a range of specificities, predominantly to F-actin (99, 100). The remainder of patients who lack ANA or SMA antibodies, but present with liver disease pathology in accordance with the IAIHG diagnosis criteria, may possess other defined autoantibodies including anti-perinuclear neutrophil cytoplasmic antibodies (pANCA), anti-liver cytosol (LC-1), anti-soluble liver antigen/liver-pancreas (SLA/LP) and/or asialoglycoprotein receptor (ASGPR). Of note, SLA/LP is present in around 30% of AIH patients and has been identified in both adults and children (101–103). SLA/LP autoantibodies are specific to the autoantigen SLA/LP/tRNP(Ser)Sec (104, 105) and is therefore the only defined autoantigen implicated in AIH-1.

AIH-2 is rarely seen as a newly-diagnosed disease in adult cohorts but is reported to represent around 30% of pediatric AIH patients (106). AIH-2 has a less varied autoantigen profile and is diagnosed predominantly by the presence of anti-liver kidney microsomal antibody (LKM-1) and to a lesser extent anti-liver cytosol antibody (LC-1), specific to the liver proteins cytochrome P450 2D6 (CYP2D6) and formiminotransferase cyclodeaminase (FTCD), respectively (74, 107). Both T cell and B cell epitope mapping studies of CYP2D6 have been published, providing evidence that CYP2D6-reactive lymphocytes circulate in AIH-2 patients but not in healthy people (74, 108). Again, neither LKM-1 or LC-1 autoantibodies are restricted to AIH-2 – notably LKM-1 antibodies are detected in 5–10% of chronic HCV patients (101, 109) with an identified homologous sequence between HCV and CYP2D6 judged to be the cause (102).

The success of antigen-specific immunotherapies in re-establishing tolerance is reliant on having strong knowledge of the autoantigens underpinning immune pathology. Therefore, with our current understanding of AIH disease, it is likely that the most appropriate immediate targets for AIH-2 are CYP2D6, FTCD and for AIH-1 SLA/LP/tRNP(Ser)Sec. To be applicable to the majority of AIH-1 patients, however, detailed antigen profiling of AMA and SMA targets is required but has proved to be extremely challenging thus far.

PBC is diagnosed by the presence of highly-specific anti-mitochondrial antibodies (AMA) against the pyruvate dehydrogenase complex (PDCE2) (110–112). Over 90% of PBC patients are positive for AMA antibodies (113). PDCE2 is expressed at detectable levels on biliary epithelial cells in PBC but not in healthy individuals (114, 115). A minority of PBC patients are AMA negative, however, histological analyses of the bile ducts reveal no difference in pathology and presentation of PDCE2 between AMA positive and AMA negative PBC patients (114). Interestingly, PBC is also associated with prior urinary tract infections which are most frequently caused by *E.coli* (116–118). It is thought that *E.coli* induces B and T cell cross reactive responses to human PDCE2 by molecular mimicry (115).

In the case of AIH and PBC the presence of reliable autoantibodies to known autoantigens, and lymphocytes specific to these autoantigens found in patients provides vital evidence that supports targeting autoreactive cells in patients could have therapeutic benefit.

CURRENT TREATMENTS

The clinical options to treat AILDs are limited once diagnosis is confirmed. The current front-line treatments center on broad immunosuppressive agents and ursodeoxycholic acid (UDCA) – a biliary protective drug of which the mechanism of action is still poorly understood.

In AIH, randomized controlled trials from the 1970's helped establish the mainstay treatment options of corticosteroids

(PRED) and azathioprine (AZA) (119–121). Today, 50 years later, the treatment plan is almost identical to these early trials. This is sufficient to obtain biochemical disease remission and to prevent further liver damage in around 80% of AIH-1 patients (122). However, this level of immunosuppression commonly causes side effects including Cushingoid features, weight gain and gastrointestinal issues. For the vast majority of patients immunosuppressive therapy is lifelong, bringing a range of side effects, including osteoporeosis (especially problematic in middle aged women), diabetes mellitus, an increased risk of infections and risk of both hepatocellular and extra-hepatic cancers (123). Despite treatment, *de novo* cirrhosis occurs in around 14% of patients increasing the likelihood patients progress to transplant or hepatocellular carcinoma (124, 125). Adolescents often display poor treatment regime compliance, leading to the highest rate of relapse of any age group; therefore, an approach which causes fewer side effects, would be particularly welcome in this cohort (126). A recent trial using the corticosteroid budesonide with AZA indicated improved efficacy to PRED and a much improved adverse effect profile (127). So far, this is yet to be translated to a change in clinical treatment practices for AIH.

The primary course of treatment for PBC is UDCA (128). UDCA slows PBC disease progression by protecting cholangiocytes and hepatocytes from damage (129). UDCA significantly improves transplant free survival (130, 131); however, up to 40% of patients treated with UDCA have an insufficient response to treatment (132, 133), therefore in the long term, a liver transplant is often required. Even with a liver transplant, PBC recurs in around 30% of patients after 10 years (134–136). A recent development in approved PBC treatment is administration of obeticholic acid, particularly in patients refractory to or intolerant of UDCA. Obeticholic acid significantly improved liver function tested by alkaline phosphatase levels in patients with insufficient UDCA responses, with 69% of treated patients achieving a 20% reduction in ALP vs. only 8% of patients treated with UDCA alone (137, 138).

There are no effective treatments for PSC that have been proven to improve transplant free survival. There is no clear evidence that UDCA can treat PSC despite multiple clinical trials (139, 140). Trials applying other immunosuppressants to PSC, including prednisolone, budesonide, azathioprine, cyclosporin, methotrexate, mycophenolate, and tacrolimus have not shown efficacy (141). Drugs that antagonize the effects of anti-TNF-α such as pentoxifylline, etanercept and anti TNF-α monoclonal antibodies are also ineffective (141). Patients may undergo several of these pharmacological interventions in an attempt to quench biliary pathology, yet for most the only long-term option is liver transplantation. The mean time from diagnosis to liver transplantation/death is 9–12 years (90, 142). Unfortunately, PSC is expected to reoccur in 20–25% of patients over a 5–10 year period (136, 143, 144).

There is certainly an unmet need for improved treatment options with increased efficacy in hard to treat groups particularly pediatric AIH patients, refractory PBC patients and PSC patients. With the current understanding of the features of PSC, it is not clear that its pathogenesis is autoimmune, thus without the identification of autoantibodies and autoantigens relevant to PSC it will not be possible to generate antigen-specific immunotherapies for these patients. For AIH and PBC patients, however, there is sufficient evidence that antigen-specific immunotherapies could have real therapeutic value, and in contrast to systemic immunosuppressive drugs these should have a more specific mechanism of action that does not threaten the general health and immune capacity of the patient. The need for antigen-specific immunotherapies becomes ever more important as the world faces highly infectious agents such as the SARS-CoV-2 virus: such pathogens clearly endanger anyone taking immunosuppressive drugs.

ANTIGEN-SPECIFIC IMMUNOTHERAPY

Antigen-specific immunotherapy has been practiced in the field of allergy for more than 100 years (145, 146). Recently, there has been increasing interest in the development of antigen-specific approaches for specific immunotherapy of autoimmune conditions (schematic summary in **Figure 3**). This follows evidence that treatment of experimental animals with antigens can lead to amelioration of disease (146). Currently these approaches target CD4 T cell recognition of self-antigens. This is because CD4 T cells control the generation of all of the tissue damaging mechanisms associated with autoimmunity including pathogenic autoantibodies, antigen-driven inflammation and self-antigen specific CD8 T cells. It is not the focus of this review to discuss the mechanisms of action underpinning each approach aiming to induce antigen-specific tolerance; as these has been described comprehensively recently elsewhere (147, 148). We have briefly summarized within **Table 2** the proposed mechanisms of action for each approach in development or in the clinic.

Allergic desensitization involves administration of increasing and repeated doses of allergen, often a crude extract of the allergen material. Early attempts to treat autoimmune diseases in a similar way were not successful with intact antigen inducing pathogenic autoantibodies (166, 167) or driving tissue damaging cytotoxic T cells (168). To ensure safety and efficacy, autoantigens must be modified in such a way as to protect the recipient from exacerbation of the autoimmune response or they must be fragmented so as to avoid engagement with pathogenic autoimmune mechanisms. A preferred approach is to use short fragments of antigens (synthetic peptides) designed to modulate CD4 T cells but lacking either the structural integrity to engage pathogenic B cells or the peptide sequences to engage CD8 T cells.

It is important to appreciate that the mammalian adaptive immune system is poised to respond to foreign antigens but in the steady-state is adapted to limit autoimmune responses to the individual's own antigens. Responsibility for distinguishing between self and foreign antigens falls primarily on dendritic cells (169). In the steady-state, these cells are capable of binding the many fragments of self-antigens that are contained within the lymphoid pool (170). Steady-state dendritic cells presenting self-antigens are tolerogenic. It is only when these cells encounter foreign antigens in the context of microbial pattern-associated molecular patterns (e.g., LPS, bacterial DNA

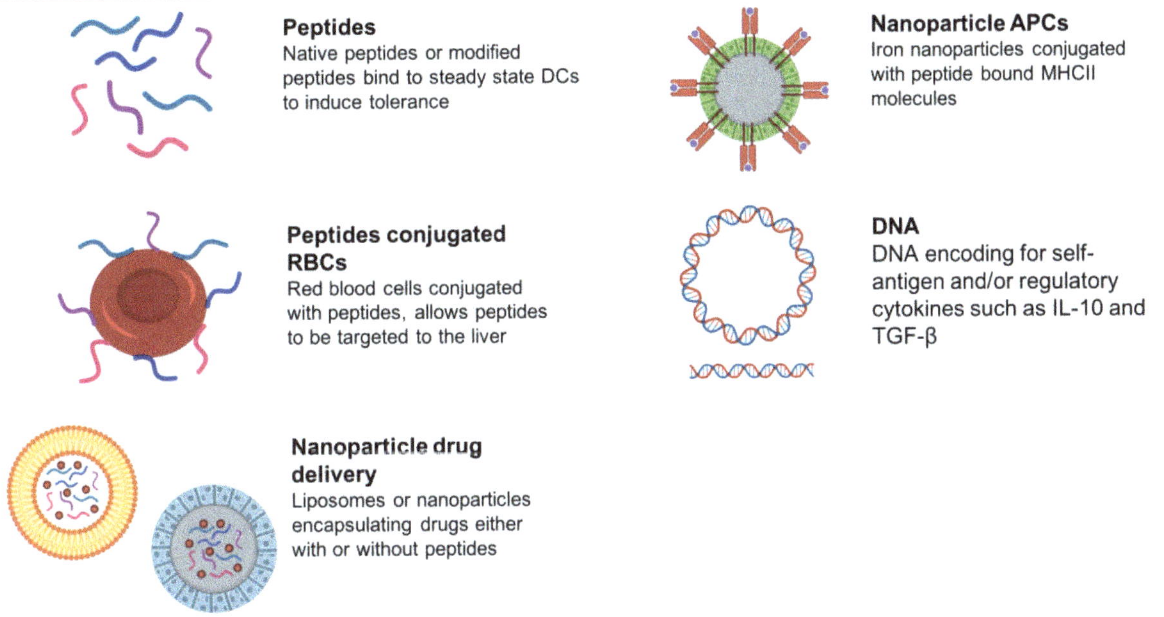

FIGURE 3 | Summary of antigen-specific immunotherapy approaches in preclinical/clinical development.

etc.) that they present antigen in an immunogenic rather than a tolerogenic fashion.

There are now a variety of clinical trials in progress that target steady-state/immature dendritic cells either *in vivo* or *in vitro*. The *in vitro* approach involves the generation of myeloid-derived dendritic cells treated with immunosuppressive agents, such as vitamin D3, to maintain a tolerogenic phenotype. The cells are then treated with peptides from self-antigens and reinjected into the patient (171–173). Alternatively, antigens can be coupled to dendritic cell targeting antibodies (e.g., anti—Dec205) for *in vivo* targeting (174). Our own work has focused on designing peptides that target steady-state dendritic cells directly. Early studies showed that some but not all known CD4 T cell epitopes induce tolerance when injected into experimental mice (175). Peptides must bind directly to MHC Class II and adopt the same conformation as the naturally processed epitope (176). Those peptides that do not mimic the naturally processed epitope fail to induce tolerance in relevant T cells. This implies that tolerogenic peptides bind directly to MHC Class II on or in steady state dendritic cells without further processing. Recent work from our laboratory has shown that such antigen-processing independent epitopes (apitopes) selectively bind to peptide receptive MHC class II molecules on steady-state dendritic cells but not to MHC Class II on the surface of B cells or monocytes. This is explained by the distinct, peptide-receptive nature of MHC Class II molecules on steady-state dendritic cells (177). Furthermore, tolerogenic peptides are detectable on steady state DCs up to 5 days after administration (178). We have shown that apitopes induce tolerance by induction of anergy in self-antigen reactive T cells and the expansion of antigen-specific Tr1 cells (179–182).

Alternative approaches for targeting "tolerogenic" APCs *in vivo* include combining antigen with liposomes, red blood cells or nanoparticles (Summarized in **Table 2**). These target different antigen-presenting cells in lymphoid organs or the liver depending on the size of the material or nanoparticle. This determines their modus operandi.

There is increasing evidence that nanoparticles of different sizes transit to and are taken up by different APCs according to their size. Berkland et al. have shown that particles > 200 nm are retained in the liver while those < 4 nm are rapidly excreted (183). This evidence would pair well with evidence from Kupffer cell studies that these cells establish tolerance by phagocytosing particulate material and presenting antigenic fragments (21, 22). Such small particles rapidly drain from sites of injection into blood and lymph and particles of 4–10 nm penetrate lymph node cortex where they can interact with steady-state DCs. In contrast, particles > 100 nm are retained in the sub-capsular space where they will be processed by macrophages.

Santamaria et al. have developed artificial APCs (Navacims) based on nanoparticles coated with MHC Class II and antigenic peptide (159). The mechanism of action is in principle the same as apitope immunotherapy, both establish immunological tolerance by inducing IL-10 expressing CD4 T cells through a negative feedback mechanism (159, 160, 181, 184, 185). The resulting Tr1 cells are characterized by the expression of the immunosuppressive genes such as IL10 and co-inhibitory receptors (186, 187). The Tr1 cells induced by Navacims, however, also express inflammatory cytokines such as TNF-α, IL5, and GM CSF (188). In contrast, Tr1 cells derived from apitope immunotherapy do not express TNF-α, IL5, or GM-CSF (182). Their recent studies serve as a valuable proof of concept, as antigenic peptides identified by *in silico* binding predictions from PDC-E2 loaded onto IAg7 MHC-nanoparticles are able to ameliorate PBC-like liver damage.

TABLE 2 | This table summarizes the current status of pre-clinical and clinical developments of antigen-specific immunotherapies for autoimmune diseases.

Company	Delivery approach	Proposed mechanism of action	Impact on T cell response	Efficacy in experimental models	Clinical trials progress
Anokion	Antigens modified with polymeric forms of either N-acetylgalactosamine or N-acetyl-glucosamine	Target hepatic antigen-presenting cells	Induce CD4+ and CD8+ T-cell deletion and anergy	EAE[A], T1D	Enrolling patients for KAN-101 trial in coeliac disease
Apitope International NV	Synthetic peptides designed as antigen processing independent CD4+ T cell epitopes (apitopes) injected in saline i.d. or s.c.	Highly soluble peptides traffic to and selectively bind to MHC II antigens on steady-state DC in lymphoid organs	Induction of anergy and generation of regulatory T cells (primarily Tr1)	EAE and Graves' disease models (149, 150)	Phase Ia in SPMS (149) Phase Ib in RRMS (151) Phase II in RRMS (151) Phase I in Graves' disease (152)
Cellerys	Red blood cells (RBC) coupled with peptides from myelin in MS	RBC target macrophages and Kupffer cells in spleen and liver	Increase in Tr1 cell response to antigen with reduced IFN-γ		Phase 1 in RRMS[B]
Cour/takeda	Antigen encapsulated in PLG [poly(lactide-co-glycolide)] nanoparticles	Ag-PLG internalized by splenic marginal zone macrophages and liver phagocytic cells via scavenger receptors (MARCO)	Increase in Foxp3 Treg cells, dependent on CTLA-4, PD-1 and IL-10	EAE, T1D and coeliac disease models (153–155)	Phase I trial of gliadin-PLG in patients with coeliac disease (unpublished)
Dendright/Janssen Biotech Inc	Antigen with calcitriol in liposomes	Liposomes (105–135 nm) target steady-state DC in draining lymph nodes	Increase in Foxp3 Treg cells	Autoimmune arthritis and experimental Goodpasture's vasculitis (156)	Phase I in ACPA+ rheumatod arthritis[C]
Imcyse	T cell epitopes modified by addition of a thioredox motif (CXXC), injected in Alum adjuvant	Promotes cytotoxic activity in T cells through increasing expression of granzyme B and FasL	Cytotoxic cells delete B cells in cognate recognition	T1D (157)	Phase I with 3 staggered doses of modified pro-insuln peptide in T1D (unpublished)
Novo nordisk	Plasmid DNA encoding proinsulin and co-expressing IL-10 and TGF-β	Promotes treg cells	Promotes Treg cell differentiation	T1D with vector expressing GAD antigen (158)	
Parvus	Nanoparticles coated with MHC II proteins and antigenic peptides	Bind directly to $CD4^+$ effector cells	Drives differentiation of Tr1 cells from Th1 precursors in mice	EAE, CIA, T1D and autoimmune liver diseases (159, 160)	In pre-clinical development for T1D and autoimmune liver diseases
Selecta	PLG nanoparticles containing rapamycin co-administered with antigen	Nanoparticles found in dendritic cells in spleen and LSEC and Kupffer cells in the liver where they mediate down-regulation of CD80, CD86, class II MHC and upregulation of PDL-1	Promotes Treg cell differentiation	EAE and anti-drug antibodies (161, 162)	Phase II study in gout designed to block the anti-drug antibody response to Pegadricase[D]
Tolerion	DNA encoding self-antigen	CpG islands in DNA replaced with GpG to reduce immunogenicity of antigen delivery	Promote immune regulatory response to self-antigen	BHT-3021 prevents T1D in mouse model (163)	Phase I trial completed and phase II enrolling (164)
Topaz	Ferromagnetic nanoparticles coupled to T cell epitopes	Nanoparticle-based autoantigen delivery to liver sinusoidal endothelial cells	Induction of $Foxp3^+$ Treg cells in the liver	EAE (165)	First patient enrolment in phase I trial of TPM203 in Pemphigus Vulgaris

Where either pre-clinical or clinical trials have been published these are referenced. Additional results are discussed in relevant conference abstracts and company websites.

[A] https://anokion.com/wp-content/uploads/2019/09/ECTRIMS_Poster_9.13.19.pdf.

[B] MULTIPLE SCLEROSIS JOURNAL Volume: 25 Special Issue: SI Supplement: 2 Pages: 894–894 Meeting Abstract: 339 Published: SEP 2019.

[C] https://acrabstracts.org/abstract/a-phase-i-randomized-double-blind-placebo-controlled-single-center-single-dose-escalation-to-investigate-the-safety-tolerability-and-pharmacodynamics-of-subcutaneously-administered-den-181-in-a/.

[D] https://selectabio.com/immtor/goutttherapy/phase2results.

These Navacims, MHCII-based nanomedicines displaying epitopes from mitochondrial, endoplasmic reticulum, or cytoplasmic antigens associated with primary biliary cholangitis or autoimmune hepatitis can suppress disease progression in various murine models in an organ- rather than disease-specific manner (160). The improvement in liver score was shown to be IL-10 and TGF-β dependent. However, none of these liver disease models fully recapitulates the human condition. Furthermore, the T cell epitopes restricted by murine MHC class II molecules are unlikely to resemble those binding HLA-DR and DQ molecules i.e., relevant to human disease

However, Navacims do not work prophylactically to prevent disease onset, this is in contrast to apitope immunotherapy which is effective before as well as after disease onset (160, 179, 182). The bystander suppression demonstrated by loading the artificial APCs with PDC-E2 peptides and supressing the response against the CYP2D6 antigen and *vice versa* is intriguing and suggests that bystander suppression can influence different autoimmune conditions within the same tissue (189).

FUTURE PROSPECTS FOR ANTIGEN-SPECIFIC IMMUNOTHERAPIES FOR AUTOIMMUNE LIVER DISEASES

At this stage, it is too early to compare the safety and efficacy of the various approaches shown in **Table 2**. It is likely that different approaches will prove more or less effective for control of different immune pathologies and diseases. It is of paramount importance, however, to apply three tests to these approaches.

1. What is the mechanism of action? It will be critical to fully understand the mechanism by which these approaches induce antigen-specific tolerance both in experimental models and in patients.
2. Which approaches induce bystander suppression? For diseases like Graves' disease, we know precisely what the target antigen is. However, for most autoimmune diseases we do not know which antigen is targeted by the immune system to initiate the disease. For many others, antibodies specific for self-antigens are associated with disease but may or may not have a role in immune pathology. Furthermore, in most autoimmune conditions, epitope spreading leads to the generation of an immune response to a range of antigens within the same tissue (190). In order to account for epitope spreading, we and others have shown that certain immune regulatory mechanisms, such as Tr1 cells, mediate bystander suppression (191). By targeting antigen A within a tissue and eliciting immunosuppressive regulatory T cells, we can control the immune response to antigens B, C, D etc. within the same tissue.
3. Which approach permits repeated antigen administration? Apitope has now conducted clinical trials in multiple sclerosis and Graves' disease. In both cases, protection from immune pathology was observed but the patients treated did not enter a permanent state of tolerance (149, 151). Protection was seen for up to 1 month after the last dose of peptide which correlates well with the duration of tolerance observed in euthymic mice (192). It may well be that humans have evolved to require continued exposure to antigens in order to maintain tolerance. For this reason, it is likely that repeated administration of the different tolerogenic materials described in **Table 2** will be required. A successful therapeutic approach must avoid induction of anti-drug antibodies or non-specific immune suppression.

There is already substantial progress in the quest for specific immunotherapies for autoimmune liver diseases. With this in mind, our laboratory is designing putative disease-altering apitopes from the dominant human autoantigens associated with PBC and type 2 AIH.

AUTHOR CONTRIBUTIONS

All authors listed have made a substantial, direct and intellectual contribution to the work, and approved it for publication.

REFERENCES

1. Benítez C, Londoño MC, Miquel R, Manzia TM, Abraldes JG, Lozano JJ, et al. Prospective multicenter clinical trial of immunosuppressive drug withdrawal in stable adult liver transplant recipients. *Hepatology.* (2013) 58:1824–35. doi: 10.1002/hep.26426
2. Takatsuki M, Uemoto S, Inomata Y, Egawa H, Kiuchi T, Fujita S, et al. Weaning of immunosuppression in living donor liver transplant recipients. *Transplantation.* (2001) 72:449–54. doi: 10.1097/00007890-200108150-00016
3. Tisone G, Orlando G, Cardillo A, Palmieri G, Manzia TM, Baiocchi L, et al. Complete weaning off immunosuppression in HCV liver transplant recipients is feasible and favourably impacts on the progression of disease recurrence. *J Hepatol.* (2006) 44:702–9. doi: 10.1016/j.jhep.2005.11.047
4. Benseler V, McCaughan GW, Schlitt HJ, Bishop GA, Bowen DG, Bertolino P. The liver: a special case in transplantation tolerance. *Semin Liver Dis.* (2007) 27:194–213. doi: 10.1055/s-2007-979471
5. Jenne CN, Kubes P. Immune surveillance by the liver. *Nat Immunol.* (2013) 14:996–1006. doi: 10.1038/ni.2691
6. Crispe IN. The liver as a lymphoid organ. *Annu Rev Immunol.* (2009) 27:147–63. doi: 10.1146/annurev.immunol.021908.132629
7. Taimr P, Higuchi H, Kocova E, Rippe RA, Friedman S, Gores GJ. Activated stellate cells express the TRAIL receptor-2/death receptor-5 and undergo TRAIL-mediated apoptosis. *Hepatology.* (2003) 37:87–95. doi: 10.1053/jhep.2003.50002
8. Ochi M, Ohdan H, Mitsuta H, Onoe T, Tokita D, Hara H, et al. Liver NK cells expressing TRAIL are toxic against self hepatocytes in mice. *Hepatology.* (2004) 39:1321–31. doi: 10.1002/hep.20204
9. Bamboat ZM, Stableford JA, Plitas G, Burt BM, Nguyen HM, Welles AP, et al. Human liver dendritic cells promote T cell hyporesponsiveness. *J Immunol.* (2009) 182:1901–11. doi: 10.4049/jimmunol.0803404
10. Goubier A, Dubois B, Gheit H, Joubert G, Villard-Truc F, Asselin-Paturel C, et al. Plasmacytoid dendritic cells mediate oral tolerance. *Immunity.* (2008) 29:464–75. doi: 10.1016/j.immuni.2008.06.017
11. Xia S, Guo Z, Xu X, Yi H, Wang Q, Cao X. Hepatic microenvironment programs hematopoietic progenitor differentiation into regulatory dendritic cells, maintaining liver tolerance. *Blood.* (2008) 112:3175–85. doi: 10.1182/blood-2008-05-159921
12. Castellaneta A, Sumpter TL, Chen L, Tokita D, Thomson AW. NOD2 ligation subverts IFN-α production by liver plasmacytoid dendritic cells and inhibits their T cell allostimulatory activity via B7-H1 up-regulation. *J Immunol.* (2009) 183:6922–32. doi: 10.4049/jimmunol.0900582

13. Takayama T, Morelli AE, Onai N, Hirao M, Matsushima K, Tahara H, et al. Mammalian and viral IL-10 enhance C-C chemokine receptor 5 but down-regulate C-C chemokine receptor 7 expression by myeloid dendritic cells: impact on chemotactic responses and *in vivo* homing ability. *J Immunol.* (2001) 166:7136–43. doi: 10.4049/jimmunol.166.12.7136
14. Knolle PA, Uhrig A, Hegenbarth S, Löser E, Schmitt E, Gerken G, et al. IL-10 down-regulates T cell activation by antigen-presenting liver sinusoidal endothelial cells through decreased antigen uptake via the mannose receptor and lowered surface expression of accessory molecules. *Clin Exp Immunol.* (1998) 114:427–33. doi: 10.1046/j.1365-2249.1998.00713.x
15. Carambia A, Freund B, Schwinge D, Heine M, Laschtowitz A, Huber S, et al. TGF-b-dependent induction of $CD4^+$ $CD25^+$ $Foxp3^+$ Tregs by liver sinusoidal endothelial cells. *J Hepatol.* (2014) 61:594–9. doi: 10.1016/j.jhep.2014.04.027
16. Limmer A, Ohl J, Kurts C, Ljunggren HG, Reiss Y, Groettrup M, et al. Efficient presentation of exogenous antigen by liver endothelial cells to CD8+ T cells results in antigen-specific T-cell tolerance. *Nat Med.* (2000) 6:1348–54. doi: 10.1038/82161
17. Diehl L, Schurich A, Grochtmann R, Hegenbarth S, Chen L, Knolle PA. Tolerogenic maturation of liver sinusoidal endothelial cells promotes B7-homolog 1-dependent CD8+ T cell tolerance. *Hepatology.* (2008) 47:296–305. doi: 10.1002/hep.21965
18. Carambia A, Frenzel C, Bruns OT, Schwinge D, Reimer R, Hohenberg H, et al. Inhibition of inflammatory CD4 T cell activity by murine liver sinusoidal endothelial cells. *J Hepatol.* (2013) 58:112–8. doi: 10.1016/j.jhep.2012.09.008
19. Tokita D, Shishida M, Ohdan H, Onoe T, Hara H, Tanaka Y, et al. Liver sinusoidal endothelial cells that endocytose allogeneic cells suppress T cells with indirect allospecificity. *J Immunol.* (2006) 177:3615–24. doi: 10.4049/jimmunol.177.6.3615
20. Kuniyasu Y, Marfani SM, Bin Inayat I, Sheikh SZ, Mehal WZ. Kupffer cells required for high affinity peptide-induced deletion, not retention, of activated $CD8^+$ T cells by mouse liver. *Hepatology.* (2004) 39:1017–27. doi: 10.1002/hep.20153
21. You Q, Cheng L, Kedl RM, Ju C. Mechanism of T cell tolerance induction by murine hepatic kupffer cells. *Hepatology.* (2008) 48:978–90. doi: 10.1002/hep.22395
22. Heymann F, Peusquens J, Ludwig-Portugall I, Kohlhepp M, Ergen C, Niemietz P, et al. Liver inflammation abrogates immunological tolerance induced by kupffer cells. *Hepatology.* (2015) 62:279–91. doi: 10.1002/hep.27793
23. Yu MC, Chen CH, Liang X, Wang L, Gandhi CR, Fung JJ, et al. Inhibition of T-cell responses by hepatic stellate cells via B7-H1-mediated T-cell apoptosis in mice. *Hepatology.* (2004) 96:17–24. doi: 10.1002/hep.20488
24. Yang HR, Hsieh CC, Wang L, Fung JJ, Lu L, Qian S. A critical role of trail expressed on cotransplanted hepatic stellate cells in prevention of islet allograft rejection. *Microsurgery.* (2010) 30:332–7. doi: 10.1002/micr.20697
25. Ichikawa S, Mucida D, Tyznik AJ, Kronenberg M, Cheroutre H. Hepatic stellate cells function as regulatory bystanders. *J Immunol.* (2011) 186:5549–55. doi: 10.4049/jimmunol.1003917
26. Dunham RM, Thapa M, Velazquez VM, Elrod EJ, Denning TL, Pulendran B, et al. Hepatic stellate cells preferentially induce $Foxp^{3+}$ regulatory T cells by production of retinoic acid. *J Immunol.* (2013) 190:2009–16. doi: 10.4049/jimmunol.1201937
27. Herkel J, Jagemann B, Wiegard C, Garcia Lazaro JF, Lueth S, Kanzler S, et al. MHC class II-expressing hepatocytes function as antigen-presenting cells and activate specific CD4 T lymphocytes. *Hepatology.* (2003) 37:1079–85. doi: 10.1053/jhep.2003.50191
28. Franco A, Barnaba V, Natali P, Balsano C, Musca A, Balsano F. Expression of class I and class II major histocompatibility complex antigens on human hepatocytes. *Hepatology.* (1988) 8:449–54. doi: 10.1002/hep.1840080302
29. Mühlbauer M, Fleck M, Schütz C, Weiss T, Froh M, Blank C, et al. PD-L1 is induced in hepatocytes by viral infection and by interferon-α and -γ and mediates T cell apoptosis. *J Hepatol.* (2006) 45:520–8. doi: 10.1055/s-2006-931751
30. Wahl C, Bochtler P, Chen L, Schirmbeck R, Reimann J. B7-H1 on hepatocytes facilitates priming of specific CD8 T cells but limits the specific recall of primed responses. *Gastroenterology.* (2008) 135:980–8. doi: 10.1053/j.gastro.2008.05.076
31. Burghardt S, Erhardt A, Claass B, Huber S, Adler G, Jacobs T, et al. Hepatocytes contribute to immune regulation in the liver by activation of the notch signaling pathway in T cells. *J Immunol.* (2013) 191:5574–82. doi: 10.4049/jimmunol.1300826
32. Lumsden AB, Henderson JM, Kutner MH. Endotoxin levels measured by a chromogenic assay in portal, hepatic and peripheral venous blood in patients with cirrhosis. *Hepatology.* (1988) 8:232–6. doi: 10.1002/hep.1840080207
33. Catalá M, Antón A, Portolés MT. Characterization of the simultaneous binding of *Escherichia coli* endotoxin to kupffer and endothelial liver cells by flow cytometry. *Cytometry.* (1999) 36:123–130. doi: 10.1002/(SICI)1097-032036:2<123::AID-CYTO6>3.0.CO;2-Y
34. Tu Z, Bozorgzadeh A, Crispe IN, Orloff MS. The activation state of human intrahepatic lymphocytes. *Clin Exp Immunol.* (2007) 149:186–93. doi: 10.1111/j.1365-2249.2007.03415.x
35. Doherty DG, O'Farrelly C. Innate and adaptive lymphoid cells in the human liver. *Immunol Rev.* (2000) 174:5–20. doi: 10.1034/j.1600-0528.2002.017416.x
36. Gao B, Jeong W II, Tian Z. Liver: an organ with predominant innate immunity. *Hepatology.* (2008) 47:729–36. doi: 10.1002/hep.22034
37. Radaeva S, Sun R, Jaruga B, Nguyen VT, Tian Z, Gao B. Natural killer cells ameliorate liver fibrosis by killing activated stellate cells in NKG2D-dependent and tumor necrosis factor related apoptosis inducing ligand-dependent manners. *Gastroenterology.* (2006) 130:435–52. doi: 10.1053/j.gastro.2005.10.055
38. Melhem A, Muhanna N, Bishara A, Alvarez CE, Ilan Y, Bishara T, et al. Anti-fibrotic activity of NK cells in experimental liver injury through killing of activated HSC. *J Hepatol.* (2006) 45:60–71. doi: 10.1016/j.jhep.2005.12.025
39. Martins EB, Graham AK, Chapman RW, Fleming KA. Elevation of γδT lymphocytes in peripheral blood and livers of patients with primary sclerosing cholangitis and other autoimmune liver diseases. *Hepatology.* (1996) 23:988–93. doi: 10.1053/jhep.1996.v23.pm0008621180
40. Hammerich L, Tacke F. Role of gamma-delta T cells in liver inflammation and fibrosis. *World J Gastrointest Pathophysiol.* (2014) 5:107–13. doi: 10.4291/wjgp.v5.i2.107
41. Schurich A, Berg M, Stabenow D, Böttcher J, Kern M, Schild H-J, et al. Dynamic regulation of CD8 T cell tolerance induction by liver sinusoidal endothelial cells. *J Immunol.* (2010) 184:4107–14. doi: 10.4049/jimmunol.0902580
42. Knoll P, Schlaak J, Uhrig A, Kempf P, zum Büschenfelde KHM, Gerken G. Human kupffer cells secrete IL-10 in response to lipopolysaccharide (LPS) challenge. *J Hepatol.* (1995) 22:226–9. doi: 10.1016/0168-8278(95)80433-1
43. Kruse N, Neumann K, Schrage A, Derkow K, Schott E, Erben U, et al. Priming of CD4+ T cells by liver sinusoidal endothelial cells induces CD25low forkhead box protein 3- regulatory T cells suppressing autoimmune hepatitis. *Hepatology.* (2009) 50:1904–13. doi: 10.1002/hep.23191
44. Schildberg FA, Hegenbarth SI, Schumak B, Limmer A, Knolle PA. Liver sinusoidal endothelial cells veto CD8 T cell activation by antigen-presenting dendritic cells. *Eur J Immunol.* (2008) 38:957–67. doi: 10.1002/eji.200738060
45. Onoe T, Ohdan H, Tokita D, Shishida M, Tanaka Y, Hara H, et al. Liver sinusoidal endothelial cells tolerize T cells across MHC barriers in mice. *J Immunol.* (2005) 175:139–46. doi: 10.4049/jimmunol.175.1.139
46. Ebe Y, Hasegawa G, Takatsuka H, Umezu H, Mitsuyama M, Arakawa M, et al. The role of kupffer cells and regulation of neutrophil migration into the liver by macrophage inflammatory protein-2 in primary listeriosis in mice. *Pathol Int.* (1999) 49:519–32. doi: 10.1046/j.1440-1827.1999.00910.x
47. Lee WY, Moriarty TJ, Wong CHY, Zhou H, Strieter RM, Van Rooijen N, et al. An intravascular immune response to borrelia burgdorferi involves kupffer cells and iNKT cells. *Nat Immunol.* (2010) 11:295–302. doi: 10.1038/ni.1855
48. Helmy KY, Katschke KJ, Gorgani NN, Kljavin NM, Elliott JM, Diehl L, et al. CRIg: A macrophage complement receptor required for phagocytosis of circulating pathogens. *Cell.* (2006) 124:915–27. doi: 10.1016/j.cell.2005.12.039
49. Chensue SW, Terebuh PD, Remick DG, Scales WE, Kunkel SL. *In vivo* biologic and immunohistochemical analysis of interleukin-1 alpha, beta and tumor necrosis factor during experimental endotoxemia. Kinetics, kuppfer cell expression, and glucocorticoid effects. *Am J Pathol.* (1991) 138:395–402.
50. Perez R V, Swanson C, Morgan M, Erickson K, Hubbard NE, German JB. Portal venous transfusion up-regulates kupffer cell cyclooxygenase activity: a mechanism of immunosuppression in organ transplantation. *Transplantation.* (1997) 64:135 9. doi: 10.1097/00007890 199707150 00023
51. Winau F, Quack C, Darmoise A, Kaufmann SH. Starring stellate cells in liver immunology. *Curr Opin Immunol.* (2008)

20:68–74. doi: 10.1016/j.coi.2007.10.006

52. Trautwein C, Friedman SL, Schuppan D, Pinzani M. Hepatic fibrosis: Concept to treatment. *J Hepatol.* (2015) 62(Suppl. 1):S15–24. doi: 10.1016/j.jhep.2015.02.039
53. Talwalkar JA, Lindor KD. Primary biliary cirrhosis. *Lancet.* (2015) 386:10003. doi: 10.1016/S0140-6736(15)00154-3
54. Karlsen TH, Boberg KM. Update on primary sclerosing cholangitis. *J Hepatol.* (2013) 59:571–82. doi: 10.1016/B978-1-4377-0881-3.00042-5
55. Geller SA. Autoimmune hepatitis: histopathology. *Clin Liver Dis.* (2014) 3:19–23. doi: 10.1002/cld.301
56. European Association for the Study of the Liver. EASL clinical practice guidelines: autoimmune hepatitis. *J Hepatol.* (2015) 63:971–1004. doi: 10.1016/j.jhep.2015.06.030
57. Alvarez F, Berg PA, Bianchi FB, Bianchi L, Burroughs AK, Cancado EL, et al. International autoimmune hepatitis group report: review of criteria for diagnosis of autoimmune hepatitis. *J Hepatol.* (1999) 31:929–38. doi: 10.1016/S0168-8278(99)80297-9
58. Hennes EM, Zeniya M, Czaja AJ, Parés A, Dalekos GN, Krawitt EL, et al. Simplified criteria for the diagnosis of autoimmune hepatitis. *Hepatology.* (2008) 48:169–76. doi: 10.1002/hep.22322
59. Boberg KM, Aadland E, Jahnsen J, Raknerud N, Stiris M, Bell H. Incidence and prevalence of primary biliary cirrhosis, primary sclerosing cholangitis, and autoimmune hepatitis in a norwegian population. *Scand J Gastroenterol.* (1998) 33:99–103. doi: 10.1080/00365529850166284
60. Ngu JH, Bechly K, Chapman BA, Burt MJ, Barclay ML, Gearry RB, et al. Population-based epidemiology study of autoimmune hepatitis: A disease of older women? *J Gastroenterol Hepatol.* (2010) 25:1681–6. doi: 10.1111/j.1440-1746.2010.06384.x
61. Van Gerven NMF, Verwer BJ, Witte BI, Van Erpecum KJ, Van Buuren HR, Maijers I, et al. Epidemiology and clinical characteristics of autoimmune hepatitis in the Netherlands. *Scand J Gastroenterol.* (2014) 49:1245–54. doi: 10.3109/00365521.2014.946083
62. Werner M, Prytz H, Ohlsson B, Almer S, Björnsson E, Bergquist A, et al. Epidemiology and the initial presentation of autoimmune hepatitis in Sweden: a nationwide study. *Scand J Gastroenterol.* (2008) 43:1232–40. doi: 10.1080/00365520802130183
63. Grønbæk L, Vilstrup H, Jepsen P. Autoimmune hepatitis in Denmark: incidence, prevalence, prognosis, and causes of death. A nationwide registry-based cohort study. *J Hepatol.* (2014) 60:612–17. doi: 10.1016/j.jhep.2013.10.020
64. Boonstra K, Beuers U, Ponsioen CY. Epidemiology of primary sclerosing cholangitis and primary biliary cirrhosis: a systematic review. *J Hepatol.* (2012) 56:1181–8. doi: 10.1016/j.jhep.2011.10.025
65. Boonstra K, Kunst AE, Stadhouders PH, Tuynman HA, Poen AC, van Nieuwkerk KMJ, et al. Rising incidence and prevalence of primary biliary cirrhosis: a large population-based study. *Liver Int.* (2014) 34:31–38. doi: 10.1111/liv.12434
66. Czaja AJ. The overlap syndromes of autoimmune hepatitis. *Dig Dis Sci.* (2013) 58:326–43. doi: 10.1007/s10620-012-2367-1
67. Card TR, Solaymani-Dodaran M, West J. Incidence and mortality of primary sclerosing cholangitis in the UK: a POPULATION-BASED COHORT STUDY. *J HEPATOL.* (2008) 48:939–44. doi: 10.1016/J.JHEP.2008.02.017
68. Liang H, Manne S, Shick J, Lissoos T, Dolin P. Incidence, prevalence, and natural history of primary sclerosing cholangitis in the United Kingdom. *Med.* (2017) 96:e7116. doi: 10.1097/MD.0000000000007116
69. Hirschfield GM, Karlsen TH, Lindor KD, Adams DH. Primary sclerosing cholangitis. *Lancet.* (2013) 382:1587–99. doi: 10.1016/S0140-6736(13)60096-3
70. Mells GF, Kaser A, Karlsen TH. Novel insights into autoimmune liver diseases provided by genome-wide association studies. *J Autoimmun.* (2013) 46:41–54. doi: 10.1016/j.jaut.2013.07.004
71. Donaldson P. Susceptibility to autoimmune chronic active hepatitis: human leukocyte antigens DR4 and A1-B8-DR3 are independent risk factors. *Hepatology.* (1991) 13:701–6. doi: 10.1002/hep.1840130415
72. Czaja AJ, Carpenter HA, Santrach PJ, Moore BS. Significance of HLA DR4 in type 1 autoimmune. *Gastroenterologylogy.* (1993) 105:1502–7. doi: 10.1016/0016-5085(93)90157-8
73. Montano-Loza AJ, Carpenter HA, Czaja AJ. Clinical significance of HLA DRB1 *03-DRB1 * 04 in type 1 autoimmune hepatitis. *Liver Int.* (2006) 26:1201–8. doi: 10.1111/j.1478-3231.2006.01387.x
74. Ma Y, Bogdanos DP, Hussain MJ, Underhill J, Bansal S, Longhi MS, et al. Polyclonal T-cell responses to cytochrome P450IID6 are associated with disease activity in autoimmune hepatitis type 2. *Gastroenterology.* (2006) 130:868–82. doi: 10.1053/j.gastro.2005.12.020
75. Gregorio G V., Portmann B, Reid F, Donaldson PT, Doherty DG, McCartney M, et al. Autoimmune hepatitis in childhood: a 20-year experience. *Hepatology.* (1997) 25:541–7. doi: 10.1002/hep.510250308
76. Teufel A, Weinmann A, Kahaly GJ, Centner C, Piendl A, Wörns M, et al. Concurrent autoimmune diseases in patients with autoimmune hepatitis. *J Clin Gastroenterol.* (2010) 44:208–13. doi: 10.1097/MCG.0b013e3181c74e0d
77. Manns MP, Bremm A, Schneider PM, Notghi A, Gerken G, Prager-Eberle M, et al. HLA DRw8 and complement C4 deficiency as risk factors in primary biliary cirrhosis. *Gastroenterology.* (1991) 101:1367–73. doi: 10.1016/0016-5085(91)90090-8
78. Invernizzi P, Selmi C, Poli F, Frison S, Floreani A, Alvaro D, et al. Human leukocyte antigen polymorphisms in Italian primary biliary cirrhosis: a multicenter study of 664 patients and 1992 healthy controls. *Hepatology.* (2008) 48:1906–12. doi: 10.1002/hep.22567
79. Spurkland A, Saarinen S, Boberg KM, Mitchell S, Broome U, Caballeria L, et al. HLA class II haplotypes in primary sclerosing cholangitis patients from five European populations. *Tissue Antigens.* (1999) 53:459–69. doi: 10.1034/j.1399-0039.1999.530502.x
80. Donaldson PT, Norris S. Immunogenetics in PSC. *Best Pract Res Clin Gastroenterol.* (2001) 15:611–27. doi: 10.1053/bega.2001.0208
81. Czaja A, Donaldson P. Genetic susceptibilities for immune expression and liver cell injury in autoimmune hepatitis. *Immunol Rev.* (2000) 174:250–9. doi: 10.1034/j.1600-0528.2002.017401.x
82. Chaouali M, Carvalho A, Tezeghdenti A, Ben Azaiez M, Cunha C, Ghazouani E, et al. Cytotoxic T lymphocyte antigen-4 gene polymorphisms and susceptibility to type 1 autoimmune hepatitis in the tunisian population. *Genes Dis.* (2018) 5:256–62. doi: 10.1016/j.gendis.2017.12.006
83. Walker EJ, Hirschfield GM, Xu C, Lu Y, Liu X, Lu Y, et al. CTLA4/ICOS gene variants and haplotypes are associated with rheumatoid arthritis and primary biliary cirrhosis in the Canadian population. *Arthritis Rheum.* (2009) 60:931–7. doi: 10.1002/art.24412
84. Juran BD, Atkinson EJ, Larson JJ, Schlicht EM, Liu X, Heathcote EJ, et al. Carriage of a tumor necrosis factor polymorphism amplifies the cytotoxic T-lymphocyte antigen 4 attributed risk of primary biliary cirrhosis: evidence for a gene-gene interaction. *Hepatology.* (2010) 52:223–9. doi: 10.1002/hep.23667
85. Ji SG, Juran BD, Mucha S, Folseraas T, Jostins L, Melum E, et al. Genome-wide association study of primary sclerosing cholangitis identifies new risk loci and quantifies the genetic relationship with inflammatory bowel disease. *Nat Genet.* (2017) 49:269–73. doi: 10.1038/ng.3745
86. Wiencke K, Boberg KM, Donaldson P, Harbo H, Ling V, Schrumpf E, et al. No major effect of the CD28/CTLA4/ICOS gene region on susceptibility to primary sclerosing cholangitis. *Scand J Gastroenterol.* (2006) 41:586–91. doi: 10.1080/00365520500377870
87. Kristiansen OP, Larsen ZM, Pociot F. CTLA-4 in autoimmune diseases - A general susceptibility gene to autoimmunity? *Genes Immun.* (2000) 1:170–84. doi: 10.1038/sj.gene.6363655
88. Zhernakova A, Withoff S, Wijmenga C. Clinical implications of shared genetics and pathogenesis in autoimmune diseases. *Nat Rev Endocrinol.* (2013) 9:646–59. doi: 10.1038/nrendo.2013.161
89. Hirschfield GM, Liu X, Xu C, Lu Y, Xie G, Lu Y, et al. Primary biliary cirrhosis associated with HLA, IL12A, and IL12RB2 variants. *N Engl J Med.* (2009) 360:2544–55. doi: 10.1056/NEJMoa0810440
90. Broomé U, Olsson R, Lööf L, Bodemar G, Hultcrantz R, Danielsson Å, et al. Natural history and prognostic factors in 305 Swedish patients with primary sclerosing cholangitis. *Gut.* (1996) 38:610–15. doi: 10.1136/gut.38.4.610
91. Lunder AK, Hov JR, Borthne A, Gleditsch J, Johannesen G, Tveit K, et al. Prevalence of sclerosing cholangitis detected by magnetic resonance cholangiography in patients with long-term inflammatory bowel disease. *Gastroenterology.* (2016) 151:660–9.e4. doi: 10.1053/j.gastro.2016.06.021
92. Schramm C, Eaton J, Ringe KI, Venkatesh S, Yamamura J. Recommendations on the use of magnetic resonance imaging in PSC-A position statement from the international PSC study group. *Hepatology.* (2017) 66:1675–88. doi: 10.1002/hep.29293
93. Kumagai J, Taida T, Ogasawara S, Nakagawa T, Iino Y, Shingyoji

A, et al. Clinical characteristics and outcomes of primary sclerosing cholangitis and ulcerative colitis in Japanese patients. *PLoS ONE.* (2018) 13:e0209352. doi: 10.1371/journal.pone.0209352
94. Hov JR, Boberg KM, Karlsen TH. Autoantibodies in primary sclerosing cholangitis. *World J Gastroenterol.* (2008) 14:3781–91. doi: 10.3748/wjg.14.3781
95. Muratori P, Lalanne C, Fabbri A, Cassani F, Lenzi M, Muratori L. Type 1 and type 2 autoimmune hepatitis in adults share the same clinical phenotype. *Aliment Pharmacol Ther.* (2015) 41:1281–7. doi: 10.1111/apt.13210
96. von Mühlen CA, Tan EM. Autoantibodies in the diagnosis of systemicrheumatic diseases. *Semin Arthritis Rheum.* (1995) 24:323–58. doi: 10.1016/S0049-0172(95)80004-2
97. McMillan SA, Haire M. The specificity of IgG- and IgM-class smooth muscle antibody in the sera of patients with multiple sclerosis and active chronic hepatitis. *Clin Immunol Immunopathol.* (1979) 14:256–63. doi: 10.1016/0090-1229(79)90148-X
98. Verstegen G, Duyck MC, Meeus P, Ravelingien I, De Vlam K. Detection and identification of antinuclear antibodies (ANA) in a large community hospital. *Acta Clin Belg.* (2009) 64:317–23. doi: 10.1179/acb.2009.049
99. Czaja AJ, Cassani F, Cataleta M, Valentini P, Bianchi FB. Frequency and significance of antibodies to actin in type 1 autoimmune hepatitis. *Hepatology.* (1996) 24:1068–73. doi: 10.1002/hep.510240515
100. Lidman K, Biberfeld G, Fagraeus A, Norberg R, Torstensson R, Utter G, et al. Anti-actin specificity of human smooth muscle antibodies in chronic active hepatitis. *Clin Exp Immunol.* (1976) 24:266–72.
101. Dalekos GN, Wedemeyer H, Obermayer-Straub P, Kayser A, Barut A, Frank H, et al. Epitope mapping of cytochrome P4502D6 autoantigen in patients with chronic hepatitis C during α-interferon treatment. *J Hepatol.* (1999) 30:366–75. doi: 10.1016/S0168-8278(99)80092-0
102. Kerkar N, Choudhuri K, Ma Y, Mahmoud A, Bogdanos DP, Muratori L, et al. Cytochrome P4502D6193-212: a new immunodominant epitope and target of virus/self cross-reactivity in liver kidney microsomal autoantibody type 1-positive liver disease. *J Immunol.* (2003) 170:1481–9. doi: 10.4049/jimmunol.170.3.1481
103. Manns M, Kyriatsoulis A, Gerken G, Staritz M, Meyer KH, Büschenfelde Z. Characterisation of a new subgroup of autoimmune chronic active hepatitis by autoantibodies against a soluble liver antigen. *Lancet.* (1987) 329:292–4. doi: 10.1016/S0140-6736(87)92024-1
104. Vitozzi S, Djilali-Saiah I, Lapierre P, Alvarez F. Anti-soluble liver antigen/liver-pancreas (SLA/LP) antibodies in pediatric patients with autoimmune hepatitis. *Autoimmunity.* (2002) 35:485–92. doi: 10.1080/0891693021000056712
105. Stechemesser E, Klein R, Berg PA. Characterization and clinical relevance of liver-pancreas antibodies in autoimmune hepatitis. *Hepatology.* (1993) 18:1–9. doi: 10.1002/hep.1840180102
106. Manns MP, Vogel A. Autoimmune hepatitis, from mechanisms to therapy. *Hepatology.* (2006) 43(2 Suppl. 1):S132–44. doi: 10.1002/hep.21059
107. Longhi MS, Ma Y, Mieli-Vergani G, Vergani D. Aetiopathogenesis of autoimmune hepatitis. *J Autoimmun.* (2010) 34:7–14. doi: 10.1016/j.jaut.2009.08.010
108. Longhi MS, Hussain MJ, Bogdanos DP, Quaglia A, Mieli-Vergani G, Ma Y, et al. Cytochrome P450IID6-specific CD8 T cell immune responses mirror disease activity in autoimmune hepatitis type 2. *Hepatology.* (2007) 46:472–84. doi: 10.1002/hep.21658
109. Cassani F, Cataleta M, Valentini P, Muratori P, Giostra F, Francesconi R, et al. Serum autoantibodies in chronic hepatitis C: comparison with autoimmune hepatitis and impact on the disease profile. *Hepatology.* (1997) 26:561–6. doi: 10.1002/hep.510260305
110. Walker JG, Doniach D, Roitt IM, Sherlock S. Serological tests in diagnosis of primary biliary cirrhosis. *Lancet.* (1965) 285:827–31. doi: 10.1016/S0140-6736(65)91372-3
111. Gershwin ME, Mackay IR, Sturgess A, Coppel RL. Identification and specificity of a cDNA encoding the 70 kd mitochondrial antigen recognized in primary biliary cirrhosis. *J Immunol.* (1987) 138:3525–31.
112. Yeaman SJ, Danner DJ, Mutimer DJ, M Fussey SP, W James OF, Bassendine MF. Primary biliary cirrhosis: identification of two major M2 mitochondrial antigens. *Lancet.* (1988) 331:1067–70. doi: 10.1016/S0140-6736(88)91894-6
113. Vergani D, Alvarez F, Bianchi FB, Cançado ELR, MacKay IR, Manns MP, et al. Liver autoimmune serology: a consensus statement from the committee for autoimmune serology of the international autoimmune hepatitis group. *J Hepatol.* (2004) 41:677–83. doi: 10.1016/j.jhep.2004.08.002
114. Tsuneyama K, Van De Water J, Van Thiel D, Coppel R, Ruebner B, Nakanuma Y, et al. Abnormal expression of PDC-E2 on the apical surface of biliary epithelial cells in patients with antimitochondrial antibody-negative primary biliary cirrhosis. *Hepatology.* (1995) 22:1440–6. doi: 10.1002/hep.1840220517
115. Van de Water J, Turchany J, Leung PSC, Lake J, Munoz S, Surh CD, et al. Molecular mimicry in primary biliary cirrhosis. Evidence for biliary epithelial expression of a molecule cross-reactive with pyruvate dehydrogenase complex-E2. *J Clin Invest.* (1993) 91:2653–64. doi: 10.1172/JCI116504
116. Gershwin ME, Selmi C, Worman HJ, Gold EB, Watnik M, Utts J, et al. Risk factors and comorbidities in primary biliary cirrhosis: a controlled interview-based study of 1032 patients. *Hepatology.* (2005) 42:1194–202. doi: 10.1002/hep.20907
117. Corpechot C, Chrétien Y, Chazouillères O, Poupon R. Demographic, lifestyle, medical and familial factors associated with primary biliary cirrhosis. *J Hepatol.* (2010) 53:162–9. doi: 10.1016/j.jhep.2010.02.019
118. Morreale M, Tsirigotis M, Hughes MD, Brumfitt W, McIntyre N, Burroughs AK. Significant bacteriuria has prognostic significance in primary biliary cirrhosis. *J Hepatol.* (1989) 9:149–58. doi: 10.1016/0168-8278(89)90045-7
119. CooK GC, Mulligan R, Sherlock S. Controlled prospective trial of corticosteroid therapy in active chronic hepatitis. *QJM.* (1971) 40:159–85. doi: 10.1093/oxfordjournals.qjmed.a067264
120. Murray-Lyon IM, Stern RB, Williams R. Controlled trial of prednisone and azathioprine in active chronic hepatitis. *Lancet.* (1973) 301:735–7. doi: 10.1016/S0140-6736(73)92125-9
121. Soloway RD, Summerskill WH, Baggenstoss AH, Geall MG, Gitnićk GL, Elveback IR, et al. Clinical, biochemical, and histological remission of severe chronic active liver disease: a controlled study of treatments and early prognosis. *Gastroenterology.* (1972) 63:820–33. doi: 10.1016/S0016-5085(19)33223-8
122. Johnson PJ, Mcfarlane IG, Williams R. Azathioprine for long-term maintenance of remission in autoimmune hepatitis. *N Engl J Med.* (1995) 333:958–63. doi: 10.1056/NEJM199510123331502
123. Werner M, Almer S, Prytz H, Lindgren S, Wallerstedt S, Björnsson E, et al. Hepatic and extrahepatic malignancies in autoimmune hepatitis. A long-term follow-up in 473 Swedish patients. *J Hepatol.* (2009) 50:388–93. doi: 10.1016/j.jhep.2008.08.022
124. Hoeroldt B, McFarlane E, Dube A, Basumani P, Karajeh M, Campbell MJ, et al. Long-term outcomes of patients with autoimmune hepatitis managed at a nontransplant center. *Gastroenterology.* (2011) 140:1980–9. doi: 10.1053/j.gastro.2011.02.065
125. Gleeson D. Long-term outcomes of autoimmune hepatitis. *Clin Liver Dis.* (2019) 14:24–8. doi: 10.1002/cld.797
126. Floreani A, Liberal R, Vergani D, Mieli-Vergani G. Autoimmune hepatitis: contrasts and comparisons in children and adults - A comprehensive review. *J Autoimmun.* (2013) 46:7–16. doi: 10.1016/j.jaut.2013.08.004
127. Manns MP, Woynarowski M, Kreisel W, Lurie Y, Rust C, Zuckerman E, et al. Budesonide induces remission more effectively than prednisone in a controlled trial of patients with autoimmune hepatitis. *Gastroenterology.* (2010) 139:1198–206. doi: 10.1053/j.gastro.2010.06.046
128. Rudic JS, Poropat G, Krstic MN, Bjelakovic G, Gluud C. Ursodeoxycholic acid for primary biliary cirrhosis. *Cochrane Database Syst Rev.* (2012) 12:CD000551. doi: 10.1002/14651858.CD000551.pub3
129. Poupon R. Ursodeoxycholic acid and bile-acid mimetics as therapeutic agents for cholestatic liver diseases: an overview of their mechanisms of action. *Clin Res Hepatol Gastroenterol.* (2012) 36(Suppl. 1):S3–12. doi: 10.1016/S2210-7401(12)70015-3
130. Ter Borg PCJ, Schalm SW, Hansen BE, Van Buuren HR. Prognosis of ursodeoxycholic acid-treated patients with primary biliary cirrhosis. Results of a 10-yr cohort study involving 297 patients. *Am J Gastroenterol.* (2006) 101:2044–50. doi: 10.1111/j.1572-0241.2006.00699.x
131. Poupon RE, Lindor KD, Cauch-Dudek K, Dickson ER, Poupon R, Heathcote EJ. Combined analysis of randomized controlled trials of ursodeoxycholic acid in primary biliary cirrhosis. *Gastroenterology.* (1997) 113:884–90. doi: 10.1016/S0016-5085(97)70183-5
132. Corpechot C, Abenavoli L, Rabahi N, Chrétien Y, Andréani T, Johanet C, et al. Biochemical response to ursodeoxycholic acid and long-term prognosis in primary biliary cirrhosis. *Hepatology.* (2008) 48:871–7. doi: 10.1002/hep.22428
133. Kuiper EMM, Hansen BE, de Vries RA, den Ouden-Muller JW, van Ditzhuijsen TJM, Haagsma EB, et al. Improved prognosis of patients with

primary biliary cirrhosis that have a biochemical response to ursodeoxycholic acid. *Gastroenterology.* (2009) 136:1281–7. doi: 10.1053/j.gastro.2009.01.003
134. Carbone M, Neuberger J. Liver transplantation in PBC and PSC: indications and disease recurrence. *Clin Res Hepatol Gastroenterol.* (2011) 35:446–54. doi: 10.1016/j.clinre.2011.02.007
135. Gilroy RK, Lynch S V., Strong RW, Kerlin P, Balderson GA, Stuart KA, et al. Confirmation of the role of the mayo risk score as a predictor of resource utilization after orthotopic liver transplantation for primary biliary cirrhosis. *Liver Transplant.* (2000) 6:749–52. doi: 10.1053/jlts.2000.9746
136. Graziadei IW, Wiesner RH, Batts KP, Marotta PJ, Larusso NF, Porayko MK, et al. Recurrence of primary sclerosing cholangitis following liver transplantation. *Hepatology.* (1999) 8:575–81. doi: 10.1002/hep.510290427
137. Hirschfield GM, Mason A, Luketic V, Lindor K, Gordon SC, Mayo M, et al. Efficacy of obeticholic acid in patients with primary biliary cirrhosis and inadequate response to ursodeoxycholic acid. *Gastroenterology.* (2015) 148:751–61.e8. doi: 10.1053/j.gastro.2014.12.005
138. Nevens F, Andreone P, Mazzella G, Strasser SI, Bowlus C, Invernizzi P, et al. A placebo-controlled trial of obeticholic acid in primary biliary cholangitis. *N Engl J Med.* (2016) 375:631–43. doi: 10.1056/NEJMoa1509840
139. Lindor KD, Kowdley K V., Luketic VAC, Harrison ME, McCashland T, Befeler AS, et al. High-dose ursodeoxycholic acid for the treatment of primary sclerosing cholangitis. *Hepatology.* (2009) 50:808–14. doi: 10.1002/hep.23082
140. Olsson R, Boberg KM, Schaffalitsky De Muckadell O, Lindgren S, Hultcrantz R, Folvik G, et al. High-dose ursodeoxycholic acid in primary sclerosing cholangitis: a 5-year multicenter, randomized, controlled study. *Gastroenterology.* (2005) 129:1464–72. doi: 10.1053/j.gastro.2005.08.017
141. Cullen SN, Chapman RW. Review article: current management of primary sclerosing cholangitis. *Aliment Pharmacol Ther.* (2005) 21:933–48. doi: 10.1111/j.1365-2036.2005.02407.x
142. Ponsioen CY, Vrouenraets SME, Prawirodirdjo W, Rajaram R, Rauws EAJ, Mulder CJJ, et al. Natural history of primary sclerosing cholangitis and prognostic value of cholangiography in a dutch population. *Gut.* (2002) 51:562–6. doi: 10.1136/gut.51.4.562
143. Campsen J, Zimmerman MA, Trotter JF, Wachs M, Bak T, Steinberg T, et al. Clinically recurrent primary sclerosing cholangitis following liver transplantation: a time course. *Liver Transplant.* (2008) 14:181–5. doi: 10.1002/lt.21313
144. Alabraba E, Nightingale P, Gunson B, Hubscher S, Olliff S, Mirza D, et al. A re-evaluation of the risk factors for the recurrence of primary sclerosing cholangitis in liver allografts. *Liver Transplant.* (2009) 15:330–40. doi: 10.1002/lt.21679
145. Noon L. Prophylactic inoculation against hay fever. *Lancet.* (1911) 177:1572–3. doi: 10.1016/S0140-6736(00)78276-6
146. Sabatos-Peyton CA, Verhagen J, Wraith DC. Antigen-specific immunotherapy of autoimmune and allergic diseases. *Curr Opin Immunol.* (2010) 22:609–15. doi: 10.1016/j.coi.2010.08.006
147. Serra P, Santamaria P. Antigen-specific therapeutic approaches for autoimmunity. *Nat Biotechnol.* (2019) 37:238–51. doi: 10.1038/s41587-019-0015-4
148. Wraith DC. Designing antigens for the prevention and treatment of autoimmune diseases. *Curr Opin Chem Eng.* (2018) 19:35–42. doi: 10.1016/j.coche.2017.12.004
149. Streeter HB, Rigden R, Martin KF, Scolding NJ, Wraith DC. Preclinical development and first-in-human study of ATX-MS-1467 for immunotherapy of MS. *Neurol Neuroimmunol Neuroinflamm.* (2015) 2:e93. doi: 10.1212/NXI.0000000000000093
150. Jansson L, Vrolix K, Jahraus A, Martin KF, Wraith DC. Immunotherapy with apitopes blocks the immune response to TSH receptor in HLA-DR transgenic mice. *Endocrinology.* (2018) 159:3446–57. doi: 10.1210/en.2018-00306
151. Chataway J, Martin K, Barrell K, Sharrack B, Stolt P, Wraith DC. Effects of ATX-MS-1467 immunotherapy over 16 weeks in relapsing multiple sclerosis. *Neurology.* (2018) 90:e955–62. doi: 10.1212/WNL.0000000000005118
152. Pearce SHS, Dayan C, Wraith DC, Barrell K, Olive N, Jansson L, et al. Antigen-specific immunotherapy with thyrotropin receptor peptides in graves' hyperthyroidism: a phase I study. *Thyroid.* (2019) 29:1003–11. doi: 10.1089/thy.2019.0036
153. Getts DR, Turley DM, Smith CE, Harp CT, Mccarthy D, Feeney EM, et al. Tolerance induced by apoptotic PD-L1+ and IL-10- producing splenic antigen-coupled leukocytes is induced by macrophages and maintained by T this information is current as regulatory cells. *J Immunol.* (2011) 187:2405–17. doi: 10.4049/jimmunol.1004175
154. Prasad S, Neef T, Xu D, Podojil JR, Getts DR, Shea LD, et al. Tolerogenic Ag-PLG nanoparticles induce tregs to suppress activated diabetogenic CD4 and CD8 T cells. *J Autoimmun.* (2018) 89:112–24. doi: 10.1016/j.jaut.2017.12.010
155. Freitag TL, Podojil JR, Pearson RM, Fokta FJ, Sahl C, Messing M, et al. Gliadin nanoparticles induce immune tolerance to gliadin in mouse models of celiac disease. *Gastroenterology.* (2020) 158:1667–81.e12. doi: 10.1053/j.gastro.2020.01.045
156. Galea R, Nel HJ, Talekar M, Liu X, Ooi JD, Huynh M, et al. PD-L1– and calcitriol-dependent liposomal antigen-specific regulation of systemic inflammatory autoimmune disease. *JCI Insight.* (2019) 4:e126025. doi: 10.1172/jci.insight.126025
157. Abrahimians EM, Elst L Vander, Carlier VA, Saint-Remy JM. Thioreductase-containing epitopes inhibit the development of type 1 diabetes in the NOD mouse model. *Front Immunol.* (2016) 7:67. doi: 10.3389/fimmu.2016.00067
158. Pagni PP, Bresson D, Rodriguez-Calvo T, Hani AB, Manenkova Y, Amirian N, et al. Combination therapy with an anti+IL-1β antibody and GAD65 DNA vaccine can reverse recent-onset diabetes in the RIP-GP mouse model. *Diabetes.* (2014) 63:2015–25. doi: 10.2337/db13-1257
159. Clemente-Casares X, Blanco J, Ambalavanan P, Yamanouchi J, Singha S, Fandos C, et al. Expanding antigen-specific regulatory networks to treat autoimmunity. *Nature.* (2016) 530:434–40. doi: 10.1038/nature16962
160. Umeshappa CS, Singha S, Blanco J, Shao K, Nanjundappa RH, Yamanouchi J, et al. Suppression of a broad spectrum of liver autoimmune pathologies by single peptide-MHC-based nanomedicines. *Nat Commun.* (2019) 10:2150. doi: 10.1038/s41467-019-09893-5
161. Maldonado RA, LaMothe RA, Ferrari JD, Zhang A-H, Rossi RJ, Kolte PN, et al. Polymeric synthetic nanoparticles for the induction of antigen-specific immunological tolerance. *Proc Natl Acad Sci USA.* (2015) 112:E156–65. doi: 10.1073/pnas.1408686111
162. Kishimoto TK, Ferrari JD, Lamothe RA, Kolte PN, Griset AP, O'Neil C, et al. Improving the efficacy and safety of biologic drugs with tolerogenic nanoparticles. *Nat Nanotechnol.* (2016) 11:890–9. doi: 10.1038/nnano.2016.135
163. Solvason N, Lou Y-P, Peters W, Evans E, Martinez J, Ramirez U, et al. Improved efficacy of a tolerizing DNA vaccine for reversal of hyperglycemia through enhancement of gene expression and localization to intracellular sites. *J Immunol.* (2008) 181:8298–307. doi: 10.4049/jimmunol.181.12.8298
164. Roep BO, Solvason N, Gottlieb PA, Abreu JR, Harrison LC, Eisenbarth GS, et al. Plasmid-encoded proinsulin preserves C-peptide while specifically reducing proinsulin-specific CD8 + T cells in type 1 diabetes. *Diabetes Technol Ther.* (2014) 5:191ra82. doi: 10.1126/scitranslmed.3006103
165. Carambia A, Freund B, Schwinge D, Bruns OT, Salmen SC, Ittrich H, et al. Nanoparticle-based autoantigen delivery to treg-inducing liver sinusoidal endothelial cells enables control of autoimmunity in mice. *J Hepatol.* (2015) 62:1349–56. doi: 10.1016/j.jhep.2015.01.006
166. Genain CP, Abel K, Belmar N, Villinger F, Rosenberg DP, Linington C, et al. Late complications of immune deviation therapy in a nonhuman primate. *Science.* (1996) 274:2054–7. doi: 10.1126/science.274.5295.2054
167. Rapoport B, Banuelos B, Aliesky HA, Hartwig Trier N, McLachlan SM. Critical differences between induced and spontaneous mouse models of graves' disease with implications for antigen-specific immunotherapy in humans. *J Immunol.* (2016) 197:4560–68. doi: 10.4049/jimmunol.1601393
168. Hanninen A, Braakhuis A, Heath WR, Harrison LC. Mucosal antigen primes diabetogenic cytotoxic T-lymphocytes regardless of dose or delivery route. *Diabetes.* (2001) 50:771–5. doi: 10.2337/diabetes.50.4.771
169. Steinman RM, Hawiger D, Nussenzweig MC. Tolerogenic dendritic cells. *Annu Rev Immunol.* (2003) 21:685–711. doi: 10.1146/annurev.immunol.21.120601.141040
170. Clement CC, Rotzschke O, Santambrogio L. The lymph as a pool of self-antigens. *Trends Immunol.* (2011) 32:6–11. doi: 10.1016/j.it.2010.10.004
171. Benham H, Nel HJ, Law SC, Mehdi AM, Street S, Ramnoruth N, et al. Citrullinated peptide dendritic cell immunotherapy in HLA risk genotype-positive rheumatoid arthritis patients. *Sci Transl Med.* (2015) 7:290ra87. doi: 10.1126/scitranslmed.aaa9301
172. Bell GM, Anderson AE, Diboll J, Reece R, Eltherington O, Harry RA, et al. Autologous tolerogenic dendritic cells for rheumatoid and inflammatory arthritis. *Ann Rheum Dis.* (2017) 76:227–34. doi: 10.1136/annrheumdis-2015-208456

173. Willekens B, Presas-Rodríguez S, Mansilla MJ, Derdelinckx J, Lee WP, Nijs G, et al. Tolerogenic dendritic cell-based treatment for multiple sclerosis (MS): a harmonised study protocol for two phase I clinical trials comparing intradermal and intranodal cell administration. *BMJ Open.* (2019) 9:1–11. doi: 10.1136/bmjopen-2019-030309
174. Bonifaz L, Bonnyay D, Mahnke K, Rivera M, Nussenzweig MC, Steinman RM. Efficient targeting of protein antigen to the dendritic cell receptor DEC-205 in the steady state leads to antigen presentation on major histocompatibility complex class I products and peripheral CD8+ T cell tolerance. *J Exp Med.* (2002) 196:1627–38. doi: 10.1084/jem.20021598
175. Anderton SM, Wraith DC. Hierarchy in the ability of T cell epitopes to induce peripheral tolerance to antigens from myelin. *Eur J Immunol.* (1998) 28:1251–61. doi: 10.1002/(SICI)1521-4141(199804)28:04<1251::AID-IMMU1251>3.0.CO;2-O
176. Anderton SM, Viner NJ, Matharu P, Lowrey PA, Wraith DC. Influence of a dominant cryptic epitope on autoimmune T cell tolerance. *Nat Immunol.* (2002) 3:175–81. doi: 10.1038/ni756
177. Santambrogio L, Sato AK, Fischer FR, Dorf ME, Stern LJ. Abundant empty class II MHC molecules on the surface of immature dendritic cells. *Proc Natl Acad Sci USA.* (1999) 96:15050–5. doi: 10.1073/pnas.96.26.15050
178. Metzler B, Anderton SM, Manickasingham SP, Wraith DC. Kinetics of peptide uptake and tissue distribution following a single intranasal dose of peptide. *Immunol Invest.* (2000) 29:61–70. doi: 10.3109/08820130009105145
179. Burkhart C, Liu GY, Anderton SM, Metzler B, Wraith DC. Peptide-induced T cell regulation of experimental autoimmune encephalomyelitis: a role for IL-10. *Int Immunol.* (1999) 11:1625–34. doi: 10.1093/intimm/11.10.1625
180. Sundstedt A, O'Neill EJ, Nicolson KS, Wraith DC. Role for IL-10 in suppression mediated by peptide-induced regulatory T cells *in vivo. J Immunol.* (2003) 170:1240–8. doi: 10.4049/jimmunol.170.3.1240
181. Gabryšová L, Nicolson KS, Streeter HB, Verhagen J, Sabatos-peyton C a, Morgan DJ, et al. Negative feedback control of the autoimmune response through antigen-induced differentiation of IL-10 – secreting Th1 cells. *Regulation.* (2009) 206:1755–67. doi: 10.1084/jem.20082118
182. Burton BR, Britton GJ, Fang H, Verhagen J, Smithers B, Sabatos-Peyton C a, et al. Sequential transcriptional changes dictate safe and effective antigen-specific immunotherapy. *Nat Commun.* (2014) 5:4741. doi: 10.1038/ncomms5741
183. Hartwell BL, Antunez L, Sullivan BP, Thati S, Sestak JO, Berkland C. Multivalent nanomaterials: learning from vaccines and progressing to antigen-specific immunotherapies. *J Pharm Sci.* (2015) 104:346–61. doi: 10.1002/jps.24273
184. Metzler B, Wraith DC. Inhibition of experimental autoimmune encephalomyelitis by inhalation but not oral administration of the encephalitogenic peptide: influence of MHC binding affinity. *Int Immunol.* (1993) 5:1159–65. doi: 10.1093/intimm/5.9.1159
185. Gabryšová L, Wraith DC. Antigenic strength controls the generation of antigen-specific IL-10-secreting T regulatory cells. *Eur J Immunol.* (2010) 40:1386–95. doi: 10.1002/eji.200940151
186. Groux H, O'Garra A, Bigler M, Rouleau M, Antonenko S, De Vries JE, et al. A CD4+ T-cell subset inhibits antigen-specific T-cell responses and prevents colitis. *Nature.* (1997) 389:737–42. doi: 10.1038/39614
187. Gagliani N, Magnani CF, Huber S, Gianolini ME, Pala M, Licona-Limon P, et al. Coexpression of CD49b and LAG-3 identifies human and mouse T regulatory type 1 cells. *Nat Med.* (2013) 19:739–46. doi: 10.1038/nm.3179
188. Singha S, Shao K, Yang Y, Clemente-Casares X, Solé P, Clemente A, et al. Peptide-MHC-based nanomedicines for autoimmunity function as T-cell receptor microclustering devices. *Nat Nanotechnol.* (2017) 12:701–10. doi: 10.1038/nnano.2017.56
189. Umeshappa CS, Mbongue J, Singha S, Mohapatra S, Yamanouchi J, Lee JA, et al. Ubiquitous antigen-specific T regulatory type 1 cells variably suppress hepatic and extrahepatic autoimmunity. *J Clin Invest.* (2020) 130:1823–9. doi: 10.1172/JCI130670
190. Vanderlugt CL, Miller SD. Epitope spreading in immune-mediated diseases: implications for immunotherapy. *Nat Rev Immunol.* (2002) 2:85–95. doi: 10.1038/nri724
191. Wraith D. Antigen-specific immunotherapy. *Nature.* (2016) 530:422–3. doi: 10.1038/nature17300
192. Metzler B, Wraith DC. Inhibition of T-cell responsiveness by nasal peptide administration: influence of the thymus and differential recovery of T-cell-dependent functions. *Immunology.* (1999) 97:257–63. doi: 10.1046/j.1365-2567.1999.00795.x

10

Metabolic Optimisation of Regulatory T Cells in Transplantation

*Mo Atif[1,2,3], Audrey Mohr[1], Filomena Conti[1,2], Olivier Scatton[2], Guy Gorochov[1] and Makoto Miyara[1]**

[1] Inserm U1135, Centre d'Immunologie et des Maladies Infectieuses (CIMI-Paris), Hôpital Pitié-Salpêtrière, AP-HP, Sorbonne Université, Paris, France, [2] Unité de Transplantation Hépatique, Hôpital Pitié-Salpêtrière, AP-HP, Paris, France, [3] Centre for Liver and Gastrointestinal Research, NIHR Birmingham Biomedical Research Centre, University of Birmingham, Birmingham, United Kingdom

***Correspondence:**
Makoto Miyara
makoto.miyara@aphp.fr;
makoto.miyara@psl.aphp.fr

Regulatory T (Treg) cells expressing the FOXP3 transcription factor are presently under investigation by many teams globally as a cellular therapy to induce tolerance in transplantation. This is primarily due to their immunosuppressive and homeostatic functions. Depending on the type of allograft, Treg cells will need to infiltrate and function in metabolically diverse microenvironments. This means that any resident and circulating Treg cells need to differentially adapt to counter acute or chronic allograft rejection. However, the links between Treg cell metabolism and function are still not entirely delineated. Current data suggest that Treg cells and their effector counterparts have different metabolite dependencies and metabolic programs. These properties could be exploited to optimize intragraft Treg cell function. In this review, we discuss the current paradigms regarding Treg cell metabolism and outline critical intracellular axes that link metabolism and function. Finally, we discuss how this knowledge could be clinically translated for the benefit of transplant patients.

Keywords: regulatory T cells, Treg, transplant, cell therapy, metabolism, metabolic, mTOR, hypoxia

INTRODUCTION

Novel immunomodulatory approaches are required to induce tolerance in solid organ transplantation (SOT) (1, 2). Although spontaneous tolerance has been reported in certain long-term patients (especially post-liver transplant), the majority continue to require ongoing immunosuppression (3, 4). These immunosuppressants have numerous side effects and do not overcome the challenges of delayed allograft dysfunction as well as infectious/neoplastic complications. Hence, there is an urgent clinical need for novel immunomodulatory strategies.

Regulatory T (Treg) cells are a CD4$^+$ T-cell subset that was first identified as having immunosuppressive effects in mice (5). In SOT, the presence of Treg cells in the periphery and the graft has been associated with allograft tolerance (6–8). These cells perform their functions through a range of effector cell contact-dependent and –independent mechanisms (9–13). However, in recent years several groups have identified that these functions are tightly linked to Treg cell metabolism and epigenome too (14–16) (**Figure 1**). These are important links to delineate as Treg cells need to survive and function in the metabolically demanding microenvironment of a chronically inflamed allograft. Moreover, novel data demonstrates that metabolites such as acetyl coenzyme A (acetyl CoA) and fatty acids do not just partake in different metabolic programs but can directly modulate the epigenome too (17, 18) (**Figure 2**). Through either DNA acetylation or DNA/histone methylation, these metabolites facilitate a complex network involving the epigenome, metabolism, and function of Treg cells. Delineating this network is important to understand Treg cell behavior in the allograft. In this review, we discuss Treg cell metabolism and interlink it with their diverse functions.

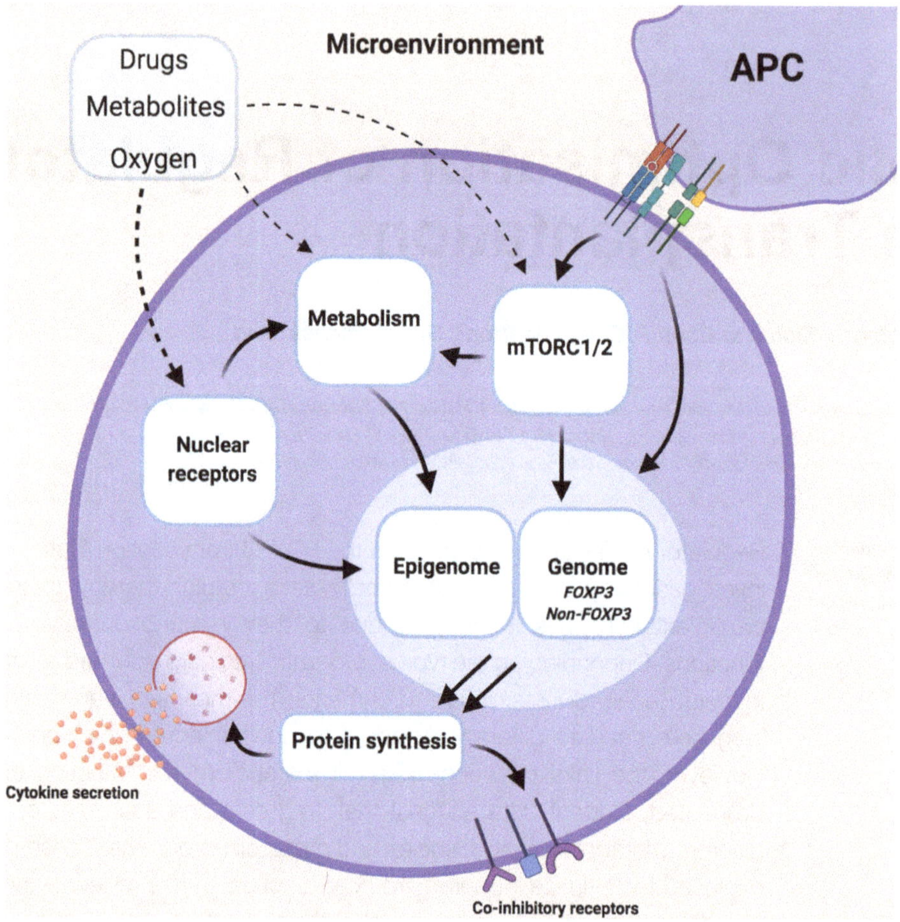

FIGURE 1 | Illustrating the influence of the microenvironment on Treg cell metabolism, epigenome and function. The inflamed tissue microenvironment consists varying concentrations of dietary metabolites, oxygen as well as concomitant immunosuppressants. These entities can individually or collectively modulate various intracellular Treg cell pathways such as mammalian transporter of rapamycin (mTOR), mitochondrial/non-mitochondrial metabolism, nuclear receptors, the epigenome and genome. This modulation has downstream consequences for the Treg cell transcriptome and overall cell function.

From a clinical perspective, the initial data from Phase I trials in transplant and non-transplant settings has shown Treg cells to be safe (1, 19–22). The current Good Manufacturing Practice (GMP) protocols center on the hypothesis that the infusion of expanded autologous Treg cells could modulate the inflamed allograft microenvironment in favor of immunoregulation instead. In parallel, Treg cells are also being modified in different ways to augment their potential activity e.g., expansion period, antigen-specificity, pharmacological agents (1, 23–25). However, metabolic modulation of Treg cells in this context has not been widely performed (26). In this review, we discuss how metabolic pathways can be exploited to improve the efficacy of Treg cell therapies in transplantation.

LINKING TREG CELL FUNCTIONS AND METABOLISM

Despite the heterogeneous phenotype of Treg cells, the expression of the Forkhead Box Protein 3 (FOXP3) transcription factor (TF) is considered as a reliable indicator of Treg cells (1, 9, 27, 28). FOXP3 in combination with T-cell receptor (TCR) activation, IL-2, mammalian transporter of rapamycin (mTOR) complexes, and others play a key role in promoting Treg cell proliferation and function.

However, to sustain these metabolically demanding processes, Treg cells rely on various stimuli, metabolites, and metabolic pathways (14, 15, 25) (**Figure 1**). These stimuli are dynamic (e.g., oxygen gradient, glucose/lipid availability) and vary depending on the type of organ and disease (29–31). In recent years, numerous publications have demonstrated how the manipulation of these metabolic factors can in turn modulate Treg cell function. This is important as Treg cells (circulating or resident) need to survive and function in diverse microenvironments (32, 33). During inflammatory diseases e.g., allograft rejection), the microenvironment is infiltrated by other effector cells, who will also start competing for metabolites to survive and function (34). From the perspective of SOT, the aim is that by exploiting cellular metabolism, one could augment Treg cell survival and function in the inflamed allograft microenvironment (**Figure 1**). This would

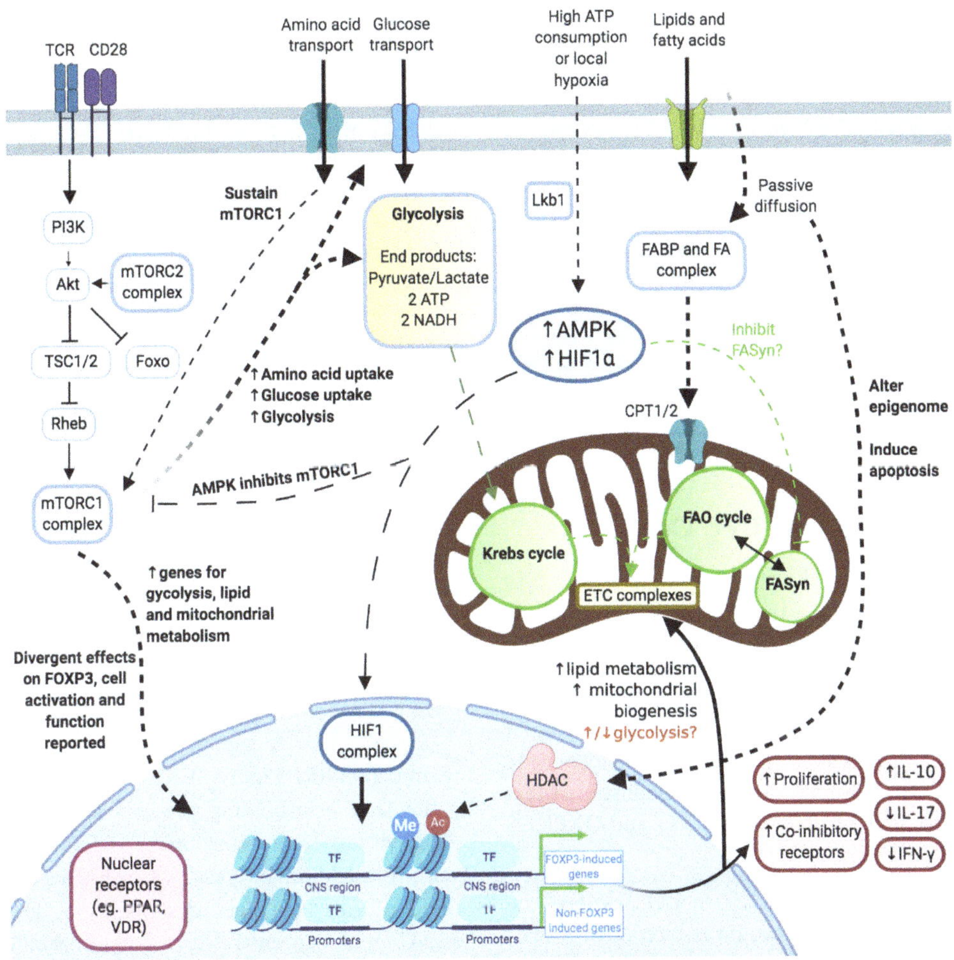

FIGURE 2 | Illustrating the complex and multiple links between Treg cell metabolism, function and the epigenome. **Activation and mTOR:** Upon acute activation, the mTORC1 complex is activated. This process is also promoted (and maintained) via amino acids. **Glucose:** Treg cells upregulate glycolysis and glucose uptake upon acute activation. **Lipids/Fatty acids:** Short- and medium-chained fatty acids are taken up into cells via passive diffusion whereas long-chain fatty acids depend on transporters. Fatty acids affect cellular survival, metabolism and epigenetics. **Hypoxia:** Hypoxia is associated with increased levels of adenosine monophosphate (AMP) and HIF1 complex. These modulate mTORC1 activity, fatty acid synthesis and the transcriptome. **Nuclear receptors:** Nuclear receptors are a key link between the steroidal and non-steroidal ligands and DNA modulation.

be an additional strategy to support either tissue-resident Treg cells or infiltrating Treg cells as part of a cellular therapy protocol.

As we discuss in the following sections, many studies into Treg cell immunometabolism have identified drugs/metabolites that mediate their roles through key intracellular axes. As these axes interlink both Treg cell metabolism and function, their modulation is a novel approach with the potential for clinical translation in SOT. In the following sections, we discuss Treg cell metabolism in-depth and contextualize this through the following three intracellular axes (**Figure 1**):

1. mTOR.
2. Hypoxia.
3. Nuclear Receptors.

For clarity, in this review we will describe naturally occurring Treg cells as thymus-derived Treg (tTreg) cells, the induced Treg cells as iTreg cells and peripheral Treg cells as pTreg cells (35).

Glycolysis in Treg Cells

Upon activation via co-stimulation of the T-cell receptor (TCR) and CD28, the signaling cascades promote glucose uptake (via Glut1 transporters) and glycolysis (Warburg effect) instead (36, 37) (**Figure 2**). This process occurs in the cytoplasm and generates 2 units of adenosine triphosphate (ATP) per mole of glucose converted to CO_2 (38). In parallel, Treg cells increase FOXP3 expression, cellular proliferation, and immunosuppressive functions (14, 15, 37, 39). It is not yet established why Treg cells switch to this less efficient ATP-generating metabolic program rather than continuing with oxidative phosphorylation (OXPHOS) – especially as cellular activation increases metabolic demands in terms of protein synthesis.

A further process to comprehend is the regulation of the end products of glycolysis (either pyruvate or lactate) (40). The balance between both of these products depends on the activity of lactate dehydrogenase (LDH) as well as the levels of nicotinamide adenine dinucleotide (reduced form; NADH and oxidized form; NAD^+) (41). This is relevant to Treg cells because FOXP3 can modulate LDH to prevent lactate formation and form pyruvate instead (40). Moreover, in a high lactate low glucose environment, Treg cells can convert lactate to pyruvate too. Whilst lactate may negatively impact on T-cell proliferation as a whole, it does not impact Treg cell immunosuppression. This is of particular relevance to tumoral microenvironments which are known to have high levels of local lactate and Treg cell accumulation (40).

If not converted to lactate, the resulting pyruvate is transported into mitochondria to be converted via pyruvate dehydrogenase into acetyl-CoA and NADH (42). This acetyl-CoA molecule subsequently enters the Krebs cycle (42).

Fatty Acid Metabolism in Treg Cells

In addition to glycolysis, Treg cells rely on lipid metabolism to meet their metabolic requirements. In the murine tumor setting, Treg cells were shown to express both genes for glycolysis and as well as the pentose phosphate pathway (PPP) (16). The end products of this pathway could be used for fatty acid synthesis (FASyn) or protein synthesis. Tumoral Treg cells also stored lipids intracellularly and preserved the ability to perform fatty acid oxidation (FAO) too. Overall, this data demonstrated that murine tumoral Tregs were capable of glycolysis and OXPHOS mediated via FASyn/FAO.

However, it is unclear why Treg cells should maintain the FASyn and FAO programs as both would theoretically at least nullify the effects of the other (**Figure 2**). Indeed, this question has been studied by a few teams in recent years (36, 43, 44). In one study involving murine T-cells, the inhibition of acetyl-CoA carboxylase (key enzyme for FASyn) in naïve $CD4^+$ T-cells, via either genetic knockout (KO) or pharmacological means, diverted the differentiation process toward $FOXP3^+$ cells instead of IL-17A-producing cells (44). These FASyn-inhibited iTregs were just as immunosuppressive *in vitro* as control iTregs. Moreover, the control iTregs and FASyn-inhibited iTregs had similarly reduced levels of genes for glycolysis and glutaminolysis. Both took up equal amounts of palmitate too. Put together, modulating fatty acid metabolic pathways could be a strategy to polarize iTreg cell differentiation and function.

A further yet important line of inquiry is regarding how FOXP3 can modulate lipid metabolism (**Figure 2**). $FOXP3^+$ tissue Treg cells take up long-chain fatty acids (lcFAs) into via the CD36 receptor (45). However, short and medium-chained fatty acids (scFAs and mcFAs, respectively) diffuse passively across the cytoplasm and mitochondrial outer/inner membranes to participate in FAO (46). In a series of eloquent experiments using a murine lymphoma cell line (EL4), Howie D. et al. demonstrated the effects of FOXP3 on lcFAs metabolism (39). They transfected EL4 cells with a FOXP3-ERT2 construct such that the administration of an estrogen modulator (4-HT) would translocate this construct to the nucleus. These transfected $FOXP3^+$ cells had an increased oxygen consumption rate (OCR) at baseline than the non-transfected controls. The OCR was further increased after being cultured with palmitate (long-chain fatty acid, C16). Interestingly, in EL4-FOXP3 cultures without palmitate, the addition of etomoxir reduced OCR rates. This demonstrated that part of the increased FOXP3-mediated OXPHOS was due to the FAO of endogenous fatty acids. These cells in parallel also increased the expression of genes for mitochondrial electron transport chain (ETC) complexes. A similar effect was demonstrated in 24 h activated human Treg cells ($CD4^+CD25^+FOXP3^+$) as they too augmented genes specific for mitochondria. This further confirmed the role of FOXP3 in promoting mitochondrial-based metabolism. The same group also studied whether FOXP3 could promote Treg cell survival in a high-fat microenvironment. They found that murine Treg cells were less apoptotic after 18 h of cultures with lcFAs compared to Teff cells. This was an interesting observation as they found that Treg cells took up more fluorescent-palmitate. This indicated that FOXP3 could indeed be inhibiting the apoptosis-inducing effects of palmitate. In their EL4-FOXP3 cells, they identified the mechanism for this effect as being due to increased FAO of palmitate. Collectively, all these data demonstrate how FOXP3 promotes OXPHOS through increasing FAO of lcFAs and mitochondrial ETS complex synthesis.

However, before Treg cells can engage lcFAs in FAO, the lcFAs need to be transported across the cytoplasm and enter the mitochondria (**Figure 2**). These two processes are facilitated by the fatty acid-binding proteins (FABP) and the carnitine palmitoyltransferase transporters (CPT1/2), respectively (47). Treg cells predominantly express the FABP5 transporter although other isoforms have been described (48, 49). Recent work by Field C. et al. demonstrated that pharmacological inhibition of FABP5 in newly differentiated iTregs switched their metabolic program from OXPHOS to glycolysis (as evidence by the extracellular acidification rates; ECAR) (48). These cells also developed an altered mitochondrial structure and synthesized fewer proteins specific for the mitochondrial ETCs. As a consequence, lcFAs were unable to engage in FAO and the Krebs cycle. However, in an interesting demonstration of the roles of lcFA metabolism in modulating Treg cell function, they also identified that FABP5 inhibition in iTregs and human Treg cells led to increased *in vitro* suppression via IL-10 secretion. The mechanism for this effect involved the release of mitochondrial DNA and subsequent increase in interferon signaling via the innate pattern recognition pathway, cycle GMP-AMP synthase (cGAS) and Stimulator of Interferon Genes (STING). Collectively, these data suggest that inhibiting lcFA-FAO metabolic pathway may be more favorable as an approach to increasing Treg cell suppressive function. They also suggest that the overall effects of FAO on Treg cells are broader than just supplementing the Krebs cycle. It is plausible that various intermediates produced during FAO such as acetyl-CoA and reduced flavin/nicotinamide adenine dinucleotides (FADH/NADH) could be interfering with Treg cell function through yet unknown mechanisms.

The actual FAO process occurs in the mitochondria and involves the formation of one acetyl-CoA molecule per cycle (50). The acylated fatty acids keep entering the FAO cycle until a

2-carbon unit can no longer be formed. Each cycle also produces an NADH and $FADH_2$ molecule that donate additional electrons to the ETCs (50). With regards to producing ATP, this is a very efficient process as the full metabolism of a 16-chain fatty acid (palmitate) leads to 106 molecules of ATP – much more than via glycolysis or glucose substrate-only OXPHOS (50). This may explain why in a glucose-deprived tumoral microenvironment, Treg cells utilize CD36 to maximize fat uptake as a fuel to meet their metabolic demands (45).

Krebs Cycle and Mitochondrial Complexes in Treg Cells

The purpose of the above pathways is to generate enough acetyl-CoA to feed into the Krebs cycle and then generate sufficient ATP through the mitochondrial ETC. This is an important process in Treg cells as links between FOXP3, ETC synthesis, and cellular functions have been described (39, 51, 52) (**Figure 2**). Although the mechanism was not uncovered, the induction of FOXP3 in iTreg cells correlated with increased expression of mitochondria-associated genes (39). Moreover, a recent manuscript involving mice demonstrated that complex III *per se* was key to promoting Treg cell suppressive function (40, 52). The Treg-specific knockout of complex III was associated with reduced immunosuppressive capacity and increased DNA methylation status – without affecting FOXP3 expression, cell frequency, or co-inhibitor receptor expression (52). These mice also developed a general inflammatory condition (similar to that of *scurfy* mice) and did not live beyond 4 weeks of life. Put together, these data identify the additional role of mitochondrial metabolism alongside FOXP3 in facilitating Treg cell function.

Do tTreg and iTreg Cells Have Different Metabolic Programs?

Although the majority of FOXP3 + Treg cells are of thymic-origin, a small proportion are induced (iTreg cells *in vitro*) from effector T (Teff) cells via exposure to different cytokines in the microenvironment (35). Through studying the conversion of effector T (Teff) cells to iTreg cells, one can identify how their metabolic phenotype changes via *de novo* FOXP3 induction. This is not possible with tTreg cells which already express FOXP3 upon entering the peripheral circulation.

Ex vivo non-activated murine tTreg cells (defined as $CD4^+FOXP3^+$) have a higher baseline proliferative status (Ki67) and express more Glut1 (glucose transporter) than Teff cells (37). Just as FOXP3 expression is a Treg cell-lineage identifier, there is increasing data that OXPHOS is their key lineage metabolic program (37) (**Figure 2**). This supported by metabolomics data of resting human tTregs (defined as $CD4^+CD25^+$ or $CD4^+CD127^{lo}CD49b^-$ in the referenced study), which found Treg cells to produce increased glycolysis- and OXPHOS-related metabolites such as lactate, α-ketoglutarate, and succinate in comparison to Teff cells or naïve $CD4^+$ T-cells (53). In comparison, another study utilizing a proteomics approach, demonstrate slightly different results (54). Although resting human Treg cells ($CD4^+CD25^+CD127^{lo}$) did indeed express a greater quantity of glycolysis-related proteins than Teff cells ($CD4^+CD25^-$), the Teff cells expressed a greater quantity of proteins related to the Krebs cycle and the mitochondrial ETC instead. Moreover, these proteomic differences did not translate into differing metabolic programs as the Treg cells consistently had a higher baseline rate of ECAR and OCR. Collectively, these datasets suggest that both glycolysis and oxidative phosphorylation are a fundamental part of the baseline tTreg cell metabolic program.

In comparison, acutely activated human tTreg cells in the *in vitro* setting initially reduce their rate of ECAR and OCR in comparison to Teff cells (43). However, after a ~1-week stimulation with anti-CD3 antibody, IL-2, and antigen-presenting cells (APCs), these Treg cells had significantly higher rates of ECAR and OCR than corresponding Teff cells. The activated Treg cells also took up more of the fluorescent glucose dye than Teff cells despite having similar levels of Glut1 expression. Moreover, the importance of FAO was demonstrated in these Treg cells too as the addition of palmitate to cultures further increased the OCR. Put together, these data suggested that tTreg cells were better equipped than Teff cells to meet their additional metabolic requirements through upregulating both glycolysis and FAO upon acute activation (**Figure 2**).

From a functional perspective, the inhibition of either glycolysis or FAO was found not to profoundly affect Treg cell immunosuppressive capacity (54). However, the data from this study contrasts with data from other published work that reported Treg cell immunosuppressive capacity to be more significantly reduced when glycolysis, FAO, or lipid/cholesterol synthesis were individually inhibited (53). When reconciling these divergent results, we noted key differences in the experimental design of the suppression assay e.g., responder cell type, the dose of metabolism inhibitors, pre-culture period, and the readout dye (thymidine/carboxyfluorescein). It is important to take these differences into account when considering the evidence base. Collectively, these data demonstrate that the link between tTreg cell metabolism and immunosuppressive function is not fully delineated.

With respect to iTreg cells, the increase in the rate of glycolysis in murine iTreg cells was less pronounced compared to *de novo* induced Th1/2/17 cells (36). These iTregs also expressed less Glut1. However, similarly to the tTreg cells from the above-discussed studies, these iTregs demonstrated dependence on lipid metabolism too. They oxidized significantly more palmitate than their non-Treg counterparts. Moreover, when the FAO inhibitor, etomoxir, was added to the culture system (albeit at a relatively high dose), both the oxidation was inhibited as well as the upregulation of FOXP3. This effect was also identified by another team studying murine iTregs as they demonstrated an association with FOXP3 upregulation and increased OXPHOS rates (40).

All in all, these data suggest that tTreg and iTreg cells depend on both glycolysis and FAO to meet their metabolic demands. These processes are upregulated during activation and their inhibition affects Treg cell proliferation and function (**Figure 2**).

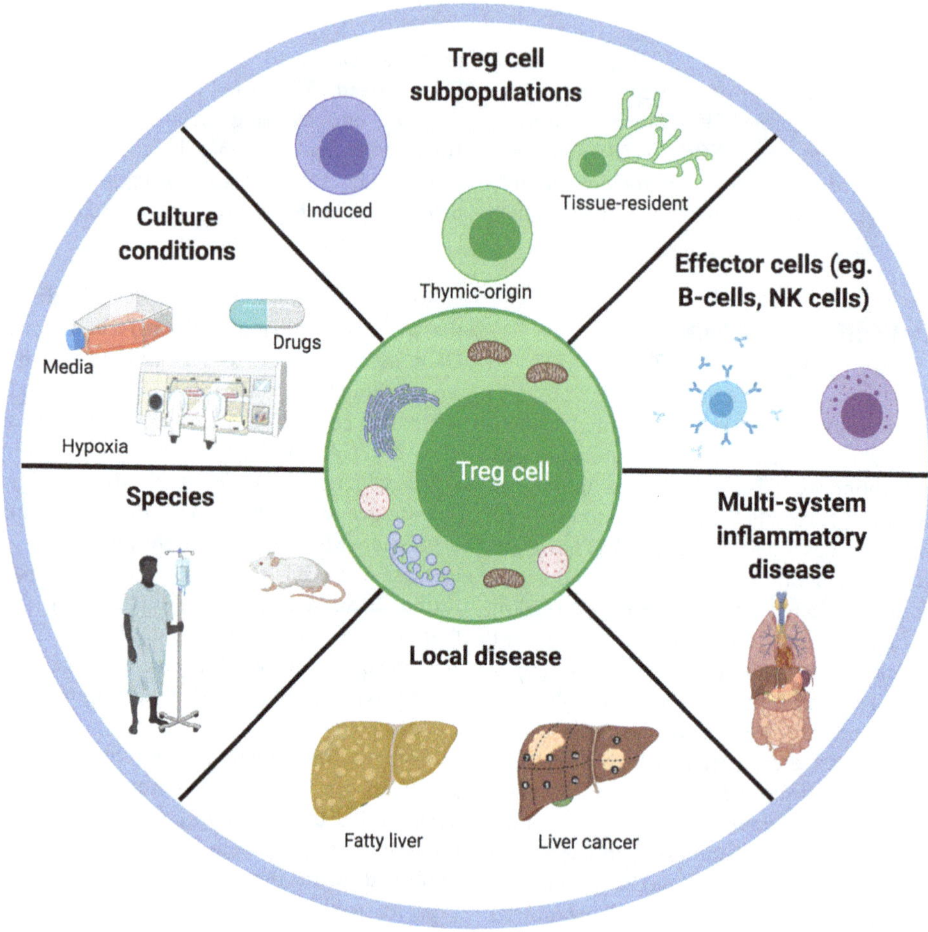

FIGURE 3 | Illustrating the range of variables that could explain differences between published data on Treg cell metabolism and function. Different teams work on Treg cells from different species, different tissue systems and disease settings. This has implications for the type of microenvironment that the Treg cells will have been adapted for. Moreover, any subsequent *in vitro* or *ex vivo* experiments are often carried out in different culture conditions involving different types of media, concomitant pharmacological agents as well as atmospheric oxygen concentrations. Furthermore, the competition for metabolites is different depending on the presence of competing effector cells as well as the constitutive Treg cell metabolic program.

Explaining the Variation in Published Experimental Literature

When considering the relevant literature on Treg cell metabolism, it is important to take into account a range of factors (**Figure 3**):

- Culture conditions (*in vivo/ex vivo/in vitro*).
- Treg cell subtype (thymic, peripheral, induced, FOXP3$^+$, and CD25$^+$CD127^{lo}).
- Disease (graft rejection, tumor, and autoimmunity) or healthy tissue.
- Species (murine and human).
- Microenvironment (competing cells, substrates, oxygen gradient, and drugs).

As is evident from our discussions above, a challenge with the current *in vitro* metabolic assays is ensuring that they reflect *in vivo* physiology. The concentrations of substrates, their competing cells, and the ongoing disease process are constantly evolving when *in vivo*. To study glycolysis, certain studies we discuss in this review have used the inhibitor, 2-deoxyglucose (2-DG) (16, 55). However, there is data demonstrating that this agent can also have off-target effects in terms of triggering kinase pathways e.g., Akt/Erk) (55, 56). Moreover, to study FAO, different studies have used different doses of palmitate (up to 1000 uM) (36, 39). The challenge here is that palmitate is not an exclusive fatty acid in the microenvironment and the concentration can be affected by albumin levels too (36, 57, 58). Finally, certain assays have used etomoxir (mitochondrial lcFA uptake inhibitor) to block CPT1 however, there is data demonstrating that etomoxir acts “independently of CPT1” instead in T-cells (59). A further issue of concern is regarding etomoxir dosing as it has off-target effects above the dose of 5 uM (60). These are only some of the extraneous variables to consider. Overall, our key message is that the relevant data must be contextualized within the limitations of the respective assays.

Having discussed Treg cell metabolism in detail, in the next sections we outline the following key internal axes that connect both metabolism and function in Treg cells (**Figure 1**):

1. mTOR.
2. Hypoxia.
3. Nuclear Receptors.

mTOR: THE IMMUNOMETABOLIC HIGHWAY

The mTOR complexes play a central role in Treg cell metabolism and function (14, 61) (**Figure 1**). Their ability to sense upstream changes in the microenvironment and subsequently modulate Treg cell metabolism/function that makes them the highway of immunometabolic modulation (61).

mTOR signaling is facilitated through mTOR being linked with other adapter proteins in the form of mTORC1 and mTORC2 complexes (61). The phosphorylation signaling cascade upstream of mTOR starts with stimulation of either the TCR complex or CD28 (62) (**Figure 2**). This triggers sequential phosphorylation of phosphoinositide 3-kinase (PI3K), phosphoinositide-dependent kinase 1 (PDK1) and then protein kinase B (Akt). Akt subsequently inhibits the heterodimeric tuberous sclerosis complex (TSC1/2) to maintain Rheb protein activity (63). Finally, Rheb can directly and indirectly increase mTORC1 activation (62, 64). This promotes Treg cell immunosuppressive function, prevents the onset of autoimmunity and maintains tissue homeostasis (14).

How Is mTOR Signaling Modulated?

From a metabolic perspective, mTORC1 activity can be modulated upstream via essential amino acids and hypoxia *(discussed in the next chapter of this review)* (65). Essential amino acids e.g., arginine, leucine, isoleucine) are known as such as they must be acquired from dietary consumption. Although these play a key role in DNA and protein synthesis, they are also vital in promoting Treg-specific mTORC1 activity (15, 66). The evolutionary reasons for this relationship remain unknown.

Amino acids are taken up through dedicated receptors such as SLC7A1, SLC7A5, SLC3A2/CD98, and ASCT2 (15, 66, 67). The expression of these receptors is further increased upon TCR stimulation to optimize amino acid uptake. This is an important mechanism as its inhibition reduces mTORC1 activation (15' 67). Upon acute cellular activation, the ongoing presence of amino acids such as arginine and leucine sustains activation of mTORC1 as well as of the Treg cell itself (via increased *cytotoxic T-cell lymphocyte antigen-4;* CTLA4 and *inducible T-cell costimulator;* ICOS) (15, 68). The inhibition of amino acid uptake receptors has been shown in murine models to reduce *in vivo* Treg cell quantity, cellular proliferation, and suppressive capacity. Moreover, this effect was specific to Treg cells and not Teff cells – thus further confirming a key role for essential amino acids in these cells. Once inside the Treg cell, amino acids activate the Rag small GTPases (such as RagA/B), which alongside the protein Rheb, recruit mTORC1 to lysosomes (15, 68). These are critical processes as murine KO models of either Rag GTPases or Rheb proteins have demonstrated the mice to have Treg cell metabolism/function and they all developed an autoimmune disease similar to that of *scurfy* mice.

How Does mTORC1 Connect Metabolism and Function?

Resting $CD4^+FOXP3^+$ (Treg cells) have higher levels of constitutive mTORC1 activity than naïve $CD4^+$ T-cells or Teff cells (68, 69). Upon activation by anti-CD3, the phosphorylation of S6 and 4E-BP1 (indicators of mTORC1 activity) was increased alongside key functional markers such as CTLA4 (68, 69). These activated Treg cells were also more immunosuppressive.

From a metabolic perspective, resting non-activated Treg cells (isolated either as $CD4^+CD25^+$ or $CD4^+CD127^{lo}CD49b^-$) were found to have higher expression levels of genes involved in glucose metabolism e.g., *Glut1, Glut3, PKM2*) and lipid metabolism (*cpt1, fasn, acc1*) than Teff cells (53). Upon Treg cell activation, the increase in mTOR signaling upregulated interferon regulatory factor 4 (IRF4) which further promoted genes for cellular growth, glycolysis, OXPHOS, fatty acid metabolism amongst others (14). Moreover, transfecting tTreg cells with Rheb to upregulate mTOR signaling further increased glucose uptake and glycolysis (53). All this data collectively indicated that promoting mTORC1 activity could also promote Treg cell activation, function, and support both the glycolysis and OXPHOS metabolic pathways.

However, numerous others have demonstrated often divergent effects of mTOR signaling on Treg cells. For example, in a Treg specific Raptor KO murine model (to inhibit mTORC1 activity), the mice demonstrated an increase in $CD4^+FOXP3^+$ (Treg cells) (69). These Treg cells were still immunosuppressive during *in vitro* assays however they were unable to inhibit colitis development or the *scurfy* phenotype of *in vivo* murine models. Furthermore, from a metabolic perspective, the Raptor KO Treg cells had lower levels of ECAR and OCR. They also downregulated genes for cholesterol and lipid biosynthesis. In particular, cholesterol biosynthesis was demonstrated mechanistically as being important in promoting Treg cell activation, proliferation, and function. Collectively, these data demonstrated that constitutive *in vivo* mTORC1 signaling was important and that mTORC1 played a critical role in promoting lipogenic metabolism and Treg cell function.

These findings were taken further by another group who developed two different murine models to delineate mTORC1 activity; Treg-specific KO of RagA/B GTPases (amino acid sensors) and Treg-specific KO of Rheb1/2 (15). As expected, mTORC1 activity was relatively reduced (not completely inhibited) upon TCR-stimulation in both models compared to wild-type mice. From a functional perspective, the cells demonstrated reduced *in vitro* immunosuppressive capacity – although FOXP3 expression was unaffected (15). Put together, these data suggest that both a combination of mTORC1-related and non-mTORC1-related effects of Rag/Rheb protein signaling could be involved in Treg cell function.

From a metabolic perspective, Treg cells from both models also had reduced rates of glycolysis and oxidative phosphorylation (15). Indeed, the RagA/B KO mice also had fewer mitochondria, reduced mitochondrial function, and superoxide levels. The analysis of the transcriptomes of activated Treg cells of both KO models compared to wild-type Treg cells demonstrated upregulation in pro-inflammatory genes e.g., interferon-gamma, tumor necrosis factor-alpha) as well as a downregulation in genes for cellular proliferation e.g., myc, G2M checkpoint) and oxidative phosphorylation (15). However, within these transcriptomic alterations, there was also a divergence in terms of the effects of metabolism. The RagA/B KO Treg cells upregulated genes involved with lysosomes and lipid metabolism and downregulated those specific for mitochondrial complexes. In comparison, the Rheb1/2 KO Treg cells downregulated genes for metabolizing fatty acids and cholesterol without any changes in mitochondrial biosynthesis/function. Collectively, these data demonstrate that mTORC1 activity plays an important role in Treg cell activation, function, and increased metabolic demands (via glycolysis and OXPHOS). However, they also demonstrate that the RagA/B and Rheb1/2 proteins differentially modulate lipid metabolism and OXPHOS. Exactly how these divergent metabolic pathways are reconciled during Treg cell activation and increased mTORC1 activity is yet unknown.

How Does mTORC2 Connect Treg Cell Metabolism and Function?

Concerning mTORC2, its role in Treg cells has been relatively less well-defined compared to mTORC1. mTORC2 activates Akt via phosphorylation at the serine residue (position 473) (70) (**Figure 2**). In response, Akt phosphorylates mTORC1 and the FOXO transcription factors (70). Phosphorylation of the FOXO TFs propagates their subsequent degradation via ubiquitination. Hence, any experiments involving mTORC2 inhibition need to take into account that the downstream effects could involve reduced mTORC1 activity as well as increased FOXO levels (**Figure 2**).

Studies into the effects of mTORC2 modulation on Treg cells have generally demonstrated mixed effects on their phenotype and function (69–71). In one study, the murine model of Treg-specific mTORC2 KO (Rictor−/−) demonstrated reduced frequencies of Treg cells in all peripheral tissue (except the thymus) (69). However, the phenotype of the Treg cells was unaltered (CTLA4, ICOS levels). They also remained immunosuppressive during *in vitro* assays. From a metabolic perspective, their mitochondrial function was also unaffected.

These findings are in contrast to those of another group who developed murine models with a Treg-specific loss-of-function modification of FOXP3 with and without an additional Rictor KO (mTORC2 inhibition) (71). Through these single- and dual-mutated mice, they were able to delineate the relationship between functional FOXP3$^+$ Treg cells and those without a functioning mTORC2 component (71). The phenotypic analysis of Treg cells from the dual-mutated mice demonstrated increased expression of markers such as *glucocorticoid-induced tumor necrosis factor receptor* (GITR) and ICOS. These cells had the capacity to secrete more IL-4, IL-10, and less IFNγ compared to the FOXP3-mutation mice (IL-17A was unchanged). They were also more immunosuppressive during *in vitro* suppression assays compared to Tregs from the FOXP3-mutation mice. However, importantly, the suppressive capacity of the FOXP3-only mutated Treg cells improved with rapamycin pre-treatment. Collectively, these data suggested that mTORC2 inhibition promoted Treg cell activation status, Th2-like differentiation, and immunosuppressive function.

From a metabolic perspective, the Treg cells of the FOXP3-mutation mice upregulated glycolysis and OXPHOS (as demonstrated via increased ECAR and OCR, respectively) (71). This was reflected by upregulation of enzymes and metabolites involved in glycolysis and the Krebs cycle. Furthermore, the inhibition of glycolysis in these cells reduced their secretion of IFNγ, IL-4, and improved their *in vitro* immunosuppressive function. However, this metabolic reprogramming was attenuated in Treg cells from mice with the additional Rictor-KO (mTORC2 inhibition). Put together, these data suggest that FOXP3 and mTORC2 have opposing effects on Treg cell phenotype, metabolism and function (71). However, it is yet unknown how this relationship is affected by other metabolites such as amino acids (which sustain mTORC1 activity) or fatty acids.

HYPOXIA

Understanding the role of hypoxia in Treg cells is especially important with regards to delineating their survival and function in the physiological hypoxia liver (72). During hypoxia or a state of high ATP consumption, there is a proportional increase in intracellular AMP as well as *hypoxia-inducing-factor-1-alpha* (HIF1α) transcription factor (HIF1α) (65). Both of these cofactors utilize different signaling pathways to modulate Treg cell functions.

The proportional increase in AMP leads to adenosine monophosphate kinase (AMPK) phosphorylation and activation by liver kinase B1 (Lkb1). This Lkb1 enzyme is crucial for Treg cell metabolism and function (65). The activated AMPK then inhibits Rheb and phosphorylates Raptor (mTOR adapter protein) to inhibit mTORC1 activity (73). Interestingly, activated AMPK also in parallel, inhibits acetyl-CoA carboxylase (ACC) to prevent fatty acid synthesis (74). Although this latter mechanism has not been demonstrated in Treg cells, it may be a potential metabolic adaptation during a low ATP state to divert available intracellular lipids toward acetyl-CoA-generating FAO instead.

In comparison, HIF1α levels increase during hypoxia as it is unable to be degraded via the proteasome-based mechanism (75). This would normally involve prolyl hydroxylation, subsequent binding to von Hippel-Lindau protein, and ubiquitination (75). Without this degradation, HIF1α forms a complex with its counterpart HIF1β, which then binds to specific hypoxic response elements (HRE) to influence Treg cell metabolism/function (**Figure 2**). However, the exact role of HIF1α in Treg cells is not clear as the data we discuss below describe contrasting effects.

FOXP3

Firstly, hypoxia appears to differentially modulate tTreg and iTreg cells. When murine tTreg cells ($CD4^+FOXP3^+$) were cultured for 5 days under acute hypoxia (1% O_2) with anti-CD3/28-based activation and IL-2, there was no change in their FOXP3 expression (76). This was also matched by *in vivo* data demonstrating that tTreg cells from murine models of CD4-specific KO of HIF1α had comparable levels of FOXP3 to control mice (76, 77). However, when $CD4^+$ T-cells from control mice were cultured under acute hypoxia with activation, IL-2 ± TGFβ, there was a proportional and significant increase in cells expressing FOXP3 (76, 78). This increase was also demonstrated *in vivo* in mice exposed to environmental hypoxia (10% O_2 for 24 h) (76). Put together, these data suggest that hypoxia does not alter FOXP3 expression on tTregs but induces it in non-Treg cells.

Immunosuppressive Function

In an *in vitro* suppression assay, the hypoxia-induced iTreg cells discussed above were cultured at different ratios with Teff cells ($CD4^+CD25^-$) and anti-CD3/28 antibodies for 72 h. These iTregs were better able to suppress Teff proliferation than their normoxic counterparts (78). In comparison, a rather different result was achieved using Treg cells from murine models of CD4-specific HIF1α KO (76). In this study, $CD4^+CD25^+$ Treg cells were only slightly less immunosuppressive at the higher ratios of Tregs:Teff cells (1:1, 1:2) compared to control Treg cells. However, there were no differences in immunosuppression between the two groups at the lower ratios. Moreover, adoptive transfer of these HIF1α KO Treg cells into a murine model of T-cell-mediated colitis demonstrated that the Treg cells were unable to inhibit weight loss or the development of colitis. Put together, these data suggest that HIF1α also differentially affects the immunosuppressive functions of tTreg/iTreg cells (76).

A further unknown question is how *in vivo* Treg cells function in hypoxic inflammatory microenvironments (79). In one study, involving tTreg cells, their acute activation was associated with an increase in HIF1α was identified compared to normoxic controls (53). The PI3K-mTOR pathway was crucial in upregulating HIF1α (53, 79). In addition, HIF1α played an important role in augmenting tTreg cell function as pre-culturing these cells for 24 h with a HIF1α-inhibitor reduced their ability to suppress naïve T-cell proliferation (53). Put together, these data suggest that tTregs could have augmented HIF1α levels and immunosuppressive function in inflammatory hypoxic microenvironments. This could have positive implications for their utilization in physiologically hypoxic liver allografts.

Treg Cell Differentiation and Stability

Concerning iTreg cells, an important question is whether hypoxia could influence the differentiation of $CD4^+$ T-cells to Th17/iTreg cells. In one study, murine splenocytes were cultured under hypoxia with anti-CD3 antibody, IL-2, TGFβ for 5 days before staining (76). The authors identified an increase in FOXP3 expression amongst the $CD4^+$ T-cells cultured under hypoxia as opposed to normoxia. Conversely, the $CD4^+$ T-cells did not change their expression levels of RORγt or secretion of IL-17A. Indeed, they found that they had to deliberately culture their splenocytes under Th17-differentiating conditions to induce these changes. This study suggested that HIF1α had an additive effect on differentiation rather than a polarizing toward Th17 or iTregs.

However, a different study using a pure naïve $CD4^+$ T-cell population identified that HIF1α was indeed the key factor in influencing differentiation to Th17 cells (80). Under Th17-differentiating conditions, they identified that *signal transducer and activator of transcription 3* (STAT3)-induced augmentation of HIF1α expression promoted transcription of RORγt. Both HIF1α and RORγt then formed a complex with the histone acetyltransferase, p300, to bind to the IL-17A promoter region. In comparison, when naïve $CD4^+$ T-cells from mice with $CD4^+$-specific HIF1α KO were cultured under Th17-differentiating conditions, they identified an increase in FOXP3 expression compared to wildtype controls. Moreover, when the same cells were cultured under iTreg-differentiating conditions instead, the $HIF1\alpha^{-/-}$ cells expressed much more FOXP3 than wildtype controls. All of this suggested that HIF1α was negatively affecting FOXP3 levels. Indeed, they confirmed this hypothesis by demonstrating that HIF1α utilized the ubiquitin-based degradation mechanism to directly target and degrade FOXP3. Overall, these studies suggest that HIF1α can modulate Th17/iTreg differentiation through epigenetic and metabolic means.

A further question is whether HIF1α can modulate Treg cell stability. This was demonstrated using a Treg-specific model of von Hippel-Lindau (VHL) KO to study the effects of HIF1α overexpression in Treg cells only (81). These mice did not survive beyond 6–11 weeks and had increased Th1 infiltrates in all tissues. Interestingly, the Treg cells from this model had no alterations in their baseline activation or functional phenotypes e.g., CD25, CTLA4, CD69). However, after 48 h of anti-CD3/28-based activation, the Treg cells secreted significantly more IFNγ, IL-4, IL-10, and other chemokines than controls (crucially no IL-2). From a functional perspective, the adoptive transfer of these cells into a RagKO murine colitis model found that the Treg cells lost FOXP3 expression after 8 weeks, there was an accumulation of IFNγ-producing Th1 cells and thus, the development of colitis was not prevented. Considering the data discussed in the previous paragraph, it is plausible that VHL KO-Treg cells were more susceptible to degradation of FOXP3 and the promotion of the effector Th1 program through binding to the HRE regions of the *IFNγ* gene. Overall, considering the data from this study of tTreg cells and studies from the above paragraphs of iTreg cells, it appears that HIF1α differentially modulates their differentiation, stability, and function. This raises additional challenges for understanding how Treg cells survive and function *in vivo* as environmental hypoxia would equally affect both cell subtypes.

Metabolism

The effect of hypoxia on Treg cells' metabolic pathways and how this influences cell function is not yet established (82). One would hypothesize that during hypoxia, Treg cells would adopt the non-oxygen-requiring glycolysis pathway to meet their metabolic demands. Indeed, the VHL KO Treg cells from the previous paragraph were found to have upregulated glycolysis-related genes. The glycolytic process also affected their function as the addition of 2-DG (glycolysis inhibitor) to these cells inhibited pro-inflammatory cytokine secretion. Collectively, this suggested that glycolysis was augmented during hypoxia, which in turn induced effector cell function in tTreg cells (81).

Regarding iTreg cells, the data suggest that hypoxia and glycolysis independently influence their metabolism (77). This was based upon several observations. Firstly, newly differentiated normoxic iTregs demonstrated a significantly lower rate of glycolysis than their newly differentiated Th1/2/17 counterparts. Secondly, the addition of 2-DG (glycolysis inhibitor) or rapamycin (mTOR inhibitor) to cultures of naïve $CD4^+$ T-cells under Th17-differentiating conditions, prevented the adoption of the Th17-like phenotype. The cells still proliferated, however, they adopted a more iTreg-like phenotype instead - as demonstrated by the induction of FOXP3 and reduced secretion of IL-17A. Moreover, the 2-DG inhibited glycolysis directly and did not modulate glycolysis-related genes. Concerning hypoxia, the iTreg cells originating from a CD4-specific HIF1α-KO murine model expressed more FOXP3 and CTLA4 than their controls. Collectively, these data demonstrated that the induction of hypoxia and glycolysis were key to influencing $CD4^+$ T-cell differentiation toward iTreg cells.

Overall, the roles of hypoxia in modulating Treg cell phenotype, function, and metabolism still need to be defined. We do not know if Treg cells still perform FAO despite hypoxia. We also do not know if by adopting glycolysis, whether they upregulate the PPP program for amino acid synthesis. Furthermore, a limitation of many studies is that they elucidated the effects of acute hypoxia only through *in vitro* experiments (**Figure 3**). In parallel, the KO models are unable to account for any tissue-specific effects of hypoxia and do not exclude the possibility of redundancy mechanisms to compensate for KO of HIF1/VHL. This issues are important for the liver allograft as its physiological hypoxia means that resident/circulating cells would have to adapt to survive/function in response to the chronically hypoxic microenvironment.

NUCLEAR RECEPTORS

The nuclear receptors are a unique family that interconnects lipophilic steroidal and non-steroidal ligands directly with DNA modulation (83) (**Figure 1**). A key difference in their mechanism is that steroidal receptors bind to DNA as homodimers whereas the non-steroidal receptors bind to DNA as heterodimers attached to the retinoid X receptor (RXR). In doing so, they collectively modulate genes responsible for cell differentiation, proliferation, function, and metabolism (83) (**Figure 2**). Whilst an in-depth discussion of these receptors is beyond the scope of this review, the ones implicated in promoting Treg cells include:

- Peroxisome proliferator-activator receptors (PPARα, β, γ).
- Liver X receptors (LXRα, β).
- Farsenoid X receptors (FXR).
- Vitamin D receptors (VDR).
- Retinoic acid receptor (RARα, β, γ).

PPAR

The PPAR receptors are activated via fatty acids or pharmacological agonists (84). As previously discussed, acute activation of Treg cells upregulates mTORC1 activity, increases glycolysis and fatty acid catabolism. However, recent work in $CD4^+$ T-cells has demonstrated that the mechanism for fatty acid catabolism is dependent on mTORC1 inducing PPARγ as well as the sterol regulatory element-binding protein 1 (SREBP1) (84). The PPARγ gene promoted the expression of genes to take-up lipids, perform fatty acid synthesis, and lipolysis too. Moreover, the induction of PPARγ was also important in promoting the proliferation and activation of $CD4^+$ T-cells (84).

The role of PPARγ in Treg cells has been particularly investigated in visceral adipose tissue (VAT). For example, the expression of both PPARγ and FOXP3 was identified as crucial to inducing the genetic signature of VAT-specific Treg cells (85). PPARy agonism via thiazolidinediones upregulated genes crucial to both Treg cell metabolism and function. For example, genes for lcFA metabolism such as CD36, CPT1 as well as fatty acid synthesis were upregulated. In parallel, there was also an increase in the expression of FOXP3 and Gata3. Most importantly, these changes were identified in VAT-resident Tregs only, which suggested a role for the lipid-rich microenvironment in local immunoregulation.

Similar effects were also identified in the tumor setting via the PPARβ receptor (45). The CD36-based triggering activated the PPARβ signaling pathway which promoted lipid metabolism and function in Treg cells. This process involved increased FOXP3 expression, mitochondrial function, and the NAD/NADH ratio. Most notably, in this tumoral setting PPARγ was not identified as being affected via CD36 signaling. This suggests that the PPAR isoforms could be differentially implicated in Treg cell metabolism/function depending on the tissue setting.

LXR

There are two forms of the LXR receptor (α, β) of which LXRβ is universally present on all tissues whereas LXRα is specific to certain tissues e.g., hepatic, adipose and gut (86, 87). LXRs are activated by oxidized cholesterol derivatives (oxysterols) and propagate a genetic response that involves increased cholesterol and lipid metabolism (86). In particular, they augment the expression of ABC-cassette transporters which are responsible for the excretion of sterols (88).

Concerning Treg cells, there is *in vitro* data demonstrating that culturing murine $CD4^+$ T-cells under iTreg-differentiating conditions with LXR agonists significantly increased the expression of FOXP3, reduced IFN-γ, and IL-17A secretion (89). These iTreg cells were also more immunosuppression during *in vitro* assays. This effect was confirmed *in vivo* with oral LXR agonists as an increase in intestinal accumulation of Treg cells was identified.

LXR agonists are presently undergoing clinical trials as anti-inflammatory agents in atherosclerosis, however, an increase in hepatic steatosis has been identified as a key side effect. From this perspective, another group developed an LXR inverse agonist which demonstrated a reduction in murine models of hepatic steatosis instead (90). Put together, these data demonstrate that we still need to further understand the implications of LXR-mediated DNA modulation before progressing to clinical trials.

FXR

The FXR receptors are particularly pertinent in liver physiology as their key ligands are biliary acids. Upon activation, FXR receptors induce the transcription of genes specific for transporters that facilitate biliary efflux and inhibit genes responsible for biliary acid synthesis (91). However, although the FXR receptor is highly expressed in hepatic tissue, very low levels of FXR mRNA have been identified in all peripheral blood mononuclear cells e.g., T/B-cells, monocytes) (92). Hence, it is likely that if biliary acids do impact Treg cell function, this occurs indirectly. The two potential mechanisms could be (1) FXR-independent modulation of Treg cells or (2) FXR modulation of non-Treg cells whose downstream effects involve Treg cells. Indeed, evidence for both such mechanisms has been recently reported.

(1) The isoallolithocholic (isoallo-LCA) biliary acid was shown to modulate Treg cells independently of FXR (93). In cultures of murine CD4$^+$ T-cells under iTreg-differentiating conditions with isoallo-LCA, the expression of FOXP3 was significantly increased compared to other biliary acids. The mechanism of action of isoallo-LCA involved interacting with the conserved nuclear sequence 3 (CNS3) on the FOXP3 gene to indirectly promote FOXP3 acetylation. Moreover, these iTregs were able to suppress colitis development upon adoptive transfer – thus demonstrating superior *in vivo* immunosuppressive capacity. From a metabolic perspective, isoallo-LCA increased the OCR and superoxide levels in iTregs. Put together, this work demonstrated how isoallo-LCA could both augment mitochondrial-based metabolism and promote iTreg cell function.

(2) In comparison, the omega-muricholic and 3β-hydroxydeoxycholic (isoDCA) acids were found to significantly increase FOXP3 expression on naïve murine CD4$^+$ T-cells when co-cultured with DCs (94). This effect was not possible when the biliary acids were cultured with naïve CD4 T-cells only – thus, indicating an indirect DC-based effect. Indeed, the mechanism involved isoDCA having an antagonistic effect upon binding to the FXR receptor on DCs and downregulating a range of pro-inflammatory genes. Through a range of innovative murine models and engineered microbes, they confirmed that these effects by demonstrating how these biliary acids could induce colonic pTreg cells. However, the exact nature of the interaction between the DCs and naïve CD4$^+$ T-cells was not identified. Moreover, the effects of these biliary acids on the metabolism of the iTreg/pTreg cells were not explored either.

VDR

The VDR receptor in T-cells is activated by the active form of vitamin D, 1,25-dihydroxyvitamin D3 (83). The receptor then forms a heterodimeric complex with RXR, which can bind to specific sections of DNA (called vitamin D response elements; VDRE) (95). This propagates the transcription of a range of protein complexes responsible for enacting T-cell functions.

The addition of active vitamin D into cultures of activated human CD4$^+$ T-cells or CD4$^+$CD25$^-$ T-cells has been shown to significantly increase FOXP3 expression compared to controls (96, 97). In parallel, it also increased expression of CTLA4 and reduced secretion of IFN-γ, IL-17A, and IL-2. These iTregs were better able to suppress the proliferation of Teff cells during *in vitro* assays and they secreted slightly more IL-10 too. However, these iTregs were unstable as FOXP3 expression declined after day 4 of activation. In a different study, VDR was also able to induce functioning iTregs from Th2 cells (98). Overall, although VDR activation can induce Treg cells, it is unknown how (and if) VDR in parallel modulates Treg cell metabolism.

RAR

The RAR group of receptors in T-cells are activated by the active form of vitamin A, all-trans retinoic acid (ATRA) (83). Similar to VDR, they form a heterodimeric complex with RXR, which then binds to the complementary sections of DNA (called retinoic acid response elements; RARE).

With respect to tTreg cells, *in vitro* cultures of ATRA and rapamycin with activated human Treg cells (defined as CD4$^+$CD25$^+$CD127^{lo} in the study) found that the combined ATRA/rapamycin group significantly increased FOXP3 expression on their Treg cells. These cells also demonstrated superior immunosuppressive capacity (99). Similar effects were also identified in experiments investigating ATRA in TGF-β-induced Tregs (100). However, it is unknown how (if at all) ATRA modulates Treg cell metabolism.

TRANSLATIONAL POTENTIAL OF TREG CELL METABOLISM

The aim of targeting Treg cell metabolism for cellular therapy applications is to induce specific metabolic pathways that augment cellular survival/function (**Figure 1**). These optimized Treg cells could outcompete Teffs metabolically in the allograft and thus, inhibit their survival and suppress their effector activity (34). Treg cells also have the potential for Th17 plasticity so combined immunometabolic optimization could prevent Treg cell interconversion in an inflammatory allograft (32, 101). A further advantage of optimizing Treg cell activity is to exploit their bystander suppressor functions and thereby reduce the effector functions of other pro-inflammatory cells (102).

This combined immunometabolic modulation could be performed either *in vivo* or *ex vivo* (**Figure 4**). Concerning the *in vivo* approach, this would involve either dietary supplementation of substrates e.g., fatty acids, amino acids) or systemic administration of substrates/drugs. This approach is clinically feasible and could be periodically delivered in response

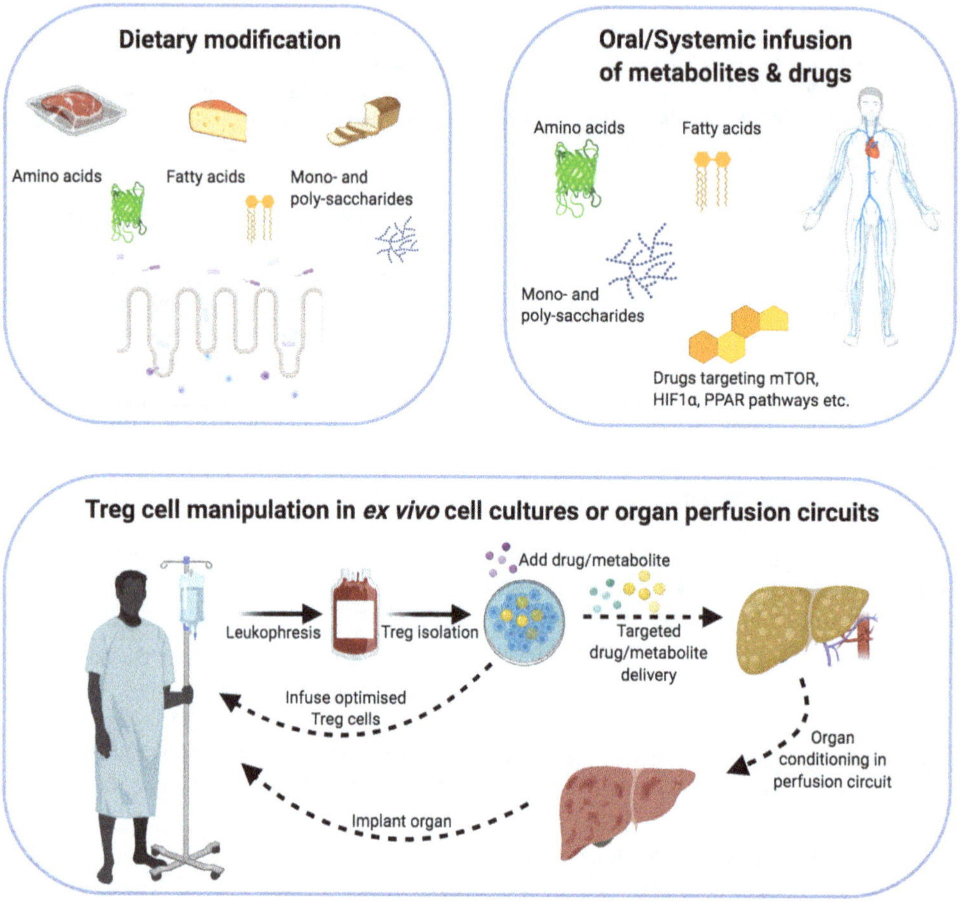

FIGURE 4 | Demonstrating how regulatory T-cells can be metabolically optimized through dietary changes, *ex vivo* cellular therapy or organ reperfusion machines. **Dietary modification/supplementation:** Different metabolites differentially modulate Treg cell metabolism and function. Treg cells metabolize mainly via non-mitochondrial (glycolysis) and mitochondrial e.g., oxidative phosphorylation and fatty acid oxidation) means. In addition, their internal cofactors such as mTOR, PPAR and HIF1α allow Treg cells to respond to substrate/oxygen changes in the microenvironment. Dietary modification or systemic infusions of drugs/metabolites could be used to augment Treg cell metabolism and function in an inflammatory allograft. **Cellular therapy:** Cell therapy involves the isolation of autologous Treg cells, which undergo expansion under sterile Good Manufacturing Principle (GMP) conditions. During this expansion process, the function and metabolism of Treg cells can be modified through drugs or change the substrate composition of metabolites. After the expansion process, the Treg cells could be returned to the patient or infused into an organ reperfusion circuit. **Organ reperfusion:** The recent introduction of organ reperfusion machines into clinical practice is changing the *modus operandi* of transplantation. Extended-criteria organs can be re-conditioned using different oxygen-delivery molecules, cytokines, drugs and metabolites to reduce their intrinsic ischemia/inflammatory burden as well as support the function of resident Treg cells. In parallel, recipient-expanded Treg cells could be infused during the reperfusion process to further optimize the reconditioning process. The recovery of an organ can then be measured through objective criteria e.g., pH, bile acid, lactate) and a decision made to implant or discard the organ.

to post-transplant protocol biopsies. However, to ensure its efficacy, there will need to be additional pharmacokinetic studies and even utilization of novel drug delivery approaches for Treg-specific targeting. In comparison, the *ex vivo* approach would involve culture media supplementation with the relevant substrates/drugs during the GMP process. In this way, the Treg cells could be specifically targeted and the substrates/drugs leftover could be washed out at the end of the culture process.

Metabolite Supplementation

Treg cells utilize glycolysis, FAO, and OXPHOS as their constitutive metabolic programs (**Figure 2**). During activation, Treg (and Teff) cells upregulate the expression of Glut1 transporters and their rate of glycolysis (ECAR). Hence, to allow Treg cells to outcompete their effector counterparts, supporting FAO could be a viable therapeutic approach instead. This would involve either direct supplementation of fatty acids, or inhibiting FASyn (via C75, soraphen) (26, 43, 44). In the past, direct supplementation with scFAs has been attempted, however, perhaps using lcFAs or polyunsaturated FAs would be more efficient in terms of ATP generation (26) (**Figure 2**). An opposite approach would involve targeting Teff cells by inhibiting glucose uptake (via Glut transporters), glycolysis e.g., 2-DG), or inhibiting fatty acid uptake (CD36), fatty acid transport (a) or mitochondrial uptake (CPT1) (60, 103–106).

However, we do not know yet which metabolic pathways are utilized or favorable to a graft experiencing acute or chronic rejection. It is also not known whether over usage of particular metabolic pathways would increase oxidative stress and propagate early apoptosis (39) (**Figure 2**). From a pharmaceutical perspective, although systemic infusion of dietary metabolites would be a route of administration, one could also utilize the oral route for improved bioavailability in intestinal and hepatic allografts (107). However, further pharmacokinetic studies are needed to assess these approaches in-depth.

Finally, a novel point of intervention could be through *ex vivo* organ machine perfusion technologies (108–110) (**Figure 4**). These are increasingly being used for conditioning to improve organ quality and subsequent patient outcomes. Upon explantation, the organ is first connected to a circulatory circuit within the perfusion machine. During the hours that follow (depending on the platform), the organ physiology can be monitored using a range of quality-control criteria such as color, pH, lactate levels, and even bile production. This period of perfusion would be optimal for metabolic-based immunomodulation.

Pharmacological Modulation

In this manuscript, we have discussed the internal immunometabolic axes of Treg cells that could be modulated to optimize both metabolic/functional pathways.

mTOR

Mammalian transporter of rapamycin inhibition via rapamycin is a part of current immunosuppression protocols as well as *ex vivo* GMP Treg cell expansion protocols (1, 19, 20, 111). This is because rapamycin improves Treg cell expansion, FOXP3 expression, and immunosuppressive function (25). Another way of inhibiting mTOR involves metformin, which is an AMPK kinase activator (73, 112). In Treg cells, it can inhibit FASyn by targeting ACC (112). This could augment FAO activity to outcompete the Teff cells.

However, the mTOR inhibitory approach is complicated by data discussed in previous sections demonstrating divergent roles of mTOR signaling in Treg cells (14, 53) (**Figure 2**). mTOR signaling improves Treg cell proliferation, glycolysis, lipid metabolism, and OXPHOS. Furthermore, essential amino acids also promote mTORC1 activity in Treg cells. Indeed, the ongoing presence of amino acids is necessary for Treg cells to sustain mTORC1 activity and Treg cell function (15, 68). To reconcile the differences in published studies, although the idea of an mTOR "oscillatory switch" has been hypothesized, it does mean that any mTOR-based modulation needs to be carefully refined for clinical benefit (113).

Hypoxia

As discussed in the Hypoxia section, the overall effects of hypoxia signaling in Treg cells are unclear. In tTreg cells, HIF1α seems to reduce (or not affect) FOXP3 expression, augments glycolysis, and induce effector activity. In comparison, HIF1α induces FOXP3 in iTregs (**Figure 2**).

In terms of manipulating tTreg cells during cell therapy or targeting allograft resident tTregs, increasing either local oxygen delivery or reducing HIF1α levels could be therapeutic approaches (**Figure 4**). Indeed, non-blood-based oxygen carriers have already been investigated in normothermic machine perfusion of the liver (114). The livers were more efficient at taking up the stored oxygen from these carrier molecules than hemoglobin. With regard to HIF1α levels, a range of HIF1α-targeting agonists/antagonists are either in trials or clinically available (115–117). These could either be systemically administered to patients or utilized in GMP culture protocols or machine perfusion technologies.

Nuclear Receptors

Nuclear receptor agonism could more precisely target Treg cell metabolism than oxygen-based or mTOR modulation. For example, PPARβ/γ agonism has been shown to jointly promote FOXP3 expression, FAO, FASyn, and mitochondrial function in Treg cells. Indeed, PPARγ agonists such as thiazolidinediones are clinically available and have been used for many years in diabetes already (118). Many patients with kidney allografts will be used to taking them too.

In comparison, although LXR agonists are being studied pre-experimentally in the settings of atherosclerosis/dyslipidemia, their noted side effect of inducing hepatic steatosis is a safety concern (119). Concerning the FXR receptor, indirect modulation via biliary acids is likely to be more challenging. There will need to be a range of pharmacokinetic studies to study their composition as well as intestinal/hepatic bioavailability. Furthermore, ensuring the specificity of their action on Treg cells only will require the use of more novel drug delivery approaches. Hence, LXR and FXR modulation is not a currently feasible Treg cell modulation strategy in transplantation.

FUTURE CHALLENGES

In summary, this review has outlined numerous ways in which Treg cell metabolism could be exploited for therapeutic benefit in transplantation. Through our discussions, we have also highlighted crucial ongoing knowledge gaps. The following themes need to be addressed in detail if we are going to move forward with translational Treg cell immunometabolism:

- When should Treg cells be administered post-transplant?
- Do antigen-specific or genetically engineered Treg cells metabolize differently?
- How can drugs and metabolites be delivered specifically to *in vivo* Tregs cells?
- At which time point post-infusion will Treg-boosting metabolites need to be administered?
- Can *in vivo* Treg cell metabolic programs be switched on/off as per clinical need?
- How can Treg cell metabolic activity be monitored in the graft?

Although the focus of this review has been on Treg cell metabolism, there is also a global cohort of teams actively researching other novel approaches such as genetic engineering, improved donor antigen-specificity, and epigenetics to optimize Treg cells. In light of the acceptable safety profile of Treg cells demonstrated in recent clinical trials, we can look forward to these novel approaches being exploited to optimize Treg cell efficacy. The coming years are indeed going to be exciting for Treg cell therapy – both for us and for our patients.

AUTHOR CONTRIBUTIONS

MA and MM designed, wrote, and revised the manuscript. AM, FC, OS, and GG advised on the editing and helped to revise the manuscript. All authors contributed to the article and approved the submitted version.

ACKNOWLEDGMENTS

All figures were created with BioRender.com.

REFERENCES

1. Atif M, Conti F, Gorochov G, Oo YH, Miyara M. Regulatory T cells in solid organ transplantation. *Clin Trans Immunol.* (2020) 9:e01099.
2. Tang Q, Vincenti F. Transplant trials with Tregs: perils and promises. *J Clin Invest.* (2017) 127:2505–12. doi: 10.1172/jci90598
3. Feng S. Spontaneous and induced tolerance for liver transplant recipients. *Curr Opin Organ Transplant.* (2016) 21:53–8. doi: 10.1097/mot.0000000000000268
4. Sasaki H, Oura T, Spitzer TR, Chen YB, Madsen JC, Allan J, et al. Preclinical and clinical studies for transplant tolerance via the mixed chimerism approach. *Hum Immunol.* (2018) 79:258–65. doi: 10.1016/j.humimm.2017.11.008
5. Sakaguchi S, Sakaguchi N, Asano M, Itoh M, Toda M. Immunologic self-tolerance maintained by activated T cells expressing IL-2 receptor alpha-chains (CD25). Breakdown of a single mechanism of self-tolerance causes various autoimmune diseases. *J Immunol.* (1995) 155:1151–64.
6. Bahmani B, Uehara M, Jiang L, Ordikhani F, Banouni N, Ichimura T, et al. Targeted delivery of immune therapeutics to lymph nodes prolongs cardiac allograft survival. *J Clin Invest.* (2018) 128:4770–86. doi: 10.1172/jci120923
7. Graca L, Cobbold SP, Waldmann H. Identification of regulatory T cells in tolerated allografts. *J Exp Med.* (2002) 195:1641–6. doi: 10.1084/jem.20012097
8. Lee I, Wang L, Wells AD, Dorf ME, Ozkaynak E, Hancock WW. Recruitment of Foxp3+ T regulatory cells mediating allograft tolerance depends on the CCR4 chemokine receptor. *J Exp Med.* (2005) 201:1037–44. doi: 10.1084/jem.20041709
9. Miyara M, Yoshioka Y, Kitoh A, Shima T, Wing K, Niwa A, et al. Functional delineation and differentiation dynamics of human CD4+ T cells expressing the FoxP3 transcription factor. *Immunity.* (2009) 30:899–911. doi: 10.1016/j.immuni.2009.03.019
10. Vignali DAA, Collison LW, Workman CJ. How regulatory T cells work. *Nat Rev Immunol.* (2008) 8:523–32. doi: 10.1038/nri2343
11. Pandiyan P, Zheng L, Ishihara S, Reed J, Lenardo MJ. CD4+CD25+Foxp3+ regulatory T cells induce cytokine deprivationâ "mediated apoptosis of effector CD4+ T cells. *Nat Immunol.* (2007) 8:1353–62. doi: 10.1038/ni1536
12. Takahashi T, Kuniyasu Y, Toda M, Sakaguchi N, Itoh M, Iwata M, et al. Immunologic self-tolerance maintained by CD25+CD4+ naturally anergic and suppressive T cells: induction of autoimmune disease by breaking their anergic/suppressive state. *Int Immunol.* (1998) 10:1969–80. doi: 10.1093/intimm/10.12.1969
13. Gondek DC, Lu LF, Quezada SA, Sakaguchi S, Noelle RJ. Cutting edge: contact-mediated suppression by CD4+CD25+ regulatory cells involves a granzyme B-dependent, perforin-independent mechanism. *J Immunol.* (2005) 174:1783–6. doi: 10.4049/jimmunol.174.4.1783
14. Chapman NM, Zeng H, Nguyen TM, Wang Y, Vogel P, Dhungana Y, et al. mTOR coordinates transcriptional programs and mitochondrial metabolism of activated Treg subsets to protect tissue homeostasis. *Nat Commun.* (2018) 9:2095.
15. Shi H, Chapman NM, Wen J, Guy C, Long L, Dhungana Y, et al. Amino acids license kinase mTORC1 activity and treg cell function via small G proteins rag and rheb. *Immunity.* (2019) 51:1012–1027e1017.
16. Pacella I, Procaccini C, Focaccetti C, Miacci S, Timperi E, Faicchia D, et al. Fatty acid metabolism complements glycolysis in the selective regulatory T cell expansion during tumor growth. *Proc Natl Acad Sci USA.* (2018) 115:E6546–55.
17. Peng M, Yin N, Chhangawala S, Xu K, Leslie CS, Li MO. Aerobic glycolysis promotes T helper 1 cell differentiation through an epigenetic mechanism. *Science.* (2016) 354:481–4. doi: 10.1126/science.aaf6284
18. Kespohl M, Vachharajani N, Luu M, Harb H, Pautz S, Wolff S, et al. The microbial metabolite butyrate induces expression of Th1-associated factors in CD4(+) T Cells. *Front Immunol.* (2017) 8:1036.
19. Sanchez-Fueyo A, Whitehouse G, Grageda N, Cramp ME, Lim TY, Romano M, et al. Applicability, safety, and biological activity of regulatory T cell therapy in liver transplantation. *Am J Transplant.* (2020) 20:1125–36. doi: 10.1111/ajt.15700
20. Mathew JM, Hv J, LeFever A, Konieczna I, Stratton C, He J, et al. A phase i clinical trial with ex vivo expanded recipient regulatory t cells in living donor kidney transplants. *Sci Rep.* (2018) 8:7428.
21. Oo YH, Ackrill S, Cole R, Jenkins L, Anderson P, Jeffery HC, et al. Liver homing of clinical grade Tregs after therapeutic infusion in patients with autoimmune hepatitis. *JHEP Rep.* (2019) 1:286–96. doi: 10.1016/j.jhepr.2019.08.001
22. Sawitzki B, Harden PN, Reinke P, Moreau Al, Hutchinson JA, Game DS, et al. Regulatory cell therapy in kidney transplantation (The ONE Study): a harmonised design and analysis of seven non-randomised, single-arm, phase 1/2A trials. *Lancet.* (2020) 395:1627–39.
23. MacDonald KN, Piret JM, Levings MK. Methods to manufacture regulatory T cells for cell therapy. *Clin Exp Immunol.* (2019) 197:52–63.
24. MacDonald KG, Hoeppli RE, Huang Q, Gillies J, Luciani DS, Orban PC, et al. Alloantigen-specific regulatory T cells generated with a chimeric antigen receptor. *J Clin Invest.* (2016) 126:1413–24. doi: 10.1172/jci82771
25. Miyara M, Chader D, Burlion A, Goldstein J, Sterlin D, Norol F, et al. Combination of IL-2, rapamycin, DNA methyltransferase and histone deacetylase inhibitors for the expansion of human regulatory T cells. *Oncotarget.* (2017) 8:104733–44. doi: 10.18632/oncotarget.10914
26. Schmidt A, Eriksson M, Shang MM, Weyd H, Tegner J. Comparative analysis of protocols to induce human CD4+Foxp3+ regulatory T Cells by combinations of IL-2, TGF-beta, retinoic acid, rapamycin and butyrate. *PLoS One.* (2016) 11:e0148474. doi: 10.1371/journal.pone.0148474
27. Nishimura E, Sakihama T, Setoguchi R, Tanaka K, Sakaguchi S. Induction of antigen-specific immunologic tolerance by in vivo and in vitro antigen-specific expansion of naturally arising Foxp3+CD25+CD4+ regulatory T cells. *Int Immunol.* (2004) 16:1189–201. doi: 10.1093/intimm/dxh122
28. Salomon B, Lenschow DJ, Rhee L, Ashourian N, Singh B, Sharpe A, et al. B7/CD28 costimulation is essential for the homeostasis of the CD4+CD25+ immunoregulatory T cells that control autoimmune diabetes. *Immunity.* (2000) 12:431–40. doi: 10.1016/s1074-7613(00)80195-8
29. Lan R, Geng H, Singha PK, Saikumar P, Bottinger EP, Weinberg JM, et al. Mitochondrial pathology and glycolytic shift during proximal tubule atrophy after ischemic AKI. *J Am Soc Nephrol.* (2016) 27:3356–67. doi: 10.1681/asn.2015020177
30. Ma C, Kesarwala AH, Eggert T, Medina-Echeverz J, Kleiner DE, Jin P, et al. NAFLD causes selective CD4(+) T lymphocyte loss and promotes hepatocarcinogenesis. *Nature.* (2016) 531:253–7. doi: 10.1038/nature16969
31. Pouyssegur J, Dayan F, Mazure NM. Hypoxia signalling in cancer and approaches to enforce tumour regression. *Nature.* (2006) 441:437–43. doi: 10.1038/nature04871
32. Ma L, Zhang H, Hu K, Lv G, Fu Y, Ayana DA, et al. The imbalance between Tregs, Th17 cells and inflammatory cytokines among renal transplant recipients. *BMC Immunol.* (2015) 16:56.
33. Jeffery HC, Jeffery LE, Lutz P, Corrigan M, Webb GJ, Hirschfield GM, et al. Low-dose interleukin-2 promotes STAT-5 phosphorylation, Treg survival and CTLA-4-dependent function in autoimmune liver diseases. *Clin Exp Immunol.* (2017) 188:394–411. doi: 10.1111/cei.12940
34. Kedia-Mehta N, Finlay DK. Competition for nutrients and its role in controlling immune responses. *Nat Commun.* (2019) 10:2123.
35. Shevach EM, Thornton AM. tTregs, pTregs, and iTregs: similarities and differences. *Immunol Rev.* (2014) 259:88–102. doi: 10.1111/imr.12160

36. Michalek RD, Gerriets VA, Jacobs SR, Macintyre AN, MacIver NJ, Mason EF, et al. Cutting edge: distinct glycolytic and lipid oxidative metabolic programs are essential for effector and regulatory CD4+ T cell subsets. *J Immunol.* (2011) 186:3299–303. doi: 10.4049/jimmunol.1003613
37. Gerriets VA, Kishton RJ, Johnson MO, Cohen S, Siska PJ, Nichols AG, et al. Foxp3 and Toll-like receptor signaling balance Treg cell anabolic metabolism for suppression. *Nat Immunol.* (2016) 17:1459–66. doi: 10.1038/ni.3577
38. Mookerjee SA, Gerencser AA, Nicholls DG, Brand MD. Quantifying intracellular rates of glycolytic and oxidative ATP production and consumption using extracellular flux measurements. *J Biol Chem.* (2017) 292:7189–207. doi: 10.1074/jbc.m116.774471
39. Howie D, Cobbold SP, Adams E, Ten Bokum A, Necula AS, Zhang W, et al. Foxp3 drives oxidative phosphorylation and protection from lipotoxicity. *JCI Insight.* (2017) 2:e89160.
40. Angelin A, Gil-de-Gomez L, Dahiya S, Jiao J, Guo L, Levine MH, et al. Foxp3 reprograms T cell metabolism to function in low-glucose, high-lactate environments. *Cell Metab.* (2017) 25:1282–1293e1287.
41. Andre ND, Barbosa DS, Munhoz E, Estevao D, Cecchini R, Watanabe MA. Measurement of cytotoxic activity in experimental cancer. *J Clin Lab Anal* (2004) 18:27–30. doi: 10.1002/jcla.20006
42. Hui S, Ghergurovich JM, Morscher RJ, Jang C, Teng X, Lu W, et al. Glucose feeds the TCA cycle via circulating lactate. *Nature.* (2017) 551:115–8. doi: 10.1038/nature24057
43. Cluxton D, Petrasca A, Moran B, Fletcher JM. Differential regulation of human treg and Th17 cells by fatty acid synthesis and glycolysis. *Front Immunol.* (2019) 10:115.
44. Berod L, Friedrich C, Nandan A, Freitag J, Hagemann S, Harmrolfs K, et al. De novo fatty acid synthesis controls the fate between regulatory T and T helper 17 cells. *Nat Med.* (2014) 20:1327–33. doi: 10.1038/nm.3704
45. Wang H, Franco F, Tsui YC, Xie X, Trefny MP, Zappasodi R, et al. CD36-mediated metabolic adaptation supports regulatory T cell survival and function in tumors. *Nat Immunol.* (2020) 21:298–308. doi: 10.1038/s41590-019-0589-5
46. Kamp F, Hamilton JA. How fatty acids of different chain length enter and leave cells by free diffusion. *Prostagland Leukot Essent Fatty Acids.* (2006) 75:149–59. doi: 10.1016/j.plefa.2006.05.003
47. Raud B, McGuire PJ, Jones RG, Sparwasser T, Berod L. Fatty acid metabolism in CD8(+) T cell memory: challenging current concepts. *Immunol Rev.* (2018) 283:213–31. doi: 10.1111/imr.12655
48. Field CS, Baixauli F, Kyle RL, Puleston DJ, Cameron AM, Sanin DE, et al. Mitochondrial integrity regulated by lipid metabolism is a cell-intrinsic checkpoint for treg suppressive function. *Cell Metab.* (2020) 31:422–437e425.
49. Frizzell H, Fonseca R, Christo SN, Evrard M, Cruz-Gomez S, Zanluqui NG, et al. Organ-specific isoform selection of fatty acid-binding proteins in tissue-resident lymphocytes. *Sci Immunol.* (2020) 5:eaay9283. doi: 10.1126/sciimmunol.aay9283
50. Lochner M, Berod L, Sparwasser T. Fatty acid metabolism in the regulation of T cell function. *Trends Immunol.* (2015) 36:81–91. doi: 10.1016/j.it.2014.12.005
51. Beier UH, Angelin A, Akimova T, Wang L, Liu Y, Xiao H, et al. Essential role of mitochondrial energy metabolism in Foxp3(+) T-regulatory cell function and allograft survival. *FASEB J.* (2015) 29:2315–26. doi: 10.1096/fj.14-268409
52. Weinberg SE, Singer BD, Steinert EM, Martinez CA, Mehta MM, Martinez-Reyes I, et al. Mitochondrial complex III is essential for suppressive function of regulatory T cells. *Nature.* (2019) 565:495–9. doi: 10.1038/s41586-018-0846-z
53. Li L, Liu X, Sanders KL, Edwards JL, Ye J, Si F, et al. TLR8-mediated metabolic control of human treg function: a mechanistic target for cancer immunotherapy. *Cell Metab.* (2019) 29:103–123e105.
54. Procaccini C, Carbone F, Di Silvestre D, Brambilla F, De Rosa V, Galgani M, et al. The proteomic landscape of human ex vivo regulatory and conventional T cells reveals specific metabolic requirements. *Immunity.* (2016) 44:406–21. doi: 10.1016/j.immuni.2016.01.028
55. Tanimine N, Germana SK, Fan M, Hippen K, Blazar BR, Markmann JF, et al. Differential effects of 2-deoxy-D-glucose on in vitro expanded human regulatory T cell subsets. *PLoS One.* (2019) 14:e0217761. doi: 10.1371/journal.pone.0217761
56. Zhong D, Xiong L, Liu T, Liu X, Liu X, Chen J, et al. The glycolytic inhibitor 2-deoxyglucose activates multiple prosurvival pathways through IGF1R. *J Biol Chem.* (2009) 284:23225–33. doi: 10.1074/jbc.m109.005280
57. Abdelmagid SA, Clarke SE, Nielsen DE, Badawi A, El-Sohemy A, Mutch DM, et al. Comprehensive profiling of plasma fatty acid concentrations in young healthy Canadian adults. *PLoS One.* (2015) 10:e0116195. doi: 10.1371/journal.pone.0116195
58. Riggio O, Merli M, Cantafora A, Di Biase A, Lalloni L, Leonetti F, et al. Total and individual free fatty acid concentrations in liver cirrhosis. *Metabolism.* (1984) 33:646–51. doi: 10.1016/0026-0495(84)90064-7
59. Raud B, Roy DG, Divakaruni AS, Tarasenko TN, Franke R, Ma EH, et al. Etomoxir actions on regulatory and memory T cells are independent of cpt1a-mediated fatty acid oxidation. *Cell Metab.* (2018) 28:504–515e507.
60. O'Connor RS, Guo L, Ghassemi S, Snyder NW, Worth AJ, Weng L, et al. The CPT1a inhibitor, etomoxir induces severe oxidative stress at commonly used concentrations. *Sci Rep.* (2018) 8:6289.
61. Pollizzi KN, Powell JD. Regulation of T cells by mTOR: the known knowns and the known unknowns. *Trends Immunol.* (2015) 36:13–20. doi: 10.1016/j.it.2014.11.005
62. Colombetti S, Basso V, Mueller DL, Mondino A. Prolonged TCR/CD28 engagement drives IL-2-independent T cell clonal expansion through signaling mediated by the mammalian target of rapamycin. *J Immunol.* (2006) 176:2730–8. doi: 10.4049/jimmunol.176.5.2730
63. Huang J, Manning BD. A complex interplay between Akt, TSC2 and the two mTOR complexes. *Biochem Soc Trans.* (2009) 37:217–22. doi: 10.1042/bst0370217
64. Manning BD, Cantley LC. Rheb fills a GAP between TSC and TOR. *Trends Biochem Sci.* (2003) 28:573–6. doi: 10.1016/j.tibs.2003.09.003
65. He N, Fan W, Henriquez B, Yu RT, Atkins AR, Liddle C, et al. Metabolic control of regulatory T cell (Treg) survival and function by Lkb1. *Proc Natl Acad Sci USA.* (2017) 114:12542–7. doi: 10.1073/pnas.1715363114
66. Ikeda K, Kinoshita M, Kayama H, Nagamori S, Kongpracha P, Umemoto E, et al. Slc3a2 mediates branched-chain amino-acid-dependent maintenance of regulatory T Cells. *Cell Rep.* (2017) 21:1824–38. doi: 10.1016/j.celrep.2017.10.082
67. Nakaya M, Xiao Y, Zhou X, Chang JH, Chang M, Cheng X, et al. Inflammatory T cell responses rely on amino acid transporter ASCT2 facilitation of glutamine uptake and mTORC1 kinase activation. *Immunity.* (2014) 40:692–705. doi: 10.1016/j.immuni.2014.04.007
68. Do MH, Wang X, Zhang X, Chou C, Nixon BG, Capistrano KJ, et al. Nutrient mTORC1 signaling underpins regulatory T cell control of immune tolerance. *J Exp Med.* (2020) 217:848.
69. Zeng H, Yang K, Cloer C, Neale G, Vogel P, Chi H. mTORC1 couples immune signals and metabolic programming to establish T(reg)-cell function. *Nature.* (2013) 499:485–90. doi: 10.1038/nature12297
70. Delgoffe GM, Pollizzi KN, Waickman AT, Heikamp E, Meyers DJ, Horton MR, et al. The kinase mTOR regulates the differentiation of helper T cells through the selective activation of signaling by mTORC1 and mTORC2. *Nat Immunol.* (2011) 12:295–303.
71. Charbonnier LM, Cui Y, Stephen-Victor E, Harb H, Lopez D, Bleesing JJ, et al. Functional reprogramming of regulatory T cells in the absence of Foxp3. *Nat Immunol.* (2019) 20:1208–19. doi: 10.1038/s41590-019-0442-x
72. Jungermann K, Kietzmann T. Oxygen: modulator of metabolic zonation and disease of the liver. *Hepatology.* (2000) 31:255–60. doi: 10.1002/hep.510310201
73. Blagih J, Coulombe F, Vincent EE, Dupuy F, Galicia-Vazquez G, Yurchenko E, et al. The energy sensor AMPK regulates T cell metabolic adaptation and effector responses in vivo. *Immunity.* (2015) 42:41–54. doi: 10.1016/j.immuni.2014.12.030
74. Galic S, Loh K, Murray-Segal L, Steinberg GR, Andrews ZB, Kemp BE. AMPK signaling to acetyl-CoA carboxylase is required for fasting- and cold-induced appetite but not thermogenesis. *Elife.* (2018) 7:e32656.
75. Semenza GL. Hypoxia-inducible factor 1 (HIF-1) pathway. *Sci Stke.* (2007) 2007:cm8. doi: 10.1126/stke.4072007cm8
76. Clambey ET, McNamee EN, Westrich JA, Glover LE, Campbell EL, Jedlicka P, et al. Hypoxia-inducible factor-1 alpha-dependent induction of FoxP3 drives regulatory T-cell abundance and function during inflammatory hypoxia of the mucosa. *Proc Natl Acad Sci USA.* (2012) 109:E2784–93.
77. Shi LZ, Wang R, Huang G, Vogel P, Neale G, Green DR, et al. HIF1alpha-dependent glycolytic pathway orchestrates a metabolic checkpoint for the differentiation of TH17 and Treg cells. *J Exp Med.* (2011) 208:1367–76. doi: 10.1084/jem.20110278
78. Ben-Shoshan J, Maysel-Auslender S, Mor A, Keren G, George J. Hypoxia

controls CD4+CD25+ regulatory T-cell homeostasis via hypoxia-inducible factor-1alpha. *Eur J Immunol.* (2008) 38:2412–8. doi: 10.1002/eji.200838318
79. Nakamura H, Makino Y, Okamoto K, Poellinger L, Ohnuma K, Morimoto C, et al. Engagement increases hypoxia-inducible factor-1 alpha protein synthesis via rapamycin-sensitive pathway under hypoxic conditions in human peripheral T cells. *J Immunol.* (2005) 174:7592–9. doi: 10.4049/jimmunol.174.12.7592
80. Dang EV, Barbi J, Yang HY, Jinasena D, Yu H, Zheng Y, et al. Control of T(H)17/T(reg) balance by hypoxia-inducible factor 1. *Cell.* (2011) 146:772–84.
81. Lee JH, Elly C, Park Y, Liu YC. E3 ubiquitin ligase VHL regulates hypoxia-inducible factor-1alpha to maintain regulatory T cell stability and suppressive capacity. *Immunity.* (2015) 42:1062–74. doi: 10.1016/j.immuni.2015.05.016
82. Semenza GL, Roth PH, Fang HM, Wang GL. Transcriptional regulation of genes encoding glycolytic enzymes by hypoxia-inducible factor 1. *J Biol Chem.* (1994) 269:23757–63.
83. Chawla A, Repa JJ, Evans RM, Mangelsdorf DJ. Nuclear receptors and lipid physiology: opening the X-files. *Science.* (2001) 294:1866–70. doi: 10.1126/science.294.5548.1866
84. Angela M, Endo Y, Asou HK, Yamamoto T, Tumes DJ, Tokuyama H, et al. Fatty acid metabolic reprogramming via mTOR-mediated inductions of PPARgamma directs early activation of T cells. *Nat Commun.* (2016) 7:13683.
85. Cipolletta D, Feuerer M, Li A, Kamei N, Lee J, Shoelson SE, et al. Gamma is a major driver of the accumulation and phenotype of adipose tissue Treg cells. *Nature.* (2012) 486:549–53. doi: 10.1038/nature11132
86. Janowski BA, Willy PJ, Devi TR, Falck JR, Mangelsdorf DJ. An oxysterol signalling pathway mediated by the nuclear receptor LXR alpha. *Nature.* (1996) 383:728–31. doi: 10.1038/383728a0
87. Bookout AL, Jeong Y, Downes M, Yu RT, Evans RM, Mangelsdorf DJ. Anatomical profiling of nuclear receptor expression reveals a hierarchical transcriptional network. *Cell.* (2006) 126:789–99. doi: 10.1016/j.cell.2006.06.049
88. Bensinger SJ, Bradley MN, Joseph SB, Zelcer N, Janssen EM, Hausner MA, et al. Signaling couples sterol metabolism to proliferation in the acquired immune response. *Cell.* (2008) 134:97–111. doi: 10.1016/j.cell.2008.04.052
89. Herold M, Breuer J, Hucke S, Knolle P, Schwab N, Wiendl H, et al. Liver X receptor activation promotes differentiation of regulatory T cells. *PLoS One.* (2017) 12:e0184985. doi: 10.1371/journal.pone.0184985
90. Griffett K, Welch RD, Flaveny CA, Kolar GR, Neuschwander-Tetri BA, Burris TP. The LXR inverse agonist SR9238 suppresses fibrosis in a model of non-alcoholic steatohepatitis. *Mol Metab.* (2015) 4:353–7. doi: 10.1016/j.molmet.2015.01.009
91. Devlin AS, Fischbach MA. A biosynthetic pathway for a prominent class of microbiota-derived bile acids. *Nat Chem Biol.* (2015) 11:685–90. doi: 10.1038/nchembio.1864
92. Schote AB, Turner JD, Schiltz J, Muller CP. Nuclear receptors in human immune cells: expression and correlations. *Mol Immunol.* (2007) 44:1436–45. doi: 10.1016/j.molimm.2006.04.021
93. Hang S, Paik D, Yao L, Kim E, Trinath J, Lu J, et al. Bile acid metabolites control TH17 and Treg cell differentiation. *Nature.* (2019) 576:143–8. doi: 10.1038/s41586-019-1785-z
94. Campbell C, McKenney PT, Konstantinovsky D, Isaeva OI, Schizas M, Verter J, et al. Bacterial metabolism of bile acids promotes generation of peripheral regulatory T cells. *Nature.* (2020). doi: 10.1038/s41586-020-2193-0 [Epub ahead of print].
95. Haussler MR, Whitfield GK, Kaneko I, Haussler CA, Hsieh D, Hsieh JC, et al. Molecular mechanisms of vitamin D action. *Calcif Tissue Int.* (2013) 92:77–98.
96. Jeffery LE, Burke F, Mura M, Zheng Y, Qureshi OS, Hewison M, et al. 1,25-Dihydroxyvitamin D3 and IL-2 combine to inhibit T cell production of inflammatory cytokines and promote development of regulatory T cells expressing CTLA-4 and FoxP3. *J Immunol.* (2009) 183:5458–67. doi: 10.4049/jimmunol.0803217
97. Urry Z, Chambers ES, Xystrakis E, Dimeloe S, Richards DF, Gabrysova L, et al. The role of 1alpha,25-dihydroxyvitamin D3 and cytokines in the promotion of distinct Foxp3+ and IL-10+ CD4+ T cells. *Eur J Immunol.* (2012) 42:2697–708. doi: 10.1002/eji.201242370
98. Lu D, Lan B, Din Z, Chen H, Chen G. A vitamin D receptor agonist converts CD4+ T cells to Foxp3+ regulatory T cells in patients with ulcerative colitis. *Oncotarget.* (2017) 8:53552–62. doi: 10.18632/oncotarget.18614
99. Golovina TN, Mikheeva T, Brusko TM, Blazar BR, Bluestone JA, Riley JL. Retinoic acid and rapamycin differentially affect and synergistically promote the ex vivo expansion of natural human T regulatory cells. *PLoS One.* (2011) 6:e15868. doi: 10.1371/journal.pone.0015868
100. Lu L, Ma J, Li Z, Lan Q, Chen M, Liu Y, et al. All-trans retinoic acid promotes TGF-beta-induced Tregs via histone modification but not DNA demethylation on Foxp3 gene locus. *PLoS One.* (2011) 6:e24590. doi: 10.1371/journal.pone.0024590
101. Itoh S, Kimura N, Axtell RC, Velotta JB, Gong Y, Wang X, et al. Interleukin-17 accelerates allograft rejection by suppressing regulatory T cell expansion. *Circulation.* (2011) 124:S187–96.
102. Thornton AM, Shevach EM. Suppressor effector function of CD4+CD25+ immunoregulatory T cells is antigen nonspecific. *J Immunol.* (2000) 164:183–90. doi: 10.4049/jimmunol.164.1.183
103. Reckzeh ES, Waldmann H. Small-molecule inhibition of glucose transporters GLUT-1-4. *Chembiochem.* (2020) 21:45–52. doi: 10.1002/cbic.201900544
104. Zhang D, Li J, Wang F, Hu J, Wang S, Sun Y. 2-Deoxy-D-glucose targeting of glucose metabolism in cancer cells as a potential therapy. *Cancer Lett.* (2014) 355:176–83. doi: 10.1016/j.canlet.2014.09.003
105. Geloen A, Helin L, Geeraert B, Malaud E, Holvoet P, Marguerie G. CD36 inhibitors reduce postprandial hypertriglyceridemia and protect against diabetic dyslipidemia and atherosclerosis. *PLoS One.* (2012) 7:e37633. doi: 10.1371/journal.pone.0037633
106. Wang YT, Liu CH, Zhu HL. Fatty acid binding protein (FABP) inhibitors: a patent review (2012-2015). *Expert Opin Ther Pat.* (2016) 26:767–76. doi: 10.1080/13543776.2016.1182500
107. Srinivas TR, Meier-Kriesche HU, Kaplan B. Pharmacokinetic principles of immunosuppressive drugs. *Am J Transplant.* (2005) 5:207–17. doi: 10.1111/j.1600-6143.2005.00748.x
108. Nasralla D, Coussios CC, Mergental H, Akhtar MZ, Butler AJ, Ceresa CDL, et al. Consortium for Organ Preservation in E. A randomized trial of normothermic preservation in liver transplantation. *Nature.* (2018) 557:50–6.
109. Bishawi M, Roan J-N, Milano CA, Daneshmand MA, Schroder JN, Chiang Y, et al. Normothermic ex vivo organ perfusion delivery method for cardiac transplantation gene therapy. *Sci Rep.* (2019) 9:8029.
110. Divithotawela C, Cypel M, Martinu T, Singer LG, Binnie M, Chow CW, et al. Long-term outcomes of lung transplant with ex vivo lung perfusion. *JAMA Surg.* (2019). doi: 10.1001/jamasurg.2019.4079 [Epub ahead of print].
111. Saunders RN, Metcalfe MS, Nicholson ML. Rapamycin in transplantation: a review of the evidence. *Kidney Int.* (2001) 59:3–16. doi: 10.1046/j.1523-1755.2001.00460.x
112. Rena G, Hardie DG, Pearson ER. The mechanisms of action of metformin. *Diabetologia.* (2017) 60:1577–85. doi: 10.1007/s00125-017-4342-z
113. Procaccini C, De Rosa V, Galgani M, Abanni L, Cali G, Porcellini A, et al. An oscillatory switch in mTOR kinase activity sets regulatory T cell responsiveness. *Immunity.* (2010) 33:929–41. doi: 10.1016/j.immuni.2010.11.024
114. Laing RW, Bhogal RH, Wallace L, Boteon Y, Neil DAH, Smith A, et al. The use of an acellular oxygen carrier in a human liver model of normothermic machine perfusion. *Transplantation.* (2017) 101:2746–56. doi: 10.1097/tp.0000000000001821
115. Yu T, Tang B, Sun X. Development of inhibitors targeting hypoxia-inducible factor 1 and 2 for cancer therapy. *Yonsei Med J.* (2017) 58:489–96. doi: 10.3349/ymj.2017.58.3.489
116. Fricker LD. Proteasome inhibitor drugs. *Ann Rev Pharmacol Toxicol.* (2020) 60:457–76. doi: 10.1146/annurev-pharmtox-010919-023603
117. Hasegawa S, Tanaka T, Nangaku M. Hypoxia-inducible factor stabilizers for treating anemia of chronic kidney disease. *Curr Opin Nephrol Hypertens.* (2018) 27:331–8. doi: 10.1097/mnh.0000000000000431
118. Cheng HS, Tan WR, Low ZS, Marvalim C, Lee JYH, Tan NS. Exploration and development of PPAR modulators in health and disease: an update of clinical evidence. *Int J Mol Sci.* (2019) 20:5055. doi: 10.3390/ijms20205055
119. Beltowski J. Liver X receptors (LXR) as therapeutic targets in dyslipidemia. *Cardiovasc Ther.* (2008) 26:297–316. doi: 10.1111/j.1755-5922.2008.00062.x

11

Effect of Hepatic Macrophage Polarization and Apoptosis on Liver Ischemia and Reperfusion Injury During Liver Transplantation

Liping Ye [1], *Saiqin He* [1,2], *Xinli Mao* [1], *Yu Zhang* [1], *Yue Cai* [1] *and Shaowei Li* [1*]

[1] *Department of Gastroenterology, Taizhou Hospital of Zhejiang Province Affiliated to Wenzhou Medical University, Linhai, China,* [2] *Endoscopy Center, Taizhou Hospital of Zhejiang Province Affiliated to Wenzhou Medical University, Linhai, China*

Correspondence:
Shaowei Li
li_shaowei81@hotmail.com

Ischemia-reperfusion (I/R) injury is injury caused by a limited blood supply and subsequent blood supply recovery during liver transplantation. Serious ischemia-reperfusion injury is the main cause of transplant failure. Hepatic I/R is characterized by tissue hypoxia due to a limited blood supply and reperfusion inducing oxidative stress and an immune response. Studies have confirmed that Kupffer cells (KCs), resident macrophages in the liver, play a key role in aseptic inflammation induced by I/R. In liver macrophage polarization, M1 macrophages activated by interferon-γ (IFN-γ) and lipopolysaccharide (LPS) exert a pro-inflammatory effect and release a variety of inflammatory cytokines. M2 macrophages activated by IL-4 have an anti-inflammatory response. M1-type KCs are the dominant players in I/R as they secrete various pro-inflammatory cytokines that exacerbate the injury and recruit other types of immune cells via the circulation. In contrast, M2-type KCs can ameliorate I/R through unregulated anti-inflammatory factors. A new notion has been proposed that KC apoptosis may influence I/R in yet another manner as well. Management of KCs is expected to help improve I/R. This review summarizes the effects of hepatic macrophage polarization and apoptosis on liver I/R.

Keywords: liver transplantation, kupffer cells, ischemia reperfusion, apoptosis, polarization

INTRODUCTION

Advances in surgical procedures and the application of immunosuppressive technologies have made liver transplantation (LT) the optimal treatment for almost all types of end-stage liver disease (1). The current technology has brought the 1-year survival rate of patients receiving LT to more than 80%, but some problems associated with LT must still be addressed.

The most important factor is I/R (2), which includes ischemic liver damage and subsequent reperfusion injury. It is a two-stage pathophysiological process that occurs during liver resection and liver transplantation (3). Hepatic ischemic injury is characterized by ATP and glycogen depletion as well as cellular metabolic stress caused by mitochondrial dysfunction, all of which lead to initial cell death (4). Subsequent reperfusion injury refers to the phenomenon wherein the liver sustains severe damage after the blood flow and reoxygenation are restored. During this process, metabolic disorders and a large number of reactive oxygen species (ROS) and cytokines or chemokines stimulate various immune cells to produce a severe inflammatory response (5).

Multiple studies have shown that I/R damage to the liver tissue involves a series of pathological processes (6–8). I/R-related macrophage activation and related inflammatory factor explosions are key to graft dysfunction and even the occurrence of primary non-function (9, 10).

The liver has several types of innate immune cells, including the inherent macrophages known as Kupffer cells (KCs) (11), dendritic cells (DCs), and natural killer T (NKT) cells. KCs are an important part of the innate immune response and the largest fixed macrophage population in the body, accounting for 40–65% of the total liver non-parenchymal cells (12). Polarization and apoptosis of KCs have been recognized as important topics concerning hepatic I/R injury.

We herein review the dual role of KC polarization and apoptosis in I/R.

QUIESCENCE AND ACTIVATION OF KCs IN I/R

KCs are liver macrophages located in the liver sinusoid and play a key role in the immune response. Under steady-state conditions, KCs have close contact with circulating blood flowing from the portal vein or hepatic artery, which allows them to devour most pathogens. In addition, they are responsible for removing other substances, including cell debris and immune complexes (13). It is now believed that KCs in healthy livers exhibit a "tolerogenic" phenotype that can maintain immune tolerance. However, in a disease state, such as IR, a phenotypic change occurs, which is involved in the immune response (14, 15). The activated KCs secrete pro-inflammatory cytokines and induce a subsequent inflammatory response. The activated KC function is, thus, enhanced, and the cells produce a number of different cytokines and chemokines, such as IL-6, TNFα, Nos2, Argl, and Mrcl (16).

POLARIZATION OF KCs IN I/R

KCs are usually polarized to the M1 type during hepatic IR damage (17). It is important that macrophage polarization be understood as a spectrum of transformation. There is no pure M1- or M2-type macrophage population, and these phenotypes undergo transformation according to the stimulation signals they receive (18). M2 macrophages can counteract the pro-inflammatory effects of M1 macrophages during the process of inhibiting pro-inflammatory signaling (19). The pathogenesis of type 2 diabetes (T2D) is chronic hyperinsulinemia caused by systemic and hepatic insulin resistance (IR). Without intervention, pancreatic β-cell failure will result. IR and T2D are commonly observed in individuals with non-alcoholic fatty liver disease (NAFLD) (20).

Hyperglycemia reduces the secretion of IL-10 by inducing the reduction of Argl and Mrcl expression and the activation of the STAT3 and STAT6 signaling pathways to inhibit M2-like KC polarization. It was demonstrated that hyperglycemia induces high inflammatory activation of KCs during liver I/R. Therefore, the hyperglycemia-induced overexpression of C/EBP homologous protein (CHOP) inhibits the polarization of M2-like KCs secreted IL-10, leading to inflammatory activation of KC during liver I/R (21).

PPAR-γ exerts a protective effect by inducing KCs to polarize to M2-type macrophages (22). Sphingosine-1-phosphate (S1P) and sphingosine-1-phosphate receptors (S1PRs) are involved in metabolic and inflammatory diseases. Hyperglycemia exacerbates I/R by promoting M1 polarization and inhibiting M2 polarization, specifically triggering S1P/S1PR3 signaling (23).

Min et al. used myeloid-specific HO-1 gene knockout (mHO-1-KO) and transgenic (mHO-1-Tg) mice to delete or overexpress HO-1, verifying that myeloid HO-1 expression improves liver IR damage by promoting macrophage M2 phenotypic polarization. Interestingly, in human liver transplantation biopsies, subjects with higher HO-1 levels showed a lower expression of M1 markers and higher expression of M2 markers as well as reduced hepatic damage and an improved prognosis (24). Soluble fibrinogen-like protein 2 (sFGL2) promotes the secretion of anti-inflammatory cytokines (IL-10, TGF-β) and the high expression of CD206 and inhibits the activity of STAT1 and NF-κB signaling pathways. sFGL2 improves the prognosis of LT by inducing KC M2 polarization in rat orthotropic liver transplantation (OLT) models (25).

APOPTOSIS OF KCs AND I/R

A transplanted liver is not only directly affected by I/R but also damaged by apoptosis during transplantation (26). At present, inhibiting and regulating the KC function has become a hot topic in protecting transplanted livers from I/R. GdCl3 induces KC apoptosis and reduces IR damage in liver transplantation (27). In the early stages of I/R, the activation of KCs and overexpression of inflammatory factors, such as TNF-α, are the main causes of graft dysfunction after transplantation (28). KC activation inhibitors are widely used drugs that reduce liver damage in donor animals (29).

KCs exert a protective effect on liver tissue I/R during transplantation (30). Upregulating the expression of IL-10 can protect against I/R in steatotic liver, and more importantly, KC still has a hepatoprotective effect in steatotic liver (31).

Mesenchymal stem cells (MSCs) have been proposed as promising treatments for certain liver diseases, and studies have found that MSCs also have a protective role in "donated after circulatory death" LT. In a mouse non-heartbeat LT model, the survival rate and cytokine, and chemokine expression of animals with and without MSC infusion were compared. It was found that the protective effect of MSCs on I/R was caused by the

---

Abbreviations: LT, liver transplantation; I/R, ischemia-reperfusion injury; KC, Kupffer cells; ROS, reactive oxygen species; TNF-α, tumor necrosis factor α; IL, interleukin; DAMPs, Damage-associated molecular patterns; sFGL2, Soluble fibrinogen-like protein 2; DC, dendritic cells.

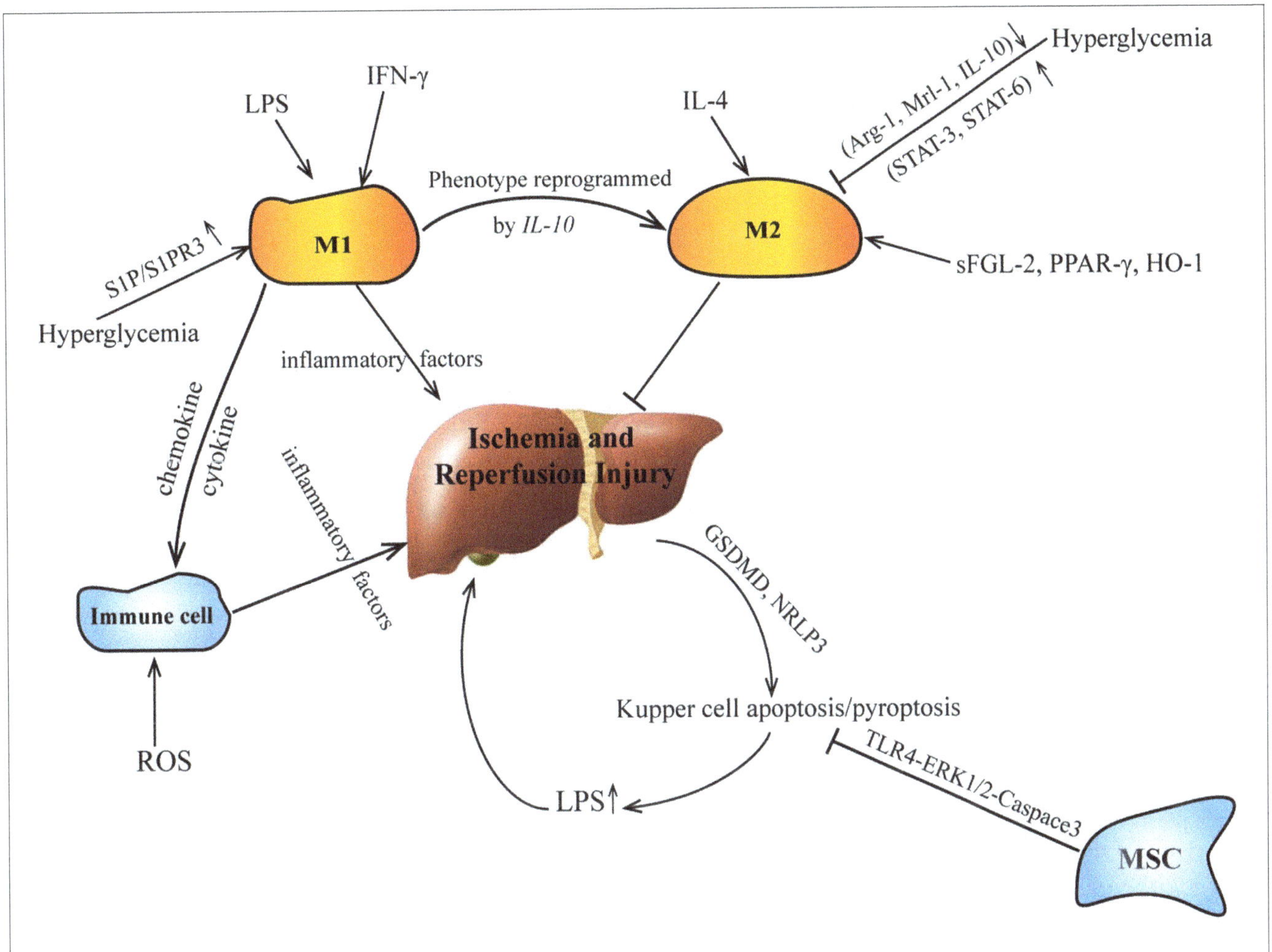

FIGURE 1 | The crosstalk of apoptosis/pyroptosis and polarization of KCs in I/R. IL, Interleukin; sFGL, soluble fibrinogen-like protein.

secretion of PGE2, which regulated the TLR4-ERK1/2-caspase3 pathway and inhibited KC apoptosis (32). KCs, as an important part of the reticuloendothelial system, are responsible for the clearance and detoxification of intestinal Lipopolysaccharide (LPS) (33). Under conditions of KC depletion, LPS is not effectively metabolized in the liver and may continue to cause damage (34). However, indiscriminately reducing KC activation is not an effective way to reduce I/R in steatosis liver (31).

CROSSTALK OF APOPTOSIS AND POLARIZATION OF KCs IN I/R

IL-10 is a key anti-inflammatory cytokine produced by immune cells when activated (35). The macrophage phenotype can be reprogrammed from M1 to M2 by upregulating endogenous IL-10 (36). M1 polarization is promoted while M2 polarization is inhibited to specifically aggravate liver I/R (23). In the absence of IL 10 signaling, mTOR can promote the accumulation of damaged mitochondria in macrophages, leading to the dysregulation of NLRP3 inflammatory bodies and production of excess IL-1β (37). In the polarization of primary human macrophages, the expression of apoptosis inhibitor (IAP) protein is different in macrophages with different polarizations. NLR family apoptosis inhibitory protein (NAIP) is highly expressed in M2 macrophages, and cellular IAP 1 (cIAP1) and cIAP2 show opposite expression patterns in M1/M2 polarized macrophages with cIAP1 expressed in M2 and cIAP2 preferentially expressed in M1. Interestingly, IAP antagonists can induce the upregulation of NAIP in M2, downregulation of cIAP1 expression in M1 and M2, and high expression of cIAP2 in M1 macrophages (38).

Cell pyrolysis (pyroptosis), also known as cell inflammatory necrosis, is a new type of programmed cell death (39). It is shown that the permeability of the cell membrane changes, resulting in the release of a large amount of cell contents; at the same time, the water outside the cell enters the cell via channels in the cell membrane. This eventually results in the cell lysing to death, triggering a strong inflammation reaction (40). Liver

I/R may promote the pyroptosis of KCs mediated by GSDMD and NRLP3 (41). M2-type KCs promote M1-type KC apoptosis through an IL-10-mediated arginase-dependent mechanism (42). The crosstalk of apoptosis/pyroptosis and polarization of KCs in I/R are shown on **Figure 1**.

CONCLUSION AND FUTURE DIRECTIONS

Because I/R during LT can increase the risk of graft dysfunction, transplant rejection, and organ failure, managing I/R remains a major problem in clinical practice. I/R activates KCs, and these activated KCs can be polarized into two subtypes. M1-type KCs play a pro-inflammatory role, and M2-type KCs play an anti-inflammatory role. The effects of KC apoptosis on I/R development are controversial at present. Interestingly, IL-10 plays a role in attenuating liver I/R, likely through regulating the apoptosis of KCs as well as modifying their polarization. However, the mechanism underlying liver I/R is not yet fully understood, highlighting the importance of continued research and clarifying the role of KCs in all factors involved in I/R. Such an understanding will aid in the development of more accurate and complete treatment strategies for LT. Future research on I/R in LT should be aimed at developing new therapeutic interventions, implementing prognostic biomarkers based on KCs, and designing clinical studies. It will be necessary to identify new technologies based on regulating the polarization and apoptosis of KCs to encourage the macrophage population to develop in a direction that results in beneficial rather than harmful inflammatory responses.

AUTHOR CONTRIBUTIONS

LY, SH, XM, YZ, YC, and SL contributed to the writing and editing of the manuscript. All authors contributed to the article and approved the submitted version.

REFERENCES

1. Russo FP, Ferrarese A, Zanetto A. Recent advances in understanding and managing liver transplantation. *F1000Res.* (2016) 5:F1000. doi: 10.12688/f1000research.8768.1
2. Cardoso L, Moreira LFP, Pinto MA, Henriques-Pons A, Alves LA. Domino hepatocyte transplantation: a therapeutic alternative for the treatment of acute liver failure. *Can J Gastroenterol Hepatol.* (2018) 2018:2593745. doi: 10.1155/2018/2593745
3. Jimenez-Castro MB, Cornide-Petronio ME, Gracia-Sancho J, Peralta C. Inflammasome-mediated inflammation in liver ischemia-reperfusion injury *Cells.* (2019) 8:1131. doi: 10.3390/cells8101131
4. Kalogeris T, Baines CP, Krenz M, Korthuis RJ. Cell biology of ischemia/reperfusion injury. *Int Rev Cell Mol Biol.* (2012) 298:229–317. doi: 10.1016/B978-0-12-394309-5.00006-7
5. Granger DN, Kvietys PR. Reperfusion injury and reactive oxygen species: the evolution of a concept. *Redox Biol.* (2015) 6:524–51. doi: 10.1016/j.redox.2015.08.020
6. Zhang W, Wang M, Xie HY, Zhou L, Meng XQ, Shi J, et al. Role of reactive oxygen species in mediating hepatic ischemia-reperfusion injury and its therapeutic applications in liver transplantation. *Transplant Proc.* (2007) 39:1332–7. doi: 10.1016/j.transproceed.2006.11.021
7. Kalogeris T, Baines CP, Krenz M, Korthuis RJ. Ischemia/Reperfusion. *Compr Physiol.* (2016) 7:113–70. doi: 10.1002/cphy.c160006
8. Soares ROS, Losada DM, Jordani MC, Evora P, Castro ESO. Ischemia/reperfusion injury revisited: an overview of the latest pharmacological strategies. *Int J Mol Sci.* (2019) 20:5034. doi: 10.3390/ijms20205034
9. Bhogal RH, Sutaria R, Afford SC. Hepatic liver ischemia/reperfusion injury: processes in inflammatory networks–a review. *Liver Transpl.* (2011) 17:95. doi: 10.1002/lt.22205
10. Datta G, Fuller BJ, Davidson BR. Molecular mechanisms of liver ischemia reperfusion injury: insights from transgenic knockout models. *World J Gastroenterol.* (2013) 19:1683–98. doi: 10.3748/wjg.v19.i11.1683
11. Lee LY, Kaizu T, Toyokawa H, Zhang M, Ross M, Stolz DB, et al. Carbon monoxide induces hypothermia tolerance in Kupffer cells and attenuates liver ischemia/reperfusion injury in rats. *Liver Transpl.* (2011) 17:1457–66. doi: 10.1002/lt.22415
12. Lee VG, Johnson ML, Baust J, Laubach VE, Watkins SC, Billiar TR. The roles of iNOS in liver ischemia-reperfusion injury. *Shock.* (2001) 16:355–60. doi: 10.1097/00024382-200116050-00006
13. Ramirez-Pedraza M, Fernandez M. Interplay between macrophages and angiogenesis: a double-edged sword in liver disease. *Front Immunol.* (2019) 10:2882. doi: 10.3389/fimmu.2019.02882
14. Heymann F, Peusquens J, Ludwig-Portugall I, Kohlhepp M, Ergen C, Niemietz P, et al. Liver inflammation abrogates immunological tolerance induced by Kupffer cells. *Hepatology.* (2015) 62:279–91. doi: 10.1002/hep.27793
15. Byun JS, Yi HS. Hepatic immune microenvironment in alcoholic and nonalcoholic liver disease. *Biomed Res Int.* (2017) 2017:6862439. doi: 10.1155/2017/6862439
16. Dong B, Zhou Y, Wang W, Scott J, Kim KH, Sun Z, et al. Vitamin D receptor activation in liver macrophages ameliorates hepatic inflammation, steatosis, and insulin resistance in mice. *Hepatology.* (2019) 71:1559–74. doi: 10.1002/hep.30937
17. Nagy LE. The role of innate immunity in alcoholic liver disease. *Alcohol Res.* (2015) 37:237-50.
18. Yang F, Wang S, Liu Y, Zhou Y, Shang L, Feng M, et al. IRE1alpha aggravates ischemia reperfusion injury of fatty liver by regulating phenotypic transformation of kupffer cells. *Free Radic Biol Med.* (2018) 124:395–407. doi: 10.1016/j.freeradbiomed.2018.06.043
19. Sica A, Mantovani A. Macrophage plasticity and polarization: *in vivo* veritas. *J Clin Invest.* (2012) 122:787–95. doi: 10.1172/JCI59643
20. Ballestri S, Nascimbeni F, Romagnoli D, Baldelli E, Targher G, Lonardo A. Type 2 diabetes in non-alcoholic fatty liver disease and hepatitis C virus infection–liver: the "musketeer" in the spotlight. *Int J Mol Sci.* (2016) 17:355. doi: 10.3390/ijms17030355
21. Rao Z, Sun J, Pan X, Chen Z, Sun H, Zhang P, et al. Hyperglycemia aggravates hepatic ischemia and reperfusion injury by inhibiting liver-resident macrophage M2 polarization via C/EBP homologous protein-mediated endoplasmic reticulum stress. *Front Immunol.* (2017) 8:1299. doi: 10.3389/fimmu.2017.01299
22. Linares I, Farrokhi K, Echeverri J, Kaths JM, Kollmann D, Hamar M, et al. PPAR-gamma activation is associated with reduced liver ischemia-reperfusion injury and altered tissue-resident macrophages polarization in a mouse model. *PLoS ONE.* (2018) 13:e0195212. doi: 10.1371/journal.pone.0195212
23. Hu Y, Yang C, Shen G, Yang S, Cheng X, Cheng F, et al. Hyperglycemia-triggered sphingosine-1-phosphate and sphingosine-1-phosphate receptor 3 signaling worsens liver ischemia/reperfusion injury by regulating M1/M2 polarization. *Liver Transpl.* (2019) 25:1074–90. doi: 10.1002/lt.25470
24. Zhang M, Nakamura K, Kageyama S, Lawal AO, Gong KW, Bhetraratana M, et al. Myeloid HO-1 modulates macrophage polarization and protects against ischemia-reperfusion injury. *JCI Insight.* (2018) 3:e120596. doi: 10.1172/jci.insight.120596
25. Pan G, Zhao Z, Tang C, Ding L, Li Z, Zheng D, et al. Soluble fibrinogen-like protein 2 ameliorates acute rejection of liver transplantation in rat via inducing Kupffer cells M2 polarization. *Cancer Med.* (2018) 7:3168–77. doi: 10.1002/cam4.1528
26. Tao T, Chen F, Bo L, Xie Q, Yi W, Zou Y, et al. Ginsenoside Rg1 protects mouse liver against ischemia-reperfusion injury through anti-inflammatory and anti-apoptosis properties. *J Surg Res.* (2014) 191:231–8. doi: 10.1016/j.jss.2014.03.067
27. Li JY, Gu X, Zhang WH, Jia S, Zhou Y. GdCl3 abates hepatic ischemia-

reperfusion injury by inhibiting apoptosis in rats. *Hepatobiliary Pancreat Dis Int.* (2009) 8:518–23.

28. Gracia-Sancho J, Casillas-Ramirez A, Peralta C. Molecular pathways in protecting the liver from ischaemia/reperfusion injury: a 2015 update. *Clin Sci.* (2015) 129:345–62. doi: 10.1042/CS20150223
29. Yamanaka K, Houben P, Bruns H, Schultze D, Hatano E, Schemmer P. A systematic review of pharmacological treatment options used to reduce ischemia reperfusion injury in rat liver transplantation. *PLoS ONE.* (2014) 10:e0122214. doi: 10.1371/journal.pone.0122214
30. Ellett JD, Atkinson C, Evans ZP, Amani Z, Balish E, Schmidt MG, et al. Murine Kupffer cells are protective in total hepatic ischemia/reperfusion injury with bowel congestion through IL-10. *J Immunol.* (2010) 184:5849–58. doi: 10.4049/jimmunol.0902024
31. Sutter AG, Palanisamy AP, Ellet JD, Schmidt MG, Schnellmann RG, Chavin KD. Intereukin-10 and Kupffer cells protect steatotic mice livers from ischemia-reperfusion injury. *Eur Cytokine Netw.* (2014) 25:69–76. doi: 10.1684/ecn.2015.0359
32. Tian Y, Wang J, Wang W, Ding Y, Sun Z, Zhang Q, et al. Mesenchymal stem cells improve mouse non-heart-beating liver graft survival by inhibiting Kupffer cell apoptosis via TLR4-ERK1/2-Fas/FasL-caspase3 pathway regulation. *Stem Cell Res Ther.* (2016) 7:157. doi: 10.1186/s13287-016-0416-y
33. Shao B, Kitchens RL, Munford RS, Rogers TE, Rockey DC, Varley AW. Prolonged hepatomegaly in mice that cannot inactivate bacterial endotoxin. *Hepatology.* (2011) 54:1051–62. doi: 10.1002/hep.24488
34. Crouser ED, Julian MW, Huff JE, Joshi MS, Bauer JA, Gadd ME, et al. Abnormal permeability of inner and outer mitochondrial membranes contributes independently to mitochondrial dysfunction in the liver during acute endotoxemia. *Crit Care Med.* (2004) 32:478–88. doi: 10.1097/01.CCM.0000109449.99160.81
35. Ouyang W, Rutz S, Crellin NK, Valdez PA, Hymowitz SG. Regulation and functions of the IL-10 family of cytokines in inflammation and disease. *Annu Rev Immunol.* (2011) 29:71–109. doi: 10.1146/annurev-immunol-031210-101312
36. Yu B, Qin SY, Hu BL, Qin QY, Jiang HX, Luo W. Resveratrol improves CCL4-induced liver fibrosis in mouse by upregulating endogenous IL-10 to reprogramme macrophages phenotype from M(LPS) to M(IL 4). *Biomed Pharmacother.* (2019) 117:109110. doi: 10.1016/j.biopha.2019.109110
37. Ip WKE, Hoshi N, Shouval DS, Snapper S, Medzhitov R. Anti-inflammatory effect of IL-10 mediated by metabolic reprogramming of macrophages. *Science.* (2017) 356:513–9. doi: 10.1126/science.aal3535
38. Moron-Calvente V, Romero-Pinedo S, Toribio-Castello S, Plaza-Diaz J, Abadia-Molina AC, Rojas-Barros DI, et al. Inhibitor of apoptosis proteins, NAIP, cIAP1 and cIAP2 expression during macrophage differentiation and M1/M2 polarization. *PLoS ONE.* (2018) 13:e0193643. doi: 10.1371/journal.pone.0193643
39. Shi J, Gao W, Shao F. Pyroptosis: gasdermin-mediated programmed necrotic cell death. *Trends Biochem Sci.* (2017) 42:245–54. doi: 10.1016/j.tibs.2016.10.004
40. Fink SL, Cookson BT. Pillars article: caspase-1-dependent pore formation during pyroptosis leads to osmotic lysis of infected host macrophages. *Cell Microbiol.* (2006) 8:1812–25. doi: 10.1111/j.1462-5822.2006.00751.x
41. Hua S, Ma M, Fei X, Zhang Y, Gong F, Fang M. Glycyrrhizin attenuates hepatic ischemia-reperfusion injury by suppressing HMGB1-dependent GSDMD-mediated kupffer cells pyroptosis. *Int Immunopharmacol.* (2019) 68:145–55. doi: 10.1016/j.intimp.2019.01.002
42. Wan J, Benkdane M, Teixeira-Clerc F, Bonnafous S, Louvet A, Lafdil F, et al. M2 Kupffer cells promote M1 Kupffer cell apoptosis: a protective mechanism against alcoholic and nonalcoholic fatty liver disease. *Hepatology.* (2014) 59:130–42. doi: 10.1002/hep.26607

12

Recent Advances in Costimulatory Blockade to Induce Immune Tolerance in Liver Transplantation

Mingjie Ding[1,2,3]*, Yuting He*[1,2]*, Shuijun Zhang*[1,2,3] *and Wenzhi Guo*[1,2,3]*

[1] *Department of Hepatobiliary and Pancreatic Surgery, The First Affiliated Hospital of Zhengzhou University, Zhengzhou, China,* [2] *Open and Key Laboratory of Hepatobiliary & Pancreatic Surgery and Digestive Organ Transplantation at Henan Universities, Zhengzhou, China,* [3] *Zhengzhou Key Laboratory of Hepatobiliary & Pancreatic Diseases and Organ Transplantation Medicine, Zhengzhou, China*

Correspondence:
Wenzhi Guo
guowz66@163.com

Liver transplantation is an effective therapy for end-stage liver disease. However, most postoperative patients must take immunosuppressive drugs to prevent organ rejection. Interestingly, some transplant recipients have normal liver function and do not experience organ rejection after the withdrawal of immunosuppressive agents. This phenomenon, called immune tolerance, is the ultimate goal in clinical transplantation. Costimulatory molecules play important roles in T cell-mediated immune responses and the maintenance of T cell tolerance. Blocking costimulatory pathways can alter T cell responses and prolong graft survival. Better understanding of the roles of costimulatory molecules has facilitated the use of costimulatory blockade to effectively induce immune tolerance in animal transplantation models. In this article, we review the state of the art in costimulatory pathway blockade for the induction of immune tolerance in transplantation and its potential application prospects for liver transplantation.

Keywords: liver transplantation, immune tolerance, costimulatory, block, induce

INTRODUCTION

Liver transplantation is the most effective treatment for end-stage liver disease. However, graft rejection seriously restricts graft function and recipient quality of life. The emergence of immunosuppressive agents has reduced the occurrence of rejection and improved transplant outcomes. However, most recipients require lifelong immunosuppression, which is expensive and increases the risk of infection; additionally, for hepatocellular carcinoma patients, immunosuppressants increase the risk of tumor recurrence after transplantation. As an "immune-privileged organ," the liver has a lower probability and degree of rejection after transplantation than many solid organs (1). Indeed, in the clinical setting, some transplant recipients develop liver graft immune tolerance-normal liver graft function in the absence of graft rejection after the withdrawal of immunosuppression. The induction of immune tolerance is the ultimate goal for transplant doctors, as it is the best way to avoid graft rejection and the toxic side effects caused by immunosuppressive agents.

Earlier studies found that approximately 20% of liver transplant patients developed immune tolerance after they stopped taking immunosuppressants (2) among those who could not successfully stop taking the drugs, some patients were able to take lower doses of their immunosuppressants. In

2012, Feng et al. (3) conducted an immunosuppressive drug withdrawal test on 20 pediatric patients who had received related-living-donor liver transplants. They found that up to 60% of the recipients successfully stopped taking immunosuppressants completely and achieved liver transplantation immune tolerance. Moreover, the later the time of drug withdrawal after surgery, the higher the probability of the recipient achieving immune tolerance. In an international multicenter study of 102 adult liver transplant patients, 41.8% of those followed for more than 5 years successfully stopped taking immunosuppressants (4). In another study of adult liver transplant patients, up to 63% successfully stopped taking immunosuppressants and achieved immune tolerance (5). Liver transplantation recipients typically achieve immune tolerance late after transplantation, whereas they mainly experience adverse reactions to immunosuppressive agents in the early period after transplantation. Therefore, it is critical to intervene early after transplant to help recipients develop immune tolerance and avoid the deleterious effects of immunosuppressive drugs. The mechanism of liver transplantation immune tolerance has not been fully elucidated, so most methods for inducing immune tolerance are still in preclinical or clinical stages of experimentation.

THE ROLES AND MECHANISMS OF T CELLS IN IMMUNE TOLERANCE

Immune tolerance is divided into central and peripheral immune tolerance. Central immune tolerance is the tolerance to autoantigens generated by exposure to those antigens during embryonic development and the development of T and B cells. Peripheral immune tolerance occurs when mature T cells and B cells are exposed to endogenous or exogenous antigens in the absence of the signals that lead to an immune response. The liver has excellent immune regulation abilities that ensure local and systemic immune tolerance to self and foreign antigens, as well as the effective immune response to pathogens, and immune tolerance is a dynamic, self-replicating state, which requires the host to recognize the graft antigen to form a stable regulatory environment (6). Liver transplant rejection is the core content of transplantation immunity research, and it is an adaptive immune response that involves the activation of T and B lymphocytes. T cells play an important role in immune responses to allografts, the activation of T cells can lead to rejection of allografts, but sometimes it will weaken in the process of liver transplantation, which can promote the acceptance of transplanted liver and even immune tolerance. The mechanism of induction and maintenance of tolerance has been the main focus of transplant immunology researchers.

After the body recognition of "non-self" antigens, immune cells can be activated and generate appropriate immune responses through a series of cell responses, including proliferation and differentiation (7). However, the immune cells showed low or no response when faced self-antigens, and this non-responsive situation or state can be considered as immune tolerance. The formation and maintenance of immune tolerance are affected by multiple immune cells, and T cells act as the most important role, which are the major player of the adaptive immune system. T cells can be divided into different subgroups according to their function, mainly including CD4+T cells (helper T cells, Th), CD8+T cells (cytotoxic T cells, Tc), suppressor T cells, etc. CD4 + cells have affinity for MHC class II, while CD8 + cells have affinity for MHC class I. Th cells can be divided into Th1 and Th2 subsets, in normal conditions, Th1/Th2 is in dynamic balance. Th1 cells mainly secrete interleukin-2 (IL-2), interferon-γ (IFN-γ), tumor necrosis factor-β (TNF-β) and other cytokines, they can activate Tc to induce delayed type hypersensitivity, and can also activate macrophages and natural killer (NK) cells to specifically kill the antigen of the grafts, and participate in the cellular immune response. Th2 cells mainly secrete cytokines such as IL-4, IL-5, IL-10 and IL-13, which participate in humoral immune responses. Meanwhile, they can also induce specific cellular immune responses through other pathways. Th1 and Th2 cells restrict each other. IL-10 can inhibit the synthesis of Th1 cytokines, especially IFN-γ, while IFN-γ can selectively inhibit the proliferation of Th2 cells. Th1 cells play an important role in the development of acute rejection after liver transplantation, while Th2 is mainly related to the formation of tolerance, and the deviation fromTh1 to Th2 is considered to be one of the mechanisms of transplantation tolerance.

Tolerance can be defined as the graft receptor cannot express the destructive immune response of the graft, which can be described as a complex process, balancing the reactivity against foreign antigens and autoantigens. T cell tolerance is an unresponsive state of T cells to self-antigens to prevent the occurrence of autoimmune diseases. Under the stimulation of T cell receptor (TCR) signal, the tolerant T cells could not effectively proliferate and secrete cytokines. There are two different mechanisms for the T cells tolerance occurs. The first is the exhaustion of self-reactive T cells during their maturation in the thymus and the other is to inhibit and/or elimination of self-reactive mature T cells in the periphery (8). T cells need to undergo negative selection and positive selection during their maturation in the thymus gland, and eventually become mature CD4+ and CD8+T cells. After negative and positive selection, mature T cells (CD4+and CD8+) are released from the thymus into the peripheral circulation and secondary lymphoid organs. Most self-reactive T cells are eliminated in the thymus by negative selection, however, it is incomplete and a certain number of self-reactive T cells that escape negative selection and migrate to the periphery. These escaped self-reactive T cells can be eliminated in the periphery through a series of tolerance mechanisms, including the induction of anergy (unresponsiveness), suppression by other immunologically active cells (Tregs) and deletion. T cells activation or tolerance is regulated by a series of costimulatory signals, on one hand, such as CD28 and inducible costimulator (ICOS) are important costimulatory molecules required for T cells activation and function, and inhibit or deficiencies in both them can lead to T cells tolerance. On the other hand, many inhibitory costimulatory molecules such as CTLA-4, PD-1, Lag-3, Tigit, B7-H3,BTLA and B7S1 can also regulate T cells activation or tolerance (9, 10). When T cells are stimulated by TCR and receive a large amount of inhibitory costimulatory signals and lack of positive costimulatory signals, it will lead to T cell tolerance, which is mainly manifested as limited cell expansion and impaired effector function (11, 12).

T-CELL ACTIVATION AND COSTIMULATORY MOLECULAR PATHWAYS

The activation of T cells is a complex process, which three signals are typically required to fully activate T cells. The first signal is specific binding of the TCR on the surface of the initial T cell to an antigen peptide: major histocompatibility complex on the surface of an antigen-presenting cell (APC) (13). The second signal is the interaction of a costimulatory receptor on the T cell membrane with its ligand on the surface of the APC; these costimulatory pairs include CD28/B7 ligands (B7-1 and B7-2), CD40/CD40 ligand (also known as CD154), tumor necrosis factor (TNF) receptor superfamily member 4 (also known as OX40)/TNF superfamily member 4 (also known as OX40L), and ICOS/ICOS ligand (ICOSLG). The balance of signals from costimulatory and coinhibitory receptors on the surface of a T cell determines the functional result of TCR signal transduction (14). TCR stimulation in the absence of the second signal can result in anergy, immune tolerance, or even programmed cell death (**Figure 1**). When the costimulatory signal exceeds the coinhibitory signal, transcription factors are activated that trigger the production of IL-2 and other proinflammatory factors, thereby promoting T cell proliferation and differentiation.

Based on their structures, costimulatory molecules can be roughly divided into 4 groups: the immunoglobulin (Ig)-related family, the TNF-related family, the hepatitis A virus cellular receptor 2 (also known as T-cell immunoglobulin mucin family member 3 [TIM]) family, and the adhesion factor family. In general, the Ig-related superfamily and TNF-related super families are particularly important for adaptive immune responses (15). These costimulatory molecular pathways play important roles in the recognition of antigens and the activation of T cells.

The inhibition of costimulatory molecules is essential for the establishment and maintenance of peripheral immune tolerance. In the absence of appropriate costimulation, the recognition of an antigen by a TCR makes the T cell non-responsive to the antigen, thereby inducing peripheral tolerance (16). Multiple mechanisms contribute to the formation of transplant tolerance, including ignorance, deletion, anergy, exhaustion, and immune regulation; nearly all of these mechanisms involve alloreactive T cells. As blocking these second signals can prevent T cell activation and acute rejection, costimulatory blockade is currently one of the most active areas of research in transplantation immunity. Studies have shown that blocking the activation of T cells can prolong graft survival time (17). So, blocking costimulatory pathways during liver transplantation may change anti-allograft immune responses and weaken rejection, and it is may be a strategy to induce immune tolerance in transplant recipients, thereby limiting toxicity from immunosuppressive drugs after transplantation (18). So, we review the current state of costimulatory pathway blockade for the induction of immune tolerance in transplantation (summarized in **Table 1**).

IG-RELATED SUPERFAMILY COSTIMULATORY PATHWAYS

CD28/B7 Costimulatory Pathway

CD28/B7 is the most important and best-studied costimulatory pathway in transplantation. CD28, the most important costimulatory molecule in the T cell membrane, is a homodimeric cell surface glycoprotein that belongs to the Ig transmembrane superfamily (38). CD80 (also known as B7-1) and CD86 (also known as B7-2), the ligands of CD28, are also members of the Ig superfamily. B7-1 exists as a dimer on the cell surface, whereas B7-2 is a monomer. CD28 binding to B7-1 and B7-2 on APCs activates CD28 signal transduction to enhance T cell responses to antigens. This signal promotes T cell proliferation through the transcription of cytokines such as IL-2 and enhances T cell survival through the transcription of Bcl2-Bclx (39). After the activation of T cells, they can express cytotoxic T-lymphocyte associated antigen 4 (CTLA4), which also binds B7-1 and B7-2. Unlike CD28,

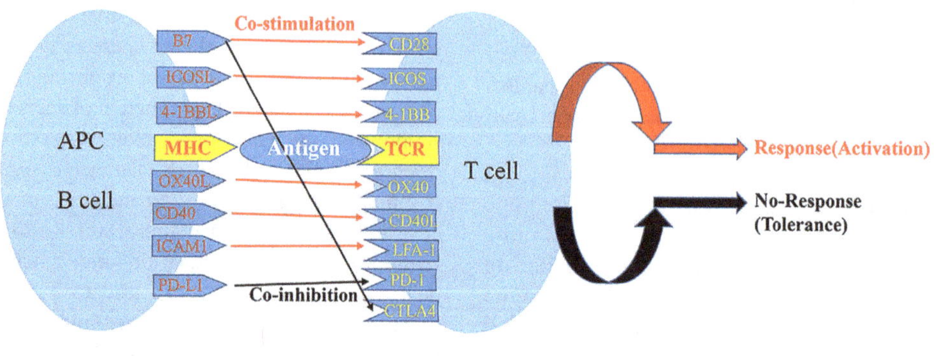

FIGURE 1 | Major costimulatory molecular pathways and their interplay.

TABLE 1 | The roles of costimulatory pathways in liver transplantation.

Costimulatory Signal	Ligand	Strategies to target	Outcome (Effects on liver transplantation immune tolerance)	References
CD28	B7	CTLA-4Ig	Suppress T cell dependent immune response and prolong the long-term survival of xenografts and allografts.	(19–22)
		(belatacept)	Animal Trials: Successfully induced immune tolerance.	(23)
			Clinical Trials: Phase II showed acute rejection and graft loss.	(24)
ICOS	ICOSL	anti- ICOS mAb	Prolong the survival of rat liver allografts and prevent acute rejection, and the combination with FK506 can induce grafts tolerance.	(25) (26)
		RNAi- ICOS	Prevents acute rejection and prolongs the survival of grafts.	(27)
CD40	CD154	anti-CD40 mAb (ASKP1240)	Animal Trials: The non-human primates showed good tolerance and increased the survival rate of liver grafts.	(28)
			The anti-CD40 mAb can prolong the survival of xenografts.	(29)
OX40	OX40L	OX40Ig	Inhibit the rejection of allografts and induce immune tolerance by reducing IL-2 expression.	(30)
4-1BB	4-1BBL	anti-4-1BB mAb	Prolong the allograft survival time and prevent allograft rejection.	(31)
		RNAi-4-1BB	Inhibiting or alleviating acute rejection of liver transplantation in rats.	(32, 33)
GITR	GITRL		Still to be explored in liver transplantation.	
Tim-1		anti-Tim-1 mAb (3B3, MT1-10)	3B3: Promote T cell proliferation and block allograft tolerance. MT1-10: No application has been found in liver transplantation.	(34, 35)
Tim-3	galectin-9	anti-Tim-3 mAb (RMT3-23)	No sufficient data.	
Tim-4		anti-Tim-4 mAb	Alleviate the acute rejection injury and down-regulate the expression of pro-inflammatory factors.	(36)
LFA-1	ICAM-1	anti-LFA-1 mAb anti-ICAM-1 mAb	Prolong the allografts survival time, but can not induce permanent tolerance.	(37)

CTLA4 is a negative regulatory factor that sends inhibitory signals to T cells, thereby limiting the T cell responses. CTLA4 shares sequence similarity with CD28, for which it is a structural analog. CTLA4 competitively binds to B7-1/B7-2 with higher affinity than CD28, thereby blocking costimulatory signals.

CTLA4Ig (belatacept) is a soluble fusion protein that was approved by the Food and Drug Administration in 2011 for use in renal transplantation patients. It blocks the CD28/B7 pathway in T cells, inhibits T cell activation, and promotes graft tolerance. *In vivo* experiments have shown that CTLA4Ig suppresses T cell-dependent immune responses and prolongs the long-term survival of xenografts and allografts (19–21). CTLA4Ig can markedly prolong the survival of allografts in non-human primates (NHPs) (22). Two phase III clinical trials found that the overall survival and graft survival rates of renal transplant recipients on belatacept were similar to those of cyclosporine-treated recipients over 3 years, but with statistically better renal function and cardiovascular/metabolic disease risk status (40–44). Schwarz et al. (45) conducted a trial of belatacept for liver transplantation in 15 patients, which was terminated due to graft dysfunction with acute rejection at approximately 10 weeks. Interestingly, in another study, belatacept was reportedly safe and effective in hepatitis C-positive patients with renal insufficiency and for use as a bridge to renal rehabilitation (46). In rat liver transplantation models, CTLA4 signaling is essential for inducing immune tolerance (23). However, in a phase II clinical trial of adult liver transplantation, belatacept treatment resulted in a higher incidence of acute rejection and graft loss (24). Perhaps the "benefits" of belatacept in liver transplantation will be shown in appropriate patient selection and trial design.

ICOS/ICOSLG Costimulatory Pathway

ICOS is an inducible T cell costimulatory molecule of the Ig superfamily with strong structural similarity to CD28 and CTLA4 (47). It is expressed on activated T cells and its expression persists in effector and memory T cells. The B7 family member ICOSLG is structurally related to B7-1/B7-2. It is expressed on B cells, macrophages and dendritic cells; its expression can also be induced on non-lymphoid cells, including endothelial and pulmonary epithelial cells (48). ICOS binds only with ICOSLG, but not B7-1 or B7-2 (49, 50). The ICOS/ICOSLG pathway is critical for T cell-dependent B cell responses (51, 52). ICOS costimulation can enhances T-cells activation, proliferation, differentiation and effector functions. Treatment with anti-ICOS antibodies can prolong the survival of cardiac allografts (53). The timing of ICOS blockade is a key factor; only delayed blockade can inhibit the production of CD8+ T cells and statistically prolong the survival time of allografts (54). Treatment with anti-ICOS antibodies in combination with anti-CD154 antibodies or CTLA4Ig can prolong the survival of heart allografts and prevent chronic rejection (55). Some studies have shown that the survival of rat liver allografts can be prolonged by injecting anti-ICOS antibody after surgery (25). When combined with FK506, an anti-ICOS antibody synergistically prevents rejection after liver transplantation and induces graft tolerance (26). In addition, activation of the ICOS pathway can be inhibited by RNA interference, which prevents acute rejection and prolongs the survival of grafts by promoting T cell apoptosis and suppressing the production of cytokines by T lymphocytes (27). Considering that ICOS appears to work independently of CD28, blocking the ICOS/ICOSLG pathway in combination with the CD28/B7 pathway may be as a potential therapeutic strategy, but the ICOS/ICOSLG blocking drugs or clinical trial have not yet been studied in human liver transplantation (56).

TNF-RELATED SUPERFAMILY COSTIMULATORY PATHWAYS

CD40/CD154 Costimulatory Pathway

CD40 is a member of the TNF receptor family, which is expressed in APCs, including B cells, macrophages, and dendritic cells (DCs), as well as in endothelial cells, fibroblasts, and smooth muscle cells (57). CD40 mainly binds to CD154, which is expressed on activated T cells. CD154 also belongs to the TNF superfamily; both CD40 and CD154 are type II transmembrane proteins. In addition to playing an important role in B cell activation and Ig class conversion, the CD40/CD154 costimulatory pathway is important for costimulating T cell immune responses (58). CD40/CD154 interactions are also critical in T cell-dependent humoral immune responses and T cell-mediated activation of DCs and macrophages (59). The interaction between CD40 on T cells and CD154 on APCs lead to the maturation of DCs, which increases the production of cytokines and costimulatory molecules and enhances their ability to promote T effector cell differentiation (60). This pathway affects the function of many immune cells that are critical to the adaptive immune response, and studies in animal transplant models have shown considerable promise. Targeting CD154 prevents acute rejection and induces tolerance in some transplant models (61). In a model of mouse skin and heart transplantation, treatment with anti-CD154 prolongs graft survival (62, 63). In an NHP model, blocking CD154 leads to long-term survival of renal allografts and the loss of donor-specific mixed lymphocyte reactivity (64). When used in combination with CTLA4Ig, CD40/CD154 blockade had synergistic effects, on the enhancement of long-term skin and heart graft survival (65, 66). However, thromboembolic complications related to the anti-CD154 antibody were later reported in NHP research (67). It is now believed that the binding of the Fc domain of the anti-CD154 antibody to the Fc receptor of platelets contributes to platelet aggregation (68). Therefore, the current approaches to targeting this pathway mainly focus on the use of CD40-blocking antibodies.

Treatment with an anti-CD40 monoclonal antibody is an effective alternative method to block the costimulatory CD40/CD154 signal without interfering with platelet aggregation. ASKP1240 is a fully humanized inhibitory monoclonal antibody against CD40, which can block the CD40/CD154 interaction and inhibit cell-mediated and humoral immune responses without immunogenic and thromboembolic complications (69). A trial in NHPs showed that monotherapy with ASKP1240 increases the survival rate of liver grafts without the occurrence of thromboembolism, and monkeys showed good tolerance (28). In a 2017 study of a liver xenotransplantation model, the use of a blocking anti-CD40 monoclonal antibody prolonged the survival of xenografts (29). Other CD40 antibodies, such as 4D11, HCD122, and 2C10R4, have been effective in heart and kidney transplantation studies, but they have not been tested in liver transplantation studies.

OX40/OX40L Costimulatory Pathway

The expression of the TNF superfamily member OX40 on activated T cells is time-dependent (70). OX40 is essential for the regulation of T cell proliferation, differentiation, survival, and cytokine production (71). The expression of its ligand OX40L is induced on activated T cells and APCs, such as DCs, macrophages, and B cells, but also some endothelia and mast T cells. OX40-OX40L costimulatory pathway has been shown to be involved in the regulation of Th cells differentiation. Although CD28 signaling up-regulates the expression of OX40 on T cells, OX40 costimulation does not depend on a complete CD28 signal (72). Blocking the OX40/OX40L pathway alone had little effect in an allograft model (73). However, OX40/OX40L pathway blockers prolonged allograft survival time in CD28/CD40 dual-gene knockouts or in transplantation models featuring CD28/B7-1 blockers (74, 75). However, OX40/OX40L costimulatory blockade inhibited skin allograft rejection not by inhibiting T cell activation and proliferation, but by preventing the trafficking of peripheral lymph node effector T cells into the grafts (76). Combination therapy using OX40L blockers with traditional costimulatory blockers effectively prevents the allo-reactive T cell responses that impede long-term graft function and survival (47). Blocking the OX40/OX40L pathway with OX40Ig inhibits the rejection of liver allografts and induces immune tolerance in rats by reducing IL-2 expression (30). However, there have been no any clinical trials of OX40/OX40L pathway blockade in transplantation.

TNF Receptor Superfamily Member 9/TNF Superfamily Member 9 Costimulatory Pathway

TNF receptor superfamily member 9 (also known as 4-1BB or CD137) is a transmembrane protein expressed on T cells, DCs, and B cells. It reaches peak expression after T cell activation. Its ligand TNF superfamily member 9 (also known as 4-1BBL or CD137L) is expressed on APCs, including mature DCs, macrophages, and activated B cells, but not on resting or activated T cells (77). The 4-1BB/4-1BBL costimulatory signal can activate T cells independently of the CD28 signal (78), and 4-1BB can provide sufficient costimulation to drive T cell activation. The role of the 4-1BB/4-1BBL costimulatory pathway in transplantation varies depending on the model, as uncovered using antagonistic or agonistic anti-4-1BB monoclonal antibodies or gene silencing of 4-1BB. In a mouse model of graft-versus-host disease, treatment with an agonistic anti-4-1BB monoclonal antibody exacerbated cytotoxic $CD8^+$ T cell-mediated tissue damage and accelerated the rate of rejection of heart allografts or skin grafts (79). However, blocking the interaction of 4-1BB/4-1BBL with an antagonistic 4-1BB monoclonal antibody prolonged allograft survival time and helped prevent allograft rejection (31). It has been reported that silencing 4-1BB with RNA interference or blocking the pathway with an anti-4-1BBL monoclonal antibody can inhibit or limit acute rejection in rat liver transplantation (32, 33).

TNF Receptor Superfamily Member 18/TNF Superfamily Member 18 Costimulatory Pathway

TNF receptor superfamily member 18 (also known as glucocorticoid induced tumor necrosis factor related receptor or GITR) is a type I transmembrane protein that can be expressed on T lymphocytes, NK cells, and APCs. Regulatory T cells highly express GITR, which can also be expressed at low levels on resting T cells; however, the expression of GITR is up-regulated when T cells are activated, especially in the presence of the CD28 signal (80). Its ligand TNF receptor superfamily member 18 (also known as GITRL) is mainly expressed on APCs after stimulation through Toll-like receptors. GITR activation is a positive costimulatory signal for $CD4^+$ and $CD8^+$ T cells, leading to enhanced proliferation, survival, and cytokine production (81). In addition, GITR-induced signaling is important for regulatory T cell-mediated inhibition of effector T cell activity and the prevention of autoimmune diseases. Shimizu J et al. (82) found that increased expression of GITR in T cells impairs allograft tolerance and self-tolerance. Wei et al. (83) showed that GITR expressed on Kupffer cells may mediate acute rejection of rat liver grafts. However, the role of the GITR/GITRL pathway in transplantation requires further investigation.

OTHER PATHWAYS

TIM Family Molecules

The TIM family of genes encodes type 1 glycoproteins that share a common Ig V-like domain, mucin-like domain, single transmembrane domain, and cytoplasmic domain (84). The TIM gene family consists of 8 members in mice; the 3 human TIM genes are most similar to mouse TIM-1, TIM-3, and TIM-4. As a novel family of costimulatory molecules, the TIM gene family plays an important role in the activation and differentiation of Th cells (85). TIM-1 (also known as HAVCR1 or KIM1) is not expressed on naive $CD4^+$ T cells, but it is expressed after TCR stimulation, preferentially on Th2 cells (34). TIM-1 is not only necessary for regulating Th1 and Th2 immune responses, it also regulates Th17 and regulatory T cells. Agonism of TIM-1 with the high-affinity monoclonal antibody 3B3 promoted the expansion of antigen-specific T cells expressing Th1 and Th17 cytokines and blocked allograft tolerance (34, 35). However, the use of the blocking monoclonal antibody MT1-10, which has a lower affinity for TIM-1, prolonged the survival of completely mismatched cardiac allografts and induced tolerance in combination with rapamycin (86).

Although it was originally identified in Th1-differentiated cells, TIM-3 has a wide range of expression and is the first among the TIM family of proteins that was discovered. In addition to its expression on Th1 and Th17 cells, it is constitutively expressed on DCs, macrophages, NK cells and mast cells (84). Like other TIM family members, TIM-3 is a phosphatidylserine receptor; it can bind multiple ligands, including galectin-9, phosphatidylserine, high mobility group box 1, and CEA cell adhesion molecule 1 (84, 87–89). As a negative costimulatory molecule, TIM-3 dampens Th1 and Th17 responses after binding galectin-9, thereby playing an important role in immune and inflammatory responses. It can promote apoptosis and inhibit the immune response mediated by Th1 cells. In a cardiac allograft transplantation model, blocking TIM-3/galectin-9 costimulatory signal transduction with an anti-TIM-3 monoclonal antibody (RMT3-23) accelerated rejection (90), in a process characterized by the promotion of Th1/Th17 polarization, inhibition of regulatory T cell differentiation, and promotion of donor-specific alloantibody production. In contrast, the application of exogenous galectin-9 prolonged the survival of skin and heart allografts (91, 92), and combination therapy with rapamycin promoted allograft tolerance (93). So far, human transplantation studies have focused on the use of Tim-3 as a marker of Th1 activation and rejection.

TIM-4 is mainly expressed on APCs, including $CD11c^+$ DCs and macrophages, but not on T cells (94). TIM-4 was originally thought to be a ligand of TIM-1 that promoted T cell proliferation; however, it was later demonstrated that direct interaction between TIM-1 and TIM-4 was achieved by bridging exosomes (95). The specific effect of TIM-4 on T cell activation remains unclear, and *in vitro* studies using the TIM-4Ig fusion protein have shown conflicting results. The use of the TIM-4Ig fusion protein can enhance TIM-4 signal transduction and increase the proliferation of activated T cells, but has the opposite effect on naive T cells (96–98). Blocking TIM-4 ameliorated acute rejection injury after liver transplantation in rats and down-regulated the expression of TNF-α, IFN-γ, CCL2, and CXCL2 in allografts. When combined with exogenous TGF-β, it further ameliorated acute rejection injury and increased graft survival time (36).

Integrin Subunit Alpha L/Intracellular Adhesion Molecule 1 Costimulatory Pathway

Integrin subunit alpha L (also known as lymphocyte function-associated antigen 1 or LFA-1) is an adhesion molecule found on the surface of T cells, which belongs to the integrin family of cell adhesion factors. When it binds intercellular adhesion molecule 1 (ICAM1) expressed on endothelial cells, LFA-1 can provide the costimulatory second signal and promote the activation and proliferation of T cells (99). Some studies have shown that blocking the interaction between LFA-1 and ICAM1 with anti LFA-1 and anti-ICAM1 monoclonal antibodies prolonged the survival time of mouse skin, heart, and islet allografts (100–102). Earlier studies showed that the use of anti-ICAM1 and anti-LFA-1 antibodies prolonged the survival of rat liver allografts, but did not induce permanent tolerance (103). When combined with donor-specific blood transfusion, LFA-1/ICAM1 blockade induced tolerance in 80% of rats (37). Currently, few clinical trials have investigated blocking this costimulatory pathway in liver transplantation, and its future role in liver transplantation remains unclear.

CONCLUSION

Traditionally, the induction of allograft tolerance has been regarded as the "holy grail" of transplantation immunology as graft can survive a long time in patients with tolerance. However, for most liver transplant recipients, it is still very difficult to withdraw immunosuppressants and achieve immune tolerance. T cell-mediated rejection after liver transplantation is a complex and dynamic process. The relative strength of the costimulatory and coinhibitory signals activated after transplant determines how T cells respond to allografts. As the key second signal, costimulatory pathways are essential in the activation of T cells, especially CD28/B7 costimulatory signal pathway. Although belatacept has achieved considerable results in clinical renal transplantation since it was approved by FDA, its clinical trials results in liver transplantation are not very satisfactory. Considering the complex mechanisms involved in the immune response to liver allograft transplantation, blocking a single costimulatory pathway may not be sufficient to induce tolerance. Besides, further clinical trials may be needed to compare different costimulatory blockers to understand their respective advantages, and we anticipate that blocking multiple costimulatory pathways in combination with coinhibitory signaling pathways may be the optimal regimen to achieve the true transplant tolerance in humans.

AUTHOR CONTRIBUTIONS

All authors listed have made a substantial, direct and intellectual contribution to the work, and approved it for publication.

ACKNOWLEDGMENTS

We would like to thank Editage (www.editage.cn) for English language editing.

REFERENCES

1. Lerut J, Sanchez-Fueyo A. An appraisal of tolerance in liver transplantation. *Am J Transpl* (2006) 6:1774–80. doi: 10.1111/j.1600-6143.2006.01396.x
2. Devlin J, Doherty D, Thomson L, Wong T, Donaldson P, Portmann B, et al. Defining the outcome of immunosuppression withdrawal after liver transplantation. *Hepatology* (1998) 27:926–33. doi: 10.1002/hep.510270406
3. Feng S, Ekong UD, Lobritto SJ, Demetris AJ, Roberts JP, Rosenthal P, et al. Complete immunosuppression withdrawal and subsequent allograft function among pediatric recipients of parental living donor liver transplants. *JAMA* (2012) 307:283–93. doi: 10.1001/jama.2011.2014
4. Benitez C, Londono MC, Miquel R, Manzia TM, Abraldes JG, Lozano JJ, et al. Prospective multicenter clinical trial of immunosuppressive drug withdrawal in stable adult liver transplant recipients. *Hepatology* (2013) 58:1824–35. doi: 10.1002/hep.26426
5. de la Garza RG, Sarobe P, Merino J, Lasarte JJ, D'Avola D, Belsue V, et al. Trial of complete weaning from immunosuppression for liver transplant recipients: factors predictive of tolerance. *Liver Transpl* (2013) 19:937–44. doi: 10.1002/lt.23686
6. Horst AK, Neumann K, Diehl L, Tiegs G. Modulation of Liver Tolerance by Conventional and Nonconventional Antigen-Presenting Cells and Regulatory Immune Cells. *Cell Mol Immunol* (2016) 13:277–92. doi: 10.1038/cmi.2015.112
7. Cui B, Lin H, Yu J, Yu J, Hu Z. Autophagy and the Immune Response. *Adv Exp Med* (2019) 1206:595–634. doi: 10.1007/978-981-15-0602-4_27
8. Alpdogan O, van den Brink MRM. Immune Tolerance and Transplantation. *Semin Oncol* (2012) 39:629–42. doi: 10.1053/j.seminoncol.2012.10.001
9. Greenwald RJ, Freeman GJ, Sharpe AH. THE B7 FAMILY REVISITED. *Annu Rev Immunol* (2005) 23:515–48. doi: 10.1146/annurev.immunol.23.021704.115611
10. Nguyen T, Yu X, Nurieva R, Martin-Orozco N, Dong C, Thomas S, et al. T-cell tolerance or function is determined by combinatorial costimulatory signals. *EMBO J* (2006) 25:2623–33. doi: 10.1038/sj.emboj.7601146
11. Wherry EJ, Kurachi M. Molecular and cellular insights into T cell exhaustion. *Nat Rev Immunol* (2015) 15:486–99. doi: 10.1038/nri3862
12. Anderson AC, Joller N, Kuchroo VK. Lag-3, Tim-3, and TIGIT: Co-inhibitory Receptors with Specialized Functions in Immune Regulation. *Immunity* (2016) 44:989–1004. doi: 10.1016/j.immuni.2016.05.001
13. Zhuang Q, Liu Q, Divito SJ, Zeng Q, Yatim KM, Hughes AD, et al. Graft-infiltrating host dendritic cells play a key role in organ transplant rejection. *Nat Commun* (2016) 7:12623. doi: 10.1038/ncomms12623
14. Chen L, Flies DB. Molecular mechanisms of T cell co-stimulation and co-inhibition. *Nat Rev Immunol* (2013) 13:227–42. doi: 10.1038/nri3405
15. Schroder PM, Fitch ZW, Schmitz R, Choi AY, Kwun J, Knechtle SJ. The past, present, and future of costimulation blockade in organ transplantation. *Curr Opin Organ Transpl* (2019) 24:391–401. doi: 10.1097/MOT.0000000000000656
16. Liu L, He C, Liu J, Lv Z, Wang G, Gao H, et al. Transplant Tolerance: Current Insights and Strategies for Long-Term Survival of Xenografts. *Arch Immunol Ther Exp (Warsz)* (2018) 66:355–64. doi: 10.1007/s00005-018-0517-7
17. Kinnear G, Jones ND, Wood KJ. Costimulation blockade: current perspectives and implications for therapy. *Transplantation* (2013) 95:527–35. doi: 10.1097/TP.0b013e31826d4672
18. Hartigan CR, Sun H, Ford ML. Memory T-cell exhaustion and tolerance in transplantation. *Immunol Rev* (2019) 292:225–42. doi: 10.1111/imr.12824
19. Linsley PS, Wallace PM, Johnson J, Gibson MG, Greene JL, Ledbetter JA, et al. Immunosuppression in vivo by a soluble form of the CTLA-4 T cell activation molecule. *Science* (1992) 257:792–5. doi: 10.1126/science.1496399
20. Lenschow DJ, Zeng Y, Thistlethwaite JR, Montag A, Brady W, Gibson MG, et al. Long-term survival of xenogeneic pancreatic islet grafts induced by CTLA4lg. *Science* (1992) 257:789–92. doi: 10.1126/science.1323143
21. Turka LA, Linsley PS, Lin H, Brady W, Leiden JM, Wei RQ, et al. T-cell activation by the CD28 ligand B7 is required for cardiac allograft rejection in vivo. *Proc Natl Acad Sci U S A* (1992) 89:11102–5. doi: 10.1073/pnas.89.22.11102
22. Larsen CP, Pearson TC, Adams AB, Tso P, Shirasugi N, Strobert E, et al. Rational development of LEA29Y (belatacept), a high-affinity variant of CTLA4-Ig with potent immunosuppressive properties. *Am J Transpl* (2005) 5:443–53. doi: 10.1111/j.1600-6143.2005.00749.x
23. Li W, Zheng XX, Kuhr CS, Perkins JD. CTLA4 engagement is required for induction of murine liver transplant spontaneous tolerance. *Am J Transpl* (2005) 5:978–86. doi: 10.1111/j.1600-6143.2005.00823.x
24. Klintmalm GB, Feng S, Lake JR, Vargas HE, Wekerle T, Agnes S, et al. Belatacept-based immunosuppression in de novo liver transplant recipients: 1-year experience from a phase II randomized study. *Am J Transpl* (2014) 14:1817–27. doi: 10.1111/ajt.12810
25. Guo L, Li XK, Funeshima N, Fujino M, Nagata Y, Kimura H, et al. Prolonged survival in rat liver transplantation with mouse monoclonal antibody against an inducible costimulator (ICOS). *Transplantation* (2002) 73:1027–32. doi: 10.1097/00007890-200204150-00003
26. Guo L, Li XK, Enosawa S, Funeshima N, Suzuki S, Kimura H, et al. Significant enhancement by anti-ICOS antibody of suboptimal tacrolimus immunosuppression in rat liver transplantation. *Liver Transpl* (2004) 10:743–7. doi: 10.1002/lt.20167
27. Chen Y, Liu H, Liu Z, Liang S, Chen J, Long F, et al. Blockade of inducible costimulator pathway to prevent acute rejection in rat liver transplantation. *Am J Surg* (2009) 198:244–9. doi: 10.1016/j.amjsurg.2008.09.014
28. Oura T, Yamashita K, Suzuki T, Fukumori D, Watanabe M, Hirokata G, et al. Long-term hepatic allograft acceptance based on CD40 blockade by ASKP1240 in nonhuman primates. *Am J Transpl* (2012) 12:1740–54. doi: 10.1111/j.1600-6143.2012.04014.x
29. Shah JA, Patel MS, Elias N, Navarro-Alvarez N, Rosales I, Wilkinson RA, et al. Prolonged Survival Following Pig-to-Primate Liver Xenotransplantation Utilizing Exogenous Coagulation Factors and Costimulation Blockade. *Am J Transpl* (2017) 17:2178–85. doi: 10.1111/ajt.14341
30. Chen ZH, Wang C, Wei FX, Xu BB, Liu J, Pu Y, et al. Adenovirus-mediated OX40Ig gene transfer induces long-term survival of orthotopic liver allograft in rats. *Transpl Immunol* (2018) 48:32–8. doi: 10.1016/j.trim.2018.02.010
31. Cho HR, Kwon B, Yagita H, La S, Lee EA, Kim JE, et al. Blockade of 4-1BB

(CD137)/4-1BB ligand interactions increases allograft survival. *Transpl Int* (2004) 17:351–61. doi: 10.1007/s00147-004-0726-3
32. Shi Y, Hu S, Song Q, Yu S, Zhou X, Yin J, et al. Gene silencing of 4-1BB by RNA interference inhibits acute rejection in rats with liver transplantation. *BioMed Res Int* (2013) 2013:192738. doi: 10.1155/2013/192738
33. Qin L, Guan HG, Zhou XJ, Yin J, Lan J, Qian HX. Blockade of 4-1BB/4-1BB ligand interactions prevents acute rejection in rat liver transplantation. *Chin Med J (Engl)* (2010) 123:212–5. doi: 10.3760/cma.j.issn.0366-6999.2010.02.017
34. Umetsu SE, Lee WL, McIntire JJ, Downey L, Sanjanwala B, Akbari O, et al. TIM-1 induces T cell activation and inhibits the development of peripheral tolerance. *Nat Immunol* (2005) 6:447–54. doi: 10.1038/ni1186
35. Degauque N, Mariat C, Kenny J, Zhang D, Gao W, Vu MD, et al. Immunostimulatory Tim-1-specific antibody deprograms Tregs and prevents transplant tolerance in mice. *J Clin Invest* (2008) 118:735–41. doi: 10.1172/JCI32562
36. Wu H, Xu X, Li J, Gong J, Li M. TIM4 blockade of KCs combined with exogenous TGFbeta injection helps to reverse acute rejection and prolong the survival rate of mice receiving liver allografts. *Int J Mol Med* (2018) 42:346–58. doi: 10.3892/ijmm.2018.3606
37. Degawa H, Watanabe K, Uchida H, Nagao T, Tomikawa S, Beck Y, et al. Blocking of ICAM-1 and LFA-1 in rat liver transplantation. *Transplant Proc* (1996) 28:1362–3.
38. Paterson AM, Vanguri VK, Sharpe AH. SnapShot: B7/CD28 costimulation. *Cell* (2009) 137:974–4.e1. doi: 10.1016/j.cell.2009.05.015
39. Malvezzi P, Jouve T, Rostaing L. Costimulation Blockade in Kidney Transplantation: An Update. *Transplantation* (2016) 100:2315–23. doi: 10.1097/TP.0000000000001344
40. Larsen CP, Grinyo J, Medina-Pestana J, Vanrenterghem Y, Vincenti F, Breshahan B, et al. Belatacept-based regimens versus a cyclosporine A-based regimen in kidney transplant recipients: 2-year results from the BENEFIT and BENEFIT-EXT studies. *Transplantation* (2010) 90:1528–35. doi: 10.1097/TP.0b013e3181ff87cd
41. Durrbach A, Pestana JM, Pearson T, Vincenti F, Garcia VD, Campistol J, et al. A phase III study of belatacept versus cyclosporine in kidney transplants from extended criteria donors (BENEFIT-EXT study). *Am J Transpl* (2010) 10:547–57. doi: 10.1111/j.1600-6143.2010.03016.x
42. Vincenti F, Charpentier B, Vanrenterghem Y, Rostaing L, Bresnahan B, Darji P, et al. A phase III study of belatacept-based immunosuppression regimens versus cyclosporine in renal transplant recipients (BENEFIT study). *Am J Transpl* (2010) 10:535–46. doi: 10.1111/j.1600-6143.2009.03005.x
43. Vincenti F, Larsen CP, Alberu J, Bresnahan B, Garcia VD, Kothari J, et al. Three-year outcomes from BENEFIT, a randomized, active-controlled, parallel-group study in adult kidney transplant recipients. *Am J Transplant* (2012) 12:210–7. doi: 10.1111/j.1600-6143.2011.03785.x
44. Pestana JO, Grinyo JM, Vanrenterghem Y, Becker T, Campistol JM, Florman S, et al. Three-year outcomes from BENEFIT-EXT: a phase III study of belatacept versus cyclosporine in recipients of extended criteria donor kidneys. *Am J Transpl* (2012) 12:630–9. doi: 10.1111/j.1600-6143.2011.03914.x
45. Schwarz C, Rasoul-Rockenschaub S, Soliman T, Berlakovich GA, Steininger R, Muhlbacher F, et al. Belatacept treatment for two yr after liver transplantation is not associated with operational tolerance. *Clin Transpl* (2015) 29:85–9. doi: 10.1111/ctr.12483
46. LaMattina JC, Jason MP, Hanish SI, Ottmann SE, Klassen DK, Potosky D, et al. Safety of belatacept bridging immunosuppression in hepatitis C-positive liver transplant recipients with renal dysfunction. *Transplantation* (2014) 97:133–7. doi: 10.1097/01.TP.0000438635.44461.2e
47. Mages HW, Hutloff A, Heuck C, Buchner K, Himmelbauer H, Oliveri F, et al. Molecular cloning and characterization of murine ICOS and identification of B7h as ICOS ligand. *Eur J Immunol* (2000) 30:1040–7. doi: 10.1002/(SICI)1521-4141(200004)30:4<1040::AID-IMMU1040<3.0.CO;2-6
48. Xiao Z, Mayer AT, Nobashi TW, Gambhir SS. ICOS Is an Indicator of T-cell–Mediated Response to Cancer Immunotherapy. *Cancer Res* (2020) 80 (14):3023–32. doi: 10.1158/0008-5472.CAN-19-3265
49. McAdam AJ, Chang TT, Lumelsky AE, Greenfield EA, Boussiotis VA, Duke-Cohan JS, et al. Mouse inducible costimulatory molecule (ICOS) expression is enhanced by CD28 costimulation and regulates differentiation of CD4+ T cells. *J Immunol* (2000) 165:5035–40. doi: 10.4049/jimmunol.165.9.5035
50. Yoshinaga SK, Whoriskey JS, Khare SD, Sarmiento U, Guo J, Horan T, et al. T-cell co-stimulation through B7RP-1 and ICOS. *Nature* (1999) 402:827–32. doi: 10.1038/45582
51. Mak TW, Shahinian A, Yoshinaga SK, Wakeham A, Boucher LM, Pintilie M, et al. Costimulation through the inducible costimulator ligand is essential for both T helper and B cell functions in T cell-dependent B cell responses. *Nat Immunol* (2003) 4:765–72. doi: 10.1038/ni947
52. Smith KM, Brewer JM, Webb P, Coyle AJ, Gutierrez-Ramos C, Garside P. Inducible costimulatory molecule-B7-related protein 1 interactions are important for the clonal expansion and B cell helper functions of naive, Th1, and Th2 T cells. *J Immunol* (2003) 170:2310–5. doi: 10.4049/jimmunol.170.5.2310
53. Ozkaynak E, Gao W, Shemmeri N, Wang C, Gutierrez-Ramos JC, Amaral J, et al. Importance of ICOS-B7RP-1 costimulation in acute and chronic allograft rejection. *Nat Immunol* (2001) 2:591–6. doi: 10.1038/89731
54. Harada H, Salama AD, Sho M, Izawa A, Sandner SE, Ito T, et al. The role of the ICOS-B7h T cell costimulatory pathway in transplantation immunity. *J Clin Invest* (2003) 112:234–43. doi: 10.1172/JCI17008
55. Kosuge H, Suzuki J, Gotoh R, Koga N, Ito H, Isobe M, et al. Induction of immunologic tolerance to cardiac allograft by simultaneous blockade of inducible co-stimulator and cytotoxic T-lymphocyte antigen 4 pathway. *Transplantation* (2003) 75:1374–9. doi: 10.1097/01.TP.0000061601.26325.82
56. Uehara M, McGrath MM. The Role of Costimulatory Pathways in Transplant Tolerance. *Clin Lab Med* (2019) 39:87–106. doi: 10.1016/j.cll.2018.10.009
57. Chatzigeorgiou A, Lyberi M, Chatzilymperis G, Nezos A, Kamper E. CD40/CD40L signaling and its implication in health and disease. *Biofactors* (2009) 35:474–83. doi: 10.1002/biof.62
58. Tseng M, Ge S, Roberts R, Kuo C, Choi J, Nissen NN, et al. Liver Transplantation in a Patient With CD40 Ligand Deficiency and Hyper-IgM Syndrome: Clinical and Immunological Assessments. *Am J Transpl* (2016) 16:1626–32. doi: 10.1111/ajt.13580
59. Yeung MY, Grimmig T, Sayegh MH. Costimulation Blockade in Transplantation. *Adv Exp Med Biol* (2019) 1189:267–312. doi: 10.1007/978-981-32-9717-3_10
60. Pinelli DF, Ford ML. Novel insights into anti-CD40/CD154 immunotherapy in transplant tolerance. *Immunotherapy-Uk* (2015) 7:399–410. doi: 10.2217/imt.15.1
61. Yamada AA, Sayegh MH. The CD154-CD40 costimulatory pathway in transplantation. *Transplantation* (2002) 73:S36–9. doi: 10.1097/00007890-200201151-00012
62. Hancock WW, Sayegh MH, Zheng XG, Peach R, Linsley PS, Turka LA. Costimulatory function and expression of CD40 ligand, CD80, and CD86 in vascularized murine cardiac allograft rejection. *Proc Natl Acad Sci U S A* (1996) 93:13967–72. doi: 10.1073/pnas.93.24.13967
63. Pinelli DF, Wagener ME, Liu D, Yamniuk A, Tamura J, Grant S, et al. An anti-CD154 domain antibody prolongs graft survival and induces Foxp3(+) iTreg in the absence and presence of CTLA-4 Ig. *Am J Transpl* (2013) 13:3021–30. doi: 10.1111/ajt.12417
64. Kirk AD, Burkly LC, Batty DS, Baumgartner RE, Berning JD, Buchanan K, et al. Treatment with humanized monoclonal antibody against CD154 prevents acute renal allograft rejection in nonhuman primates. *Nat Med* (1999) 5:686–93. doi: 10.1038/9536
65. Zhu P, Chen YF, Chen XP, Li D, Cheng Q, Huang ZY, et al. Mechanisms of survival prolongation of murine cardiac allografts using the treatment of CTLA4-Ig and MR1. *Transplant Proc* (2008) 40:1618–24. doi: 10.1016/j.transproceed.2008.03.148
66. Larsen CP, Elwood ET, Alexander DZ, Ritchie SC, Hendrix R, Tucker-Burden C, et al. Long-term acceptance of skin and cardiac allografts after blocking CD40 and CD28 pathways. *Nature* (1996) 381:434–8. doi: 10.1038/381434a0
67. Koyama I, Kawai T, Andrews D, Boskovic S, Nadazdin O, Wee SL, et al. Thrombophilia associated with anti-CD154 monoclonal antibody treatment and its prophylaxis in nonhuman primates. *Transplantation* (2004) 77:460–2. doi: 10.1097/01.TP.0000110291.29370.C0
68. Robles-Carrillo L, Meyer T, Hatfield M, Desai H, Davila M, Langer F, et al. Anti-CD40L immune complexes potently activate platelets in vitro and cause thrombosis in FCGR2A transgenic mice. *J Immunol* (2010) 185:1577–83. doi: 10.4049/jimmunol.0903888
69. Okimura K, Maeta K, Kobayashi N, Goto M, Kano N, Ishihara T, et al. Characterization of ASKP1240, a fully human antibody targeting human CD40

with potent immunosuppressive effects. *Am J Transpl* (2014) 14:1290–9. doi: 10.1111/ajt.12678

70. Webb GJ, Hirschfield GM, Lane PJ. OX40, OX40L and Autoimmunity: a Comprehensive Review. *Clin Rev Allergy Immunol* (2016) 50:312–32. doi: 10.1007/s12016-015-8498-3
71. Willoughby J, Griffiths J, Tews I, Cragg MS. OX40: Structure and function - What questions remain? *Mol Immunol* (2017) 83:13–22. doi: 10.1016/j.molimm.2017.01.006
72. Walker LS, Gulbranson-Judge A, Flynn S, Brocker T, Raykundalia C, Goodall M, et al. Compromised OX40 function in CD28-deficient mice is linked with failure to develop CXC chemokine receptor 5-positive CD4 cells and germinal centers. *J Exp Med* (1999) 190:1115–22. doi: 10.1084/jem.190.8.1115
73. Yuan X, Salama AD, Dong V, Schmitt I, Najafian N, Chandraker A, et al. The role of the CD134-CD134 ligand costimulatory pathway in alloimmune responses in vivo. *J Immunol* (2003) 170:2949–55. doi: 10.4049/jimmunol.170.6.2949
74. Demirci G, Amanullah F, Kewalaramani R, Yagita H, Strom TB, Sayegh MH, et al. Critical role of OX40 in CD28 and CD154-independent rejection. *J Immunol* (2004) 172:1691–8. doi: 10.4049/jimmunol.172.3.1691
75. Croft M, So T, Duan W, Soroosh P. The significance of OX40 and OX40L to T-cell biology and immune disease. *Immunol Rev* (2009) 229:173–91. doi: 10.1111/j.1600-065X.2009.00766.x
76. Kinnear G, Wood KJ, Fallah-Arani F, Jones ND. A diametric role for OX40 in the response of effector/memory CD4+ T cells and regulatory T cells to alloantigen. *J Immunol* (2013) 191:1465–75. doi: 10.4049/jimmunol.1300553
77. Futagawa T, Akiba H, Kodama T, Takeda K, Hosoda Y, Yagita H, et al. Expression and function of 4-1BB and 4-1BB ligand on murine dendritic cells. *Int Immunol* (2002) 14:275–86. doi: 10.1093/intimm/14.3.275
78. Teschner D, Wenzel G, Distler E, Schnurer E, Theobald M, Neurauter AA, et al. In vitro stimulation and expansion of human tumour-reactive CD8+ cytotoxic T lymphocytes by anti-CD3/CD28/CD137 magnetic beads. *Scand J Immunol* (2011) 74:155–64. doi: 10.1111/j.1365-3083.2011.02564.x
79. Shuford WW, Klussman K, Tritchler DD, Loo DT, Chalupny J, Siadak AW, et al. 4-1BB costimulatory signals preferentially induce CD8+ T cell proliferation and lead to the amplification in vivo of cytotoxic T cell responses. *J Exp Med* (1997) 186:47–55. doi: 10.1084/jem.186.1.47
80. Kwon B, Yu KY, Ni J, Yu GL, Jang IK, Kim YJ, et al. Identification of a novel activation-inducible protein of the tumor necrosis factor receptor superfamily and its ligand. *J Biol Chem* (1999) 274:6056–61. doi: 10.1074/jbc.274.10.6056
81. Tone M, Tone Y, Adams E, Yates SF, Frewin MR, Cobbold SP, et al. Mouse glucocorticoid-induced tumor necrosis factor receptor ligand is costimulatory for T cells. *Proc Natl Acad Sci U S A* (2003) 100:15059–64. doi: 10.1073/pnas.2334901100
82. Shimizu J, Yamazaki S, Takahashi T, Ishida Y, Sakaguchi S. Stimulation of CD25(+)CD4(+) regulatory T cells through GITR breaks immunological self-tolerance. *Nat Immunol* (2002) 3:135–42. doi: 10.1038/ni759
83. Wei S, Li J, Lian Z, Chen Y, Liu Z, You H, et al. Expression of glucocorticoid-induced tumor necrosis factor receptor ligand in rat graft after liver transplantation. *Transplant Proc* (2011) 43:1971–5. doi: 10.1016/j.transproceed.2011.03.054
84. Freeman GJ, Casasnovas JM, Umetsu DT, DeKruyff RH. TIM genes: a family of cell surface phosphatidylserine receptors that regulate innate and adaptive immunity. *Immunol Rev* (2010) 235:172–89. doi: 10.1111/j.0105-2896.2010.00903.x
85. Rodriguez-Manzanet R, DeKruyff R, Kuchroo VK, Umetsu DT. The costimulatory role of TIM molecules. *Immunol Rev* (2009) 229:259–70. doi: 10.1111/j.1600-065X.2009.00772.x
86. Ueno T, Habicht A, Clarkson MR, Albin MJ, Yamaura K, Boenisch O, et al. The emerging role of T cell Ig mucin 1 in alloimmune responses in an experimental mouse transplant model. *J Clin Invest* (2008) 118:742–51. doi: 10.1172/JCI32451
87. Huang YH, Zhu C, Kondo Y, Anderson AC, Gandhi A, Russell A, et al. Corrigendum: CEACAM1 regulates TIM-3-mediated tolerance and exhaustion. *Nature* (2016) 536:359. doi: 10.1038/nature17421
88. Chiba S, Baghdadi M, Akiba H, Yoshiyama H, Kinoshita I, Dosaka-Akita H, et al. Tumor-infiltrating DCs suppress nucleic acid-mediated innate immune responses through interactions between the receptor TIM-3 and the alarmin HMGB1. *Nat Immunol* (2012) 13:832–42. doi: 10.1038/ni.2376
89. Zhu C, Anderson AC, Schubart A, Xiong H, Imitola J, Khoury SJ, et al. The Tim-3 ligand galectin-9 negatively regulates T helper type 1 immunity. *Nat Immunol* (2005) 6:1245–52. doi: 10.1038/ni1271
90. Boenisch O, D'Addio F, Watanabe T, Elyaman W, Magee CN, Yeung MY, et al. TIM-3: a novel regulatory molecule of alloimmune activation. *J Immunol* (2010) 185:5806–19. doi: 10.4049/jimmunol.0903435
91. Wang F, He W, Yuan J, Wu K, Zhou H, Zhang W, et al. Activation of Tim-3-Galectin-9 pathway improves survival of fully allogeneic skin grafts. *Transpl Immunol* (2008) 19:12–9. doi: 10.1016/j.trim.2008.01.008
92. He W, Fang Z, Wang F, Wu K, Xu Y, Zhou H, et al. Galectin-9 significantly prolongs the survival of fully mismatched cardiac allografts in mice. *Transplantation* (2009) 88:782–90. doi: 10.1097/TP.0b013e3181b47f25
93. Cai L, Zhou H, Fang Z, Yuan J, Niki T, Hirashima M, et al. Galectin-9 in combination with rapamycin induces cardiac allograft tolerance in mice. *Transplantation* (2013) 96:379–86. doi: 10.1097/TP.0b013e31829b07b5
94. Meyers JH, Chakravarti S, Schlesinger D, Illes Z, Waldner H, Umetsu SE, et al. TIM-4 is the ligand for TIM-1, and the TIM-1-TIM-4 interaction regulates T cell proliferation. *Nat Immunol* (2005) 6:455–64. doi: 10.1038/ni1185
95. Kobayashi N, Karisola P, Pena-Cruz V, Dorfman DM, Jinushi M, Umetsu SE, et al. TIM-1 and TIM-4 glycoproteins bind phosphatidylserine and mediate uptake of apoptotic cells. *Immunity* (2007) 27:927–40. doi: 10.1016/j.immuni.2007.11.011
96. Rodriguez-Manzanet R, Meyers JH, Balasubramanian S, Slavik J, Kassam N, Dardalhon V, et al. TIM-4 expressed on APCs induces T cell expansion and survival. *J Immunol* (2008) 180:4706–13. doi: 10.4049/jimmunol.180.7.4706
97. Mizui M, Shikina T, Arase H, Suzuki K, Yasui T, Rennert PD, et al. Bimodal regulation of T cell-mediated immune responses by TIM-4. *Int Immunol* (2008) 20:695–708. doi: 10.1093/intimm/dxn029
98. Cao W, Ryan M, Buckley D, O'Connor R, Clarkson MR. Tim-4 inhibition of T-cell activation and T helper type 17 differentiation requires both the immunoglobulin V and mucin domains and occurs via the mitogen-activated protein kinase pathway. *Immunology* (2011) 133:179–89. doi: 10.1111/j.1365-2567.2011.03424.x
99. Van Seventer GA, Shimizu Y, Horgan KJ, Shaw S. The LFA-1 ligand ICAM-1 provides an important costimulatory signal for T cell receptor-mediated activation of resting T cells. *J Immunol* (1990) 144:4579–86.
100. Isobe M, Suzuki J, Yamazaki S, Sekiguchi M. Acceptance of primary skin graft after treatment with anti-intercellular adhesion molecule-1 and anti-leukocyte function-associated antigen-1 monoclonal antibodies in mice. *Transplantation* (1996) 62:411–3. doi: 10.1097/00007890-199608150-00019
101. Grazia TJ, Gill RG, Gelhaus HJ, Doan AN, Sleater ML, Pietra BA. Perturbation of leukocyte function-associated antigen-1/intercellular adhesion molecule-1 results in differential outcomes in cardiac vs islet allograft survival. *J Heart Lung Transpl* (2005) 24:1410–4. doi: 10.1016/j.healun.2004.09.004
102. Arai K, Sunamura M, Wada Y, Takahashi M, Kobari M, Kato K, et al. Preventing effect of anti-ICAM-1 and anti-LFA-1 monoclonal antibodies on murine islet allograft rejection. *Int J Pancreatol* (1999) 26:23–31. doi: 10.1385/IJGC:26:1:23
103. Degawa H, Watanabe K, Beck Y, Tomikawa S, Nagao T, Uchida H. Effect of anti-ICAM-1 and anti-LFA-1 antibodies on rat liver transplantation. *Surg Today* (1995) 25:474–6. doi: 10.1007/BF00311833

13

Transplant Tolerance Induction: Insights from the Liver

Helong Dai[1,2,3*], *Yawen Zheng*[1,2,3,4], *Angus W. Thomson*[4,5†] *and Natasha M. Rogers*[4,6,7,8*]

[1] *Department of Kidney Transplantation, The Second Xiangya Hospital of Central South University, Changsha, China,* [2] *Clinical Research Center for Organ Transplantation in Hunan Province, Changsha, China,* [3] *Clinical Immunology Center, Central South University, Changsha, China,* [4] *Department of Surgery, Thomas E. Starzl Transplantation Institute, University of Pittsburgh School of Medicine, Pittsburgh, PA, United States,* [5] *Department of Immunology, University of Pittsburgh School of Medicine, Pittsburgh, PA, United States,* [6] *Center for Transplant and Renal Research, Westmead Institute for Medical Research, Westmead, NSW, Australia,* [7] *Renal Division, Westmead Hospital, Westmead, NSW, Australia,* [8] *Westmead Clinical School, University of Sydney, Westmead, NSW, Australia*

***Correspondence:**
Helong Dai
helong68888@csu.edu.cn
Natasha M. Rogers
natasha.rogers@sydney.edu.au

†*Senior author*

A comparison of pre-clinical transplant models and of solid organs transplanted in routine clinical practice demonstrates that the liver is most amenable to the development of immunological tolerance. This phenomenon arises in the absence of stringent conditioning regimens that accompany published tolerizing protocols for other organs, particularly the kidney. The unique immunologic properties of the liver have assisted our understanding of the alloimmune response and how it can be manipulated to improve graft function and survival. This review will address important findings following liver transplantation in both animals and humans, and how these have driven the understanding and development of therapeutic immunosuppressive options. We will discuss the liver's unique system of immune and non-immune cells that regulate immunity, yet maintain effective responses to pathogens, as well as mechanisms of liver transplant tolerance in pre-clinical models and humans, including current immunosuppressive drug withdrawal trials and biomarkers of tolerance. In addition, we will address innovative therapeutic strategies, including mesenchymal stem cell, regulatory T cell, and regulatory dendritic cell therapy to promote liver allograft tolerance or minimization of immunosuppression in the clinic.

Keywords: liver transplantation, immune tolerance, mechanisms, cell therapy, immunosuppression withdrawal

INTRODUCTION

The location and anatomy of the liver, positioned between the gastrointestinal tract and the systemic circulation, allows it to conduct its functions of digestion, synthesis of plasma proteins and detoxification (1). Circulating blood from the gastrointestinal tract enriched with food antigens (Ags) and environmental microbial products, including endotoxin, converge in the liver portal vein (2). The hepatic artery, which provides about 20% of the liver blood supply, and the hepatic portal vein mix in the liver to create sinusoids. Liver sinusoidal endothelial cells (LSEC) are located in the space of Dissé and form an immediate barrier between the hepatocytes and the bloodstream (1, 3). The non-parenchymal cell populations including dendritic cells (DC), Kupffer cells (KC), and LSEC constitute the hepatic reticulo-endothelial system, which is responsible for clearing Ags and degradation of toxins from sinusoidal blood by uptake through endocytic receptors (1). The cross-talk between T cells and liver parenchymal cells, including LSEC, hepatocytes, hepatic stellate cells, and cholangiocytes, plays a crucial role in tolerance induction (4).

"Spontaneous" liver transplant tolerance has been demonstrated in both animals and humans, however, the mechanisms that underlie development of tolerance to the liver but not to other solid organ grafts are still not well-understood. We will summarize recent research findings, focusing on (i) the specific contributions of immune cells, mesenchymal stem cells (MSC) and parenchymal cell subsets that promote a tolerogenic microenvironment within the liver, (ii) mechanisms of organ-specific tolerance, and (iii) novel strategies to predict and promote liver transplant tolerance.

INTRAHEPATIC IMMUNE CELLS INTERACT WITH LIVER PARENCHYMAL CELLS TO GENERATE A TOLEROGENIC MICROENVIRONMENT

Unlike conventional DC in secondary lymphoid tissue, both mouse and human liver DC display tolerogenic properties (5–8). Liver DC express comparatively low levels of Toll-like receptor 4 (TLR4) that limits their response to specific ligands, leading to reduced hepatic adaptive immune response (8). Similarly, freshly-isolated, unmanipulated murine liver non-conventional plasmacytoid DC (pDC) express low levels of co-stimulatory molecules and weakly stimulate T cell responses (9, 10). Liver pDC prevent oral T cell priming through inducing anergy or deletion of circulating T cells via a CD4$^+$ T cell-independent mechanism (11). Monocytes cultured with hepatocyte growth factor or liver epithelial cells can differentiate into DC that release high levels of IL-10 (12, 13), suggesting that the hepatic microenvironment modulates DC differentiation into regulatory subsets (14).

KC located in the hepatic sinusoids are recognized as tissue-resident macrophages, originally derived from the blood monocytes (2). KC can phagocytose apoptotic cells and microorganisms, and therefore function similarly to other organ-based macrophages (2, 15). KC are also involved in portal venous tolerance, where Ag administration into the portal vein induces specific tolerance to that Ag. The mechanism for this type of tolerance appears to be KC-based release of IFN-γ-stimulated nitric oxide (NO) that inhibits T cell proliferation (16). KC treated with gadolinium chloride prevented the induction of portal venous tolerance by inhibiting Ag presentation to lymphocytes, supporting the notion that both Ag presentation to and stimulation of lymphocyte proliferation are necessary for tolerance induction (17). In human studies, a greater number of KC typically found in younger living donors predicts better hepatic allograft survival compared to elderly living donors, suggesting that KC in the donor liver are a relevant prognostic factor influencing post-transplant outcomes (18). Graft- infiltrating DC and KC were also shown to be increased during and after rat liver transplant tolerance induction, again suggesting a possible important role for these cells in shaping the host immune response toward tolerance (19).

Mouse LSEC express the mannose receptor and the scavenger receptor to enhance Ag uptake, and also express co-stimulatory molecules, including CD40, CD80, and CD86 that facilitate Ag presentation and T cell stimulatory function (20). Human LSEC constitutively express CD40, but CD80/CD86 is inducible and expressed during inflammation (21). Therefore, murine and human LSECs might function differently. Mouse LSEC can present circulating exogenous Ags to CD4$^+$ T and CD8$^+$ T cells, resulting in Ag-specific T cell tolerance, but not Th1 responses (22, 23). LSEC synthetic and endocytic function has been shown to be greater in spontaneously tolerant rat liver allografts compared to those that were rejected (24). LSEC lectin uniquely recognizes activated T cells and negatively regulates their responses (25). In addition, the threshold of Ag expression within the liver is the dominant factor determining T cell fate, rather than Ag cross-presentation, since low-level hepatocyte expression of cognate Ag generates an effector response that becomes functionally silenced at a high level of the same Ag (26).

Regarding lymphocytes, the hepatic CD8$^+$: CD4$^+$ T cell ratio is higher compared to peripheral blood (27), and both natural killer (NK) and natural killer T (NKT) cells are present at a higher percentage (of total cells) compared to that in secondary lymphoid organs. In contrast to T cells activated by splenocytes, T cells activated by hepatocytes lose cytolytic function after 3 days of co-culture and fail to survive (28). The mechanism of hepatocyte-induced T cell death is neither Fas (CD95)- nor tumor necrosis factor (TNF) receptor-dependent, suggesting a type of apoptosis known as passive cell death (29). In both murine and human liver transplantation, T cell infiltration into allografts is followed by their apoptosis (30, 31). Mouse liver CD8$^+$ T cells are also programmed to die following intrahepatic activation in a pro-apoptotic protein Bim-dependent manner (32). However, the molecular recognition events that induce apoptosis of graft-infiltrating T cells, and the reason why this phenomenon occurs within the liver, but not other allografts is unclear (30, 33).

Mesenchymal stem (stromal) cells (MSC) display unique immunosuppressive and anti-inflammatory properties that may modulate allograft outcomes. Adult liver-derived MSC are negative for human leukocyte Ag class II (HLA-II) and the co-stimulatory molecules, including CD80 and CD86, which can inhibit the proliferation of T cells activated by mitogen (34). Interestingly, liver graft-derived MSC have greater capacity to suppress allo-reactive T cell proliferation and cytotoxic degranulation than bone marrow-derived MSC (BM-MSC) (35), as well as significantly higher levels of immune-regulatory genes than adipose tissue-derived MSC and BM-MSC, that depend on programmed cell death ligand 1(PDL1) expression (36) for their ability to subvert T cell response.

COMPARING THE INTRINSIC TOLEROGENICITY OF THE LIVER GRAFTS IN ANIMALS AND HUMANS

In the first report showing spontaneous tolerance induction by liver transplantation, pig hepatic allografts demonstrated long-term survival without immunosuppression, protecting other donor-specific tissue but not third-party organs from rejection (37). This phenomenon was subsequently replicated in pre-sensitized rats that failed to reject donor liver grafts, inducing

TABLE 1 | A comparison of the intrinsic tolerogenicity of liver grafts with other transplanted organs in animals and humans.

Species	Donor/recipient	Graft survival time						References
		Liver	Kidney	Heart	Skin	Co-D-Skin	Co-T-Skin	
Mouse	C57BL/6→BALB/c	70% > 100 d	39.3 ± 3.1 d	8.3 ± 1.6	<10 d	80% > 100 d	18 ± 5 d	(42, 44–48)
	BALB/c→CBA	57% > 100 d	7.5 ± 1.5 d	8.6 ± 0.9	8.5 ± 1.5 d	/	/	
	C57BL/6→C3H/HeN	73% > 100 d	7.5 ± 1.5 d	8.1 ± 0.8	10.6 ± 0.9	/	/	
Rat	DA→PVG	80% > 100 d	12 d	8 d	6 ± 2 d	75% > 100 d	8 ± 1	(38, 49–52)
Pig	Landrace→Landrace	>18 month	7 d	6.5 ± 1.5d	9 ± 3 d	>24d	11 ± 4 d	(37, 53, 54)
NHPs	Cynomolgus monkeys→cynomolgus monkeys	<7 months	<2 wks	<2 wks	6 ± 1 d	/	/	(55–58)
Human		Liver allograft achieved "operational tolerance"						(59–63)
		Advantage of liver co-transplant: protection to kidney and heart grafts						(64–67)

Co-D-Skin, Co-transplant donor derived skin with liver; Co-T-Skin, Co-transplant third party skin with liver; d, days; NHPs, non-human primates; wks, weeks.

Ag-specific tolerance in 50% of recipients (38). To avoid the toxicities of irradiation in a sick liver failure recipient, delayed tolerance induction has been promoted when the recipients have recovered post-operatively. An ACI-to-Lewis rat (allogeneic) liver transplant model developed chronic rejection, however, in the same strain combination, liver recipients receiving 100×10^6 T cell-depleted donor BM cells at 3–4 weeks post-transplant followed by tacrolimus withdrawal became tolerant. Mechanistically, this delayed tolerance induction is associated with increased mixed chimerism, Treg generation, and decreased donor-specific antibody (DSA). However, the authors did not investigate key mechanisms underlying the development of delayed tolerance (39). Allogeneic liver transplantation from DA-to-Lewis rats receiving post-transplant total lymphoid irradiation, which is a non myeloablative regimen to induce graft-infiltrating T cell apoptosis and subsequent accumulation of Treg, also induced tolerance (40). The micro RNA (miRNA) profile in these tolerant allografts was similar to syngeneic grafts, indicating that tolerance potentially returned recipients to a state of immunological quiescence (40). Tolerance to liver transplants in rats can subsequently induce tolerance to intestinal allografts by hampering the expression of IL-2 receptor on recipient $CD8\alpha\beta^+$ lymphocytes in the lamina propria and reducing recruitment of NK cell and macrophages (41).

Spontaneous liver transplant tolerance between MHC-disparate murine strain combinations is significantly higher than that seen with kidney or heart allografts (42–44), and is summarized in **Table 1**. In the murine orthotopic liver transplantation model (68), allografts were accepted in 13 mouse strain combinations that showed evidence of donor cell chimerism (42). Mouse liver allografts can rescue donor-specific skin transplants from rejection, either pre- or post-liver transplant (42).

Human liver allograft "operational tolerance" has also been described and reviewed by many investigators (59–63, 69). Hepatic allografts protect simultaneously transplanted kidney allografts from the same donor from chronic cell- and antibody-mediated immune injury, resulting in better graft function compared with kidney transplant alone (64, 65). Combined liver and heart transplantation shows less evidence of cardiac allograft vasculopathy than isolated heart transplantation when detected by coronary three-dimensional volumetric intravascular ultrasound (66). Simultaneous liver-heart transplantation also showed reduced T cell-mediated rejection compared with cardiac transplantation alone (67).

The question of why only the liver displays inherent tolerogenicity is worthy of consideration. The naïve mouse liver has a greater number of DC than other parenchymal organs, such as heart, kidney, and pancreas (70). Recent findings reveal that DBA2J pDC are more powerful in inducing forkhead box p3 (Foxp3) expression in C57BL6 T cells and promoting kidney graft tolerance than the reverse combination. This suggests that the organ- and strain-specific differences exist that determines tolerance (71). In human studies, donor-reactive T cell clones were reduced in three tolerant combined kidney and BM transplant recipients, but not in non-tolerant patients (72). However, the same group further reported that donor-reactive T cell clone reduction was not associated with liver graft tolerance or failure, again highlighting organ-specific tolerance mechanisms in patients (73).

UNDERSTANDING THE MECHANISMS OF EXPERIMENTAL LIVER TRANSPLANT TOLERANCE

The literature on mechanisms that underlie liver allograft acceptance in rodent models is extensive, but centers on immunoregulation, and an intrinsic balance between leukocyte, non-parenchymal-parenchymal cell ratios, effector, and regulatory T cells, Ag-presenting cell phenotype, and function, as well as cross-talk between cellular compartments. The identification of molecular pathways that alter immunoregulation provides promising potential therapeutic avenues for clinical application. Liver transplant acceptance is also characterized by donor-specific hypo-responsiveness, mimicking the tolerance arising from chimerism following BM transplantation. The development of liver allograft tolerance

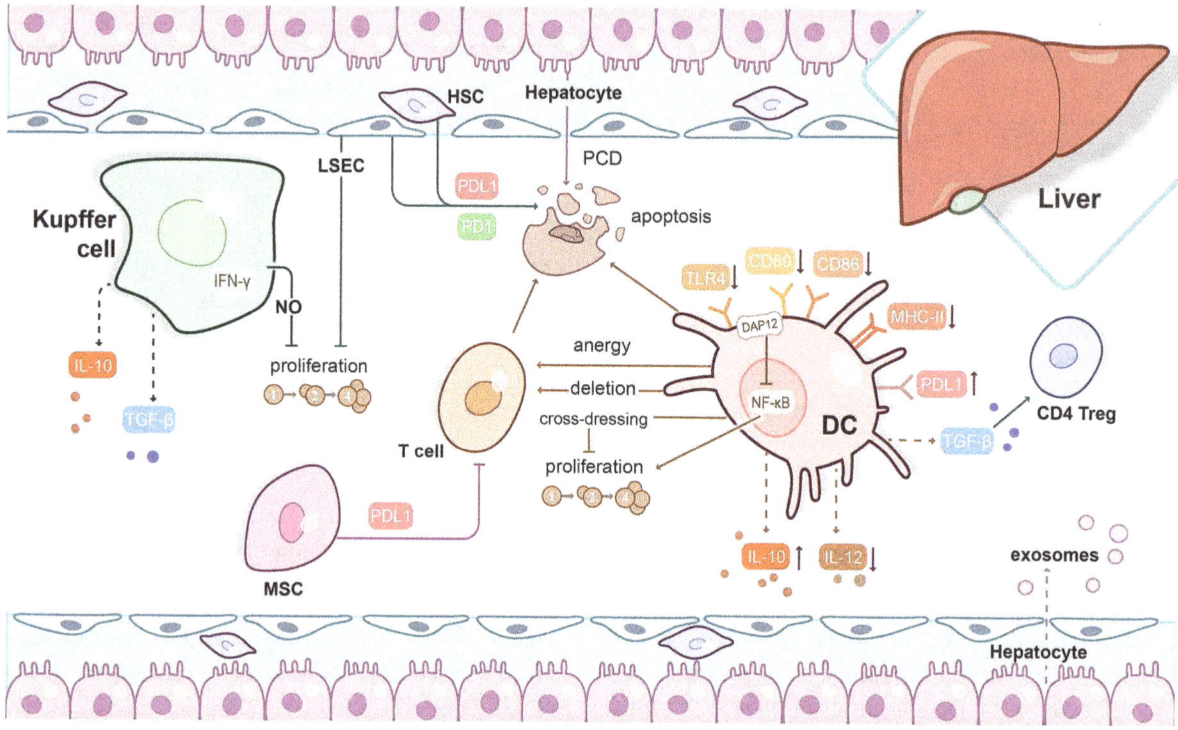

FIGURE 1 | Mechanisms underlying experimental liver transplant tolerance. Hepatic immune and parenchymal cells interact with each other to generate a tolerogenic microenvironment. Liver dendritic cells (DC) express low levels of Toll-like receptor 4 (TLR4) and co-stimulatory molecules, but high levels of PDL1, weakly stimulate T cell responses, and promote regulatory CD4^{+} T cells (CD4 Treg) induction through TGF-β. Liver DC release high levels of IL-10, but low bioactive IL-12. Liver DC prevent T cell priming of orally-administered Ag through anergy or deletion of circulating T cells. Graft-infiltrating, cross-dressed DC over-express PDL1 and subvert anti-donor T cell proliferation to promote liver graft tolerance. The DNAX-activating protein of 12 kDa (DAP12) negatively regulates liver DC IL-12 production, but positively regulates liver DC IL-10 production and T cell allostimulatory capability. Kupffer cells can release IFN-γ-stimulated nitric oxide (NO) to inhibit T cell proliferation and produce IL-10 and TGF-β to promote tolerance. Liver sinusoidal endothelial cells (LSEC) present circulating exogenous antigens to T cells, resulting in Ag-specific T cell tolerance. LSEC and hepatic stellate cells (HSC) induce T cell apoptosis through PDL1/PD1 pathway interactions. The mechanism of hepatocyte-induced T cell death occurs through a type of apoptosis known as passive cell death (PCD). Exosomes derived from hepatocytes may also be critical to a tolerogenic phenotype. Mesenchymal stromal cells (MSC) suppress T cell proliferation and differentiation through cell-cell contact that is mediated by PDL1.

appears to be independent on the thymus (74, 75). Current experimental results favor deletion of alloreactive T cells occurring within the organ and secondary lymphoid tissue, leading to a reduced burden of effector cells. Hepatic DC differ in their maturation state and allostimulatory capacity compared to DC isolated from other solid organs (76), and their capacity to modulate T cell function is well-known. However, the relative contribution of innate immune subsets like DC and NK cells has not been characterized.

Regardless of strain combination in rodent liver transplantation models, spontaneous tolerance appears to be induced by the graft itself, with liver-derived cell populations silencing the host immune response (77) (**Figure 1**). This feature is strain- and organ-specific: Lewis rat liver allografts demonstrate prolonged survival in DA recipients, although the reverse combination results in acute rejection. Rejection has been characterized by hepatocyte death, but allograft acceptance is associated with apoptotic mononuclear cells and upregulated FasL parenchymal expression. Irradiated Lewis rat donor livers lost tolerogenic capacity highlighting the role of hepatic passenger leukocytes (77). Donor passenger leukocytes, particularly T cells, but not B cells and macrophages, prolong irradiated donor liver allograft survival in the PVG-to-DA combinations, but reject transplanted heart grafts (78). Adoptive transfer of donor leukocytes or splenocytes re-establishes recipient tolerance, but not following T cell depletion. Interestingly, when two kidneys and two hearts of PVG rats were transplanted into each DA recipient, along with adoptive transfer of high dose donor leukocytes (1.5×10^{8}), transplanted organs were accepted, suggesting that liver-derived spontaneous transplant tolerance may be determined by the ratio of donor leukocytes to the quantity of donor tissues (78). Donor passenger leukocytes from transplanted liver grafts migrate rapidly into recipient lymphoid tissues, but their numbers decrease dramatically within the first 48 h (79), accompanied by deletion of alloreactive CD8^{+} T cells. Higher levels of apoptosis of infiltrating leukocytes within liver allografts are seen compared to renal allografts in the same rat strain combination (PVG-to-DA) (80). T cell clonal deletion (81, 82) was initially proposed as the cause of liver allograft acceptance. However, lymphocytes from long-term survival recipients demonstrate vigorous Ag-specific responses *in vitro* (83). Donor liver leukocyte-induced recipient T cell death by neglect also appears to be responsible for liver acceptance (77, 84). Deletion of donor passenger leukocytes by irradiation of the donor rat followed by liver transplantation breaks allograft acceptance (85). However, other studies have failed to confirm that the presence of donor passenger leukocytes is associated with allograft tolerance (86).

T cell apoptosis in the liver graft plays a crucial role in tolerance. Interferon (IFN)-γ is a key inflammatory cytokine produced by effector T cells. Surprisingly, IFN-γ knockout liver allografts are acutely rejected (87), suggesting that intact signaling is necessary for graft tolerance. T cell-derived IFN-γ signaling results in hepatic stellate cell and LSEC expression of PDL1, inducing T cell apoptosis through the PDL1/PD1 pathway (88). Functional assessment of these cells isolated from tolerated liver grafts demonstrated inhibition of T cell proliferative responses, particularly those of $CD8^+$ T cells. These findings were replicated in human $CD45^-$ non-parenchymal cells that limited peripheral blood mononuclear cell (PBMC)-derived T cell proliferation. Blocking this pathway using anti-PDL1 antibody (Ab) or using PDL1 knockout mice as donors resulted in allograft rejection, highlighting the essential role of PDL1 expression in the liver parenchyma to regulate apoptosis of alloreactive cells (89). Cytotoxic T-lymphocyte-associated protein 4 (CTLA4) blockade prevents T cell apoptosis and induces acute rejection, suggesting such signaling is also a pre-requisite for spontaneous mouse liver transplant tolerance (90). Anti-CTLA4 treatment enhances NK cell cytotoxicity, and augments IL-2 and IFN-γ in both graft and recipient spleen, in keeping with lack of alloreactive T cell death. Galectin-1, an endogenous lectin expressed in lymphoid organs, is upregulated in liver allografts and administration of recombinant protein significantly prolongs liver allografts. This was associated with enhanced $CD4^+$ and $CD8^+$ T cell apoptosis in the graft itself and recipient spleen and suppression of Th1/Th17 cell responses. There was no suggestion of modulation of regulatory effects by altering $CD4^+CD25^+FoxP3^+$ T cell numbers (91). Overexpression of galectin-1 in T cells promotes the activation of hepatic stellate cells that contribute to tolerance (92).

Regulatory T cells ($CD4^+CD25^+FoxP3^+$ Treg) have been demonstrated to increase significantly in the recipient liver graft and spleen. Moreover, depletion of recipient $CD4^+CD25^+$ T cells using anti-CD25 (IL-2Rα) Ab reduces apoptosis of graft-infiltrating $CD4^+$ and $CD8^+$ T cells, leading ultimately to liver allograft rejection (93). These findings highlight the roles of both $CD4^+$ Tregs (94, 95) and apoptosis of graft-infiltrating T cells in liver transplant tolerance induction. The $CD8^+CD103^+$ T cell subset possess suppressive function and also contributes to spontaneous liver graft tolerance, but the specific mechanism of action remains unclear (96). IFN-γ deficient liver allografts that reject around day 15 post-transplant show similar levels of Tregs but less T cell apoptosis compared to wild-type allografts, suggesting that T cell elimination may be the more critical factor (88). These data are further supported by observations in a B10-to-C3H mouse liver transplant model which showed that T cell deletion, not regulation, was responsible for spontaneous graft acceptance (30).

The role of NK cells in organ transplantation is still controversial (97–100). NK cells have been identified as a potential predictor of liver transplant tolerance (101). There are multiple potential mechanisms of action including direct lysis of recipient $CD4^+$ and $CD8^+$ T cells (102), deletion of Ag-presenting cells (103), and $CD8^+$ T cell hypo-responsiveness (104) which have been summarized elsewhere (99). However, NK cells in rat liver allografts can also promote rejection by producing IFN-γ in the early post-transplant period (105).

Host DC acquire donor major histocompatibility complex (MHC) molecules after mouse orthotopic liver transplant, to appear as "cross-dressed" DC (CD-DC). Graft-infiltrating CD-DC expressed PDL1 and IL-10 that subvert anti-donor T cell responses and promote death of graft-infiltrating $CD8^+$ T cells to promote liver graft tolerance (106). The transmembrane immuno-adaptor DNAX-activating protein of 12 kDa (DAP12) has been shown to negatively regulate conventional liver myeloid DC maturation, migration to host lymphoid tissue, and T cell allo-stimulatory capability (107, 108). $DAP12^{-/-}$ liver grafts exhibit low levels of Tregs and fail to induce liver transplant tolerance (107).

The balance of pro- and anti-inflammatory cytokines as well as other molecules within the hepatic microenvironment can crucially influence adaptive immune responses. Intrahepatic IL-4 transcripts were significantly lower in tolerated rat liver allografts compared to rejected allografts, however, no significant differences were observed for other cytokines (including IL-1α, IL-2, IL-6, IL-10, TNF-α, TNF-β, and transforming growth factor β (TGF-β) (109). IL-4 injection after rat liver transplantation converts allograft tolerance to rejection partially through a graft-specific antibody response (110). In the murine tolerant liver allograft, expression of miRNA-146a, 15b, 223, 23a, 27a, 34a, and 451 is upregulated compared to syngeneic grafts, suggesting a role for miRNA in tolerance induction (111). Expression of lectin galactose-binding soluble 1, fibrinogen-like protein 2 (Fgl2), the ectoenzyme CD39, phosphodiesterase 3B, killer cell lectin-like receptor G1 (Klrg1), Foxp3, and TGF-β, have all been shown to increase at 8–14 days following murine liver transplantation and promote tolerance to the allografts (112). However, the cellular origins of these factors are non-specific and may represent a combined signal from hepatocytes, infiltrating leukocytes, and non-parenchymal cells. The use of cutting-edge single-cell sequencing techniques will allow us to improve on these preliminary findings.

MONITORING AND PREDICTION OF CLINICAL LIVER TRANSPLANT TOLERANCE

Development of non-invasive biomarkers as diagnostic tools to define graft tolerance remains an important area of research in liver transplantation (113). Reliable, non-invasive biomarkers to predict graft rejection are not currently available, but are urgently needed (63). A prospective, longitudinal, international multi-center cohort study on immune monitoring after pediatric liver transplant is ongoing (114), and will provide much-needed data discovery and validation.

In order to investigate immunologic mechanisms elicited by immunosuppression (IS) withdrawal, 24 operationally tolerant recipients and 14 non-tolerant recipients were selected for analysis of T cell subset infiltration and gene expression pattern in protocol liver biopsy specimens prior to weaning, as well as 1 and 3 years after IS withdrawal. Treg reduction to baseline levels in liver biopsies, in addition to down-regulation of immune activation-associated genes at 3 years post-withdrawal in the context of no graft damage, suggested a balanced immune response in tolerant recipients (115). The dynamic profile of Treg in liver transplant recipients during IS weaning was explored by monitoring the frequency of Treg and Foxp3 mRNA expression in PBMC in 12 liver transplant patients undergoing IS withdrawal. A progressive increase in circulating $CD4^{+}CD25^{+}Foxp3^{+}$ Treg and Foxp3 mRNA expression was associated with operational tolerance in liver transplant recipients (14, 116). The expression of adenosine deaminase, which degrades adenosine to evoke stronger Treg activation, was higher in five tolerant liver transplant patients compared to the 12 non-tolerant recipients. These data indirectly indicate that adenosine deaminase potentially predicts liver transplant tolerance through targeting Treg (117). Using single-cell mass cytometry to detect immune profiles in peripheral blood of seven operational tolerant pediatric recipients and eight pediatric recipients on low dose single agent IS, a specific $CD4^{+}$ T cell subset that is $CD4^{+}CD5^{+}CD25^{+}CD38^{-/low}CD45RA^{-}$, distinct from Treg, correlated with liver allograft tolerance. This specific T cell subset lacks both CD45RA and stable Foxp3 expression, but expresses CD5 that has been shown to be crucial in promoting Treg induction (118).

Immune cell ratios and their balance can predict tolerance vs. rejection. A comparison of 19 liver transplant patients on IS, operationally tolerant liver transplant recipients or 24 age-matched healthy volunteers demonstrated an increased frequency of $CD4^{+}CD25^{+}$ T cells and B cells, altered $V\delta1/V\delta2\gamma\delta$ T cell ratio, but decreased NK cells in PBMC in operationally tolerant patients (119). The ratios of Treg/Th17, Th1/Th17, and $CD8^{+}$/Th17 cells were increased in tolerant patients compared with non-tolerant patients during immunosuppression tapering. The elevated Treg/Th17 ratio continued over 60 months follow-up in tolerant patients, indicating a reciprocal balance between Treg and Th17 that may contribute to the development and maintenance of tolerance (120). Tolerant liver recipients also exhibit greater numbers of $CD4^{+}CD25^{+}$ T cells and $V\delta1^{+}$ T cells in the circulation compared to non-tolerant patients and healthy individuals (121). Adult liver allografts also contain a small population of hematopoietic stem/progenitor cells ($Lin^{-}CD34^{+}CD38^{-}CD90^{+}$) that may promote long-term (6 months to 8 years) chimerism in the graft (122). The ratio of DC precursors $CD11c^{-}CD123^{hi}$ (pDC2) to $CD11c^{+}CD123^{-/low}$ (pDC1) was also significantly higher in 36 patients undergoing successful drug weaning compared to those 21 patients on maintenance immunosuppression, regardless of the dose of prednisone or tacrolimus. These data suggest that pDC2 that can polarize naïve Th cell toward a Th2 phenotype may drive tolerance induction (123). In a further study, 13 tolerant liver transplant recipients showed an elevated ratio of plasmacytoid DC (pDC) to myeloid DC compared to those 12 patients remaining on immunosuppression. Additionally, a high PDL1/CD86 ratio on pDC correlated with increased Treg and correlated with pediatric liver allograft tolerance (124).

Gene expression of sentrin-specific peptidase 6 (SENP6) and Fem-1 homolog C (FEM1C) were shown to be predictive biomarkers of liver transplant tolerance in a single cohort of 17 liver transplant recipients (125). At least 13 unique gene sets, including SENP6 that is associated with NK cells, were significantly expressed in adult and pediatric liver transplant patients, which showed a prediction for tolerance (126). This conclusion was supported by previous findings of differential gene expression between tolerant and non-tolerant transplant recipients within the NK cell compartment despite no clear differences in absolute cell number between these patient groups (101). The intra-liver allograft gene expression involved in the regulation of iron homeostasis is more active in operationally tolerant patients compared to non-tolerant recipients and independent of baseline immunosuppression (127). However, the iron-related markers were poor predictors for drug withdrawal in hepatitis C virus (HCV)-infected liver transplant recipients (128), which could be due to inhibition of hepcidin expression by HCV (129). Regardless, the blood gene expression was not sensitive enough to distinguish rejection vs. HCV-infection (130). However, type I IFN-stimulated gene overexpression within liver allografts of HCV-positive recipients, along with circulating PD1/CTLA4/2B4-positive HCV-specific $CD8^{+}$ exhausted T cells, were associated with liver graft operational tolerance induction (128).

Single-cell RNA sequencing (scRNAseq) can provide a comprehensive map to characterize human hepatic immune cell populations and also non-parenchymal cells (131), and it is anticipated that it may prove helpful in predicting liver transplant rejection vs. tolerance capacity in the near future. However, before validated accurate, non-invasive biomarkers are available, histopathological findings remain the gold standard to determine the management of immunosuppression (132).

ONGOING AND NOVEL THERAPEUTIC APPROACHES TO PROMOTE LIVER TRANSPLANT TOLERANCE IN PATIENTS

Life-long immunosuppression and its accompanying burden of increased morbidity and mortality has prompted interest in immunosuppressive drug withdrawal (133). In the first multi-center trial of drug withdrawal in adult liver transplant recipients, 41.84% of evaluated recipients were successfully weaned from immunosuppression at least 3 years post-transplantation (134). In the first multi-center immunosuppression withdrawal trial in pediatric recipients of parental living donor liver transplantation, complete cessation of immunosuppressive agents for at least 1 year showed normal graft function and stable liver graft biopsies (60). The majority of these promising clinical trials have been documented in detail elsewhere (132, 135).

TABLE 2 | Strategies to promote liver transplant tolerance using cell therapy in the clinic.

Cell type: Authors	Phase	NCT number	Date*	Donor	Number of Patients	Infusion time	Cell dose(s)	Cell source	Outcomes/status	References[&]
MSC										
Popp et al. (149)	I	NCT01841632	Nov. 2011	DD	3–24	POD 0 and 3	2 doses, 300×10^6	Third Party BM-MAPC	The study objective is to evaluate the safety and clinical feasibility	(149)
Detry etal. (150)	I–II	NCT01429038	Mar. 2012	DD	10	POD 3 ± 2	3 doses, $1.5–3 \times 10^6$/kg BW	Third Party MSC	No side effect of infusion. Tolerance was not observed	(150)
Zhang etal. (151)	I	NCT02223897	Jan. 2013	&	12 with ITBL	Weeks 1, 2, 4, 8, 12, 16 after recruitment	6 doses, 1×10^6/kg BW	UC-MSC	No MSC-related side effects. Better graft survival than the control group	(151)
Qi Zhang et al.	I–II	NCT01844063	Jul. 2013	&	210 with graft failure	&	&	UC-MSC	Recruiting	&
Yang et al.	I–II	NCT02706132	Feb. 2014	&	15	&	6 doses, 1×10^6/kg BW	MSC	Recruiting	&
Lorini et al.	I	NCT02260375	Oct. 2014	&	20	&	1 dose, $1–2 \times 10^6$/kg BW	Third Party BM derived MSC	Recruiting	&
Soeder et al. (152)	I	NCT01841632	Jun. 2015	Living	1	POD 0 and 2	2 doses, 300×10^6	MAPC	No acute complications with cell infusion. Normal liver function.	(152)
Rutgers et al.	I	NCT02557724	Sep. 2015	Living	&	&	&	&	Recruitment completed	&
Sturm et al.	I	NCT02957552	Mar. 2017	Living	7	POD 0 and 2	2 doses, 1×10^6/kg BW	Donor BM-MSC	Recruiting	(153)
Shi et al. (154)	I–II	NCT01690247	Sep. 2017	DD	13 with ACR	Rejection time	1 dose, 1×10^6/kg BW	UC-MSC	No side effects. ALT decreased with increased Treg/Th17 ratio in the grafts compared with no infusion control	(154)
Treg										
Todo et al. (155)	I–II	UMIN000015789	Nov. 2010	Living	10	POD 13	1 dose, $0.23–6.37 \times 10^6$/kg BW	Donor Lymphocytes	No side effects; Normal graft function in all patients. Seven patients withdrew IS and three patients developed ACR during weaning IS. No control group data.	(155)
Lombardi et al.	I–II	NCT02129881	May. 2014	Living	15	POD 5	1 dose, 1×10^6/kg BW	Host blood derived Treg	Recruitment completed	&
Feng et al.	I	NCT02188719	Dec. 2014	&	15	&	&	darTregs	Terminated	&
Lu et al. (96)	I	NCT01624077	Dec. 2014	Living	1	POD 0–2 years	1×10^6/kg BW	Host blood derived Treg	Active, not recruiting	&
Feng et al.	II–III	NCT02474199	Jun. 2016	Living	14	POM 24–84	300-500 $\times 10^6$/kg BW	Host blood derived Treg	Recruitment completed	&
Curry et al.	II	NCT02739412	Nov. 2016	&	7	&	&	&	Active, not recruiting	&
Sanchez-Fueyo et al. (156)	IV	NCT02949492	Dec. 2017	&	6	POY 2–6	&	&	Terminated	&

(Continued)

TABLE 2 | Continued

Cell type: Authors	Phase	NCT number	Date*	Donor	Number of Patients	Infusion time	Cell dose(s)	Cell source	Outcomes/status	References[&]
Sanchez-Fueyo, et al. (156)	I	NCT02166177	Nov. 2019	DBD/DCD	9	POM 3–16	1–4.5 × 10^6/kg BW	Host blood polyclonal Treg	Infusion is safe. Increased circulating Tregs and reduced allo-reactive T cell response	(156)
DCreg										
Thomson et al.	I–II	NCT03164265	Aug. 2017	Living	15	POD-7	1 dose, 2.5–10 × 10^6/kg BW	Donor blood monocyte-derived DCreg	Enrolling	&

ACR, acute cellular rejection; BM, bone marrow; BM-MAPC, bone marrow-derived-multipotent adult progenitor cells; BM-MSC, bone marrow-derived mesenchymal stem cells; BW, body weight; darTregs, donor-alloAg-reactive regulatory T cells; DBD, donation after brain death; DCD, donation after circulatory death; DCreg, regulatory dendritic cells; DD, deceased donation; IS, immunosuppression; ITBL, ischemic-type biliary lesions; Kg, Kilogram; M, million; MAPC, multipotent adult progenitor cells; MSC, mesenchymal stem cell; N, number; NCT, National Clinical Trial; NIAID, National Institute of Allergy and Infectious Diseases; POD, post-operative days. POM, post-operative months; POY, post-operative years; Ref, reference; UC-MSC, umbilical cord derived mesenchymal stem cell.

&means data not available or unpublished.

**Date means the trials released date or patient enrolled date or paper published date as reference indicated.*

[&]Unpublished data come from ClinicalTrials.gov or UMIN Clinical Trials Registry.

Several factors could potentially affect the outcomes of drug withdrawal. The interval between transplantation and initiation of drug withdrawal appears to be one of the most powerful clinical predictors of success (136, 137), as a longer post-transplant period (131 ± 43 vs. 83 ± 40 months) may establish better host-graft adaptation (134). Over 60% of liver transplant recipients with a longer time interval (156 months post-transplant) and a lower lymphocyte proliferation index became clinically tolerant at a median of 14 months of follow-up (138). Younger recipients at the time of transplantation had better outcomes and a higher possibility of successful weaning compared to older recipients (139, 140), suggesting that an "adapted" or "inexperienced" immune system was important in drug withdrawal (141). Immunosuppression, including high-dose antithymocyte globulin (ATG) induction followed by short-term rapamycin withdrawal at an early time-point (4 month post-transplant) failed to induce operational liver transplant tolerance, which was associated with $CD8^+$ memory T cell expansion and elevated IL-17^+ cell infiltration in liver grafts (142). Moreover, fewer donor-recipient human leukocyte antigen (HLA)-A-, B-, and DR-mismatches, and a lower incidence of early rejection were associated with successful drug withdrawal in a 3 year follow-up of 18 liver transplant recipients (143).

Due to immunosuppressive drug non-specificity, drug toxicity, inconsistent outcomes, and the difficulty of early complete immunosuppression withdrawal, other strategies, including the use of stem cells, regulatory dendritic cells (DCreg) and Treg therapy have emerged to promote liver allograft tolerance (144–148). Published trials are summarized in **Table 2**. The pivotal role of many of these cellular subsets in immunomodulation makes them ideal candidates for use as therapeutic agents. Mesenchymal stem cells have the advantage of being sourced from diverse tissues, but they lack a definitive marker to enable isolation. They display low immunogenicity and have been shown to modulate other immune and non-parenchymal cells (157, 158). Immature or regulatory DC have a well-established capacity to induce Ag-specific hypo-responsiveness, Th1 cell apoptosis, and Treg development. Indeed, this phenotype may be enhanced in hepatic DC (6). Treg have the capacity to migrate to sites of inflammation and exert immunosuppressive effects on $CD4^+$ and $CD8^+$ T cells directly or through elaboration of inhibitory cytokine production. Several studies have reported increased frequency of Tregs in operationally tolerant liver transplant recipients (121) and following weaning of immunosuppression (116). Chimeric Ag receptor or CRISPR/Cas9 technology has recently been applied to modify Treg to enhance their regulatory function *in vitro* (159, 160), and their safety and longevity *in vivo* (161).

A phase I–II study enrolled 10 liver transplant recipients who received 1.5–3 × 10^6/kg third-party MSC on post-operative day 3 ± 2, and were compared with 10 liver transplants without MSC. This study demonstrated safety, but did not promote tolerance (150). A phase I study of MSC in liver transplantation showed that two infusions of 1.5 × 10^8 third-party, multi-potent adult progenitor cells into a living-related liver transplant recipient at day 0 and 2 post-transplant was feasible and safe. However, no further follow-up data was reported (152). An open-label, prospective pilot trial of two intravenous infusions of 1×10^6 cells/kg of donor-derived MSC in pediatric living-donor transplant recipients who will receive standard immunosuppression is currently ongoing (153).

A first-in-human clinical trial of donor-derived DCreg infusion to achieve early complete immunosuppression withdrawal and potentially tolerance induction in living donor liver transplant patients is ongoing at the University of Pittsburgh (146, 162, 163) and shows no side effects of cell infusion (published as an abstract in the American Journal of Transplantation 2019). Five registered clinical trials of Treg cell therapy have previously been detailed (144) and are summarized in **Table 2**. Infusion of *ex vivo*-generated host-derived donor Ag alloreactive Tregs into 10 consecutive adult recipients early post-liver transplant following cyclophosphamide showed safety and efficacy for immunosuppression withdrawal and clinical tolerance induction in 7 out of 10 patients (155).

In vitro study shows that targeting primary human hepatocytes by silencing their HLA class I expression can alleviate alloreactive T cell proliferation without impairing metabolic function (164). In contrast to this human finding, adeno-associated viral vector transfer of donor MHC-I molecule to recipient hepatocytes can induce allospecific $CD8^+$ Treg expansion, and promote allogeneic pancreatic islet graft tolerance (165). However, targeting of HLA expression is currently far from progressing to clinical practice.

CONCLUSIONS

The liver, an atypical immune and metabolic organ, may be accepted spontaneously following transplantation in experimental animals. In humans, it may be possible to withdraw immunosuppression in carefully selected stable patients without rejection and liver grafts may also confer protection on other grafts from the same donor (strain). Current information on liver allograft acceptance suggests hepatic resident immune cells (DC, T cells, KC, and potentially NK cells) cross-talk with parenchymal LSEC and hepatocytes, in conjunction with specific anti-inflammatory cytokines and signaling molecules to create a tolerogenic microenvironment. The phenomena of infiltrating T cell apoptosis in liver transplant recipients may be crucial to operational allograft tolerance, but underlying mechanisms are not well-understood. Recent findings reveal that MSC, especially liver graft-derived MSC, can suppress T cell-based immune responses. Fundamental differences in immune cell number, subset proportions, and responsiveness to tolerogenic cues may offer some explanation as to why liver allografts, but not other solid organ transplants, are readily accepted, and deserve further investigation.

Currently, non-invasive biomarkers to predict liver graft tolerance or rejection are promising. However, there are no definitive diagnostic criteria that have been widely validated and approved. Cutting-edge technologies, such as scRNAseq, provide a potential novel approach to predict liver transplant tolerance vs. rejection in the future. However, until accurate and non-invasive biomarkers are available, histopathological findings remain the gold standard to monitor the status of liver allografts.

To minimize side effects related to life-long immunosuppression, drug withdrawal has been advocated. Yet, drug withdrawal is not suitable for every patient. The development of novel cellular therapeutics, including MSC and regulatory cell therapy, is currently under evaluation in multiple trials worldwide to establish feasibility, safety, and efficacy. However, there are significant limitations to this approach, including cost, low cell yield, unpredictable function *in vivo*, and the dependence on the immunological status of each recipient. A combinatorial approach of CRISP/Cas9, chimeric Ag-receptor or gene-edited cellular therapy, combined with immunosuppression minimization is a possible strategy to promote clinical liver transplant tolerance, but will require the presence of adequate monitoring tools.

AUTHOR CONTRIBUTIONS

HD wrote the manuscript and designed the figure. YZ generated the tables. AT designed the outline of the manuscript and revised the manuscript. NR wrote and revised the manuscript. All authors have contributed to the editing of the manuscript.

ACKNOWLEDGMENTS

The authors' work is supported by the National Science Foundation of China (81800664, 81970655 and 81900370), Natural Science Foundation of Hunan Province of China (2019JJ50842), and Huxiang Young Talents of Hunan Province (2019RS2013) to HD, National Institutes of Health grants R01 AI118777 to AT, National Health and Medical Research Council Career Development Fellowship (GNT1158977), and Project Grant (GNT1138372) to NR.

REFERENCES

1. Thomson AW, Knolle PA. Antigen-presenting cell function in the tolerogenic liver environment. *Nat Rev Immunol.* (2010) 10:753–66. doi: 10.1038/nri2858
2. Crispe IN. Hepatic T cells and liver tolerance. *Nat Rev Immunol.* (2003) 3:51–62. doi: 10.1038/nri981
3. Shetty S, Lalor PF, Adams DH. Liver sinusoidal endothelial cells - gatekeepers of hepatic immunity. *Nat Rev Gastroenterol Hepatol.* (2018) 15:555–67. doi: 10.1038/s41575-018-0020-y
4. Lei H, Reinke P, Volk HD, Lv Y, Wu R. Mechanisms of immune tolerance in liver transplantation-crosstalk between alloreactive T cells and liver cells with therapeutic prospects. *Front Immunol.* (2019) 10:2667. doi: 10.3389/fimmu.2019.02667
5. Thomson AW, Lu L. Are dendritic cells the key to liver transplant tolerance? *Immunol Today.* (1999) 20:27–32. doi: 10.1016/S0167-5699(98)01378-4
6. Bamboat ZM, Stableford JA, Plitas G, Burt BM, Nguyen HM, Welles AP, et al. Human liver dendritic cells promote T cell hyporesponsiveness. *J Immunol.* (2009) 182:1901–11. doi: 10.4049/jimmunol.0803404
7. Abe M, Tokita D, Raimondi G, Thomson AW. Endotoxin modulates the capacity of CpG-activated liver myeloid DC to direct Th1-type responses. *Eur J Immunol.* (2006) 36:2483–93. doi: 10.1002/eji.200535767

8. De Creus A, Abe M, Lau AH, Hackstein H, Raimondi G, Thomson AW. Low TLR4 expression by liver dendritic cells correlates with reduced capacity to activate allogeneic T cells in response to endotoxin. *J Immunol.* (2005) 174:2037–45. doi: 10.4049/jimmunol.174.4.2037
9. Kingham TP, Chaudhry UI, Plitas G, Katz SC, Raab J, DeMatteo RP. Murine liver plasmacytoid dendritic cells become potent immunostimulatory cells after Flt-3 ligand expansion. *Hepatology.* (2007) 45:445–54. doi: 10.1002/hep.21457
10. Pillarisetty VG, Shah AB, Miller G, Bleier JI, DeMatteo RP. Liver dendritic cells are less immunogenic than spleen dendritic cells because of differences in subtype composition. *J Immunol.* (2004) 172:1009–17. doi: 10.4049/jimmunol.172.2.1009
11. Goubier A, Dubois B, Gheit H, Joubert G, Villard-Truc F, Asselin-Paturel C, et al. Plasmacytoid dendritic cells mediate oral tolerance. *Immunity.* (2008) 29:464–75. doi: 10.1016/j.immuni.2008.06.017
12. Rutella S, Bonanno G, Procoli A, Mariotti A, de Ritis DG, Curti A, et al. Hepatocyte growth factor favors monocyte differentiation into regulatory interleukin (IL)-10^{++}IL-$12^{low/neg}$ accessory cells with dendritic-cell features. *Blood.* (2006) 108:218–27. doi: 10.1182/blood-2005-08-3141
13. Cabillic F, Rougier N, Basset C, Lecouillard I, Quelvennec E, Toujas L, et al. Hepatic environment elicits monocyte differentiation into a dendritic cell subset directing Th2 response. *J Hepatol.* (2006) 44:552–9. doi: 10.1016/j.jhep.2005.08.010
14. Baroja-Mazo A, Revilla-Nuin B, Parrilla P, Martinez-Alarcon L, Ramirez P, Pons JA. Tolerance in liver transplantation: Biomarkers and clinical relevance. *World J Gastroenterol.* (2016) 22:7676–91. doi: 10.3748/wjg.v22.i34.7676
15. Shi J, Fujieda H, Kokubo Y, Wake K. Apoptosis of neutrophils and their elimination by Kupffer cells in rat liver. *Hepatology.* (1996) 24:1256–63. doi: 10.1002/hep.510240545
16. Roland CR, Walp L, Stack RM, Flye MW. Outcome of Kupffer cell antigen presentation to a cloned murine Th1 lymphocyte depends on the inducibility of nitric oxide synthase by IFN-gamma. *J Immunol.* (1994) 153:5453–64.
17. Roland CR, Mangino MJ, Duffy BF, Flye MW. Lymphocyte suppression by Kupffer cells prevents portal venous tolerance induction: a study of macrophage function after intravenous gadolinium. *Transplantation.* (1993) 55:1151–8. doi: 10.1097/00007890-199305000-00041
18. Hidaka M, Eguchi S, Takatsuki M, Soyama A, Ono S, Adachi T, et al. The Kupffer cell number affects the outcome of living donor liver transplantation from elderly donors. *Transplant Direct.* (2016) 2:e94. doi: 10.1097/TXD.0000000000000608
19. Meyer D, Loffeler S, Otto C, Czub S, Gassel HJ, Timmermann W, et al. Donor-derived alloantigen-presenting cells persist in the liver allograft during tolerance induction. *Transpl Int.* (2000) 13:12–20. doi: 10.1111/j.1432-2277.2000.tb01030.x
20. Lohse AW, Knolle PA, Bilo K, Uhrig A, Waldmann C, Ibe M, et al. Antigen-presenting function and B7 expression of murine sinusoidal endothelial cells and Kupffer cells. *Gastroenterology.* (1996) 110:1175–81. doi: 10.1053/gast.1996.v110.pm8613007
21. Leifeld L, Trautwein C, Dumoulin FL, Manns MP, Sauerbruch T, Spengler U. Enhanced expression of CD80 (B7-1), CD86 (B7-2), and CD40 and their ligands CD28 and CD154 in fulminant hepatic failure. *Am J Pathol.* (1999) 154:1711–20. doi: 10.1016/S0002-9440(10)65427-2
22. Knolle PA, Schmitt E, Jin S, Germann T, Duchmann R, Hegenbarth S, et al. Induction of cytokine production in naive $CD4^{+}$ T cells by antigen-presenting murine liver sinusoidal endothelial cells but failure to induce differentiation toward Th1 cells. *Gastroenterology.* (1999) 116:1428–40. doi: 10.1016/S0016-5085(99)70508-1
23. Limmer A, Ohl J, Kurts C, Ljunggren HG, Reiss Y, Groettrup M, et al. Efficient presentation of exogenous antigen by liver endothelial cells to $CD8^{+}$ T cells results in antigen-specific T-cell tolerance. *Nat Med.* (2000) 6:1348–54. doi: 10.1038/82161
24. Ge X, Nowak G, Ericzon BG, Sumitran-Holgersson S. Liver sinusoidal endothelial cell function in rejected and spontaneously accepted rat liver allografts. *Transpl Int.* (2008) 21:49–56. doi: 10.1111/j.1432-2277.2007.00569.x
25. Tang L, Yang J, Liu W, Tang X, Chen J, Zhao D, et al. Liver sinusoidal endothelial cell lectin, LSECtin, negatively regulates hepatic T-cell immune response. *Gastroenterology.* (2009) 137:1498–508.e1–5. doi: 10.1053/j.gastro.2009.07.051
26. Tay SS, Wong YC, McDonald DM, Wood NA, Roediger B, Sierro F, et al. Antigen expression level threshold tunes the fate of CD8 T cells during primary hepatic immune responses. *Proc Natl Acad Sci U S A.* (2014) 111:E2540–9. doi: 10.1073/pnas.1406674111
27. Norris S, Collins C, Doherty DG, Smith F, McEntee G, Traynor O, et al. Resident human hepatic lymphocytes are phenotypically different from circulating lymphocytes. *J Hepatol.* (1998) 28:84–90. doi: 10.1016/S0168-8278(98)80206-7
28. Bertolino P, Trescol-Biemont MC, Rabourdin-Combe C. Hepatocytes induce functional activation of naive $CD8^{+}$ T lymphocytes but fail to promote survival. *Eur J Immunol.* (1998) 28:221–36. doi: 10.1002/(SICI)1521-4141(199801)28:01<221::AID-IMMU221>3.0.CO;2-F
29. Bertolino P, Trescol-Biemont MC, Thomas J, Fazekas de St Groth B, Pihlgren M, Marvel J, et al. Death by neglect as a deletional mechanism of peripheral tolerance. *Int Immunol.* (1999) 11:1225–38. doi: 10.1093/intimm/11.8.1225
30. Qian S, Lu L, Fu F, Li Y, Li W, Starzl TE, et al. Apoptosis within spontaneously accepted mouse liver allografts: evidence for deletion of cytotoxic T cells and implications for tolerance induction. *J Immunol.* (1997) 158:4654–61.
31. Meyer D, Thorwarth M, Otto C, Gassel HJ, Timmermann W, Ulrichs K, et al. Apoptosis of alloreactive T cells in liver allografts during tolerance induction. *Transplant Proc.* (1999) 31:474. doi: 10.1016/S0041-1345(98)01714-X
32. Holz LE, Benseler V, Bowen DG, Bouillet P, Strasser A, O'Reilly L, et al. Intrahepatic murine CD8 T-cell activation associates with a distinct phenotype leading to Bim-dependent death. *Gastroenterology.* (2008) 135:989–97. doi: 10.1053/j.gastro.2008.05.078
33. Sharland A, Yan Y, Wang C, Bowen DG, Sun J, Sheil AG, et al. Evidence that apoptosis of activated T cells occurs in spontaneous tolerance of liver allografts and is blocked by manipulations which break tolerance. *Transplantation.* (1999) 68:1736–45. doi: 10.1097/00007890-199912150-00018
34. Raicevic G, Najar M, Najimi M, El Taghdouini A, van Grunsven LA, Sokal E, et al. Influence of inflammation on the immunological profile of adult-derived human liver mesenchymal stromal cells and stellate cells. *Cytotherapy.* (2015) 17:174–85. doi: 10.1016/j.jcyt.2014.10.001
35. de Mare-Bredemeijer EL, Mancham S, Verstegen MM, de Ruiter PE, van Gent R, O'Neill D, et al. Human graft-derived mesenchymal stromal cells potently suppress alloreactive T-cell responses. *Stem Cells Dev.* (2015) 24:1436–47. doi: 10.1089/scd.2014.0485
36. Taner T, Abrol N, Park WD, Hansen MJ, Gustafson MP, Lerman LO, et al. Phenotypic, transcriptional and functional analysis of liver mesenchymal stromal cells and their immunomodulatory properties. *Liver Transpl.* (2020) 26:549–63. doi: 10.1002/lt.25718
37. Calne RY, Sells RA, Pena JR, Davis DR, Millard PR, Herbertson BM, et al. Induction of immunological tolerance by porcine liver allografts. *Nature.* (1969) 223:472–6. doi: 10.1038/223472a0
38. Kamada N, Davies HS, Roser B. Reversal of transplantation immunity by liver grafting. *Nature.* (1981) 292:840–2. doi: 10.1038/292840a0
39. Xie Y, Wu Y, Xin K, Wang JJ, Xu H, Ildstad ST, et al. Delayed donor bone marrow infusion induces liver transplant tolerance. *Transplantation.* (2017) 101:1056–66. doi: 10.1097/TP.0000000000001684
40. Vitalone MJ, Wei L, Fujiki M, Lau AH, Littau E, Esquivel C, et al. Liver microRNA profile of induced allograft tolerance. *Transplantation.* (2016) 100:781–90. doi: 10.1097/TP.0000000000001105
41. Sarnacki S, Nakai H, Calise D, Azuma T, Brousse N, Revillon Y, et al. Decreased expression of the interleukin 2 receptor on CD8 recipient lymphocytes in intestinal grafts rendered tolerant by liver transplantation in rats. *Gut.* (1998) 43:849–55. doi: 10.1136/gut.43.6.849
42. Qian S, Demetris AJ, Murase N, Rao AS, Fung JJ, Starzl TE. Murine liver allograft transplantation: tolerance and donor cell chimerism. *Hepatology.* (1994) 19:916–24. doi: 10.1002/hep.1840190418
43. Tse GH, Hughes J, Marson LP. Systematic review of mouse kidney transplantation. *Transpl Int.* (2013) 26:1149–60. doi: 10.1111/tri.12129
44. Zhang Z, Zhu L, Quan D, Garcia B, Ozcay N, Duff J, et al. Pattern of liver, kidney, heart, and intestine allograft rejection in different mouse strain combinations. *Transplantation.* (1996) 62:1267–72. doi: 10.1097/00007890-199611150-00016
45. Zhai Y, Meng L, Gao F, Wang Y, Busuttil RW, Kupiec-Weglinski JW. $CD4^{+}$ T regulatory cell induction and function in transplant recipients

after CD154 blockade is TLR4 independent. *J Immunol.* (2006) 176:5988–94. doi: 10.4049/jimmunol.176.10.5988
46. Mayumi H, Good RA. Long-lasting skin allograft tolerance in adult mice induced across fully allogeneic (multimajor H-2 plus multiminor histocompatibility) antigen barriers by a tolerance-inducing method using cyclophosphamide. *J Exp Med.* (1989) 169:213–38. doi: 10.1084/jem.169.1.213
47. Gerlag PG, Koene RA, Hagemann JF, Wijdeveld PG. Hyperacute rejection of skin allografts in the mouse. Sensitivity of ingrowing skin grafts to the action of alloantibody and rabbit complement. *Transplantation.* (1975) 20:308–13. doi: 10.1097/00007890-197510000-00007
48. Perez MI, Edelson RL, John L, Laroche L, Berger CL. Inhibition of antiskin allograft immunity induced by infusions with photoinactivated effector T lymphocytes (PET cells). *Yale J Biol Med.* (1989) 62:595–609.
49. Kamada N, Brons G, Davies HS. Fully allogeneic liver grafting in rats induces a state of systemic nonreactivity to donor transplantation antigens. *Transplantation.* (1980) 29:429–31. doi: 10.1097/00007890-198005000-00021
50. White E, Hildemann WH. Allografts in genetically defined rats: difference in survival between kidney and skin. *Science (New York, NY).* (1968) 162:1293–5. doi: 10.1126/science.162.3859.1293
51. Taylor AC, Lehrfeld JW. Determination of survival time of skin homografts in the rat by observation of vascular changes in the graft. *Plast Reconstr Surg (1946).* (1953) 12:423–31. doi: 10.1097/00006534-195312000-00005
52. Bistoni G, Calvitti M, Mancuso F, Arato I, Falabella G, Cucchia R, et al. Prolongation of skin allograft survival in rats by the transplantation of microencapsulated xenogeneic neonatal porcine Sertoli cells. *Biomaterials.* (2012) 33:5333–40. doi: 10.1016/j.biomaterials.2012.04.020
53. Calne RY, Bitter-Suermann H, Davis DR, Dunn DC, Herbertson BM, Reiter FH, et al. Orthotopic heart transplantation in the pig. *Nature.* (1974) 247:140–2. doi: 10.1038/247140b0
54. Kalden JR, Guthy EA. Prolonged skin allograft survival in vitamin C-deficient guinea-pigs. Preliminary communication. *Eur Surg Res.* (1972) 4:114–9. doi: 10.1159/000127607
55. Oura T, Yamashita K, Suzuki T, Fukumori D, Watanabe M, Hirokata G, et al. Long-term hepatic allograft acceptance based on CD40 blockade by ASKP1240 in nonhuman primates. *Am J Transplant.* (2012) 12:1740–54. doi: 10.1111/j.1600-6143.2012.04014.x
56. Calne RY, Davis DR, Pena JR, Balner H, de Vries M, Herbertson BM, et al. Hepatic allografts and xenografts in primates. *Lancet (London, England).* (1970) 1:103–6. doi: 10.1016/S0140-6736(70)90462-9
57. Thomas JM, Carver FM, Thomas FT. Enhanced allograft survival in rhesus monkeys treated with anti-human thymocyte globulin and donor lymphoid cells. *Surg Forum.* (1979) 30:282–3.
58. Elster EA, Xu H, Tadaki DK, Montgomery S, Burkly LC, Berning JD, et al. Treatment with the humanized CD154-specific monoclonal antibody, hu5C8, prevents acute rejection of primary skin allografts in nonhuman primates. *Transplantation.* (2001) 72:1473–8. doi: 10.1097/00007890-200111150-00001
59. Sanchez-Fueyo A, Strom TB. Immunologic basis of graft rejection and tolerance following transplantation of liver or other solid organs. *Gastroenterology.* (2011) 140:51–64. doi: 10.1053/j.gastro.2010.10.059
60. Feng S, Ekong UD, Lobritto SJ, Demetris AJ, Roberts JP, Rosenthal P, et al. Complete immunosuppression withdrawal and subsequent allograft function among pediatric recipients of parental living donor liver transplants. *JAMA.* (2012) 307:283–93. doi: 10.1001/jama.2011.2014
61. Mazariegos GV, Reyes J, Marino IR, Demetris AJ, Flynn B, Irish W, et al. Weaning of immunosuppression in liver transplant recipients. *Transplantation.* (1997) 63:243–9. doi: 10.1097/00007890-199701270-00012
62. Orlando G, Soker S, Wood K. Operational tolerance after liver transplantation. *J Hepatol.* (2009) 50:1247–57. doi: 10.1016/j.jhep.2009.03.006
63. Taner T. Liver transplantation: rejection and tolerance. *Liver Transpl.* (2017) 23:S85–S8. doi: 10.1002/lt.24840
64. Taner T, Heimbach JK, Rosen CB, Nyberg SL, Park WD, Stegall MD. Decreased chronic cellular and antibody-mediated injury in the kidney following simultaneous liver-kidney transplantation. *Kidney Int.* (2016) 89:909–17. doi: 10.1016/j.kint.2015.10.016
65. Rasmussen A, Davies HF, Jamieson NV, Evans DB, Calne RY. Combined transplantation of liver and kidney from the same donor protects the kidney from rejection and improves kidney graft survival. *Transplantation.* (1995) 59:919–21. doi: 10.1097/00007890-199503000-00025
66. Topilsky Y, Raichlin E, Hasin T, Boilson BA, Schirger JA, Pereira NL, et al. Combined heart and liver transplant attenuates cardiac allograft vasculopathy compared with isolated heart transplantation. *Transplantation.* (2013) 95:859–65. doi: 10.1097/TP.0b013e31827eef7e
67. Wong TW, Gandhi MJ, Daly RC, Kushwaha SS, Pereira NL, Rosen CB, et al. Liver allograft provides immunoprotection for the cardiac allograft in combined heart-liver transplantation. *Am J Transplant.* (2016) 16:3522–31. doi: 10.1111/ajt.13870
68. Yokota S, Yoshida O, Ono Y, Geller DA, Thomson AW. Liver transplantation in the mouse: insights into liver immunobiology, tissue injury, and allograft tolerance. *Liver Transpl.* (2016) 22:536–46. doi: 10.1002/lt.24394
69. Demetris AJ, Lunz JG 3rd, Randhawa P, Wu T, Nalesnik M, Thomson AW. Monitoring of human liver and kidney allograft tolerance: a tissue/histopathology perspective. *Transpl Int.* (2009) 22:120–41. doi: 10.1111/j.1432-2277.2008.00765.x
70. Steptoe RJ, Patel RK, Subbotin VM, Thomson AW. Comparative analysis of dendritic cell density and total number in commonly transplanted organs: morphometric estimation in normal mice. *Transpl Immunol.* (2000) 8:49–56. doi: 10.1016/S0966-3274(00)00010-1
71. Oh NA, O'Shea T, Ndishabandi DK, Yuan Q, Hong S, Gans J, et al. Plasmacytoid dendritic cell-driven induction of treg is strain specific and correlates with spontaneous acceptance of kidney allografts. *Transplantation.* (2020) 104:39–53. doi: 10.1097/TP.0000000000002867
72. Morris H, DeWolf S, Robins H, Sprangers B, LoCascio SA, Shonts BA, et al. Tracking donor-reactive T cells: evidence for clonal deletion in tolerant kidney transplant patients. *Sci Transl Med.* (2015) 7:272ra10. doi: 10.1126/scitranslmed.3010760
73. Savage TM, Shonts BA, Lau S, Obradovic A, Robins H, Shaked A, et al. Deletion of donor-reactive T cell clones after human liver transplant. *Am J Transplant.* (2020) 20:538–45. doi: 10.1111/ajt.15592
74. Kobayashi E, Kamada N, Delriviere L, Lord R, Goto S, Walker NI, et al. Migration of donor cells into the thymus is not essential for induction and maintenance of systemic tolerance after liver transplantation in the rat. *Immunology.* (1995) 84:333–6.
75. Bishop GA, Sun J, DeCruz DJ, Rokahr KL, Sedgwick JD, Sheil AG, et al. Tolerance to rat liver allografts. III. Donor cell migration and tolerance-associated cytokine production in peripheral lymphoid tissues. *J Immunol.* (1996) 156:4925–31.
76. Dai H, Thomson AW, Rogers NM. Dendritic cells as sensors, mediators, and regulators of ischemic injury. *Front Immunol.* (2019) 10:2418. doi: 10.3389/fimmu.2019.02418
77. Dresske B, Lin X, Huang DS, Zhou X, Fandrich F. Spontaneous tolerance: experience with the rat liver transplant model. *Hum Immunol.* (2002) 63:853–61. doi: 10.1016/S0198-8859(02)00448-2
78. Sun J, Sheil AG, Wang C, Wang L, Rokahr K, Sharland A, et al. Tolerance to rat liver allografts: IV. Acceptance depends on the quantity of donor tissue and on donor leukocytes. *Transplantation.* (1996) 62:1725–30. doi: 10.1097/00007890-199612270-00005
79. Tay SS, Lu B, Sierro F, Benseler V, McGuffog CM, Bishop GA, et al. Differential migration of passenger leukocytes and rapid deletion of naive alloreactive CD8 T cells after mouse liver transplantation. *Liver Transpl.* (2013) 19:1224–35. doi: 10.1002/lt.23720
80. Sharland A, Shastry S, Wang C, Rokahr K, Sun J, Sheil AG, et al. Kinetics of intragraft cytokine expression, cellular infiltration, and cell death in rejection of renal allografts compared with acceptance of liver allografts in a rat model: early activation and apoptosis is associated with liver graft acceptance. *Transplantation.* (1998) 65:1370–7. doi: 10.1097/00007890-199805270-00015
81. Kamada N, Shinomiya T. Clonal deletion as the mechanism of abrogation of immunological memory following liver grafting in rats. *Immunology.* (1985) 55:85–90.
82. Kamada N, Teramoto K, Baguerizo A, Ishikawa M, Sumimoto R, Ohkouchi Y. Cellular basis of transplantation tolerance induced by liver grafting in the rat. Extent of clonal deletion among thoracic duct lymphocytes, spleen, and lymph node cells. *Transplantation.* (1988) 46:165–7. doi: 10.1097/00007890-198807000-00034
83. Dahmen U, Qian S, Rao AS, Demetris AJ, Fu F, Sun H, et al. Split tolerance

induced by orthotopic liver transplantation in mice. *Transplantation.* (1994) 58:1–8. doi: 10.1097/00007890-199407000-00001
84. Bishop GA, Wang C, Sharland AF, McCaughan G. Spontaneous acceptance of liver transplants in rodents: evidence that liver leucocytes induce recipient T-cell death by neglect. *Immunol Cell Biol.* (2002) 80:93–100. doi: 10.1046/j.1440-1711.2002.01049.x
85. Sun J, McCaughan GW, Gallagher ND, Sheil AG, Bishop GA. Deletion of spontaneous rat liver allograft acceptance by donor irradiation. *Transplantation.* (1995) 60:233–6. doi: 10.1097/00007890-199508000-00004
86. Kreisel D, Petrowsky H, Krasinskas AM, Krupnick AS, Szeto WY, McLean AD, et al. The role of passenger leukocyte genotype in rejection and acceptance of rat liver allografts. *Transplantation.* (2002) 73:1501–7. doi: 10.1097/00007890-200205150-00022
87. Mele TS, Kneteman NM, Zhu LF, Ramassar V, Urmson J, Halloran B, et al. IFN-γ is an absolute requirement for spontaneous acceptance of liver allografts. *Am J Transplant.* (2003) 3:942–51. doi: 10.1034/j.1600-6143.2003.00153.x
88. Morita M, Joyce D, Miller C, Fung JJ, Lu L, Qian S. Rejection triggers liver transplant tolerance: involvement of mesenchyme-mediated immune control mechanisms in mice. *Hepatology.* (2015) 62:915–31. doi: 10.1002/hep.27909
89. Morita M, Fujino M, Jiang G, Kitazawa Y, Xie L, Azuma M, et al. PD-1/B7-H1 interaction contribute to the spontaneous acceptance of mouse liver allograft. *Am J Transplant.* (2010) 10:40–6. doi: 10.1111/j.1600-6143.2009.02859.x
90. Li W, Zheng XX, Kuhr CS, Perkins JD. CTLA4 engagement is required for induction of murine liver transplant spontaneous tolerance. *Am J Transplant.* (2005) 5:978–86. doi: 10.1111/j.1600-6143.2005.00823.x
91. Ye Y, Yan S, Jiang G, Zhou L, Xie H, Xie X, et al. Galectin-1 prolongs survival of mouse liver allografts from Flt3L-pretreated donors. *Am J Transplant.* (2013) 13:569–79. doi: 10.1111/ajt.12088
92. Jiang ZJ, Shen QH, Chen HY, Yang Z, Shuai MQ, Zheng S. Galectin-1 restores immune tolerance to liver transplantation through activation of hepatic stellate cells. *Cell Physiol Biochem.* (2018) 48:863–79. doi: 10.1159/000491955
93. Li W, Kuhr CS, Zheng XX, Carper K, Thomson AW, Reyes JD, et al. New insights into mechanisms of spontaneous liver transplant tolerance: the role of Foxp3-expressing $CD25^+CD4^+$ regulatory T cells. *Am J Transplant.* (2008) 8:1639–51. doi: 10.1111/j.1600-6143.2008.02300.x
94. Jiang X, Morita M, Sugioka A, Harada M, Kojo S, Wakao H, et al. The importance of $CD25^+$ $CD4^+$ regulatory T cells in mouse hepatic allograft tolerance. *Liver Transpl.* (2006) 12:1112–8. doi: 10.1002/lt.20787
95. Demirkiran A, Bosma BM, Kok A, Baan CC, Metselaar HJ, Ijzermans JN, et al. Allosuppressive donor $CD4^+CD25^+$ regulatory T cells detach from the graft and circulate in recipients after liver transplantation. *J Immunol.* (2007) 178:6066–72. doi: 10.4049/jimmunol.178.10.6066
96. Lu L, Yu Y, Li G, Pu L, Zhang F, Zheng S, et al. $CD8^+CD103^+$ regulatory T cells in spontaneous tolerance of liver allografts. *Int Immunopharmacol.* (2009) 9:546–8. doi: 10.1016/j.intimp.2009.01.021
97. van der Touw W, Bromberg JS. Natural killer cells and the immune response in solid organ transplantation. *Am J Transplant.* (2010) 10:1354–8. doi: 10.1111/j.1600-6143.2010.03086.x
98. Moroso V, Metselaar HJ, Mancham S, Tilanus HW, Eissens D, van der Meer A, et al. Liver grafts contain a unique subset of natural killer cells that are transferred into the recipient after liver transplantation. *Liver Transpl.* (2010) 16:895–908. doi: 10.1002/lt.22080
99. Harmon C, Sanchez-Fueyo A, O'Farrelly C, Houlihan DD. Natural killer cells and liver transplantation: orchestrators of rejection or tolerance? *Am J Transplant.* (2016) 16:751–7. doi: 10.1111/ajt.13565
100. Fahrner R, Dondorf F, Ardelt M, Settmacher U, Rauchfuss F. Role of NK, NKT cells and macrophages in liver transplantation. *World J Gastroenterol.* (2016) 22:6135–44. doi: 10.3748/wjg.v22.i27.6135
101. Martinez-Llordella M, Lozano JJ, Puig-Pey I, Orlando G, Tisone G, Lerut J, et al. Using transcriptional profiling to develop a diagnostic test of operational tolerance in liver transplant recipients. *J Clin Invest.* (2008) 118:2845–57. doi: 10.1172/JCI35342
102. Cerboni C, Zingoni A, Cippitelli M, Piccoli M, Frati L, Santoni A. Antigen-activated human T lymphocytes express cell-surface NKG2D ligands via an ATM/ATR-dependent mechanism and become susceptible to autologous NK- cell lysis. *Blood.* (2007) 110:606–15. doi: 10.1182/blood-2006-10-052720
103. Cooper MA, Fehniger TA, Fuchs A, Colonna M, Caligiuri MA. NK cell and DC interactions. *Trends Immunol.* (2004) 25:47–52. doi: 10.1016/j.it.2003.10.012
104. de Mare-Bredemeijer EL, Shi XL, Mancham S, van Gent R, van der Heide-Mulder M, de Boer R, et al. Cytomegalovirus-induced expression of CD244 after liver transplantation is associated with $CD8^+$ T cell hyporesponsiveness to alloantigen. *J Immunol.* (2015) 195:1838–48. doi: 10.4049/jimmunol.1500440
105. Obara H, Nagasaki K, Hsieh CL, Ogura Y, Esquivel CO, Martinez OM, et al. IFN-γ, produced by NK cells that infiltrate liver allografts early after transplantation, links the innate and adaptive immune responses. *Am J Transplant.* (2005) 5:2094–103. doi: 10.1111/j.1600-6143.2005.00995.x
106. Ono Y, Perez-Gutierrez A, Nakao T, Dai H, Camirand G, Yoshida O, et al. Graft-infiltrating PD-L1(hi) cross-dressed dendritic cells regulate antidonor T cell responses in mouse liver transplant tolerance. *Hepatology.* (2018) 67:1499–515. doi: 10.1002/hep.29529
107. Yoshida O, Kimura S, Dou L, Matta BM, Yokota S, Ross MA, et al. DAP12 deficiency in liver allografts results in enhanced donor DC migration, augmented effector T cell responses and abrogation of transplant tolerance. *Am J Transplant.* (2014) 14:1791–805. doi: 10.1111/ajt.12757
108. Nakao T, Ono Y, Dai H, Nakano R, Perez-Gutierrez A, Camirand G, et al. DNAX activating protein of 12 kDa/triggering receptor expressed on myeloid cells 2 expression by mouse and human liver dendritic cells: functional implications and regulation of liver ischemia-reperfusion injury. *Hepatology.* (2019) 70:696–710. doi: 10.1002/hep.30334
109. Farges O, Morris PJ, Dallman MJ. Spontaneous acceptance of rat liver allografts is associated with an early downregulation of intragraft interleukin-4 messenger RNA expression. *Hepatology.* (1995) 21:767–75. doi: 10.1002/hep.1840210326
110. Wang C, Li J, Cordoba SP, McLeod DJ, Tran GT, Hodgkinson SJ, et al. Posttransplant interleukin-4 treatment converts rat liver allograft tolerance to rejection. *Transplantation.* (2005) 79:1116–20. doi: 10.1097/01.TP.0000161249.20922.16
111. Morita M, Chen J, Fujino M, Kitazawa Y, Sugioka A, Zhong L, et al. Identification of microRNAs involved in acute rejection and spontaneous tolerance in murine hepatic allografts. *Sci Rep.* (2014) 4:6649. doi: 10.1038/srep06649
112. Xie L, Ichimaru N, Morita M, Chen J, Zhu P, Wang J, et al. Identification of a novel biomarker gene set with sensitivity and specificity for distinguishing between allograft rejection and tolerance. *Liver Transpl.* (2012) 18:444–54. doi: 10.1002/lt.22480
113. Vionnet J, Sanchez-Fueyo A. Biomarkers of immune tolerance in liver transplantation. *Hum Immunol.* (2018) 79:388–94. doi: 10.1016/j.humimm.2018.02.010
114. Goldschmidt I, Karch A, Mikolajczyk R, Mutschler F, Junge N, Pfister ED, et al. Immune monitoring after pediatric liver transplantation - the prospective ChilSFree cohort study. *BMC Gastroenterol.* (2018) 18:63. doi: 10.1186/s12876-018-0795-x
115. Taubert R, Danger R, Londono MC, Christakoudi S, Martinez-Picola M, Rimola A, et al. Hepatic infiltrates in operational tolerant patients after liver transplantation show enrichment of regulatory T cells before proinflammatory genes are downregulated. *Am J Transplant.* (2016) 16:1285–93. doi: 10.1111/ajt.13617
116. Pons JA, Revilla-Nuin B, Baroja-Mazo A, Ramirez P, Martinez-Alarcon L, Sanchez-Bueno F, et al. FoxP3 in peripheral blood is associated with operational tolerance in liver transplant patients during immunosuppression withdrawal. *Transplantation.* (2008) 86:1370–8. doi: 10.1097/TP.0b013e318188d3e6
117. Baroja-Mazo A, Revilla-Nuin B, de Bejar A, Martinez-Alarcon L, Herrero JI, El-Tayeb A, et al. Extracellular adenosine reversibly inhibits the activation of human regulatory T cells and negatively influences the achievement of the operational tolerance in liver transplantation. *Am J Transplant.* (2019) 19:48–61. doi: 10.1111/ajt.15023
118. Lau AH, Vitalone MJ, Haas K, Shawler T, Esquivel CO, Berquist WE, et al. Mass cytometry reveals a distinct immunoprofile of operational tolerance in pediatric liver transplantation. *Pediatr Transplant.* (2016) 20:1072–80. doi: 10.1111/petr.12795
119. Li Y, Koshiba T, Yoshizawa A, Yonekawa Y, Masuda K, Ito A, et al. Analyses of peripheral blood mononuclear cells in operational tolerance after pediatric living donor liver transplantation. *Am J Transplant.* (2004) 4:2118–25. doi: 10.1111/j.1600-6143.2004.00611.x
120. Jhun J, Lee SH, Lee SK, Kim HY, Jung ES, Kim DG, et al. Serial monitoring of immune markers being represented regulatory

T cell/T helper 17 cell ratio: indicating tolerance for tapering immunosuppression after liver transplantation. *Front Immunol.* (2018) 9:352. doi: 10.3389/fimmu.2018.00352

121. Martinez-Llordella M, Puig-Pey I, Orlando G, Ramoni M, Tisone G, Rimola A, et al. Multiparameter immune profiling of operational tolerance in liver transplantation. *Am J Transplant.* (2007) 7:309–19. doi: 10.1111/j.1600-6143.2006.01621.x
122. Wang XQ, Lo CM, Chen L, Cheung CK, Yang ZF, Chen YX, et al. Hematopoietic chimerism in liver transplantation patients and hematopoietic stem/progenitor cells in adult human liver. *Hepatology.* (2012) 56:1557–66. doi: 10.1002/hep.25820
123. Mazariegos GV, Zahorchak AF, Reyes J, Chapman H, Zeevi A, Thomson AW. Dendritic cell subset ratio in tolerant, weaning and non-tolerant liver recipients is not affected by extent of immunosuppression. *Am J Transplant.* (2005) 5:314–22. doi: 10.1111/j.1600-6143.2004.00672.x
124. Tokita D, Mazariegos GV, Zahorchak AF, Chien N, Abe M, Raimondi G, et al. High PD-L1/CD86 ratio on plasmacytoid dendritic cells correlates with elevated T-regulatory cells in liver transplant tolerance. *Transplantation.* (2008) 85:369 77. doi: 10.1097/TP.0b013e3181612ded
125. Perez-Sanz F, Revilla-Nuin B, Martinez-Alarcon L, Herrero JI, Ramirez P, Pons JA, et al. Tolerance biomarkers in liver transplantation: independent external validation of the predictive strength of SENP6 and FEM1C gene expression. *Transplantation.* (2019) 103:1887–92. doi: 10.1097/TP.0000000000002587
126. Li L, Wozniak LJ, Rodder S, Heish S, Talisetti A, Wang Q, et al. A common peripheral blood gene set for diagnosis of operational tolerance in pediatric and adult liver transplantation. *Am J Transplant.* (2012) 12:1218–28. doi: 10.1111/j.1600-6143.2011.03928.x
127. Bohne F, Martinez-Llordella M, Lozano JJ, Miquel R, Benitez C, Londono MC, et al. Intra-graft expression of genes involved in iron homeostasis predicts the development of operational tolerance in human liver transplantation. *J Clin Invest.* (2012) 122:368–82. doi: 10.1172/JCI59411
128. Bohne F, Londono MC, Benitez C, Miquel R, Martinez-Llordella M, Russo C, et al. HCV-induced immune responses influence the development of operational tolerance after liver transplantation in humans. *Sci Transl Med.* (2014) 6:242ra81. doi: 10.1126/scitranslmed.3008793
129. Girelli D, Pasino M, Goodnough JB, Nemeth E, Guido M, Castagna A, et al. Reduced serum hepcidin levels in patients with chronic hepatitis C. *J Hepatol.* (2009) 51:845–52. doi: 10.1016/j.jhep.2009.06.027
130. Bonaccorsi-Riani E, Pennycuick A, Londono MC, Lozano JJ, Benitez C, Sawitzki B, et al. Molecular characterization of acute cellular rejection occurring during intentional immunosuppression withdrawal in liver transplantation. *Am J Transplant.* (2016) 16:484–96. doi: 10.1111/ajt.13488
131. MacParland SA, Liu JC, Ma XZ, Innes BT, Bartczak AM, Gage BK, et al. Single cell RNA sequencing of human liver reveals distinct intrahepatic macrophage populations. *Nat Commun.* (2018) 9:4383. doi: 10.1038/s41467-018-06318-7
132. Feng S, Bucuvalas J. Tolerance after liver transplantation: where are we? *Liver Transpl.* (2017) 23:1601–14. doi: 10.1002/lt.24845
133. Kawai T, Leventhal J, Wood K, Strober S. Summary of the third international workshop on clinical tolerance. *Am J Transplant.* (2019) 19:324–30. doi: 10.1111/ajt.15086
134. Benitez C, Londono MC, Miquel R, Manzia TM, Abraldes JG, Lozano JJ, et al. Prospective multicenter clinical trial of immunosuppressive drug withdrawal in stable adult liver transplant recipients. *Hepatology.* (2013) 58:1824–35. doi: 10.1002/hep.26426
135. Mastoridis S, Martinez-Llordella M, Sanchez-Fueyo A. Immunotolerance in liver transplantation. *Semin Liver Dis.* (2017) 37:95–108. doi: 10.1055/s-0037-1602762
136. Sanchez-Fueyo A. Tolerance profiles and immunosuppression. *Liver Transpl.* (2013) 19 Suppl 2:S44–8. doi: 10.1002/lt.23749
137. Levitsky J, Feng S. Tolerance in clinical liver transplantation. *Hum Immunol.* (2018) 79:283–7. doi: 10.1016/j.humimm.2017.10.007
138. de la Garza RG, Sarobe P, Merino J, Lasarte JJ, D'Avola D, Belsue V, et al. Trial of complete weaning from immunosuppression for liver transplant recipients: factors predictive of tolerance. *Liver Transpl.* (2013) 19:937–44. doi: 10.1002/lt.23686
139. Talisetti A, Hurwitz M, Sarwal M, Berquist W, Castillo R, Bass D, et al. Analysis of clinical variables associated with tolerance in pediatric liver transplant recipients. *Pediatr Transplant.* (2010) 14:976–9. doi: 10.1111/j.1399-3046.2010.01360.x
140. Murphy MS, Harrison R, Davies P, Buckels JA, Mayer AD, Hubscher S, et al. Risk factors for liver rejection: evidence to suggest enhanced allograft tolerance in infancy. *Arch Dis Child.* (1996) 75:502–6. doi: 10.1136/adc.75.6.502
141. Demetris AJ, Isse K. Tissue biopsy monitoring of operational tolerance in liver allograft recipients. *Curr Opin Organ Transplant.* (2013) 18:345–53. doi: 10.1097/MOT.0b013e3283615d48
142. Donckier V, Craciun L, Miqueu P, Troisi RI, Lucidi V, Rogiers X, et al. Expansion of memory-type $CD8^+$ T cells correlates with the failure of early immunosuppression withdrawal after cadaver liver transplantation using high-dose ATG induction and rapamycin. *Transplantation.* (2013) 96:306–15. doi: 10.1097/TP.0b013e3182985414
143. Devlin J, Doherty D, Thomson L, Wong T, Donaldson P, Portmann B, et al. Defining the outcome of immunosuppression withdrawal after liver transplantation. *Hepatology.* (1998) 27:926–33. doi: 10.1002/hep.510270406
144. Tang Q, Vincenti F. Transplant trials with Tregs: perils and promises. *J Clin Invest.* (2017) 127:2505–12. doi: 10.1172/JCI90598
145. Wood KJ, Bushell A, Hester J. Regulatory immune cells in transplantation. *Nat Rev Immunol.* (2012) 12:417–30. doi: 10.1038/nri3227
146. Thomson AW, Ezzelarab MB. Regulatory dendritic cells: profiling, targeting, and therapeutic application. *Curr Opin Organ Transplant.* (2018) 23:538–45. doi: 10.1097/MOT.0000000000000565
147. Whitehouse GP, Hope A, Sanchez-Fueyo A. Regulatory T-cell therapy in liver transplantation. *Transpl Int.* (2017) 30:776–84. doi: 10.1111/tri.12998
148. Kholodenko IV, Kholodenko RV, Lupatov AY, Yarygin KN. Cell therapy as a tool for induction of immunological tolerance after liver transplantation. *Bull Exp Biol Med.* (2018) 165:554–63. doi: 10.1007/s10517-018-4213-8
149. Popp FC, Fillenberg B, Eggenhofer E, Renner P, Dillmann J, Benseler V, et al. Safety and feasibility of third-party multipotent adult progenitor cells for immunomodulation therapy after liver transplantation–a phase I study (MISOT-I). *J Transl Med.* (2011) 9:124. doi: 10.1186/1479-5876-9-124
150. Detry O, Vandermeulen M, Delbouille MH, Somja J, Bletard N, Briquet A, et al. Infusion of mesenchymal stromal cells after deceased liver transplantation: a phase I-II, open-label, clinical study. *J Hepatol.* (2017) 67:47–55. doi: 10.1016/j.jhep.2017.03.001
151. Zhang YC, Liu W, Fu BS, Wang GY, Li HB, Yi HM, et al. Therapeutic potentials of umbilical cord-derived mesenchymal stromal cells for ischemic-type biliary lesions following liver transplantation. *Cytotherapy.* (2017) 19:194–9. doi: 10.1016/j.jcyt.2016.11.005
152. Soeder Y, Loss M, Johnson CL, Hutchinson JA, Haarer J, Ahrens N, et al. First-in-human case study: multipotent adult progenitor cells for immunomodulation after liver transplantation. *Stem Cells Transl Med.* (2015) 4:899–904. doi: 10.5966/sctm.2015-0002
153. Hartleif S, Schumm M, Doring M, Mezger M, Lang P, Dahlke MH, et al. Safety and tolerance of donor-derived mesenchymal stem cells in pediatric living-donor liver transplantation: the MYSTEP1 study. *Stem Cells Int.* (2017) 2017:2352954. doi: 10.1155/2017/2352954
154. Shi M, Liu Z, Wang Y, Xu R, Sun Y, Zhang M, et al. A pilot study of mesenchymal stem cell therapy for acute liver allograft rejection. *Stem Cells Transl Med.* (2017) 6:2053–61. doi: 10.1002/sctm.17-0134
155. Todo S, Yamashita K, Goto R, Zaitsu M, Nagatsu A, Oura T, et al. A pilot study of operational tolerance with a regulatory T-cell-based cell therapy in living donor liver transplantation. *Hepatology.* (2016) 64:632–43. doi: 10.1002/hep.28459
156. Sanchez-Fueyo A, Whitehouse G, Grageda N, Cramp ME, Lim TY, Romano M, et al. Applicability, safety, and biological activity of regulatory T cell therapy in liver transplantation. *Am J Transplant.* (2020) 20:1125–36. doi: 10.1111/ajt.15700
157. Casiraghi F, Perico N, Remuzzi G. Mesenchymal stromal cells for tolerance induction in organ transplantation. *Hum Immunol.* (2018) 79:304–13. doi: 10.1016/j.humimm.2017.12.008
158. Podesta MA, Remuzzi G, Casiraghi F. Mesenchymal stromal cells for transplant tolerance. *Front Immunol.* (2019) 10:1287. doi: 10.3389/fimmu.2019.01287
159. Wagner DL, Amini L, Wendering DJ, Burkhardt LM, Akyuz L, Reinke P, et al. High prevalence of *Streptococcus pyogenes* Cas9-reactive T cells within the adult human population. *Nat Med.* (2019) 25:242–8. doi: 10.1038/s41591-018-0204-6
160. MacDonald KG, Hoeppli RE, Huang Q, Gillies J, Luciani DS, Orban PC, et al. Alloantigen-specific regulatory T cells generated with a chimeric antigen

receptor. *J Clin Invest.* (2016) 126:1413–24. doi: 10.1172/JCI82771

161. Thomson AW. A view of the future of regulatory immune cell therapy in organ transplantation. *Curr Opin Organ Transplant.* (2018) 23:507–8. doi: 10.1097/MOT.0000000000000570
162. Thomson AW, Humar A, Lakkis FG, Metes DM. Regulatory dendritic cells for promotion of liver transplant operational tolerance: rationale for a clinical trial and accompanying mechanistic studies. *Hum Immunol.* (2018) 79:314–21. doi: 10.1016/j.humimm.2017.10.017
163. Thomson AW, Zahorchak AF, Ezzelarab MB, Butterfield LH, Lakkis FG, Metes DM. Prospective clinical testing of regulatory dendritic cells in organ transplantation. *Front Immunol.* (2016) 7:15. doi: 10.3389/fimmu.2016.00015
164. Figueiredo C, Oldhafer F, Wittauer EM, Carvalho-Oliveira M, Akhdar A, Beetz O, et al. Silencing of HLA class I on primary human hepatocytes as a novel strategy for reduction in alloreactivity. *J Cell Mol Med.* (2019) 23:5705–14. doi: 10.1111/jcmm.14484
165. Le Guen V, Judor JP, Boeffard F, Gauttier V, Ferry N, Soulillou JP, et al. Alloantigen gene transfer to hepatocytes promotes tolerance to pancreatic islet graft by inducing $CD8^{+}$ regulatory T cells. *J Hepatol.* (2017) 66:765–77. doi: 10.1016/j.jhep.2016.11.019

14

Strategies for Deliberate Induction of Immune Tolerance in Liver Transplantation: From Preclinical Models to Clinical Application

Naoki Tanimine [1], Masahiro Ohira [1,2], Hiroyuki Tahara [1], Kentaro Ide [1], Yuka Tanaka [1], Takashi Onoe [1,3] and Hideki Ohdan [1]*

[1] Department of Gastroenterological and Transplant Surgery, Graduate School of Biomedical and Health Sciences, Hiroshima University, Hiroshima, Japan, [2] Medical Center for Translational and Clinical Research Hiroshima University Hospital, Hiroshima, Japan, [3] Kure Medical Center and Chugoku Cancer Center, National Hospital Organization, Kure, Japan

***Correspondence:**
Hideki Ohdan
hohdan@hiroshima-u.ac.jp

The liver exhibits intrinsic immune regulatory properties that maintain tolerance to endogenous and exogenous antigens, and provide protection against pathogens. Such an immune privilege contributes to susceptibility to spontaneous acceptance despite major histocompatibility complex mismatch when transplanted in animal models. Furthermore, the presence of a liver allograft can suppress the rejection of other solid tissue/organ grafts from the same donor. Despite this immune privilege of the livers, to control the undesired alloimmune responses in humans, most liver transplant recipients require long-term treatment with immune-suppressive drugs that predispose to cardiometabolic side effects and renal insufficiency. Understanding the mechanism of liver transplant tolerance and crosstalk between a variety of hepatic immune cells, such as dendritic cells, Kupffer cells, liver sinusoidas endothelial cells, hepatic stellate cells and so on, and alloreactive T cells would lead to the development of strategies for deliberate induction of more specific immune tolerance in a clinical setting. In this review article, we focus on results derived from basic studies that have attempted to elucidate the immune modulatory mechanisms of liver constituent cells and clinical trials that induced immune tolerance after liver transplantation by utilizing the immune-privilege potential of the liver.

Keywords: tolerance, liver, transplantation, immunosuppression, immunomonitoring

INTRODUCTION

Liver transplantation is currently a highly successful treatment for end-stage liver disease. It is well-known that liver allografts are tolerogenic, and stable grafts can be maintained across major histocompatibility complex (MHC) barriers without immunosuppression (IS) in some species (1–3). Furthermore, the presence of a liver allograft can suppress the rejection of other solid tissue grafts (e.g., heart and skin) from the same donor; hence, the liver favors introduction of immune tolerance rather than immunity (2, 4). Such a capacity of the transplanted liver to establish tolerance in an allogeneic host has been ascribed to the unique features and anatomical structure of hepatic constituent cells. In a clinical setting, however, the majority of liver transplant (LT) recipients require long-term immunosuppressive drug treatment to control the alloimmune responses. The undesired adverse effects of life-long IS remain a concern, that is, an increased risk of chronic kidney disease, metabolic disorders, infection and malignancy in LT recipients.

Safely minimizing or discontinuing IS without compromising liver allograft can be an attractive strategy to improve long-term survival after liver transplantation. For this purpose, significant efforts have been made to identify sensitive and specific biomarkers of immune tolerance in LT recipients or to establish reliable immune monitoring methods. Understanding the mechanism of the inherently tolerogenic nature of the liver would lead to the development of strategies for deliberate induction of more specific immune tolerance in clinical liver transplantation. Immune regulation in the liver is mainly controlled by a variety of antigen presenting cells (APCs), which spatiotemporally react with alloreactive T cells in LT recipients. In addition to professional APCs, such as dendritic cells (DCs), unique populations of non-professional APCs consisting of Kupffer cells, liver sinusoidal endothelial cells (LSECs), and hepatic stellate cells (HSCs) that express low levels of MHC class I/II and co-stimulatory molecules are resident in a steady-state liver. These cells are likely involved in fine-tuning the modulation of local and systemic tolerance and/or immunity after liver transplantation. In this review article, we focus on studies that attempted to elucidate the immune modulatory mechanisms of these APCs, and clinical trials that induced immune tolerance after liver transplantation by enjoying the immune-privilege potential of the liver.

ROLE OF APCs IN IMMUNE TOLERANCE IN LIVER TRANSPLANTATION

Dendritic Cells

In mice, liver, but not other organ allografts, are accepted permanently and with donor specificity between many strain combinations, without the requirement for IS (3). It has been demonstrated that donor-derived DC precursors of liver allografts can be propagated in granulocyte macrophage colony-stimulating factor (GMC-SF) from the bone marrow (BM) or spleen of unmodified LT recipients in mouse model, suggesting that bidirectional leukocyte migration and donor cell chimerism contribute to liver graft acceptance and acquired transplantation tolerance (5). A recent study supported the assumption that DCs contribute to tolerance by demonstrating that recipients of DC-depleted liver allograft showed acute rejection while those receiving non-manipulated liver allograft showed indefinite acceptance in a transgenic mouse model (6).

It has been previously shown that Flt3 ligand administration, which increases interstitial DCs and their interleukin (IL)-12 production, abrogated the acceptance of transplanted liver, and IL-12 neutralization markedly prolonged graft survival in mice receiving the Flt3 ligand (7, 8). In addition, it has been reported that the transmembrane adaptor protein, DNAX-activating protein of 12 kDa (DAP12), negatively regulates liver myeloid DC maturation and stimulation ability, and *DAP12*$^{-/-}$ livers are rejected in relation to increased pro-inflammatory cytokines including IL-12p40 (9). These results suggest that DAP12 expression by liver DCs may be critical for the induction of tolerance. Hence, donor-derived DCs assuredly contribute to tolerance status; however, it likely depends on the DC subset and inflammatory status after transplantation. Recently, it has been reported that DCs contribute to tolerance in another mechanism in context of regulatory T cells (Tregs) IS, i.e., antigen (Ag)-specific Tregs that are formed strong interactions with DCs, result in the removal of the Ag and MHC class II complex from DC surface and reducing DC's Ag-presenting capacity (10). This might be one mechanism of tolerance induction by DCs. Based on such knowledge obtained in the preclinical models, clinical trial for operational tolerance using regulatory DCs has been conducted (11). As a result, it has been shown that infusion of donor-derived, *ex-vivo* generated regulatory DCs can achieve operational tolerance in patients after liver transplantation, encouraging tolerance induction strategy with regulatory DCs in the future.

Liver Sinusoidal Endothelial Cells

The sinusoids correspond to the capillaries of the liver, and have a more complex structure than ordinary capillaries. The diameter of the sinusoids is 5–7 μm, which is narrow enough to allow circulating lymphocytes to contact LSECs closely with effective immune interaction. In fact, LSECs constitutively express the molecules necessary for Ag presentation (CD80, CD86, CD40, and MHC classes I and II), and have the capacity for Ag presentation, which is not observed in endothelial cells of other organs (12). Furthermore, LSECs express Fas-ligand and programmed death-ligand (PD-L) 1, which has been recently attracted due to Nobel-prize winning checkpoint inhibitor studies (13–15). These molecules on LSECs induce apoptosis of reactive T cells, and suppress allo-reactive and Ag-specific T cells in a mouse model (12, 16–18). LSECs can also endocytose foreign Ag and suppress cognate T cells in allogeneic, exogenous, and cancer Ag models (16, 19, 20). The immunological suppressive capacity of LSECs was reported in an *in vitro* model (12, 21) as well as *in vivo* models (22). In these studies, chimeric livers, produced by adoptive transfer of allogeneic LSECs, induced suppression of allo-specific T cells *in vivo*; however, the suppressive effect of LSECs was attenuated by anti-PD-L1 antibody (Ab) during engraftment of allogeneic LSECs. Another study using a similar model, proved that LSECs have the ability to induce tolerance of carbohydrate reactive B cells through the PD-L1 pathway by demonstrating that chimeric α1,3-galactosyltransferase gene knockout (GalT) mice in which Gal-deficient LSECs were replaced with wild-type LSECs by adoptive transfer, lost the ability to produce anti-Gal Abs even after repeated immunization (23). This result suggests that LSECs also contribute to establishment of spontaneous tolerization of B cells in ABO-blood type incompatible liver transplantation. In a mouse orthotopic liver transplantation model, it has been reported that PD-L1 mediates the immune regulatory function of graft non-hematopoietic non-parenchymal cells including LSECs (24, 25). In this model, liver allografts from chimeric mice with *PD-L1*$^{+/+}$ hematopoietic cells and *PD-L1*$^{-/-}$ non-hematopoietic cells were rejected, whereas those from wild-type mice with *PD-L1*$^{+/+}$ hematopoietic cells and *PD-L1*$^{+/+}$ non-hematopoietic

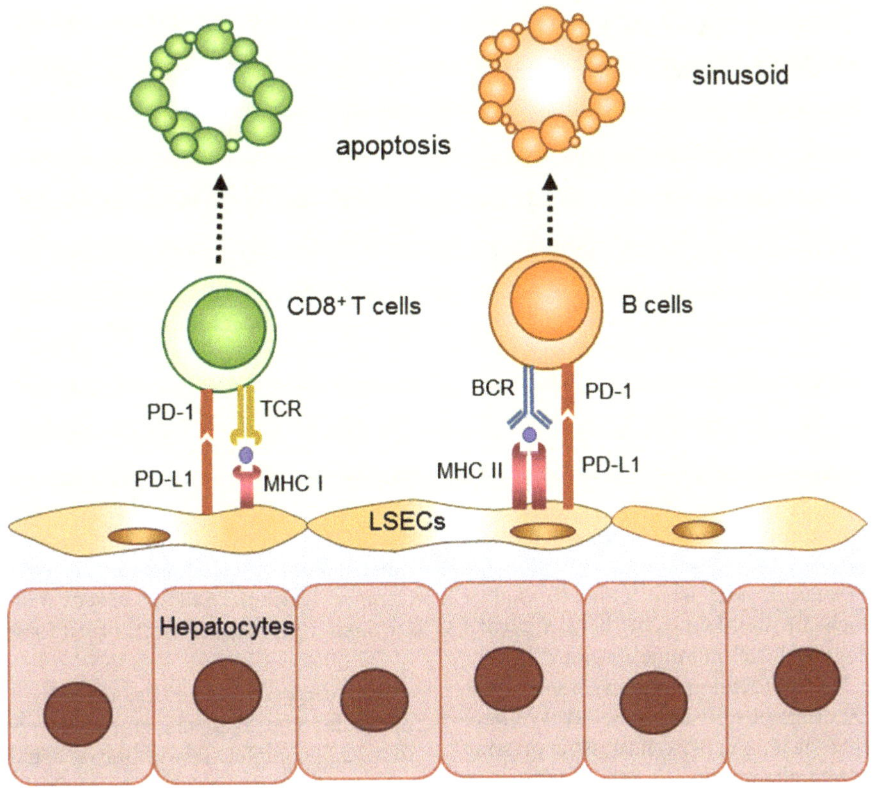

FIGURE 1 | Mechanism implicated in regulating anti-donor immune cells by LSECs in grafted liver. LSECs constitutively express classes I and II and have the capacity for Ag presentation. LSECs contribute to the establishment of immunological tolerance in grafted liver by promoting apoptosis of donor-MHC reactive T and B cells through Ag-presentation and PD-1/PD-L1 signaling.

cells were accepted *in vivo*, suggesting that *PD-L1*$^{+/+}$ non-hematopoietic cells, such as LSECs or stellate cells, likely contribute to the tolerogenicity of the liver via the PD-L1/PD-1 axis. In summary, these results suggest that LSECs contribute to the establishment of immunological tolerance in grafted liver by promoting apoptosis of donor-MHC reactive T and B cells through Ag-presentation and PD-1/PD-L1 signaling (**Figure 1**).

Notably, both in a mouse model and clinical living related liver transplantation, we have recently reported that portal hypertension enhances alloimmune responses, likely due to the impaired immune-suppression capacity of LSECs (26). In these studies, we demonstrated that expression of molecules necessary for Ag presentation and PD-L1, and the suppressive capacities of LSECs were decreased in portal hypertension. These results also strongly imply that LSECs contribute to the establishment of tolerance status after liver transplantation and importance of control of portal hypertension for achieving tolerance in liver transplantation.

Heptic Stellate Cells (HSCs)

HSCs are pericytes found in the Disse space, which is a space between the sinusoid s and hepatocytes. HSCs are classified as fibroblasts, and are well-described for their important role for hepatic fibrosis and storage of vitamin A. It has been recently shown that HSCs also function as APCs (27). HSCs express CD1d, MHC class II, and CD86, which are integral for APC, and present Ag to reactive T cells. It has been reported that mouse and human HSCs express PD-L1, and activated HSCs markedly upregulate PD-L1 expression and induce T cell-hyporesponsiveness *in vitro* (28, 29). This immune-suppressive effect of HSCs is triggered by IFN-γ and regulates the MEK/ERK pathway (30). Furthermore, it has been recently reported that HSCs preferentially induce Foxp3^{+} Tregs by the production of retinoic acid (31). In an *in vivo* model, co-transplantation of HSCs effectively protects islet allograft from rejection through PD-L1 signaling (32). These results suggest that HSCs have immune suppressive features similar to LSECs and play an important role in tolerogenic status in the liver. Of note, HSCs may be related to pericytes or mesenchymal stem/stromal cells *in vivo* due to their genetic proximity and similarities of phenotype and differentiation potency (33–35). These cells have been shown to elicit very elaborate immunoregulatory effects (36–38). In fact, a phase I-II clinical study of infusion of MSC after deceased liver transplantation to achieve operational tolerance has been reported (39). This study also might encourage a clinical application of HSC.

OTHER BASIC MECHANISMS OF IMMUNE TOLERANCE IN LIVER TRANSPLANTATION INVOLVING BREG CELLS AND NKT CELLS

Regulatory B Cells

Recent studies have shown the existence of a distinct subset of B cells with immunomodulatory properties, which have been termed regulatory B cells (Bregs), analogous to Tregs. Bregs have been found to play a pivotal role in regulating immune responses involved in inflammation, autoimmunity, and malignancy (40). Their main mechanism of action is by promoting the development of Tregs while suppressing effector $CD4^+$ and $CD8^+$ T cells, primarily by secreting IL-10, IL-35, and transforming growth factor β (TGFβ), which produce donor-specific antibodies and induce antibody-mediated rejection. However, recent studies have indicated that Bregs, which possess antibody-independent effector functions, have the capacity to control or regulate immune responses to a transplanted organ (41, 42).

As one part of Breg cells, B cells were found to express PD-L1 and PD-L2, which are well-known to have a pivotal role in regulating autologous T cell-immune response in self-immunity by engaging PD-1, providing immune homeostasis and mediating the mechanisms of tolerance (43, 44). We have recently demonstrated that the unique B-1 cell subset expressing PD-L1 and PD-L2 inhibits alloimmune T cell responses in mice (45).

Although the role of Breg cells in immune tolerance in clinical liver transplantation remains to be elucidated, one study revealed that sirolimus could amplify Bregs and Tregs among LT recipients, which might be beneficial in mitigating the immune response (46). The role of Breg cells in liver transplantation is becoming increasingly understood, and tolerization relevant to Breg cells might be expected to be applied clinically.

Natural Killer T Cells

Invariant natural killer T cells (iNKT cells), which express an invariant T cell receptor (TCR) α-chain and recognize lipids present on CD1d, secrete diverse cytokines (such as interferon-γ, IL-4, IL-5, IL-10, and IL-13) and influence many types of immune responses (47). In general, iNKT cells are non-circulating, tissue-resident lymphocytes, but the prevalence of different iNKT cell subsets differs markedly between tissues, that is, the liver, lungs, adipose tissue, and intestine (48). Among these tissues, iNKT cells are most frequent in the liver in both mice and humans.

In organ/tissue transplantation, iNKT cells play a significant immune-regulatory role in the maintenance of transplant tolerance to allografts (49–51). It has been demonstrated that CD40L/CD28 blockade fails to maintain tolerance to allograft in iNKT cell-deficient recipients mice, while peripheral transplant tolerance can be induced in wild-type recipients by that treatment (51). Consistently, it has been shown that liver allografts lacking iNKT cells manifested infiltration, hemorrhage and necrosis with significant reduction of graft survival and much less induction of tolerance compared with wild-type liver allograft in mice (52). Hence, iNKT cells, particularly donor-liver resident iNKT cells, are found to be immune regulatory cells that play a vital role in inducing spontaneous tolerance after allogeneic liver transplantation. In addition, we have also demonstrated that iNKT cells play a significant role in the immunosuppressive effects induced by LSECs on T cells with indirect allospecificity (53).

IMMUNOSUPPRESSION WITHDRAWAL TRIALS

In 1993, Reyes et al. in the Pittsburgh group reported the first series of operational tolerant recipients whose allograft did not show functional deterioration after cessation of immunosuppressants (ISs) due to their mandatory requirements such as severe infection and malignancy (54). Operational tolerance is separately understood from immunological tolerance that is observed as no proof of immunological activity in the experimental model. After the Pittsburgh report, a total of 17 groups have reported their experience and trials (11 adult/4 pediatric/2 mix population) to pursue the ideal goal, transplant tolerance, which may allow the return of natural immunity and free them from the side effects of IS (**Table 1**) (54–75).

Two early trials at Pittsburgh by Dr. Starzl and King's college by Dr. Williams and their colleagues revealed that attempting complete IS withdrawal could be successful in some recipients (19 and 27.7%, respectively), and long-surviving LT recipients were generally over-immunosuppressed (55–57). Since several experimental models have shown that donor chimerism can induce transplant tolerance (76–78), these trials and a randomized control trial (RCT) in Miami by Tryphonopoulos et al. (63) have assessed micro- and macro-chimerism as mechanisms of operational tolerance. However, donor-chimerism was not proven to be a mechanism of clinical operational tolerance. Later, Eason et al. at the New Orleans tried early induction of operational tolerance and showed that it seemed difficult to succeed, but still feasible with regard to reversal rejection events and subsequent graft survival (62). A similar finding has been shown in a recent multicenter trial with strict selection criteria and withdrawal protocol (75). As another risk factor for failure of complete IS withdrawal, recent episodes of rejection, autoimmune-related original disease were reported in early studies, and these factors are recognized as standard exclusion criteria for recent IS withdrawal trials (57, 67). Operational tolerance in pediatric recipients presented by Dr. Feng and her colleagues in San Francisco seems to show a relatively higher success rate compared to adult cases. This may be because of their immature immune system, but one of the other reasons could be more living donor cases, particularly parents who share the haplotype of HLA. Actually, data from living donor-related recipients are limited in adults. It may be a good candidate for investigating the mechanism of operational tolerance.

Currently, two IS withdrawal trails supported by the Immune Tolerance Network (ITN) leaded by Dr. Nepom are in operation. Recent trials achieving relatively high success rates of withdrawal by using strict selection criteria (69–72) showed that time after transplantation and age of recipients are the most impactful

TABLE 1 | Studies for spontaneous tolerance in liver transplantation.

Institution	Published year	Living/ Cadaver	Pediatric/ Adult	Study design	*n*	Patient with S.E.	Baseline biopsy	Time since LT (criteria) yr	IS regimen	Success rate	Acute rejection (Chronic rejection)	Graft loss	Remarks
Pittsburgh	1993 (54)	–	–	Case series reports	6	Yes	No	NA	NA	NA	NA	NA	First series report from Pittsburgh
	1995 (55) 1997 (56)	NA	Mix	Prospective	59 95	No	Yes	Mean 8.4 (>5)	14% Aza, 12% Tac 74% CsA	18/95 (19%)	25.4% (NR)	0	Two of PBC developed recurrence
King's College	1998 (57)	Cadaver	Adults	Prospective	18	Yes	No	Median 7 (–)	CsA and Aza	5/18 (27.7%)	28% (5.6%)	1/18 (5.6%)	Fewer HLA mismatch was associated with successful withdrawal. Previous rejection history and autoimmune original disease are risk factor
Kyoto	2001 (58)	Living	Pediatric	Partially prospective	26 (63)	Partially yes	No	NA (>2)	Tac	24/63 (38.1%)	12% (NR)	0	Biopsy at 4 year after weaning showed that 2 of 11 tolerant recipients had substantial bile duct atrophy and recovered by tacrolimus reinduction
	2002 (59)	Living	Mix	Prospective + retrospective	115	Partially yes	No	NA (>2)	Tac	16/67 (23.9%)	Non-protocol 25% Protocol 11.9%	0	None of clinical characteristics was identified as predictor of successful weaning
Marcia	2003 (60)	Cadaver	Adult	Prospective	9	No	Yes	Median 5.1 (>2)	CyA	3/9 (33%)	22% (NR)	0	Endothelial cell chimerism seems to have nothing to do with the induction of clinical tolerance in liver transplant patients
Stanford	2004 (61)	NA	Pediatric	Retrospective	38	Yes	No	NA	Steroid+CNI (Tac92%, CyA 8%)	8/38 (20.5%)	55.3% (5.3%)	2/38 (5.3%)	Two patients were retransplanted for chronic rejection
New Orleans	2005 (62)	Cadaver	Adult	Prospective	18	No	No	(>0.5)	Tac	1/18 (5.6%)	61% (NR)	0	Early induction of operational tolerance seems to be difficult
Miami	2005 (63)	Cadaver	Adult	RCT (donor BM)	105	No	No	Mean 4 (>3)	85% Tac 14% CsA	0%	67% (1.9%)	1/105 (0.95%)	Donor bone marrow infusion did not help successful completion of withdrawal
Rome	2006 (64) 2008 (65) 2013 (66)	Cadaver	Adult	Prospective	34	No	Yes	Mean 5.3 (>1)	CsA monotherapy	8/34 (23.4%)	76.4% (NR)	0	All HCV related recipients
Israel	2007 (67)	NA	Adult	RCT	26	No	No	Mean 4.3 vs. 5.0 (>2)	CsA +/–Aza, (Plednisone)	2/26 (7.7%)	UDCA+ 43% UDCA– 75%	0	3/4 AIH recipients had recurrence
Korea	2009 (68)	Mix	Pediatric	Retrospective	5	Yes	No	Median 3.8	NA	–	NR	0	Long term stable graft function and no rejection >1 yr were favorable findings for successful withdrawal

(Continued)

TABLE 1 | Continued

Institution	Published year	Living/ Cadaver	Pediatric/ Adult	Study design	*n*	Patient with S.E.	Baseline biopsy	Time since LT (criteria) yr	IS regimen	Success rate	Acute rejection (Chronic rejection)	Graft loss	Remarks
UCSF	2012 (69)	Living	Pediatric	Multi-center prospective	20	No	Yes	Mean 7.7 (>3)	CNI monotherapy	12/20 (60%)	36.8% (NR)	0	Later initiation of IS withdrawal after transplantation and less portal inflammation and total C4d score on screening biopsy were associated with successful withdrawal
Pamplona	2013 (70)	Cadaver	Adult	Prospective	24	Yes	Yes	Median 9.3 (>3)	NA	15/24(62.5%)	4.1% (41%)	0	Tolerant patients had a longer median interval between transplantation and inclusion in the study (156 vs. 71 months)
Barcelona	2013 (71)	Cadaver	Adult	Multi-center prospective	102	No	Yes	Median 8.6 (>3)	CNI mTOR inhibitor CSB	41/102 (40.2%)	56% (NR)	0	Time since transplantation, recipient age, and male gender were independent factor for successful withdrawal
	2014 (72)	Cadaver	Adult	Multi-center prospective	32	No	Yes	Median 7.2 (>3)	CNI +/–MMF or CBS	17/34 (50%)	44.1% (NR)	0	Persistent viral infections exert immunoregulatory effects that could contribute to the restraining of alloimmune responses
Taipei	2015 (73)	Mix	Pediatric	Single center retrospective	16	No	Yes	(>1 for Tx < 1, > 2 for Tx > 1)	Tac monotherapy	5/15 (33%)	46.7% (NR)	0	Early recruitment was favorable factor predicting operational tolerance
Chicago	2019 (74)	Cadaver	Adult	Prospective	15	No	Yes	Mean 6.7 (>3)	Silorimus	8/15 (53.3%)	40% (NR)	0	mTOR inhibitor withdrawal had similarly succeeded in comparison with CNI withdrawal
Pennsylvania	2019 (75)	Cadaver	Adult	Multi-center RCT	77	No	Yes	Median 18 (>3)	Tac (91) CsA (2), MMF(2)	10/77 (13%)	40.3% (NR)	0	Withdrawal showed likely less eventful than maintenance group

S.E., side effect; Aza, azathioprine; Tac, tacrolimus; CsA, cyclosporine A; NR, not reported; NA, not assessed; CNI, calcineurin inhibitor; RCT, randomized control study; CSB, costimulatory blockade; MMF, mycophenolate mofetil.

and common clinical factors of operational tolerance. These studies also suggested that exhausted T cells against hepatitis C virus (HCV) in HCV-related recipients and hyporesponsive T cells against polyclonal stimulation prior to withdrawal could contribute to the establishment of tolerance (70, 72). Based on these findings, multicenter IS withdrawal trial is currently being conducted by Dr. Markmann and his colleagues in Boston (NCT02533180, OPTIMAL) for evaluating donor-specific immune senescence and exhaustion as biomarker of operational tolerance in adults. Dr. Sanchez-Fueyo and his colleagues in Spain is conducting another trial (NCT02498977, LIFT) with a similar structure, but focused on exploring biomarkers in transcriptional signatures to identify operational tolerant recipients. The results of both trials could open a new gate to understand the mechanism of operational tolerance.

IMPACT OF DSA ON IMMUNOSUPPRESSION WITHDRAWAL

The deleterious effect of donor-specific antibody (DSA) on LT recipients is increasingly recognized, but has not been well-defined. The DSA may cause two types of antibody-mediated rejection (AMR): one is acute AMR resulting in immunologically adverse consequence because of preformed DSA usually accompanied by cellular rejection in the early postoperative period, and the other is chronic AMR causing progressive fibrosis in the late phase after liver transplantation. A retrospective cohort study has shown that *de novo* DSA (dnDSA) is associated with rejection, graft loss, and patient death after liver transplantation, and one of the risk factors for developing dnDSA is inadequate IS (79). However, a recent IS withdrawal trial in adult primary LT patients (A-WISH trial, NCT00135694) has shown that there was no difference in the prevalence of dnDSA (especially HLA class II dnDSA) between IS maintenance and IS minimization (44.4% vs. 51.7%, respectively), and the prevalence was the highest after IS withdrawal was completed (66.7%) (75, 80). Interesting findings in prevalence have been reported that the majority (78.7%) of dnDSA was developed against HLA-DQ Ags, which included DQB1 (57.4%) and DQA1 (21.3%) chains independent of IS status, and dnDSA against HLA class I Ags increased only when patients were free of IS. From the view of pathogenicity, dnDSA detected in patients who failed IS withdrawal may be highly pathogenic compared to that in patients under IS maintenance and IS-free according to the prevalence of acute rejection rate (71.4, 25.0, and 16.7%, respectively) (80).

It is well-recognized that different IgG subclasses have unique characteristics, such as complement fixation potential or cellular binding capacity through Fc receptors (FcRs), which may affect their pathologic potential. IgG3 is known as the strongest complement activating capacity, followed by IgG1 and IgG2, while IgG4 is the only subclass that fail to fix complement. IgG3 and IgG1 bind to all three classes of FcRs (FcRI, FcRII, and FcRIII), while IgG4 binds to FcRII and FcRIII, and IgG2 binds only FcRII (81). These binding abilities have the potential to trigger functions such as antibody-dependent cell cytotoxicity, cytokine production, intracellular signaling, and initiation of cell recruitment and degranulation with various immune mediators (macrophages, NK cells, neutrophils, and B cells) (82). Jackson et al. recently examined whether DSA IgG subclass characteristics could identify subjects whose liver allografts exhibit subclinical graft injury with samples from a multicenter IS withdrawal study for pediatric LT recipients (iWITH, NCT01638559) (83). They reported that the HLA-class II IgG4 DSA profile was associated with a higher HLA mismatch, a subclinical histopathological phenotype characterized by interface activity, and a tissue transcriptional profile of rejection. Substantial IgG subclass analysis for DSA in a prospective study is expected for better understanding and management of the dynamic evolution of DSA maturation, mechanisms of injury, and entry points for intervention (84). DSA is produced against HLA mismatches and HLA Ags has been reported to have structural epitope that dominate the strength and specificity of binding antibody (85). Recently, it has been reported that HLA class II epitope mismatch, which was analyzed by HLA Matchmaker or the predicted indirectly recognizable human leukocyte antigen epitopes algorithm (PIRCHE-II), is correlated with a high risk of dnDSA formation after liver transplantation (86, 87). By using more detail data on HLA class II epitope mismatch related to donor recipients, the eligibility criteria for patient selection in early IS minimization or IS withdrawal trials may be sophisticated (12).

IMMUNE MONITORING TO PERSONALIZE IMMUNOSUPPRESSION TOWARD TOLERANCE

Liver transplant recipients receive immunosuppressive therapy according to empirical protocols. Immune monitoring comprises candidate biomarkers capable of reflecting the donor-specific and non-specific net-activating state of the immune system, and can be dissected into tissue, cell, protein, and gene profiles with graft or systemic samples (**Figure 2**). Here, we summarize the potential tool for immune monitoring to personalize immunosuppressive therapy potentially toward operational tolerance.

As clinical information, histological findings regarding inflammation and fibrosis are the gold standard for the diagnosis of rejection. Intensive molecular analyses of biopsy specimens have shown that immune regulatory markers, such as IL-10, PD1, PDL1, BATF, TGFβ, and Foxp3 were significantly higher in tolerant patients (72). Intra-graft iron metabolism has also been identified in tolerant samples (88). Immunofluorescence staining revealed transient accumulation of $CD4^{+}FOXP3^{+}$ cells in tolerant recipients, along with the upregulation of immune regulatory genes (89). Although biopsy-based assessments are a valuable source of information on immunological status, it can be harmful because of their potential risk of complications. As candidates of safer biomarkers for successful withdrawal, the immune phenotype of peripheral blood has also been diligently investigated. Pittsburgh group reported that the increase in the ratio of plasmacytoid DCs to monocytoid DCs in peripheral blood was associated with successful withdrawal (90). Consistent

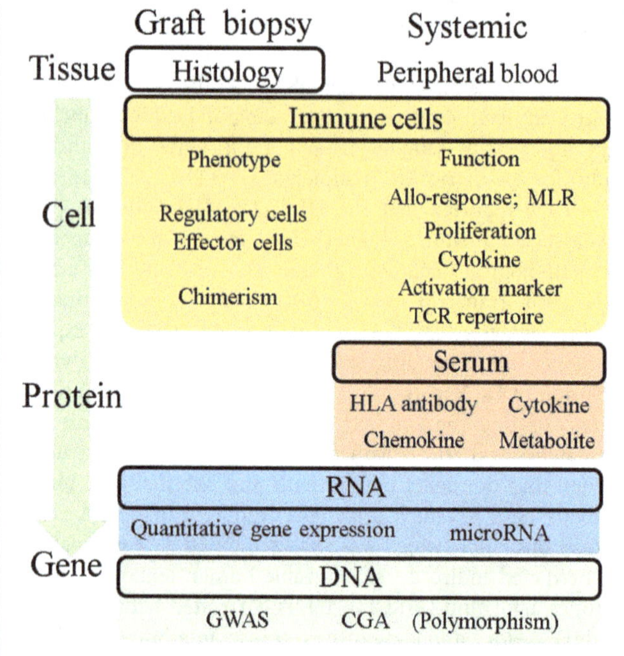

FIGURE 2 | Potential immune monitoring application for tolerance in liver transplantation. This figure summarizes the readouts being investigated for their potential use for immune monitoring to understand what is happening in the allograft and predict tolerance. Histological assessment is a direct readout of allografts, but it is not enough to predict tolerance. Systemic information from peripheral blood has been investigated as an alternative because of its less invasive availability. The readouts were categorized into four groups based on their level of information, tissue, cell, protein, and gene. MLR, mixed lymphocyte reaction; GWAS, genome-wide association study; CGA, candidate gene approach.

with this finding, a study with a mammalian target of rapamycin (mTOR) inhibitor showed a higher proportion of tolerogenic DCs in tolerant recipients (74). An increasing number of regulatory T cell subsets (Tregs and gamma-delta T cells) and NK cells in peripheral blood are associated with tolerant recipients, which is consistent with their gene signatures (58, 65, 74, 91). A recent report has shown the kinetics of increasing Tregs/Th17 cell ratio over the clinical course as a predictor of the development of tolerance (92). These have the potential to be monitoring tools for tolerance, but further investigations are needed to validate their capacities. Pioneering studies for transplant tolerance has been conducted by "The One Study" consortium leading by Dr. Geissler and his colleagues. This consortium conducted harmonized cell therapy studies by multi-center to induce tolerance with standard immunosuppressive regimen and immune monitoring protocol, which allow to analyze different trial data under same platform. These approach also would be great helpful to build solid and universal foundation in clinical tolerance, which is observed to a limited extent.

Along with the immune phenotype, functional assays have been investigated mainly using mixed lymphocyte reaction (MLR) assays with various readouts. One-way MLR with whole peripheral blood mononuclear cells (PBMCs) has been often attempted to use as clinical assay monitoring donor specific response. However, MLR readout with tritiated thymidine incorporation shows little predictive value because of its low level of reproducibility (93). ELISPOT and qPCR-based detection of cytokines in MLR assay showed sensitive results, but readout of limited cytokines from bulk cultured cells may be difficult to interpret as representative of the entire alloresponse (94–96). Non-toxic intracellular fluorescent dyes such as carboxyfluorescein diacetate succinimidyl ester (CFSE) stably stain intracellular proteins, and the fluorescence of each stained cell segregates equally to daughter cells upon cell division, resulting in sequential halving of cellular fluorescence intensity with each successive generation (97). This sequential halving of fluorescence can be analyzed to track cell division in populations of proliferating cells using intensity based analysis by flow cytometry (FACS) even in alloresponse which is comparatively lower incidence. Additionally, FACS analysis provides opportunity to assess detail phenotype of proliferating cell along with number of cells originally proliferated, that is halving of fluorescence is visualized as distinct peaks or populations of cells and can be used to track cell division in populations of proliferating cells. This allows phenotypic analysis of proliferating cells in addition to determining the number of cells produced in each generation by multicolor FACS analysis, that is, the precursor frequency of each CD4$^+$ and CD8, the precursor frequency of each CD4$^+$ and CD8$^+$ T cell (and others) can be quantified separately (**Figure 3A**). The lack of proliferation in anti-donor MLR reflects the suppression of the anti-donor response (99). We have previously reported that optimization of immunosuppressive therapy based on the CFSE-MLR assay provides a low incidence of acute rejection, reduction of infectious complications, and helps in monitoring anti-self-response of CD4$^+$ T cells, which predicts the recurrence of autoimmune liver diseases after LT (98, 100–102) (**Figure 3B**). In addition, CFSE-MLR-based immune monitoring has been proven to be a useful tool to personalize IS therapy, especially for LT patients with impaired renal function and HBV-infected LT patients requiring post-transplant HBV vaccination (103, 104). The benefit of CFSE-MLR immune-monitoring can be applied to T cell receptor (TCR) repertoire analysis by high-throughput sequencing. The Colombia group developed a TCR sequencing-based analysis of responding T cells in CFSE-MLR to identify and track a significant fraction of alloreactive T cell repertoire in any donor-recipient pair (105, 106). They have shown that liver-induced clonal deletion detected by tracking alloreactive TCR clones in pre-transplant MLR may contribute to achieving tolerance in LT recipients (107). Furthermore, another potentially beneficial application of MLR is the detection of activating induced markers and cytokines. CD154 (CD40L) has been reported to rapidly upregulate Ag-specific activating markers of T cells (108, 109). Upregulation of CD154 in T cells in MLR with donor stimulator was reported as a risk factor for rejection in pediatric liver transplant recipients (110). Like CD154, CD137 (4-1BB) has been reported as a specific activation-induced molecule on T cells (111). Interestingly, their combination, CD154^{neg}CD137$^+$, in CD4$^+$ T cells have been reported to be representative of activated Tregs under Ag stimulation, including allo-stimulation, suggesting that it could be a candidate for monitoring alloreactive T cell responses in LT recipients (112, 113).

IMMUNE TOLERANCE MEDIATED BY TREGS

Applicability of Treg Cell Therapy in Liver Transplantation

Since the discovery of suppressive T cells and markers, Tregs (mostly defined as $CD4^{+}CD25^{+}FOXP3^{+}$) have been shown to be key mediators in the induction and maintenance of immune tolerance through multiple mechanisms (114–116). Together with these accumulating findings in basic science and clinically reported footprints e.g., the number of Tregs are increasing in tolerant recipients, Treg-based cell therapy has been attempted for tolerance in the field of transplantation. Initial attempts have been made in the field of bone marrow transplantation and have shown the feasibility of transferring polyclonally expanded Tregs for graft vs. host disease (GVHD) prophylaxis (117–119). Together with promising rationale, several clinical trials have been conducted in LT recipients. Key considerations of this cell therapy are: (1) timing to infuse the cell product, (2) induction therapy to make space for adoptive Tregs, (3) cell component, whether Treg-enriched cell product or isolated Tregs for culturing, and (4) Ag specificity during expansion, polyclonal or donor specific (**Table 2**). In 2016, the Hokkaido University group demonstrated the impact of Treg-enriched cell therapy for inducing operational tolerance in 10 living donor LT patients (120). Autologous Treg-enriched cells were cultured in MLR in the presence of CD80/86 costimulatory blockade, and the cell product was administered after pre-conditioning with cyclophosphamide at early post-transplant period. Although three recipients with autoimmune liver disease developed cellular rejection during immunosuppressant weaning, the other seven (70%) recipients were successfully weaned off immunosuppressive drugs 18 months after liver transplantation. In spite of a small cohort, the result that all tolerant patients maintained normal graft function without immunosuppressive drugs for over 5 years is promising for Treg cell therapy for tolerance induction (121). Currently, clinical studies with isolated Tregs, rather than bulk cultured cells, are in operation. The King's college group is running a phase I/II clinical trial with a polyclonal expanded Treg isolated by a magnetic isolation system in LT patients with anti-thymocyte globulin (ATG) pre-conditioning (NCT02166177). No serious adverse events have been observed to date (122). The UCSF group conducted clinical trials using donor allo-Ag reactive Tregs (darTregs) cultured with donor-derived stimulators (NCT02188719). The protocol includes the use of ATG before the infusion of donor allo-Ag reactive Tregs (123). The Massachusetts General Hospital (MGH) group is employing costimulatory blockade-induced allospecific Tregs that are generated in short-term MLR with belatacept and isolated by magnetic isolation before administration. These three trials reduced the calcineurin inhibitor (CNI) regimen with the

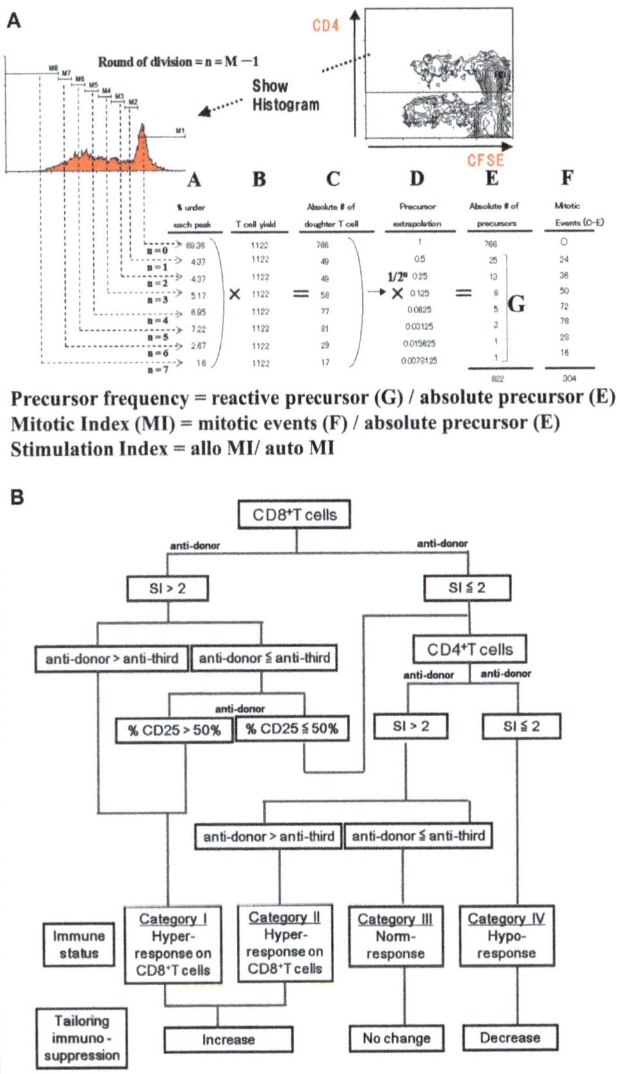

FIGURE 3 | CFSE-MLR for immune monitoring in transplantation. **(A)** Intensity-based analysis of mixed lymphocyte reaction assay with CFSE dye (CFSE-MLR) provide quantitative estimation of the alloresponse. In brief, the plot and histogram show the gating strategy for $CD4^{+}$ proliferating cells. Cell division are gated by the rationale that the CFSE fluorescence intensity shows the half-value from former generation. (A) Percentage of CD4+ T cell events in each division, (B) T cell yield, (C) the number of daughter T cells that had divided *n* times (A multiply B), (D) precursor extrapolation Using mathematical relationship, the number of division precursors (E,G) is extrapolated from the number of daughter cells of each division and from mitotic events (F). These values are used to calculate precursor frequency and mitotic index (MI). As normalized quantitative estimation, stimulation index are calculated by dividing MIs of allogeneic combinations by MIs of autologous controls. **(B)** Algorithm to estimate anti-donor alloreactivity in liver transplant recipients. The immune reactivity of liver transplantation recipients is classified into four categories. By analyzing the proliferation and CD25 expression of the $CD4^{+}$ and $CD8^{+}$ T-cell subsets in response to anti-donor and anti-third party stimuli, the immune status is categorized as hypo-, normo-, or hyper-responsive. In recipients with hyper-response on either $CD4^{+}$ or $CD8^{+}$ T cells, immunosuppressants consider to be increased. In patients with normo-response, immunosuppressant tapering is abandoned. Only in patients with hypo-response, immunosuppressant therapy can be tapered off (98). SI, stimulation index.

TABLE 2 | Trials of Treg cell therapy for liver transplantation.

Institution	Trial ID	Type of trial	*n*	Timing of infusion after transplantation	Induction therapy	Cell isolation	Specificity	Type of Tregs	Current status
Hokkaido	UMIN000015789	Phase I/II	10	2 weeks	Cyclophosphamide	No	Donor specific	Treg enriched donor-specific-anergic T cells	Published in 2016
UCSF	NCT02188719	Phase I	15	2–6 months	ATG	Yes	Donor specific	Donor alloantigen reactive Treg	Terminated
Beth Israel	NCT02739412	Phase II	7	2–4 years	–	–	–	Endogenous Treg by low dose IL-2 injection	Active, not recruiting
Nanjing	NCT 01624077	Phase I	1	–	–	No	Polyclonal	*In vitro* induced Treg	Unknown
UCSF	NCT02474199	Phase I/II	14	2–6 years	ATG	Yes	Donor specific	Donor-alloantigen reactive Treg	Completed
King's College	NCT02166177	Phase I/II	9	2 months	ATG	Yes	Polyclonal	Autologous Treg	Completed
MGH	NCT03577431	Phase I/II	9	2-6 months	Cyclophosphamide	Yes	Donor specific	Alloantigen-reactive Treg	Recruiting

Treg, regulatory T cell; UCSF, University of California, San Francisco; ATG, anti-thymocyte globulin; MGH, Massachusetts General Hospital.

addition of an mTOR inhibitor before attempting complete IS withdrawal. Since clinical-grade manufactured Tregs cells are challenging, the King's college group treated 3 recipients finally out of the initial 23 and the USCF group's trial was terminated because of the manufacturing problem. USCF is conducting another trial, the ARTEMIS trial (NCT02474199), which has a different design, to aim at the reduction of CNI in patients with stable liver graft function in 2–6 years after LT with darTregs (123). It remains unclear when and what kind of Treg cell therapy is beneficial for LT recipients. Ongoing trials may clarify some points, but a systematic approach to investigate the best option may be needed.

mTOR Inhibitor for Tolerance and Treg Expansion

Currently, a CNI-based regimen is widely employed as standard IS therapy for the management of liver transplantation. One of the most problematic side effects is nephrotoxicity of CNIs because LT candidates frequently have a variety of degrees of renal dysfunction, and chronic renal failure has a negative impact on long-term outcomes. The strategy of early CNI minimization and mTOR inhibitor maintenance has been attempted to achieve better renal function after liver transplantation. Meta-analysis and recent RCTs have shown a protective effect on renal function by converting CNIs into mTOR inhibitor, but also high frequency of rejection compared to conventional CNI-based therapy, suggesting that selected patients could receive the benefit of mTOR inhibitor conversion (124–126). The mTOR signaling pathway through PI3K/AKT is widely utilized in the regulation of cellular activity in immune cells and cancer cells. mTOR inhibitors have been reported to have therapeutic effects on hepatocellular carcinoma (HCC) through multiple mechanisms, including direct antitumor effects and immune regulation (127–129). According to the antitumor effect, LT recipients with HCC may be good candidates for mTOR inhibitor regimen (130). Another topic in the transplantation field of mTOR signaling is the impact on Treg stability and function, usually mTOR inhibition recognized as favorable effects (131). One recent IS withdrawal trial has been conducted expecting this "Treg friendly effect" to induce operational tolerance (74). Further investigation is required to elucidate the clinical application of mTOR inhibitors for transplantation tolerance.

OUTLOOK ON EMPLOYING SNPs AND miRNAs FOR TOLERANCE

Genetic factors have been reported to be involved in the mechanisms of transplant tolerance and rejection (132). Here, we summarize recent advances in genetics and genomics, particularly single nucleotide polymorphisms (SNPs) and microRNAs (miRNAs), and their roles intolerance after LT.

Genome-Wide Association Studies (GWAS)

Recent GWAS have established the genes and variants associated with outcomes in transplantation patients. Multiple GWAS have been conducted since 2016 on solid-organ transplantation, including acute rejection in renal transplantation, post-transplant malignancy in heart or renal transplantation, long-term allograft function, and new-onset diabetes mellitus after renal transplantation; however, there are no GWASs on liver transplantation (96, 132).

Candidate Gene Approaches (CGA)

The candidate gene approach has been applied in liver transplantation by conducting genetic association studies focusing on associations between immune-associated genetic variation and graft survival/rejection incidence. HLA-G, a non-classical HLA-class, has been associated with increased graft survival and decreased number of rejection cases (133–135). It is also known that HLA-G is capable of inducing a new generation of regulatory Tregs (136). A recent study has demonstrated that 14-bp ins/ins and +3142GG genotypes of HLA-G, which seem to be of serious importance for HLA-G expression, in LT recipients are involved in a low risk of acute rejection in liver transplantation, suggesting that LT recipients with a lower for developing an acute rejection may be identified by application of these genotypes as biomarkers (137). Another report has shown that the donor liver tissue-derived CYP3A5 rs776746 and small ubiquitin-like modifier 4 (SUMO4) rs237025 SNPs are associated with tacrolimus pharmacokinetics in the early period after LT, suggesting that combined evaluation of these donor genotypes may help determine the withdrawal or elimination of tacrolimus (138). We have also reported that the FOXP3 gene rs3761548 A/C SNP in living donor LT recipients is significantly concerned with susceptibility to steroid-resistant acute rejection and dnDSA formation, suggesting that the IS regime and/or anti-rejection treatment regimen should be adjusted on an individual basis by identifying FOXP3 SNPs (139). These genetic association studies may hopefully provide immune-related SNPs that can be useful markers to reduce or withdraw immunosuppressive drugs.

miRNAs as Biomarkers

miRNAs, which are ~20–22 nucleotide single-stranded RNA species, and play a central role in the regulation of protein-coding genes, are also emerging as robust biomarkers for assessing allograft status. Millán et al. have reported that plasma miRNAs can serve as early non-invasive prognostic and diagnostic biomarkers for T-cell mediated acute rejection in LT recipients, that is, miR-155-5p regulates the differentiation of $CD4^+$ T cells into Th cells and IFN-γ production in human T and NK cells, and miR-181a levels modulate T cell receptor sensitivity and intensity of signaling (140). Hence, the plasma levels of miR-155-5p and miR-181a-5p after LT potentially help identify patients for IS minimization. Revilla-Nuin et al. have reported a set of differentially expressed miRNAs in tolerant recipients after liver transplantation that might promote and control the activation of Tregs necessary to develop operational tolerance (141). Their study showed that miR95, miR24, miR31, miR146a, and miR155 were expressed more in tolerant than in non-tolerant recipients, and were positively correlated with activated Treg markers. These five miRNAs were upregulated in the peripheral blood of LT recipients, and the transcription factor Foxp3 was associated with the miRNA profiles. miR155 is constitutively expressed in Tregs; Foxp3 binds to the promoter of miR155 in the B cell integration cluster and maintains the elevated levels of miR155 required for Treg proliferation. Furthermore, Vitalone et al. reported increased expression of miR-142-5p and miR-181a in tolerant livers in an allogeneic rat LT model (142). Morita et al. have also identified miRNAs involved in acute rejection and spontaneous tolerance in murine hepatic allografts (143). They found that miR-146a, 15b, 223, 23a, 27a, 34a, and 451 were upregulated in the allogenic liver grafts compared with the expression observed in the syngeneic grafts, whereas miR-101a, 101b, and 148a were downregulated, demonstrating the change of miRNAs in the allografts and may suggest the role of miRNAs in the induction of tolerance after liver transplantation.

CONCLUSION

Progresses in immunosuppressive therapy have efficiently reduced the incidence of acute rejection of liver allograft. However, life-long IS has inevitably led to substantial morbidity and mortality. Thus far, trial and error have been attempted to minimize or even withdraw immunosuppressants in select patients. These attempts would be more successful through the establishment of reliable immune-monitoring methods and biomarkers. In addition, deliberate immunomodulatory interventions would further improve the outcome of these attempts. This review has summarized our knowledge of mechanisms underlying immune-tolerance induced after liver transplantation and prospective strategies to intentionally complete withdrawal of IS treatment.

AUTHOR CONTRIBUTIONS

NT participated in the role of drafting and revising. MO, HT, KI, YT, and TO participated in roles of writing original draft. HO participated in roles of concepts, design, and drafting and revising. All authors contributed to the article and approved the submitted version.

ACKNOWLEDGMENTS

We thank all the current and former clinical and research staffs in Department of Gastroenterological and Transplantation Surgery.

REFERENCES

1. Calne RY, Sells RA, Pena JR, Davis DR, Millard PR, Herbertson BM, et al. Induction of immunological tolerance by porcine liver allografts. *Nature.* (1969) 223:472–6. doi: 10.1038/223472a0

2. Zimmermann FA, Davies HS, Knoll PP, Gokel JM, Schmidt T. Orthotopic liver allografts in the rat. The influence of strain combination on the fate of the graft. *Transplantation.* (1984) 37:406–10. doi: 10.1097/00007890-198404000-00019
3. Qian S, Demetris AJ, Murase N, Rao AS, Fung JJ, Starzl TE. Murine liver allograft transplantation: tolerance and donor cell chimerism. *Hepatology.* (1994) 19:916–24. doi: 10.1002/hep.1840190418
4. Kamada N, Davies HS, Roser B. Reversal of transplantation immunity by liver grafting. *Nature.* (1981) 292:840–2. doi: 10.1038/292840a0
5. Lu L, Rudert WA, Qian S, McCaslin D, Fu F, Rao AS, et al. Growth of donor-derived dendritic cells from the bone marrow of murine liver allograft recipients in response to granulocyte/macrophage colony-stimulating factor. *J Exp Med.* (1995) 182:379–87. doi: 10.1084/jem.182.2.379
6. Yokota S, Yoshida O, Ono Y, Geller DA, Thomson AW. Liver transplantation in the mouse: insights into liver immunobiology, tissue injury, and allograft tolerance. *Liver Transpl.* (2016) 22:536–46. doi: 10.1002/lt.24394
7. Steptoe RJ, Fu F, Li W, Drakes ML, Lu L, Demetris AJ, et al. Augmentation of dendritic cells in murine organ donors by Flt3 ligand alters the balance between transplant tolerance and immunity. *J Immunol.* (1997) 159:5483–91.
8. Li W, Lu L, Wang Z, Wang L, Fung JJ, Thomson AW, et al. Il-12 antagonism enhances apoptotic death of T cells within hepatic allografts from Flt3 ligand-treated donors and promotes graft acceptance. *J Immunol.* (2001) 166:5619–28. doi: 10.4049/jimmunol.166.9.5619
9. Yoshida O, Kimura S, Dou L, Matta BM, Yokota S, Ross MA, et al. DAP12 deficiency in liver allografts results in enhanced donor DC migration, augmented effector T cell responses and abrogation of transplant tolerance. *Am J Transplant.* (2014) 14:1791–805. doi: 10.1111/ajt.12757
10. Akkaya B, Oya Y, Akkaya M, Al Souz J, Holstein AH, Kamenyeva O, et al. Regulatory T cells mediate specific suppression by depleting peptide-MHC class II from dendritic cells. *Nat Immunol.* (2019) 20:218–31. doi: 10.1038/s41590-018-0280-2
11. Thomson AW, Humar A, Lakkis FG, Metes DM. Regulatory dendritic cells for promotion of liver transplant operational tolerance: rationale for a clinical trial and accompanying mechanistic studies. *Hum Immunol.* (2018) 79:314–21. doi: 10.1016/j.humimm.2017.10.017
12. Onoe T, Ohdan H, Tokita D, Shishida M, Tanaka Y, Hara H, et al. Liver sinusoidal endothelial cells tolerize T cells across MHC barriers in mice. *Immunol.* (2005) 175:139–46. doi: 10.4049/jimmunol.175.1.139
13. Nishimura H, Nose M, Hiai H, Minato N, Honjo T. Development of lupus-like autoimmune diseases by disruption of the PD-1 gene encoding an ITIM motif-carrying immunoreceptor. *Immunity.* (1999) 11:141–51. doi: 10.1016/S1074-7613(00)80089-8 J
14. Leach DR, Krummel MF, Allison JP. Enhancement of antitumor immunity by CTLA-4 blockade. *Science.* (1996) 271:1734–6. doi: 10.1126/science.271.5256.1734
15. Ishida Y, Agata Y, Shibahara K, Honjo T. Induced expression of PD-1, a novel member of the immunoglobulin gene superfamily, upon programmed cell death. *Embo J.* (1992) 11:3887–95. doi: 10.1002/j.1460-2075.1992.tb05481.x
16. Tokita D, Shishida M, Ohdan H, Onoe T, Hara H, Tanaka Y, et al. Liver sinusoidal endothelial cells that endocytose allogeneic cells suppress T cells with indirect allospecificity. *J Immunol.* (2006) 177:3615–24. doi: 10.4049/jimmunol.177.6.3615
17. Knolle PA, Limmer A. Neighborhood politics: the immunoregulatory function of organ-resident liver endothelial cells. *Trends Immunol.* (2001) 22:432–7. doi: 10.1016/S1471-4906(01)01957-3
18. Iwai Y, Terawaki S, Ikegawa M, Okazaki T, Honjo T. PD-1 inhibits antiviral immunity at the effector phase in the liver. *J Exp Med.* (2003) 198:39–50. doi: 10.1084/jem.20022235
19. Limmer A, Ohl J, Kurts C, Ljunggren HG, Reiss Y, Groettrup M, et al. Efficient presentation of exogenous antigen by liver endothelial cells to CD8+ T cells results in antigen-specific T-cell tolerance. *Nat Med.* (2000) 6:1348–54. doi: 10.1038/82161
20. Hochst B, Schildberg FA, Bottcher J, Metzger C, Huss S, Turler A, et al. Liver sinusoidal endothelial cells contribute to CD8 T cell tolerance toward circulating carcinoembryonic antigen in mice. *Hepatology.* (2012) 56:1924–33. doi: 10.1002/hep.25844
21. Schurich A, Berg M, Stabenow D, Bottcher J, Kern M, Schild HJ, et al. Dynamic regulation of CD8 T cell tolerance induction by liver sinusoidal endothelial cells. *J Immunol.* (2010) 184:4107–14. doi: 10.4049/jimmunol.0902580
22. Banshodani M, Onoe T, Shishida M, Tahara H, Hashimoto S, Igarashi Y, et al. Adoptive transfer of allogeneic liver sinusoidal endothelial cells specifically inhibits T-cell responses to cognate stimuli. *Cell Transplant.* (2013) 22:1695–708. doi: 10.3727/096368912X657738
23. Igarashi Y, Onoe T, Ohdan H. The role of liver sinusoidal endothelial cells in induction of carbohydrate reactive B cells tolerance through the programmed death 1/programmed death ligand 1 pathway. *Transplantation.* (2015) 99:2325–36. doi: 10.1097/TP.0000000000000831
24. Morita M, Joyce D, Miller C, Fung JJ, Lu L, Qian S. Rejection triggers liver transplant tolerance: involvement of mesenchyme-mediated immune control mechanisms in mice. *Hepatology.* (2015) 62:915–31. doi: 10.1002/hep.27909
25. Morita M, Fujino M, Jiang G, Kitazawa Y, Xie L, Azuma M, et al. PD-1/B7-H1 interaction contribute to the spontaneous acceptance of mouse liver allograft. *Am J Transplant.* (2010) 10:40–6. doi: 10.1111/j.1600-6143.2009.02859.x
26. Hashimoto S, Onoe T, Banshodani M, Taguchi K, Tanaka Y, Ohdan H. Postoperative portal hypertension enhances alloimmune responses after living-donor liver transplantation in patients and in a mouse model. *J Immunol.* (2019) 203:1392–403. doi: 10.4049/jimmunol.1701147
27. Winau F, Hegasy G, Weiskirchen R, Weber S, Cassan C, Sieling PA, et al. Ito cells are liver-resident antigen-presenting cells for activating T cell responses. *Immunity.* (2007) 26:117–29. doi: 10.1016/j.immuni.2006.11.011
28. Yu MC, Chen CH, Liang X, Wang L, Gandhi CR, Fung JJ, et al. Inhibition of T-cell responses by hepatic stellate cells via B7-H1-mediated T-cell apoptosis in mice. *Hepatology.* (2004) 40:1312–21. doi: 10.1002/hep.20488
29. Charles R, Chou HS, Wang L, Fung JJ, Lu L, Qian S. Human hepatic stellate cells inhibit T-cell response through B7-H1 pathway. *Transplantation.* (2013) 96:17–24. doi: 10.1097/TP.0b013e318294caae
30. Gu X, Wang Y, Xiang J, Chen Z, Wang L, Lu L, et al. Interferon-gamma triggers hepatic stellate cell-mediated immune regulation through MEK/ERK signaling pathway. *Clin Dev Immunol.* (2013) 2013:389807. doi: 10.1155/2013/389807
31. Dunham RM, Thapa M, Velazquez VM, Elrod EJ, Denning TL, Pulendran B, et al. Hepatic stellate cells preferentially induce Foxp3+ regulatory T cells by production of retinoic acid. *J Immunol.* (2013) 190:2009–16. doi: 10.4049/jimmunol.1201937
32. Chen CH, Kuo LM, Chang Y, Wu W, Goldbach C, Ross MA, et al. *In vivo* immune modulatory activity of hepatic stellate cells in mice. *Hepatology.* (2006) 44:1171–81. doi: 10.1002/hep.21379
33. Kordes C, Sawitza I, Müller-Marbach A, Ale-Agha N, Keitel V, Klonowski-Stumpe H, et al. CD133+ hepatic stellate cells are progenitor cells. *Biochem Biophys Res Commun.* (2007) 352:410–7. doi: 10.1016/j.bbrc.2006.11.029
34. Kordes C, Sawitza I, Götze S, Häussinger D. Hepatic stellate cells support hematopoiesis and are liver-resident mesenchymal stem cells. *Cell Physiol Biochem.* (2013) 31:290–304. doi: 10.1159/000343368
35. Covas DT, Panepucci RA, Fontes AM, Silva WA Jr., Orellana MD, Peres LC, et al. Multipotent mesenchymal stromal cells obtained from diverse human tissues share functional properties and gene-expression profile with CD146+ perivascular cells and fibroblasts. *Exp Hematol.* (2008) 36:642–54. doi: 10.1016/j.exphem.2007.12.015
36. Aggarwal S, Pittenger MF. Human mesenchymal stem cells modulate allogeneic immune cell responses. *Blood.* (2005) 105:1815–22. doi: 10.1182/blood-2004-04-1559
37. Krampera M, Glennie S, Dyson J, Scott D, Laylor R, Simpson E, et al. Bone marrow mesenchymal stem cells inhibit the response of naive and memory antigen-specific T cells to their cognate peptide. *Blood.* (2003) 101:3722–9. doi: 10.1182/blood-2002-07-2104
38. He Y, Zhou S, Liu H, Shen B, Zhao H, Peng K, et al. Indoleamine 2, 3-dioxgenase transfected mesenchymal stem cells induce kidney allograft tolerance by increasing the production and function of regulatory T cells. *Transplantation.* (2015) 99:1829–38. doi: 10.1097/TP.0000000000000856
39. Detry O, Vandermeulen M, Delbouille MH, Somja J, Bletard N, Briquet A, et al. Infusion of mesenchymal stromal cells after deceased liver transplantation: a phase I-II, open-label, clinical study. *J Hepatol.* (2017) 67:47–55. doi: 10.1016/j.jhep.2017.03.001
40. Rosser EC, Mauri C. Regulatory B cells: origin, phenotype, and function. *Immunity.* (2015) 42:607–12. doi: 10.1016/j.immuni.2015.04.005
41. Alhabbab RY, Nova-Lamperti E, Aravena O, Burton HM, Lechler RI, Dorling A, et al. Regulatory B cells: development, phenotypes, functions, and role in transplantation. *Immunol Rev.* (2019) 292:164–79. doi: 10.1111/imr.12800
42. Peng B, Ming Y, Yang C. Regulatory B cells: the cutting edge of

immune tolerance in kidney transplantation. *Cell Death Dis.* (2018) 9:109. doi: 10.1038/s41419-017-0152-y

43. Khan AR, Hams E, Floudas A, Sparwasser T, Weaver CT, Fallon PG. PD-L1hi B cells are critical regulators of humoral immunity. *Nat Commun.* (2015) 6:5997. doi: 10.1038/ncomms6997
44. Riccomi A, Palma C. B cells and programmed death-ligand 2 signaling are required for maximal interferon-gamma recall response by splenic $CD4^+$ memory T cells of mice vaccinated with mycobacterium tuberculosis Ag85B. *PLoS ONE.* (2015) 10:e0137783. doi: 10.1371/journal.pone.0137783
45. Hirose T, Tanaka Y, Tanaka A, Sakai H, Sasaki Y, Shinohara N, et al. PD-L1/PD-L2-expressing B-1 cells inhibit alloreactive T cells in mice. *PLoS ONE.* (2017) 12:e0178765. doi: 10.1371/journal.pone.0178765
46. Song J, Du G, Chen W, Bao P, Li B, Lu Q, et al. The advantage of sirolimus in amplifying regulatory B cells and regulatory T cells in liver transplant patients. *Eur J Pharmacol.* (2020) 869:172872. doi: 10.1016/j.ejphar.2019.172872
47. Taniguchi M, Harada M, Kojo S, Nakayama T, Wakao H. The regulatory role of Valpha14 NKT cells in innate and acquired immune response. *Annu Rev Immunol.* (2003) 21:483–513. doi: 10.1146/annurev.immunol.21.120601.141057
48. Crosby CM, Kronenberg M. Tissue-specific functions of invariant natural killer T cells. *Nat Rev Immunol.* (2018) 18:559–74. doi: 10.1038/s41577-018-0034-2
49. Sonoda KH, Taniguchi M, Stein-Streilein J. Long-term survival of corneal allografts is dependent on intact CD1d-reactive NKT cells. *J Immunol.* (2002) 168:2028–34. doi: 10.4049/jimmunol.168.4.2028
50. Ikehara Y, Yasunami Y, Kodama S, Maki T, Nakano M, Nakayama T, et al. $CD4^+$ Valpha14 natural killer T cells are essential for acceptance of rat islet xenografts in mice. *J Clin Invest.* (2000) 105:1761–7. doi: 10.1172/JCI8922
51. Seino KI, Fukao K, Muramoto K, Yanagisawa K, Takada Y, Kakuta S, et al. Requirement for natural killer T (NKT) cells in the induction of allograft tolerance. *Proc Natl Acad Sci USA.* (2001) 98:2577–81. doi: 10.1073/pnas.041608298
52. Morita M, Fujino M, Li XK, Kimura H, Nakayama T, Taniguchi M, et al. Spontaneous tolerance involving natural killer T cells after hepatic grafting in mice. *Transpl Immunol.* (2007) 18:142–5. doi: 10.1016/j.trim.2007.05.015
53. Shishida M, Ohdan H, Onoe T, Tanaka Y, Igarashi Y, Banshodani M, et al. Role of invariant natural killer T cells in liver sinusoidal endothelial cell-induced immunosuppression among T cells with indirect allospecificity. *Transplantation.* (2008) 85:1060–4. doi: 10.1097/TP.0b013e31816a3372
54. Reyes J, Zeevi A, Ramos H, Tzakis A, Todo S, Demetris AJ, et al. Frequent achievement of a drug-free state after orthotopic liver transplantation. *Transplant Proc.* (1993) 25:3315–9.
55. Ramos HC, Reyes J, Abu-Elmagd K, Zeevi A, Reinsmoen N, Tzakis A, et al. Weaning of immunosuppression in long-term liver transplant recipients. *Transplantation.* (1995) 59:212–7. doi: 10.1097/00007890-199501270-00010
56. Mazariegos GV, Reyes J, Marino IR, Demetris AJ, Flynn B, Irish W, et al. Weaning of immunosuppression in liver transplant recipients. *Transplantation.* (1997) 63:243–9. doi: 10.1097/00007890-199701270-00012
57. Devlin J, Doherty D, Thomson L, Wong T, Donaldson P, Portmann B, et al. Defining the outcome of immunosuppression withdrawal after liver transplantation. *Hepatology.* (1998) 27:926–33. doi: 10.1002/hep.510270406
58. Takatsuki M, Uemoto S, Inomata Y, Egawa H, Kiuchi T, Fujita S, et al. Weaning of immunosuppression in living donor liver transplant recipients. *Transplantation.* (2001) 72:449–54. doi: 10.1097/00007890-200108150-00016
59. Oike F, Yokoi A, Nishimura E, Ogura Y, Fujimoto Y, Kasahara M, et al. Complete withdrawal of immunosuppression in living donor liver transplantation. *Transpl Proc.* (2002) 34:1521. doi: 10.1016/S0041-1345(02)02980-9
60. Pons JA, Yelamos J, Ramirez P, Oliver-Bonet M, Sanchez A, Rodriguez-Gago M, et al. Endothelial cell chimerism does not influence allograft tolerance in liver transplant patients after withdrawal of immunosuppression. *Transplantation.* (2003) 75:1045–7. doi: 10.1097/01.TP.0000058472.71775.7D
61. Hurwitz M, Desai DM, Cox KL, Berquist WE, Esquivel CO, Millan MT. Complete immunosuppressive withdrawal as a uniform approach to post-transplant lymphoproliferative disease in pediatric liver transplantation. *Pediatr Transplant.* (2004) 8:267–72. doi: 10.1111/j.1399-3046.2004.00129.x
62. Eason JD, Cohen AJ, Nair S, Alcantera T, Loss GE. Tolerance: is it worth the risk? *Transplantation.* (2005) 79:1157–9. doi: 10.1097/01.TP.0000162084.46555.10
63. Tryphonopoulos P, Tzakis AG, Weppler D, Garcia-Morales R, Kato T, Madariaga JR, et al. The role of donor bone marrow infusions in withdrawal of immunosuppression in adult liver allotransplantation. *Am J Transplant.* (2005) 5:608–13. doi: 10.1111/j.1600-6143.2004.00743.x
64. Tisone G, Orlando G, Cardillo A, Palmieri G, Manzia TM, Baiocchi L, et al. Complete weaning off immunosuppression in HCV liver transplant recipients is feasible and favourably impacts on the progression of disease recurrence. *J Hepatol.* (2006) 44:702–9. doi: 10.1016/j.jhep.2005.11.047
65. Martinez-Llordella M, Lozano JJ, Puig-Pey I, Orlando G, Tisone G, Lerut J, et al. Using transcriptional profiling to develop a diagnostic test of operational tolerance in liver transplant recipients. *J Clin Invest.* (2008) 118:2845–57. doi: 10.1172/JCI35342
66. Manzia TM, Angelico R, Baiocchi L, Toti L, Ciano P, Palmieri G, et al. The tor vergata weaning of immunosuppression protocols in stable hepatitis C virus liver transplant patients: the 10-year follow-up. *Transpl Int.* (2013) 26:259–66. doi: 10.1111/tri.12023
67. Assy N, Adams PC, Myers P, Simon V, Ghent CN. A randomised controlled trial of total immunosuppression withdrawal in stable liver transplant recipients. *Gut.* (2007) 56:304–6. doi: 10.1136/gut.2006.107862
68. Lee JH, Lee SK, Lee HJ, Seo JM, Joh JW, Kim SJ, et al. Withdrawal of immunosuppression in pediatric liver transplant recipients in Korea. *Yonsei Med J.* (2009) 50:784–8. doi: 10.3349/ymj.2009.50.6.784
69. Feng S, Ekong UD, Lobritto SJ, Demetris AJ, Roberts JP, Rosenthal P, et al. Complete immunosuppression withdrawal and subsequent allograft function among pediatric recipients of parental living donor liver transplants. *JAMA.* (2012) 307:283–93. doi: 10.1001/jama.2011.2014
70. de la Garza RG, Sarobe P, Merino J, Lasarte JJ, D'Avola D, Belsue V, et al. Trial of complete weaning from immunosuppression for liver transplant recipients: factors predictive of tolerance. *Liver Transpl.* (2013) 19:937–44. doi: 10.1002/lt.23686
71. Benitez C, Londono MC, Miquel R, Manzia TM, Abraldes JG, Lozano JJ, et al. Prospective multicenter clinical trial of immunosuppressive drug withdrawal in stable adult liver transplant recipients. *Hepatology.* (2013) 58:1824–35. doi: 10.1002/hep.26426
72. Bohne F, Londono MC, Benitez C, Miquel R, Martinez-Llordella M, Russo C, et al. HCV-induced immune responses influence the development of operational tolerance after liver transplantation in humans. *Sci Transl Med.* (2014) 6:242ra81. doi: 10.1126/scitranslmed.3008793
73. Lin NC, Wang HK, Yeh YC, Liu CP, Loong CC, Tsai HL, et al. Minimization or withdrawal of immunosuppressants in pediatric liver transplant recipients. *J Pediatr Surg.* (2015) 50:2128–33. doi: 10.1016/j.jpedsurg.2015.08.043
74. Levitsky J, Burrell BE, Kanaparthi S, Turka LA, Kurian S, Sanchez-Fueyo A, et al. Immunosuppression withdrawal in liver transplant recipients on sirolimus. *Hepatology.* (2019) doi: 10.1002/hep.31036. [Epub ahead of print].
75. Shaked A, DesMarais MR, Kopetskie H, Feng S, Punch JD, Levitsky J, et al. Outcomes of immunosuppression minimization and withdrawal early after liver transplantation. *Am J Transplant.* (2019) 19:1397–409. doi: 10.1111/ajt.15205
76. Billingham RE, Brent L, Medawar PB. Actively acquired tolerance of foreign cells. *Nature.* (1953) 172:603–6. doi: 10.1038/172603a0
77. Slavin S, Strober S, Fuks Z, Kaplan HS. Induction of specific tissue transplantation tolerance using fractionated total lymphoid irradiation in adult mice: long-term survival of allogeneic bone marrow and skin grafts. *J Exp Med.* (1977) 146:34–48. doi: 10.1084/jem.146.1.34
78. Ildstad ST, Sachs DH. Reconstitution with syngeneic plus allogeneic or xenogeneic bone marrow leads to specific acceptance of allografts or xenografts. *Nature.* (1984) 307:168–70. doi: 10.1038/307168a0
79. Kaneku H, O'Leary JG, Banuelos N, Jennings LW, Susskind BM, Klintmalm GB, et al. *De novo* donor-specific HLA antibodies decrease patient and graft survival in liver transplant recipients. *Am J Transplant.* (2013) 13:1541–8. doi: 10.1111/ajt.12212
80. Jucaud V, Shaked A, DesMarais M, Sayre P, Feng S, Levitsky J, et al. Prevalence and Impact of *de novo* donor-specific antibodies during a multicenter immunosuppression withdrawal trial in adult liver transplant recipients. *Hepatology.* (2019) 69:1273–86. doi: 10.1002/hep.30281
81. Schroeder HW Jr., Cavacini L. Structure and function of immunoglobulins. *J Allergy Clin Immunol.* (2010) 125(Suppl. 2):S41–52. doi: 10.1016/j.jaci.2009.09.046

82. O'Leary JG, Kaneku H, Banuelos N, Jennings LW, Klintmalm GB, Terasaki PI. Impact of IgG3 subclass and C1q-fixing donor-specific HLA alloantibodies on rejection and survival in liver transplantation. *Am J Transplant.* (2015) 15:1003–13. doi: 10.1111/ajt.13153
83. Jackson AM, Kanaparthi S, Burrell BE, Lucas DP, Vega RM, Demetris AJ, et al. IgG4 donor-specific HLA antibody profile is associated with subclinical rejection in stable pediatric liver recipients. *Am J Transplant.* (2020) 20:513–24. doi: 10.1111/ajt.15621
84. Feng S, Bucuvalas JC, Demetris AJ, Burrell BE, Spain KM, Kanaparthi S, et al. Evidence of chronic allograft injury in liver biopsies from long-term pediatric recipients of liver transplants. *Gastroenterology.* (2018) 155:1838–51.e7. doi: 10.1053/j.gastro.2018.08.023
85. Duquesnoy RJ. HLA epitopes and tolerance induction protocols. *Am J Transplant.* (2014) 14:2667. doi: 10.1111/ajt.12960
86. Meszaros M, Dubois V, Niemann M, Ursic-Bedoya J, Faure S, Guillaud O, et al. Class II human leukocyte antigen epitope mismatch predicts *de novo* donor-specific antibody formation after liver transplantation. *Liver Transpl.* (2019) 25:184–5. doi: 10.1002/lt.25357
87. Kubal CA, Mangus R, Ekser B, Mihaylov P, Ceballos B, Higgins N, et al. Class II human leukocyte antigen epitope mismatch predicts *de novo* donor-specific antibody formation after liver transplantation. *Liver Transpl.* (2018) 24:1101–8. doi: 10.1002/lt.25286
88. Bohne F, Martinez-Llordella M, Lozano JJ, Miquel R, Benitez C, Londono MC, et al. Intra-graft expression of genes involved in iron homeostasis predicts the development of operational tolerance in human liver transplantation. *J Clin Invest.* (2012) 122:368–82. doi: 10.1172/JCI59411
89. Taubert R, Danger R, Londono MC, Christakoudi S, Martinez-Picola M, Rimola A, et al. Hepatic infiltrates in operational tolerant patients after liver transplantation show enrichment of regulatory T cells before proinflammatory genes are downregulated. *Am J Transplant.* (2016) 16:1285–93. doi: 10.1111/ajt.13617
90. Mazariegos GV, Zahorchak AF, Reyes J, Ostrowski L, Flynn B, Zeevi A, et al. Dendritic cell subset ratio in peripheral blood correlates with successful withdrawal of immunosuppression in liver transplant patients. *Am J Transplant.* (2003) 3:689–96. doi: 10.1034/j.1600-6143.2003.00109.x
91. Li L, Wozniak LJ, Rodder S, Heish S, Talisetti A, Wang Q, et al. A common peripheral blood gene set for diagnosis of operational tolerance in pediatric and adult liver transplantation. *Am J Transplant.* (2012) 12:1218–28. doi: 10.1111/j.1600-6143.2011.03928.x
92. Jhun J, Lee SH, Lee SK, Kim HY, Jung ES, Kim DG, et al. Serial monitoring of immune markers being represented regulatory T Cell/T helper 17 cell ratio: indicating tolerance for tapering immunosuppression after liver transplantation. *Front Immunol.* (2018) 9:352. doi: 10.3389/fimmu.2018.00352
93. Segall M, Noreen H, Edwins L, Haake R, Shu XO, Kersey J. Lack of correlation of MLC reactivity with acute graft-versus-host disease and mortality in unrelated donor bone marrow transplantation. *Hum Immunol.* (1996) 49:49–55. doi: 10.1016/0198-8859(96)00055-9
94. Thomson AW, Mazariegos GV, Reyes J, Donnenberg VS, Donnenberg AD, Bentlejewski C, et al. Monitoring the patient off immunosuppression. Conceptual framework for a proposed tolerance assay study in liver transplant recipients. *Transplantation.* (2001) 72(Suppl. 8):S13–22.
95. Truong DQ, Cornet A, Wieers G, Robert A, Reding R, Latinne D. Pre- and post-transplant monitoring of granzyme B enzyme-linked immunosorbent spot assay in pediatric liver recipients. *Transpl Immunol.* (2008) 19:215–9. doi: 10.1016/j.trim.2008.06.001
96. Nasr M, Sigdel T, Sarwal M. Advances in diagnostics for transplant rejection. *Expert Rev Mol Diagn.* (2016) 16:1121–32. doi: 10.1080/14737159.2016.1239530
97. Wells AD, Gudmundsdottir H, Turka LA. Following the fate of individual T cells throughout activation and clonal expansion. Signals from T cell receptor and CD28 differentially regulate the induction and duration of a proliferative response. *J Clin Invest.* (1997) 100:3173–83. doi: 10.1172/JCI119873
98. Tanaka Y, Tashiro H, Onoe T, Ide K, Ishiyama K, Ohdan H. Optimization of immunosuppressive therapy based on a multiparametric mixed lymphocyte reaction assay reduces infectious complications and mortality in living donor liver transplant recipients. *Transplant Proc.* (2012) 44:555–9. doi: 10.1016/j.transproceed.2012.01.038
99. Tanaka Y, Ohdan H, Onoe T, Asahara T. Multiparameter flow cytometric approach for simultaneous evaluation of proliferation and cytokine-secreting activity in T cells responding to allo-stimulation. *Immunol Invest.* (2004) 33:309–24. doi: 10.1081/IMM-120038079
100. Tanaka Y, Ohdan H, Onoe T, Mitsuta H, Tashiro H, Itamoto T, et al. Low incidence of acute rejection after living-donor liver transplantation: immunologic analyses by mixed lymphocyte reaction using a carboxyfluorescein diacetate succinimidyl ester labeling technique. *Transplantation.* (2005) 79:1262–7. doi: 10.1097/01.TP.0000161667.99145.20
101. Sakai H, Ishiyama K, Tanaka Y, Ide K, Ohira M, Tahara H, et al. Potential benefit of mixed lymphocyte reaction assay-based immune monitoring after living donor liver transplantation for recipients with autoimmune hepatitis. *Transplant Proc.* (2014) 46:785–9. doi: 10.1016/j.transproceed.2013.11.123
102. Takeda K, Sawada Y, Kumamoto T, Matsuyama R, Tanaka Y, Ohdan H, et al. Successful multidisciplinary treatment of refractory cytomegalovirus infection after living donor liver transplantation using mixed lymphocyte reactions: report of a case. *Clin J Gastroenterol.* (2016) 9:38–42. doi: 10.1007/s12328-016-0627-x
103. Tahara H, Tanaka Y, Ishiyama K, Ide K, Shishida M, Irei T, et al. Successful hepatitis B vaccination in liver transplant recipients with donor-specific hyporesponsiveness. *Transpl Int.* (2009) 22:805–13. doi: 10.1111/j.1432-2277.2009.00864.x
104. Ide K, Tanaka Y, Onoe T, Banshodani M, Tazawa H, Igarashi Y, et al. Evidence for the immunosuppressive potential of calcineurin inhibitor-sparing regimens in liver transplant recipients with impaired renal function. *J Transplant.* (2011) 2011:483728. doi: 10.1155/2011/483728
105. Morris H, DeWolf S, Robins H, Sprangers B, LoCascio SA, Shonts BA, et al. Tracking donor-reactive T cells: evidence for clonal deletion in tolerant kidney transplant patients. *Sci Transl Med.* (2015) 7:272ra10. doi: 10.1126/scitranslmed.3010760
106. DeWolf S, Sykes M. Alloimmune T cells in transplantation. *J Clin Invest.* (2017) 127:2473–81. doi: 10.1172/JCI90595
107. Savage TM, Shonts BA, Lau S, Obradovic A, Robins H, Shaked A, et al. Deletion of donor-reactive T cell clones after human liver transplant. *Am J Transplant.* (2020) 20:538–45. doi: 10.1111/ajt.15592
108. Chattopadhyay PK, Yu J, Roederer M. A live-cell assay to detect antigen-specific CD4+ T cells with diverse cytokine profiles. *Nat Med.* (2005) 11:1113–7. doi: 10.1038/nm1293
109. Frentsch M, Arbach O, Kirchhoff D, Moewes B, Worm M, Rothe M, et al. Direct access to CD4+ T cells specific for defined antigens according to CD154 expression. *Nat Med.* (2005) 11:1118–24. doi: 10.1038/nm1292
110. Ashokkumar C, Talukdar A, Sun Q, Higgs BW, Janosky J, Wilson P, et al. Allospecific CD154+ T cells associate with rejection risk after pediatric liver transplantation. *Am J Transplant.* (2009) 9:179–91. doi: 10.1111/j.1600-6143.2008.02459.x
111. Wolfl M, Kuball J, Ho WY, Nguyen H, Manley TJ, Bleakley M, et al. Activation-induced expression of CD137 permits detection, isolation, and expansion of the full repertoire of CD8+ T cells responding to antigen without requiring knowledge of epitope specificities. *Blood.* (2007) 110:201–10. doi: 10.1182/blood-2006-11-056168
112. Schoenbrunn A, Frentsch M, Kohler S, Keye J, Dooms H, Moewes B, et al. A converse 4-1BB and CD40 ligand expression pattern delineates activated regulatory T cells (Treg) and conventional T cells enabling direct isolation of alloantigen-reactive natural Foxp3+ treg. *J Immunol.* (2012) 189:5985–94. doi: 10.4049/jimmunol.1201090
113. Nowak A, Lock D, Bacher P, Hohnstein T, Vogt K, Gottfreund J, et al. CD137+CD154- expression as a regulatory T cell (Treg)-specific activation signature for identification and sorting of stable human tregs from *in vitro* expansion cultures. *Front Immunol.* (2018) 9:199. doi: 10.3389/fimmu.2018.00199
114. Sakaguchi S, Fukuma K, Kuribayashi K, Masuda T. Organ-specific autoimmune diseases induced in mice by elimination of T cell subset. I. Evidence for the active participation of T cells in natural self-tolerance; deficit of a T cell subset as a possible cause of autoimmune disease. *J Exp Med.* (1985) 161:72–87. doi: 10.1084/jem.161.1.72
115. Sakaguchi S, Sakaguchi N, Asano M, Itoh M, Toda M. Immunologic self-tolerance maintained by activated T cells expressing IL-2 receptor alpha-chains (CD25). Breakdown of a single mechanism of self-tolerance causes various autoimmune diseases. *J Immunol.* (1995) 155:1151–64.
116. Hori S, Nomura T, Sakaguchi S. Control of regulatory T cell development by the transcription factor Foxp3. *Science.* (2003) 299:1057–61. doi: 10.1126/science.1079490
117. Brunstein CG, Miller JS, Cao Q, McKenna DH, Hippen KL, Curtsinger J,

et al. Infusion of *ex vivo* expanded T regulatory cells in adults transplanted with umbilical cord blood: safety profile and detection kinetics. *Blood.* (2011) 117:1061–70. doi: 10.1182/blood-2010-07-293795
118. Di Ianni M, Falzetti F, Carotti A, Terenzi A, Castellino F, Bonifacio E, et al. Tregs prevent GVHD and promote immune reconstitution in HLA-haploidentical transplantation. *Blood.* (2011) 117:3921–8. doi: 10.1182/blood-2010-10-311894
119. Edinger M, Hoffmann P. Regulatory T cells in stem cell transplantation: strategies and first clinical experiences. *Curr Opin Immunol.* (2011) 23:679–84. doi: 10.1016/j.coi.2011.06.006
120. Todo S, Yamashita K, Goto R, Zaitsu M, Nagatsu A, Oura T, et al. A pilot study of operational tolerance with a regulatory T-cell-based cell therapy in living donor liver transplantation. *Hepatology.* (2016) 64:632–43. doi: 10.1002/hep.28459
121. Todo S, Yamashita K. Anti-donor regulatory T cell therapy in liver transplantation. *Hum Immunol.* (2018) 79:288–93. doi: 10.1016/j.humimm.2017.12.010
122. Safinia N, Grageda N, Scotta C, Thirkell S, Fry LJ, Vaikunthanathan T, et al. Cell therapy in organ transplantation: our experience on the clinical translation of regulatory T cells. *Front Immunol.* (2018) 9:354. doi: 10.3389/fimmu.2018.00354
123. Tang Q, Vincenti F. Transplant trials with tregs: perils and promises. *J Clin Invest.* (2017) 127:2505–12. doi: 10.1172/JCI90598
124. Buchholz BM, Ferguson JW, Schnitzbauer AA, Nightingale P, Schlitt HJ, Geissler EK, et al. Randomized sirolimus-based early calcineurin inhibitor reduction in liver transplantation: impact on renal function. *Transplantation.* (2019) 104:1003–18. doi: 10.1097/TP.0000000000002980
125. Saliba F, Duvoux C, Gugenheim J, Kamar N, Dharancy S, Salame E, et al. Efficacy and safety of everolimus and mycophenolic acid with early tacrolimus withdrawal after liver transplantation: a multicenter randomized trial. *Am J Transplant.* (2017) 17:1843–52. doi: 10.1111/ajt.14212
126. Glover TE, Watson CJ, Gibbs P, Bradley JA, Ntzani EE, Kosmoliaptsis V. Conversion from calcineurin to mammalian target of rapamycin inhibitors in liver transplantation: a meta-analysis of randomized controlled trials. *Transplantation.* (2016) 100:621–9. doi: 10.1097/TP.0000000000001006
127. Wu YM, Joseph B, Gupta S. Immunosuppression using the mTOR inhibition mechanism affects replacement of rat liver with transplanted cells. *Hepatology.* (2006) 44:410–9. doi: 10.1002/hep.21277
128. Semela D, Piguet AC, Kolev M, Schmitter K, Hlushchuk R, Djonov V, et al. Vascular remodeling and antitumoral effects of mTOR inhibition in a rat model of hepatocellular carcinoma. *J Hepatol.* (2007) 46:840–8. doi: 10.1016/j.jhep.2006.11.021
129. Villanueva A, Chiang DY, Newell P, Peix J, Thung S, Alsinet C, et al. Pivotal role of mTOR signaling in hepatocellular carcinoma. *Gastroenterology.* (2008) 135:1972–198411. doi: 10.1053/j.gastro.2008.08.008
130. Grigg SE, Sarri GL, Gow PJ, Yeomans ND. Systematic review with meta-analysis: sirolimus- or everolimus-based immunosuppression following liver transplantation for hepatocellular carcinoma. *Aliment Pharmacol Ther.* (2019) 49:1260–73. doi: 10.1111/apt.15253
131. Tanimine N, Turka LA, Priyadharshini B. Navigating T cell immunometabolism in transplantation. *Transplantation.* (2017) 102:230–9. doi: 10.1097/TP.0000000000001951
132. Yang JY, Sarwal MM. Transplant genetics and genomics. *Nat Rev Genet.* (2017) 18:309–26. doi: 10.1038/nrg.2017.12
133. Brugiere O, Thabut G, Krawice-Radanne I, Rizzo R, Dauriat G, Danel C, et al. Role of HLA-G as a predictive marker of low risk of chronic rejection in lung transplant recipients: a clinical prospective study. *Am J Transplant.* (2015) 15:461–71. doi: 10.1111/ajt.12977
134. Qiu J, Terasaki PI, Miller J, Mizutani K, Cai J, Carosella ED. Soluble HLA-G expression and renal graft acceptance. *Am J Transplant.* (2006) 6:2152–6. doi: 10.1111/j.1600-6143.2006.01417.x
135. Lila N, Carpentier A, Amrein C, Khalil-Daher I, Dausset J, Carosella ED. Implication of HLA-G molecule in heart-graft acceptance. *Lancet.* (2000) 355:2138. doi: 10.1016/S0140-6736(00)02386-2
136. Naji A, Le Rond S, Durrbach A, Krawice-Radanne I, Creput C, Daouya M, et al. CD3+CD4low and CD3+CD8low are induced by HLA-G: novel human peripheral blood suppressor T-cell subsets involved in transplant acceptance. *Blood.* (2007) 110:3936–48. doi: 10.1182/blood-2007-04-083139
137. Thude H, Janssen M, Sterneck M, Nashan B, Koch M. 14-bp ins/del polymorphism and +3142C>G SNP of the HLA-G gene have a significant impact on acute rejection after liver transplantation. *Hum Immunol.* (2016) 77:1159–65. doi: 10.1016/j.humimm.2016.09.009
138. Zhang T, Liu Y, Zeng R, Ling Q, Wen P, Fan J, et al. Association of donor small ubiquitin-like modifier 4 rs237025 genetic variant with tacrolimus elimination in the early period after liver transplantation. *Liver Int.* (2018) 38:724–32. doi: 10.1111/liv.13597
139. Verma S, Tanaka Y, Shimizu S, Tanimine N, Ohdan H. Significant association between FOXP3 gene polymorphism and steroid-resistant acute rejection in living donor liver transplantation. *Hepatol Commun.* (2017) 1:406–20. doi: 10.1002/hep4.1052
140. Millan O, Ruiz P, Orts L, Ferre P, Crespo G, Santana M, et al. Monitoring of miR-181a-5p and miR-155-5p plasmatic expression as prognostic biomarkers for acute and subclinical rejection in *de novo* adult liver transplant recipients. *Front Immunol.* (2019) 10:873. doi: 10.3389/fimmu.2019.00873
141. Revilla-Nuin B, de Bejar A, Martinez-Alarcon L, Herrero JI, Martinez-Caceres CM, Ramirez P, et al. Differential profile of activated regulatory T cell subsets and microRNAs in tolerant liver transplant recipients. *Liver Transpl.* (2017) 23:933–45. doi: 10.1002/lt.24691
142. Vitalone MJ, Wei L, Fujiki M, Lau AH, Littau E, Esquivel C, et al. Liver microRNA profile of induced allograft tolerance. *Transplantation.* (2016) 100:781–90. doi: 10.1097/TP.0000000000001105
143. Morita M, Chen J, Fujino M, Kitazawa Y, Sugioka A, Zhong L, et al. Identification of microRNAs involved in acute rejection and spontaneous tolerance in murine hepatic allografts. *Sci Rep.* (2014) 4:6649. doi: 10.1038/srep06649

15

Progress in Liver Transplant Tolerance and Tolerance-Inducing Cellular Therapies

Xiaoxiao Du[1]*, Sheng Chang*[2]*, Wenzhi Guo*[1]*, Shuijun Zhang*[1] *and Zhonghua Klaus Chen*[2*]

[1] Henan Key Laboratory of Digestive Organ Transplantation, Open and Key Laboratory of Hepatobiliary & Pancreatic Surgery and Digestive Organ Transplantation at Henan Universities, ZhengZhou Key Laboratory of Hepatobiliary & Pancreatic Diseases and Organ Transplantation, Department of Hepatobiliary and Pancreatic Surgery, The First Affiliated Hospital of Zhengzhou University, Zhengzhou, China, [2] Key Laboratory of Organ Transplantation, Institute of Organ Transplantation, Tongji Hospital, Tongji Medical College, Huazhong University of Science and Technology, Ministry of Education, NHC Key Laboratory of Organ Transplantation, Key Laboratory of Organ Transplantation, Chinese Academy of Medical Sciences, Wuhan, China

Correspondence:
Zhonghua Klaus Chen
zc104126@126.com

Liver transplantation is currently the most effective method for treating end-stage liver disease. However, recipients still need long-term immunosuppressive drug treatment to control allogeneic immune rejection, which may cause various complications and affect the long-term survival of the recipient. Many liver transplant researchers constantly pursue the induction of immune tolerance in liver transplant recipients, immunosuppression withdrawal, and the maintenance of good and stable graft function. Although allogeneic liver transplantation is more tolerated than transplantation of other solid organs, and it shows a certain incidence of spontaneous tolerance, there is still great risk for general recipients. With the gradual progress in our understanding of immune regulatory mechanisms, a variety of immune regulatory cells have been discovered, and good results have been obtained in rodent and non-human primate transplant models. As immune cell therapies can induce long-term stable tolerance, they provide a good prospect for the induction of tolerance in clinical liver transplantation. At present, many transplant centers have carried out tolerance-inducing clinical trials in liver transplant recipients, and some have achieved gratifying results. This article will review the current status of liver transplant tolerance and the research progress of different cellular immunotherapies to induce this tolerance, which can provide more support for future clinical applications.

Keywords: tolerance, liver transplantation, operational tolerance, cell therapy, hematopoietic stem cell transplantation, regulatory T cells, regulatory dendritic cells

INTRODUCTION

Liver transplantation has been a preferred option for patients with end-stage liver disease. Since Dr. Starzl performed the first human liver transplantation in 1963, the short-term survival rate of liver transplant recipients has improved significantly, which can be attributed to advances in surgical techniques and immunosuppression (IS) agents (1). However, owing to the long-term use of IS agents, complications concerning the cardiovascular and cerebrovascular systems, diabetes, chronic renal insufficiency, infection, or tumors seriously affect the long-term survival of liver transplant recipients (2, 3).

Immunological self-tolerance refers to the ability of a healthy immune system to produce a protective immune response to pathogens and foreign antigens while maintaining tolerance to its own tissues. Therefore, transplant tolerance refers to accepting organs without the need for long-term IS and maintaining protective immunity (4). Tolerance is usually classified as complete immune tolerance, operational tolerance (OT), and prope tolerance, referred to a condition with a low, non-toxic dose of IS (5). In clinical applications, the focus of the study is OT, that is, long-term functional graft survival in a patient not requiring maintenance IS (6).

The liver is an immunologically privileged organ compared to other transplant organs such as the heart, kidney, or pancreas (7). Liver transplant recipients generally maintain a low level of IS and the hepatic graft can provide immunological protection when transplanted in combination with other solid organs (8). Since Calne first recognized the liver tolerance effect (8) in 1969, people have been enthusiastic about the induction of liver immune tolerance.

As the body's largest digestive organ, the liver has two sets of blood supplies, the portal vein and the hepatic artery. It is constantly exposed to enterically-derived blood-borne pathogens, which gives the liver a unique form of immune privilege (9). Numerous sinuses constitute the largest reticuloendothelial system in the human body and contain the largest number of specialized and non-specialized antigen-presenting cells (APC) and cells that maintain liver immune tolerance, including resident macrophages (also known as Kupffer cells), dendritic cells, hepatocytes, hepatic sinusoidal endothelial cells (LSECs), and hepatic stellate cells (HSCs) (10). When pathogen-derived products such as lipopolysaccharides pass through the liver, like an immune filter, their concentration could be reduced 100-fold, enabling the hepatic immune microenvironment to have sufficient capacity to regulate the nature and intensity of its response (11). Numerous immune regulatory mechanisms in the liver, including downregulation of co-stimulatory molecules, secretion of inhibitory cytokines, inhibition of effector T cell activation, and induction of regulatory T cells, predispose the immune response of the liver to tolerance rather than activation (12).

CURRENT STATE IN SPONTANEOUS TOLERANCE

Factually, in liver transplantation, spontaneous tolerance initially came from the casual clinical observation. Owing to poor compliance, infection complications, posttransplant lymphoproliferative disease (PTLD) or doctor's advice, some liver transplant recipients developed spontaneous tolerance after discontinuing IS, which has aroused great interest of transplant researchers. In 1993, Reyes et al. in Pittsburgh reported that 8 liver transplant recipients with poor compliance ceased IS from 0.5 to 11 years after transplantation, but unexpectedly developed OT. Among them, after weaving from IS, 7 recipients maintained good allograft function for 1 to 14.3 years. The remaining recipient underwent liver retransplantation after 7.7 years of IS withdrawal for viral hepatitis. In addition, 6 recipients were shown to have systemic chimerism (13).

Over nearly three decades, many liver transplant centers have conducted clinical trials of IS withdrawal in both adult and pediatric liver transplant recipients. It has been reported that normal liver function was successfully maintained in adult and child liver transplant recipients, with ~20% of patients (6–63%) achieving complete immunosuppressive withdrawal (**Tables 1, 2**) (14–33).

Sanchez-Fueyo et al. of the Hospital Clinic of Barcelona conducted a prospective and multicenter IS withdrawal clinical trial in 98 liver transplant recipients (NCT00647283). Of these, 41 achieved clinical tolerance (41.8%) and 57 developed mild rejection (58.2%), which was followed by remission within 5.6 months. During the 3-year follow-up after IS withdrawal, no significant histological damage was found in liver biopsies of the tolerant recipients. Statistical analysis showed that years post-transplantation correlated positively with tolerance induction and could be the strongest predictor (27).

Comparing with calcineurin inhibitors (CNI), sirolimus, a kind of rapamycin inhibitor (mTOR-I), has no significant drug toxicity, such as nephrotoxicity, hypertension, diabetes, infections and neoplasms (34). Another advantage of sirolimus is its immunomodulatory ability that could facilitate safe IS withdrawal (35). To assess if sirolimus could increase the tolerability in liver transplant recipients, Levitsky et al., at Northwestern University, performed a prospective clinical trial of single sirolimus withdrawal (NCT02062944). They recruited 15 recipients with non-viral or immunological hepatitis more than 3 years after liver transplantation. After 12 months from sirolimus withdraw, it showed that 8 recipients (53%) achieved OT. Of the other 7 patients, 3 failed IS withdrawal, 3 developed moderate cellular rejection (TCMR) on liver biopsies at the end of the study, and 1 was withdrawn from the trial owing to adrenal metastasis of hepatocellular carcinoma (32). The current result showed the OT rate of sirolimus was comparable to CNI-withdrawal studies. Except for free CNI toxicity, whether liver recipients can benefit more from sirolimus withdrawal, it still needs more and larger trials.

For pediatric liver transplant recipients, Feng et al. in the University of California conducted a multicenter, prospective clinical trial of IS withdrawal (WISP-R, NCT00320606). A total of 12 (60%) of the 20 enrolled pediatric recipients achieved clinical tolerance, and during follow-up for more than 2 years after IS withdrawal, the graft function was normal and there was no significant change in biopsy compared with baseline. A total of 3 recipients underwent acute rejection ($n = 2$) or uncertain rejection ($n = 1$) during IS withdrawal, and 4 recipients failed to achieve clinical tolerance owing to uncertain acute rejection within 1 year of drug withdrawal. Their graft function

Abbreviations: IS, immunosuppression; OT, operational tolerance; APC, antigen-presenting cells; NK cells, natural killer cells; PBMC, peripheral blood mononuclear cells; HSCs, hematopoietic stem cells; HSCT, hematopoietic stem cell transplantation; GVHD, graft vs. host disease; Tregs, regulatory T cells; DC, dendritic cells; regDC, regulatory dendritic cells; tolDC, tolerogenic dendritic cells; GM-CSF, granulocyte-macrophage colony-stimulating factor; GMP, Good manufacturing practice.

TABLE 1 | Immunosuppression withdrawal trials (≥10 recipients, single center).

ID	Year	Author	Transplant center	Adult or pediatric	No. of recipients	Donor (DD or LD)	HCV+ or AIH ?	IS	Time from LT to IS withdraw (Years)	Follow-up after IS withdraw (Months)	OT N (%)	Rejecton N (%)	References
/	1997	Mazariegos	Pittsburgh	Both	95	DD	Yes	CsA/AZA/ Pred	8.4 ± 4.7	35.5 (10.1–57.2)	18 (19%)	18 (19%)	(14)
/	1998 2005	Devlin; Girlanda	London	Adult	18	DD	Yes	CsA/AZA/ Pred	7 (5~11)	120	2 (11%)	7 (39%)	(15, 16)
/	2001	Takatsuki	Kyoto University	Pediatric	26	LD	No	TAC	>2	25 (3~69)	6(23%)	16 (25.4%)	(17)
/	2002	Oike	Kyoto University	Pediatric	115	LD	No	TAC	/	4~96	49(42%)	20 (17%)	(18)
/	2005	Eason	New Orleans	Adult	18		Yes	TAC	>0.5	6~12	1 (6%)	11 (61%)	(19)
/	2005 2010	Tryphonopoulos	Miami	Adult	104	DD	Yes	TAC/CsA/ SRL	4.1 ± 0.3	7.27 ± 0.28	23(22%)	71 (68%)	(20, 21)
/	2006 2008	Tisone; Orlando	University of Rome	Adult	34	DD	only HCV+	CsA	5.3 ± 1.7	63.5 ± 20.1	7 (20%)	26 (76.5%)	(22, 23)
/	2007	Assy	Western Ontario	Adult	26	DD	Yes	CsA/AZA	4.6 ± 1.8	12	2(8%)	15 (58%)	(24)
/	2009	Pons	Murcia	Adult	20	DD	No	CsA	40.8 ± 26.4	47.5 (10–131)	8(40%)	6 (30%)	(25)
/	2013	de la Garza	Pamplona	Adult	24	DD	No	TAC/CsA/ SRL	9.3 (6~13.3)	14(8.5~22.5)	15 (63%)	2 (8.3%)	(28)
2011-02-003IA	2015	Lin	Taipei	Pediatric	16	Both	Yes	TAC	7.8 ± 5.4	40.75 ± 5.98	5 (31%)	6 (38%)	(29)
NCT02062944	2019	Levitsky	Transplant Center	Adult	15	Both	No	SRL	8.1 (4.5~12)	18 (12~24)Months	8 (53%)	6 (40%)	(32)

CNI, calcineurin inhibitor; CsA, Cyclosporine A; Pred, prednisone; SRL, sirolimus; DD, deceased donor; LD, living donor; LT, liver transplant; IS, immunosuppression; OT, operational tolerance.

TABLE 2 | Immunosuppression withdrawal trials (≥10 recipients, Mul-Center).

ID	Year	Author	Country	Adult or pediatric	No. of recipients	Donor (DD or LD)	HCV+ or AIH ?	IS	Time from LT to IS withdraw (Years)	Follow-up after IS withdraw (Months)	OT N (%)	Rejection N (%)	References
NCT00647283	2012	Benitez	Spain/UK/Italy	Adults	98	Not mention	No AIH, HCV+ included	TAC/CsA/AZA	8.6 ± 3.9	48.9 ± 7.7	41 (42%)	57 (58%)	(27)
WISP-R, NCT00320606	2012 2017	Feng S	U.S.	Pediatric	20	LD	No	TAC/CsA	8.5 (6.4 ~ 10.75)	48(1 quit at 33.3 Months)	12(60%)	2(10%); 5(25%)not certain rejection	(26, 30)
ITN030ST	2019	Jucaud	U.S.	Adults	31	Not mention	No AIH, HCV+ included	Single CNI	1	14(12.3~24.3)	9(29%)	13(42%)	(31)
ITN030ST A-WISH NCT00135694	2019	Shaked	U.S.	Adults	77	DD	No AIH, HCV+ included	single CNI or antimetabolite	1~2	24	10(18%)	32(42%)	(33)

CNI, calcineurin inhibitor; CsA, Cyclosporine A; Pred, prednisone; SRL, sirolimus; DD, deceased donor; LD, living donor; LT, liver transplant; IS, immunosuppression; OT, operational tolerance.

recovered to normal after increased or restarted IS. Another recipient was withdrawn from the study after IS withdrawal for violating exclusion criteria. Similar to the results of the adult study, the time after transplantation was significantly longer in the tolerance group than in the non-tolerance group, suggesting that the time after transplantation is an important predictor of tolerance formation (26). Of 12 OT recipients followed for 5 years, 9 cases were positive for class I or class II DSA, but no cases resulted in chronic rejection, graft loss, or death. According to the graft biopsy, there was no progressive increase in inflammation or fibrosis, suggesting that liver grafts after immune retreat can maintain stability during a certain period of time (30).

There are also many studies focused on biomarkers that can predict immune tolerance. Bohne, et al. found that recipients with spontaneous tolerance show an increased number of natural killer (NK) cells and γδT cells in peripheral blood. High levels of hepcidin in liver tissues and ferritin in the serum, increased iron deposits in hepatocytes, and high expression of the related liver tissue genes can accurately predict the outcome for a group of independent patients with IS withdrawal (36). Mazariegos et al. showed that the ratio of monocytoid dendritic cells (mDC) and plasmacytoid dendritic cells (pDC) precursors in the peripheral blood of patients with tolerance increased significantly compared to the healthy control group and the IS maintenance group (37). Levitsky et al. also found that, compared with the baseline, the tolerogenic dendritic cells (tolDC), regulatory B cells (Breg), and cell phenotypes associated with chronic antigen presentation in peripheral blood of the OT group was significantly higher than that of the non-OT group. In addition, gene signatures in peripheral blood/biopsy tissue showed that 12/14 LTR could accurately predict tolerance (32). Chruscinski et al. performed a clinical trial (NCT02541916) for the predictive value of gene signatures in peripheral blood/biopsy tissue. Preliminary results suggest that 5 of the 9 patients, consistent with the inclusion criteria, had discontinued IS for more than 2 years (38). However, the feasibility of this method still needs to be verified by adequate prospective, multicenter, large-scale follow-up trials.

Long-term studies on the safety of immunosuppressive IS withdrawal regimens are inconclusive, and most of them lack evidence of invasive liver biopsy. However, direct comparisons of these trials are difficult because of the lack of standardization. According to the current research results, the acute rejection rate after IS withdrawal varies from 12 to 76% (**Tables 1**, **2**), but it is generally moderate and almost reversible. Chronic rejection is rare (0–6%), and the incidence of graft loss owing to rejection is extremely low (39, 40). Over time, however, the prevalence and severity of chronic graft injury such as subclinical rejection, chronic portal inflammation, borderline hepatitis, and/or fibrosis (periportal and/or perivenous) would increase (41–51). Ten years after transplantation, most studies report that normal histology is present in up to 30% of allografts; bridging fibrosis and/or cirrhosis may be equally common, accounting for about 60% (42, 45, 52). The transcriptome analysis of liver tissue revealed an expression profile very similar to that of T-cell mediated rejection (53). Notably, more than 90 percent of patients who stopped IS 20 years after the transplant did not experience rejection (27). To date, there is no definitive data suggesting that progressively abnormal histology leads to loss of liver graft or death of recipient. However, the OT is not a permanent stable state, still needed regular inspection and to deal with in time.

Because of the difficulty to conduct prospective, multicenter, and longitudinal long-term studies on clinical transplant tolerance, the risk of IS withdrawal in liver transplant recipients remains uncertain. However, based upon a broad understanding of liver disease, increased fibrosis in the allograft indicates the development of portal hypertension and associated complications. IS withdrawal alone could make recipients at the risk of re-transplantation after some years, especially for pediatric recipients. Therefore, there is a wide area of research for the development of induced liver tolerance, especially with cell therapies.

HEMATOPOIETIC STEM CELL TRANSPLANTATION (HSCT) FOR THE INDUCTION OF LIVER TRANSPLANTATION TOLERANCE

Mixed hematopoietic chimerism is associated with alloantigen tolerance, a phenomenon first identified by Owen in freemartin cattle (fraternal twins sharing placental circulation retain allogeneic tolerance to each other after birth) in 1945 (54). Subsequently, Kashiwagi and Starzl discovered donor immunoglobulin in the peripheral blood of liver recipients in 1969, proposing the concept of chimerism in human transplantation (55).

In a series of pioneering studies that began in 1961, Till and McCulloch demonstrated that bone marrow consists of a group of cells, known as hematopoietic stem cells (HSCs), which have the ability to self-renew and differentiate into multiple myeloid cell types (56–58). Afterward, Starzl et al. observed persistent multilineage hematopoietic microchimera (defined as <1% donor cells) in both lymphoid and non-lymphoid tissues of long-lived liver or kidney transplant recipients, including patients on IS for many years after transplantation in 1993 (59). Over the past 30 years, many researchers have been exploring ways to induce tolerance of solid organ transplantation (SOT) using HSCT. Both autologous and allogeneic HSCT have been applied to induce transplant tolerance clinically (60–63).

Clinically, hematopoietic stem cells were first harvested from the bone marrow of the ilium (64). In the 1990s, the protocol to mobilize stem cells into peripheral circulation with granulocyte colony-stimulating factor (G-CSF) and isolate from PBMC by magnetic activated cell sorting (MACS) or flow sorting, thereby separating CD34+ cells, greatly amplified the clinical application of HSCT. Subsequent studies show that combination with chemokine receptor 4 antagonist (AMD3100) and G-CSF can mobilize stem cells more effectively (65).

Allogeneic HSCT Inducing Chimerism

After lymphoablation of the recipient, transfusion of allogeneic donor bone marrow can lead to mixed hematopoietic chimerism, where genetically different donor HSCs are implanted into the host and differentiate into donor-derived lymphocytes that coexist with the host. Central tolerance is a key mechanism of allograft tolerance induced by long-term HSCs (66). When donor bone marrow is injected into the host that has undergone lymphoablation, such as total lymphoid irradiation (TLI) and anti-thymocyte globulin (ATG), HSCs are implanted into the recipient bone marrow and thymus for differentiation, and the host immune system is repopulated with various lymphocyte cells from the donor following by the immunoreconstitution. The presence of donor progenitor cells in the thymus leads to the apoptosis of T cells that recognize the donor antigen expressed by the transplanted organ itself without developing and donor-reactive T cells would undergo clonal deletion, so the host can tolerate the allograft (67). The coexistence of host and donor hematopoietic cells is called chimera, and it is this chimera state in the host that drives central tolerance. According to the percentage of hematopoietic cells of donor origin, the chimerism was divided into microchimerism (donor <1%) and two forms of macrochimerism: full chimerism (donor ~100%) and mixed chimerism (donor >1% but <100%) (68). Although central tolerance is the primary mechanism for HSCs-induced tolerance to homo-antigens, it may be incomplete, in part because not all donor antigens are expressed by HSCs in the host thymus. Furthermore, T lymphocytes with low affinity for their own antigens may escape the selection process, thereby entering the peripheral lymphocyte cycle. In fact, peripheral mechanisms are needed to maintain immune tolerance when the self-reactive T cell subsets evade the thymus selection process. In the transplant environment, a mild pre-treatment regimen designed to induce chimerism can also control the survival of mature alloreactive T cells through peripheral regulation mechanisms, resulting in clone deletion, anergy, or apoptosis of the extra-thymic alloreactive T lymphocytes (66, 67, 69–71). Persistent microchimerism may also be an important determinant for long-term graft survival and transplant tolerance (72, 73).

Since the mid-twentieth century, scientists have used HSC transfusion by injecting donor bone marrow to alter host immune responses in a variety of autoimmunity diseases and solid organ transplantation (SOT) (74, 75). The ideal state of clinical transplant tolerance is to combine HSCT with SOT from the same donor to form a stable hematopoietic chimera of donor and recipient (76). However, myeloablative therapy carries significant risks, most notably graft vs. host disease (GVHD) and severe infections, which are too high-risk to be applied in liver transplants routinely. Therefore, researchers investigated protocols for non-myeloablative bone marrow transplant, including co-stimulatory molecules blockade, low dose irradiation, T cell depletion by monoclonal antibody, etc. (77–79). Chimerism has always been the main method of inducing tolerance in renal transplantation. Clinical studies on transplant tolerance induced by bone marrow chimerism in renal allografts have also achieved gratifying results. In 2008, Kawai et al. reported the first successful application of mixed chimerism tolerance in human kidney transplantation without long-term maintenance of IS (80). The authors then reported that 5 out of 10 kidney recipients had achieved transplant tolerance. Although the detectable duration of chimerism was transient, it was observed that donor-specific mixed lymphocyte response

(MLR) and CTL activity decreased *in vitro* and FOXP3 mRNA level increased *in vivo* (81). Based on the enriching of HSC with tolerogenic CD8+/TCR− facilitating cells (FC) and the depleting of GVHD-producing cells, Leventhal et al. performed a clinical trial in 19 patients with uremia undergoing combined HLA-mismatched hematopoietic stem cell/kidney transplantation. Then 12 of them achieved stable chimerism and OT status of 8–48 months without GVHD after IS withdraw (82). Scandling et al. reported that 16 of 22 HLA-matched patients who had received the same treatment regimen established a persistent mixed chimera (>12 months), with successful withdrawal from immunosuppressants. Renal graft function was stable for up to 7 years after withdrawal, and no incidence of GVHD or rejection was observed (83).

In the field of liver transplantation, there have been some case reports and clinical trials with HSCT transfusion. Ringden et al. reported a liver cancer patient who received HSCT from the same donor after liver transplantation, underwent preoperative myeloablation, achieved chimerism, but subsequently died of opportunistic infection (84). Donckier et al. recruited 5 patients with advanced hepatocellular carcinoma (HCC) who underwent living liver transplantation and received donor CD34+ stem cell transfusion based on the induction regimen of non-myeloablative therapy. Two patients successfully stopped IS without allograft rejection. Three patients developed acute cellular rejection after immunosuppressant withdrawal, two of which were given steroid pulse therapy, whereas the other was reintroduced to calcineurin inhibitor (CNI) immunosuppressive therapy, with no observation of macrochimerism (85, 86).

Tryphonopoulos et al. recruited 45 adults who received cadaver livers and subsequently underwent transfusion of donor bone marrow cells on the day of the transplant. IS were discontinued for more than 3 years, starting 3 years after surgery. Acute rejection occurred in 69% of the treated patients, and immunosuppressive therapy was successfully withdrawn in 22.2% of the treated recipients. However, there was no significant increase in the success of withdrawal and chimerism levels, compared to patients who did not receive bone marrow transplants (20). Liver transplantation is mainly performed from cadaver donors, and recipients generally suffer from severe diseases during the perioperative period, as well as postoperative coagulation and circulatory dysfunction, which may lead to serious infection and tumor recurrence.

Surprisingly, Alexander et al. reported a successful case that a 9-year-old girl with type O, RhD negative underwent RhD blood type conversion to positive after receiving the liver graft of a male donor with type O, RhD positive. Furthermore, CD19 + B cells (XY) were found in the sample of bone marrow puncture. Peripheral blood lymphocyte analysis showed that 94% of T cells came from male and 6% from female; 98% of the B cells came from male and 2% from female; 100% of the granulocytes and NK cells came from male. These results support the formation of chimera. When IS was withdrawn 14 months after transplantation, both the graft and the recipient were healthy for 5 years without GVHD or acute rejection. This indicates that fully tolerated chimera can still occur under certain conditions (87).

For the application of allogeneic HSCT in liver transplant tolerance and chimerism, there are some challenges to overcome, e.g., the risk of serious infection, coagulation and circulatory dysfunction following the myeloablative, the tumor recurrence and the permanence of existence in recipient.

Autologous HSCT Inducing Chimerism

Autologous HSCT is performed by pre-collecting and cryo-preserving autologous bone marrow or peripheral blood stem cells isolated from the patient and then re-transfusing after myeloablative treatment to reconstruct the immune system, which could lead to a more tolerant immune system (88, 89). In autologous stem cell transplantation, the cells come from the recipient, which theoretically prevents the possibility of immune rejection or GVHD. Moreover, autologous bone marrow or peripheral stem cells are easier to obtain and store.

Although there are some differences between allogeneic and autologous HSCT with regard to tolerance mechanisms, they both attempt to reconstruct the recipient immune system and achieve immune tolerance through "re-education." The basic principle of autologous HSCT is to first eliminate reactive and memory immunity and then regenerate the immune system; that is, to exhaust autoreactive and memory T and B cells through a myeloablative or non-myeloablative regimen, followed by reconstruction of immune tolerance (89, 90). The immune monitoring analyses have shown that this can recreate new auto-tolerant immune T and B cell banks, enhance immune regulation mechanisms, and induce changes in the recipient's anti-inflammatory environment (63, 91–95). Muraro et al. found a large number of new T cell clones emerged after autologous HSCT in patients with multiple sclerosis (MS), substituting for the original T cell receptor (TCR) bank and showing a greater diversity of TCR spectrum (63). The immune cell gene expression profiles showed that the number of CD3 + cells remained low after autologous HSCT, and the number of CD8 + cells could return to normal after 3 months postoperatively (92). Another important phenotypic observation is that the recipient's CD4 + CD25 + FoxP3 + regulatory T cells (Tregs) were significantly increased (96–98) and so were the CD8 + Foxp3 + Tregs (99), compared to the preoperative state. The ratio of Bregs increased briefly after autologous HSCT and remained at a higher level for at least 2 years after transplantation, suggesting that Bregs may be involved in the reconstruction of self-tolerance after AHSCT (95, 100). In addition, a variety of cells, such as IL-2, IL-4, IL-6, IL-8, IL-10, IL-17, IL-18, IFN-γ, TNF-α, and TGF-β play an essential role in immune reconstruction and regulation (95, 97).

In recent years, autologous HSCT has been used in clinical trials to eliminate various types of refractory autoimmune diseases such as multiple sclerosis, systemic sclerosis (SSc), systemic lupus erythematous (SLE), rheumatoid arthritis (RA), Crohn's disease, juvenile arthritis, and type 1 diabetes (T1D), presenting better results than traditional therapies and showing promising prospects for long-term remission of autoimmune diseases without IS (90, 93, 95, 101–105). At present, autologous HSCT has also been widely used in various types of liver cirrhosis, improving liver function in varying degrees (106–109). Coupled with the study of transplant animal models, these studies provide abundant theoretical basis for expanding autologous HSCT application in organ transplantation (110–112).

In Toronto University (Canada), Levy et al. have performed a clinical trial on autologous HSCT for allogeneic organ transplant tolerance (ASCOTT) (NCT02549586) (38). Six liver transplant recipients were recruited, five of whom were enrolled. The HSCs of patients were mobilized, purified, and cryopreserved ahead of liver transplant. After immune ablation (Busulfan + Cyclophosphamide + rabbit anti-thymocyte globulin), the patients received autologous HSCT and liver transplantation. IS was withdrawn in five patients with evidence of deletion of alloreactive T cell clones. Two of them were still healthy at 406 and 518 days after HSCT; one died of heart failure at 212 days, one patient received re-transplantation at 166 days after HSCT owing to complications of venous occlusive disease, and one patient died of erythrocytic syndrome at 87 days after HSCT. However, non-hematological toxicity in grades 3–4 was found in almost all patients. It is suggested that there is a certain application prospect of HSCT-induced immune tolerance after liver transplantation, but the potential toxicity is an important problem to be solved.

CD4 + REGULATORY T CELLS IN LIVER TRANSPLANT TOLERANCE

Under physiological conditions, Tregs account for 5–10% of CD4 + T cells in peripheral blood. Tregs are characterized by high stable expression of CD25 and FoxP3, and are divided into natural regulatory T cells (nTreg) produced in the thymus and peripherally induced regulatory T cells (iTreg) (113). Modern research shows that CD4 + Treg is the key to control self-tolerance. The combination can induce peripheral tolerance to autoantigens and alloantigens through a variety of mechanisms, mainly cell-to-cell contact-induced cell lysis, local depletion of IL-2, inhibition of DC maturity, downregulation of DC function, secretion of immunosuppressive cytokines (such as IL-10, IL-35, and TGF-β), etc. (114). In addition, Tregs can migrate to the inflammation site, and their inhibitory activity is usually located in the inflammation site, without significant effects on overall immunity (115).

In rodent models of liver transplantation tolerance, Tregs are present in increased proportion in liver grafts and are involved in the induction of liver tolerance (116, 117). Relevant clinical studies have also shown that, in OT liver transplantation recipients, the proportion of Tregs in peripheral blood and liver, increases, which shows a protective effect on liver allografts (118 119). Therefore, the use of Tregs to mediate transplant tolerance is an important part of transplant immunology research.

Treg adoptive infusion is a method to induce tolerance, where the principle is to tilt the immune response toward Treg dominance, rather than to cause rejection of T effector cells, in order to reduce the dependence of patients receiving solid organ transplantation on immunosuppressant drugs.

It is now generally accepted that the best method to make Treg clinically is to effectively expand it *in vitro* and maintain high purity and inhibitory activity (115). Under certain culture conditions, human Treg can be expanded to 100–1,000 times in 2 weeks (120, 121). The required cell dose varies depending on the type of disease and the presence or absence of combination therapy (115, 122, 123). Treg separation and purification methods mainly include MACS and flow cytometry sorting.

Some researchers have used the chimeric antigen receptor (CAR) technology to produce donor antigen-specific Treg (CAR-Treg) and can overcome the limitation of alloantigen-stimulation-based protocols *in vitro*. In these studies, CARs could be developed to redirect Tregs toward a specific donor leucocyte antigen (HLA) class I molecule (HLA-A2). Unlike HLA class II, the selected donor HLA class I is expressed ubiquitously in grafts. Compared with polyclonal Tregs, CAR-Treg could have better safety, stability, and effectiveness in theory and have strong therapeutic potential to protect allograft (124–127).

Clinical trials of various autoimmune diseases and GVHD have confirmed the safety and feasibility of adoptive Treg infusions (128–131). Clinical reports of adoptive infusion of Treg in kidney transplant recipients have demonstrated the safety of this method in solid organ transplantation, and, through the method of isotope plutonium labeling (^{3}H), it has been found that Tregs can still be detectable for up to 1 year after infusion (132, 133).

Currently, multiple transplant centers around the world are conducting clinical trials of liver transplantation Treg treatment. Todo et al. from the Hokkaido University in Japan, studied 10 liver transplant recipients who received a single dose of donor antigen-specific Treg. Tregs from recipient lymphocytes were amplified by co-culture with irradiated donor cells in the presence of anti-CD80/86 monoclonal antibodies *in vitro* for 2 weeks. CD4 + CD25 + FoxP3 + Tregs were amplified 3–6-fold to 28.1% of CD4 + cells and still maintained inhibitory activity. On the 13th day after the operation, the cells were infused back to the recipient with $0.23\sim6.37 \times 10^6$ cell/Kg intravenously. IS was gradually reduced during 6 months and withdrawn 18 months postoperatively. These recipients were subjected to rigorous monitoring, including liver biopsies, T cell activity assessments, and level of donor-specific antibodies. After 16 to 33 months of follow-up, 7 patients achieved OT without rejection and 4 remained IS-free for 24 months. Mild rejection occurred in 3 patients, and low dose IS was maintained afterward (121).

Safinia et al., at London University (UK), performed a combined I/IIa clinical trial ThRIL (NCT02166177) for the application of Treg immunotherapy in the field of liver transplantation. Tregs were isolated from liver transplant recipients by Good manufacturing practice (GMP) separation technology based on CliniMACS sorting. IL-2 and rapamycin were used for Tregs expansion *in vitro*. A stable Treg population (purity of CD4 + CD25 + FOXP3 + > 95%) can be obtained in 36 days, reaching a sufficient number for its clinical application (120). With stimulation by rapamycin, the amplified Tregs could maintain high levels of FOXP3, CD127lo, and CTLA4, and, with continued expression of CD62L and CXCR3, ensure the stability and functionality of Treg amplification, which could prevent Treg from transforming into Th17 cells in the presence of pro-inflammatory cytokines (134). Nine liver transplant recipients have received autologous polyclonal Treg infusions, showing that the procedure is safe, does not increase the incidence of infection or cancer, and can temporarily increase circulating Treg pools and reduce anti-donor T cell reaction (135).

The current research has opened the door for adoptive infusion of Treg in liver transplantation induction therapy, showing good application prospects. Subsequent research may need to focus on isolation purity, functional induction, CAR-Treg, and clinical induction protocols for OT of Treg *in vitro*.

REGULATORY DENDRITIC CELLS IN LIVER TRANSPLANT TOLERANCE

In 1973, Steinman et al. found a cell type with a "star shape," or dendritic morphology, found in the preparation of adherent spleen cells and named dendritic cell (DC) (136). It has been recognized that DCs are a group of highly heterogeneous cell populations derived from the myeloid or lymphoid, which are widely distributed in all tissues and organs and are the most powerful APC in the body, regulating both innate and adaptive immunity and playing an important role in promoting self-tolerance in healthy homeostasis (137, 138). In humans, according to their cell morphology and function, DCs are divided into two mean lineages of CD11c + conventional DCs (cDCs) (HLA-DR + CD11c +) and CD11c- plasmocyte-like DCs (pDCs) (HLA-DR + CD123 +) (139).

In 1996, Steptoe and Thomson defined the DC population that can induce immune tolerance *in vivo* as tolerogenic DC (tolDC) (140). However, it is still unclear whether tolDCs constitute a particular lineage or just reflect a specific activation state of DCs (141). In 2003, Sato et al. named the tolerogenic DCs they cultured *in vitro* as "regulatory DCs (regDC)," because they had the ability to inhibit T cell activation, induce T cell anergy, and induce Tregs. They could also maintain strong immunoregulatory properties in inflammatory conditions and have the potential to resist multiple immune diseases (142, 143). This nomenclature has also been widely used in classic tolerogenic DCs and their derivatives (144–148). Currently, two methods of naming such tolerant DCs are both widely used. Over the past 20 years, a large number of studies have found that regDCs could be used to treat various autoimmune diseases in animal models, such as T1D, SSc, RA, Cohn's Disease, etc. (149–152), and to induce tolerance of in GVHD and allografts (115, 143, 153, 154). They also have good clinical application prospects in the field of liver transplant tolerance (139, 155).

The phenotypic characteristics of regDC include low expression of MHC class I and II molecules and T cell co-stimulatory molecules (CD80/B7.1, CD86/B7.2, CD40, OX40L), T cell co-inhibition of ligands (such as programmed death Ligand 1 PD-L1), high expression of death-inducing ligands (FasL), and low expression of adhesion molecules (156, 157). Unlike immature DCs, there are indications that tolerability of regDCs is the result of a specific transcription program, rather than the preservation of immature status (158).

RegDCs retain the ability to present antigens to specific T cells, and they can also build up peripheral tolerance through different immunoregulatory mechanisms. These related promotion mechanisms include the following:

- T cell anergy and T cell clonal deletion (159, 160);
- Apoptosis in naive and memory T cells through increased expression of Fas (CD95)/FasL and indoleamine 2,3-dioxygenase (IDO) (161, 162);
- Inducing and expanding regulatory lymphocytes, including Tregs (163, 164) and Bregs (165);
- Producing double negative (CD3 [+] CD4 [−] CD8 [−]) T cells (166);
- Development of tolerance by increasing the expression and release of immune regulatory molecules, such as the anti-inflammatory cytokines IL-10, TGF-b, NO, and HO-1 (167–170), the apoptosis-inducing PD-L 1, PD-L2, and human leukocytes Ag-G (HLA-G), and the tumor necrosis factor (TNF) (161, 164, 171, 172).

Recent studies have shown that exosomes released by regDCs are also involved in the induction and maintenance of peripheral T cell tolerance (172–174).

Although DCs are widely distributed in tissues, their proportion is very low. Immature DCs (imDCs) are tolerogenic in the body, but they are also unstable and may differentiate into immunogenic DCs in inflammatory conditions. Therefore, it is very important to establish a mature system for regDC culture *in vitro* to obtain a sufficient number of functional and stable regDCs.

DCs in the immune system act as "immune checkpoints," with the key role of turning immune signals on or off. A large number of anti-inflammatory and immunosuppressive mediators can promote tolerogenic phenotypes by interfering with DC differentiation or activating checkpoints (157). Researchers have explored different strategies for generating stable regDCs, some of which have been performed in clinical trials, but a consensus hasn't been reached on the best approach yet (115, 157, 172, 175, 176).

Currently, regDCs *in vitro* are mainly derived from rodent bone marrow cells and human peripheral blood mononuclear cells, as it is easier and less invasive than to operate in humans, and abundant DC precursors are also available. Granulocyte-macrophage colony-stimulating factor (GM-CSF) ± IL-4 can be added to fresh or frozen blood mononuclear cells or their precursors to promote the differentiation of myeloid tolDCs (143, 175). Then, one or more anti-inflammatory and immunosuppressive agents should also be added to inhibit their maturation and promote tolerance. These agents include anti-inflammatory cytokines (such as IL-10, TGF-β, TNF-α), anti-inflammatory/IS drugs (CNI, rapamycin, mycophenolate, corticosteroids, or aspirin), Vitamin D3, Prostaglandin E2, retinoids, and HLA-G, tissue factors, such as hepatocyte growth factor (HGF) and vasoactive intestinal peptide (VIP), etc. (139, 143, 153, 177–180).

In rodent and non-human primate transplantation models, adoptive infusion of DCreg prior to transplantation can prolong the survival of allografts and promote specific tolerance to the graft either alone, or in combination with short-term IS (144, 154, 181–183). Clinical trials on the safety and effectiveness of regDC have been conducted for a variety of autoimmune diseases, including T1D, RA, multiple sclerosis (MS), Crohn's Disease (184–188) (NCT02618902, NCT02903537, NCT01352858, NCT00445913), and renal transplant rejection (137) (NCT 0364265, NCT02252055). So far, although there are no long-term results, it has been confirmed that a regDC regimen is safe and feasible without significant side effects, and that the patient's compliance is good. These results provide a good theoretical guide for a regDC therapeutic schedule for liver transplantation.

In Pittsburgh University (USA), Thomson et al. performed a single-center, phase I/II clinical trial on regDC in living donor liver transplantation (NCT03164265). The study recruited low-risk living donor liver transplantation (LDLT) recipients, isolated monocytes from peripheral blood from potential living organ donors, and cultured cells with GM-CSF, IL-4, VitD3, and IL-10 for 7 days *in vitro*. GMP-grade donor-derived regDCs could be induced (153, 189), and a single intravenous infusion of 2.5–10 × 10 ^{6} donor-derived regDCs/kg was administered 7 days before the surgery. Meanwhile, half a dose of mycophenolic acid (MPA) was given, without ATG or Ab. MPA and Tac were administrated within 6 months after transplantation. At 6 months after transplantation, recipients who meet specific criteria [non-rejection and liver function allowance tests (LFTs)] may gradually discontinue MPA. TAC withdrawal assessments are performed 1 year after transplantation and then discontinued gradually to achieve complete IS withdrawal 18 months after liver transplantation. The recipients will be followed up for 3 years from IS withdrawal. During the follow-up period, clinical data and peripheral blood were regularly collected and analyzed to evaluate changes in liver function, renal function, donor-specific antigen (DSA) levels, cardiovascular risk factors, and quality of life. Meanwhile, liver biopsy is to be performed after 1 and 3 years from the withdrawal of IS (146). This study is still in the research stage, but we are looking forward to the results.

Autologous DCs seem to be more feasible than donor-derived DCs, especially for liver transplantation from deceased donors, as it can avoid the risk of sensitization. Autologous regDC infusion with or without donor antigen pulse has shown good tolerogenic effects in animal transplant model studies (179, 190). Some studies have shown that autologous tolDC is more effective than donor DC in delayed transplant rejection (180, 191). Under the leadership of the European Union, in Nantes University (France), Moreau A. et al. conducted a Phase I/II (feasibility/safety) "one study" (www. onestudy.org) on kidney transplant recipients with autologous tolDCs infusion (NCT0225055) (192), and its clinical effects are still being observed.

There are few clinical trials about regDC in the induction of liver transplantation tolerance, and still in the observation stage up to now. As a kind of powerful immune-regulating cell, the prospect of regDC is still thrilling in liver transplantation tolerance. For the successful conversion from preclinical researches to clinical application, researches still have many issues to be studied extensively, such as the further optimization of the regDC induction scheme to extend its half-life, the stability of immunomodulatory function, and the administration scheme of IS. However, the further exploration of methods to induce immune tolerance will also improve our understanding of the biological characteristics of DC and the mechanisms of tolerance.

SUMMARY AND FUTURE DEVELOPMENT

Immune tolerance has always been the "holy grail" in the field of organ transplantation. On the basis of a large number of preclinical studies, various cell therapies could hold promising prospects for inducing liver tolerance. This article reviews the related research and progress regarding spontaneous tolerance and the HSCT, Tregs, and regDCs strategies in the field of liver transplant tolerance. There are many other cells not reviewed that may also have the potential to induce liver transplant tolerance, such as mesenchymal stem cells, regulatory macrophages, regulatory B cells, and bone marrow-derived immunosuppressive cells. At present, the clinical trials of various cell therapies are still in the early stages, and most of them are single-center studies. Thus, there is no clear clinical effect, the purity and stability of cell-induced therapy and its safety for long-term recipients should still be explored for a long time, as many issues need to be observed.

The immune system is extremely delicate and complex. It may be difficult to achieve immune tolerance using only one type of tolerant cell or one mechanism. It may be necessary to consider different mechanisms in combination with different immune cells or drugs. The development of immunologic surveillance and tolerance markers is also critical. This could develop personalized tolerance induction programs for transplant recipients and could guide the timing of immunosuppressive drug withdrawal or early detection of rejection, infection, or tumors.

With the in-depth development of multi-field, multi-disciplinary, and multi-level research, the application of various new experimental methods can provide more possibilities and theoretical guidance for liver transplant tolerance. With the development of multi-center clinical trials, we are optimistic about the good prospects for liver transplant tolerance.

AUTHOR CONTRIBUTIONS

ZC devised this topic. XD wrote the manuscript. ZC, SC, WG, and SZ helped to revise the manuscript. All authors contributed to the article and approved the submitted version.

REFERENCES

1. Starzl TE. The long reach of liver transplantation. *Nat Med.* (2012) 18:1489–92. doi: 10.1038/nm.2927
2. Rabkin JM, de La Melena V, Orloff SL, Corless CL, Rosen HR, Olyaei AJ. Late mortality after orthotopic liver transplantation. *Am J Surg.* (2001) 181:475–9. doi: 10.1016/S0002-9610(01)00595-5
3. Dopazo C, Bilbao I, Castells LL, Sapisochin G, Moreiras C, Campos-Varela I,

et al. Analysis of adult 20-year survivors after liver transplantation. *Hepatol Int.* (2015) 9:461–70. doi: 10.1007/s12072-014-9577-x
4. Lechler RI, Sykes M, Thomson AW, Turka LA. Organ transplantation–how much of the promise has been realized? *Nat Med.* (2005) 11:605–13. doi: 10.1038/nm1251
5. Calne RY. Prope tolerance–the future of organ transplantation from the laboratory to the clinic. *Int Immunopharmacol.* (2005) 5:163–7. doi: 10.1016/j.intimp.2004.09.026
6. Calne RY. The future of organ transplantation: from the laboratory to the clinic. *Philos Trans R Soc Lond B Biol Sci.* (2001) 356:767–71. doi: 10.1098/rstb.2001.0848
7. Crispe IN. Immune tolerance in liver disease. *Hepatology.* (2014) 60:2109–17. doi: 10.1002/hep.27254
8. Calne RY, Sells RA, Pena JR, Davis DR, Millard PR, Herbertson BM, et al. Induction of immunological tolerance by porcine liver allografts. *Nature.* (1969) 223:472–6. doi: 10.1038/223472a0
9. Jenne CN, Kubes P. Immune surveillance by the liver. *Nat Immunol.* (2013) 14:996–1006. doi: 10.1038/ni.2691
10. Thomson AW, Knolle PA. Antigen-presenting cell function in the tolerogenic liver environment. *Nat Rev Immunol.* (2010) 10:753–66. doi: 10.1038/nri2858
11. Lumsden AB, Henderson JM, Kutner MH. Endotoxin levels measured by a chromogenic assay in portal, hepatic and peripheral venous blood in patients with cirrhosis. *Hepatology.* (1988) 8:232–6. doi: 10.1002/hep.1840080207
12. Feng S. Spontaneous and induced tolerance for liver transplant recipients. *Curr Opin Organ Transplant.* (2016) 21:53–8. doi: 10.1097/MOT.0000000000000268
13. Reyes J, Zeevi A, Ramos H, Tzakis A, Todo S, Demetris AJ, et al. Frequent achievement of a drug-free state after orthotopic liver transplantation. *Transplant Proc.* (1993) 25:3315–9.
14. Mazariegos GV, Reyes J, Marino I, Flynn B, Fung JJ, Starzl TE. Risks and benefits of weaning immunosuppression in liver transplant recipients: long-term follow-up. *Transplant Proc.* (1997) 29:1174–7. doi: 10.1016/S0041-1345(96)00535-0
15. Devlin J, Doherty D, Thomson L, Wong T, Donaldson P, Portmann B, et al. Defining the outcome of immunosuppression withdrawal after liver transplantation. *Hepatology.* (1998) 27:926–33. doi: 10.1002/hep.510270406
16. Girlanda R, Rela M, Williams R, O'Grady JG, Heaton ND. Long-term outcome of immunosuppression withdrawal after liver transplantation. *Transplant Proc.* (2005) 37:1708–9. doi: 10.1016/j.transproceed.2005.03.070
17. Takatsuki M, Uemoto S, Inomata Y, Egawa H, Kiuchi T, Fujita S, et al. Weaning of immunosuppression in living donor liver transplant recipients. *Transplantation.* (2001) 72:449–54. doi: 10.1097/00007890-200108150-00016
18. Oike F, Yokoi A, Nishimura E, Ogura Y, Fujimoto Y, Kasahara M, et al. Complete withdrawal of immunosuppression in living donor liver transplantation. *Transplant Proc.* (2002) 34:1521. doi: 10.1016/S0041-1345(02)02980-9
19. Eason JD, Cohen AJ, Nair S, Alcantera T, Loss GE. Tolerance: is it worth the risk? *Transplantation.* (2005) 79:1157–9. doi: 10.1097/01.TP.0000162084.46555.10
20. Tryphonopoulos P, Tzakis AG, Weppler D, Garcia-Morales R, Kato T, Madariaga JR, et al. The role of donor bone marrow infusions in withdrawal of immunosuppression in adult liver allotransplantation. *Am J Transplant.* (2005) 5:608–13. doi: 10.1111/j.1600-6143.2004.00743.x
21. Tryphonopoulos P, Ruiz P, Weppler D, Nishida S, Levi DM, Moon J, et al. Long-term follow-up of 23 operational tolerant liver transplant recipients. *Transplantation.* (2010) 90:1556–61. doi: 10.1097/TP.0b013e3182003db7
22. Tisone G, Orlando G, Cardillo A, Palmieri G, Manzia TM, Baiocchi L, et al. Complete weaning off immunosuppression in HCV liver transplant recipients is feasible and favourably impacts on the progression of disease recurrence. *J Hepatol.* (2006) 44:702–9. doi: 10.1016/j.jhep.2005.11.047
23. Orlando G, Manzia T, Baiocchi L, Sanchez-Fueyo A, Angelico M, Tisone G. The Tor Vergata weaning off immunosuppression protocol in stable HCV liver transplant patients: the updated follow up at 78 months. *Transplant Immunol.* (2008) 20:43–7. doi: 10.1016/j.trim.2008.08.007
24. Assy N, Adams PC, Myers P, Simon V, Minuk GY, Wall W, et al. Randomized controlled trial of total immunosuppression withdrawal in liver transplant recipients: role of ursodeoxycholic acid. *Transplantation.* (2007) 83:1571–6. doi: 10.1097/01.tp.0000266678.32250.76
25. Pons JA, Ramirez P, Revilla-Nuin B, Pascual D, Baroja-Mazo A, Robles R, et al. Immunosuppression withdrawal improves long-term metabolic parameters, cardiovascular risk factors and renal function in liver transplant patients. *Clin Transplant.* (2009) 23:329–36. doi: 10.1111/j.1399-0012.2008.00944.x
26. Feng S, Ekong UD, Lobritto SJ, Demetris AJ, Roberts JP, Rosenthal P, et al. Complete immunosuppression withdrawal and subsequent allograft function among pediatric recipients of parental living donor liver transplants. *JAMA.* (2012) 307:283–93. doi: 10.1001/jama.2011.2014
27. Benitez C, Londono MC, Miquel R, Manzia TM, Abraldes JG, Lozano JJ, et al. Prospective multicenter clinical trial of immunosuppressive drug withdrawal in stable adult liver transplant recipients. *Hepatology.* (2013) 58:1824–35. doi: 10.1002/hep.26426
28. de la Garza RG, Sarobe P, Merino J, Lasarte JJ, D'Avola D, Belsue V, et al. Trial of complete weaning from immunosuppression for liver transplant recipients: factors predictive of tolerance. *Liver Transpl.* (2013) 19:937–44. doi: 10.1002/lt.23686
29. Lin NC, Wang HK, Yeh YC, Liu CP, Loong CC, Tsai HL, et al. Minimization or withdrawal of immunosuppressants in pediatric liver transplant recipients. *J Pediatr Surg.* (2015) 50:2128–33. doi: 10.1016/j.jpedsurg.2015.08.043
30. Feng S, Demetris AJ, Spain KM, Kanaparthi S, Burrell BE, Ekong UD, et al. Five-year histological and serological follow-up of operationally tolerant pediatric liver transplant recipients enrolled in WISP-R. *Hepatology.* (2017) 65:647–60. doi: 10.1002/hep.28681
31. Jucaud V, Shaked A, DesMarais M, Sayre P, Feng S, Levitsky J, et al. Prevalence and impact of de novo donor-specific antibodies during a multicenter immunosuppression withdrawal trial in adult liver transplant recipients. *Hepatology.* (2019) 69:1273–86. doi: 10.1002/hep.30281
32. Levitsky J, Burrell BE, Kanaparthi S, Turka LA, Kurian S, Sanchez-Fueyo A, et al. Immunosuppression withdrawal in liver transplant recipients on sirolimus. *Hepatology.* (2019). doi: 10.1002/hep.31036. [Epub ahead of print].
33. Shaked A, DesMarais MR, Kopetskie H, Feng S, Punch JD, Levitsky J, et al. Outcomes of immunosuppression minimization and withdrawal early after liver transplantation. *Am J Transplant.* (2019) 19:1397–409. doi: 10.1111/ajt.15205
34. Fairbanks KD, Eustace JA, Fine D, Thuluvath PJ. Renal function improves in liver transplant recipients when switched from a calcineurin inhibitor to sirolimus. *Liver Transpl.* (2003) 9:1079–85. doi: 10.1053/jlts.2003.50183
35. Turnquist HR, Raimondi G, Zahorchak AF, Fischer RT, Wang Z, Thomson AW. Rapamycin-conditioned dendritic cells are poor stimulators of allogeneic CD4+ T cells, but enrich for antigen-specific Foxp3+ T regulatory cells and promote organ transplant tolerance. *J Immunol.* (2007) 178:7018–31. doi: 10.4049/jimmunol.178.11.7018
36. Bohne F, Martinez-Llordella M, Lozano JJ, Miquel R, Benitez C, Londono MC, et al. Intra-graft expression of genes involved in iron homeostasis predicts the development of operational tolerance in human liver transplantation. *J Clin Invest.* (2012) 122:368–82. doi: 10.1172/JCI59411
37. Mazariegos GV, Zahorchak AF, Reyes J, Ostrowski L, Flynn B, Zeevi A, et al. Dendritic cell subset ratio in peripheral blood correlates with successful withdrawal of immunosuppression in liver transplant patients. *Am J Transplant.* (2003) 3:689–96. doi: 10.1034/j.1600-6143.2003.00109.x
38. Taner T, Martins PN, Ling Q, Ng KT, Huang KT, Eymard C, et al. What is hot and new in basic and translational science in liver transplantation in 2019? Report of the basic and translational research committee of the international liver transplantation society. *Transplantation.* (2019) 104:516–21. doi: 10.1097/TP.0000000000003058
39. Lerut J, Sanchez-Fueyo A. An appraisal of tolerance in liver transplantation. *Am J Transplant.* (2006) 6:1774–80. doi: 10.1111/j.1600-6143.2006.01396.x
40. Londono MC, Rimola A, O'Grady J, Sanchez-Fueyo A. Immunosuppression minimization vs. complete drug withdrawal in liver transplantation. *J Hepatol.* (2013) 59:872–9. doi: 10.1016/j.jhep.2013.04.003
41. Fouquet V, Alves A, Branchereau S, Grabar S, Debray D, Jacquemin E, et al. Long-term outcome of pediatric liver transplantation for biliary atresia: a 10-year follow-up in a single center. *Liver Transpl.* (2005) 11:152–60. doi: 10.1002/lt.20358
42. Evans HM, Kelly DA, McKiernan PJ, Hubscher S. Progressive histological damage in liver allografts following pediatric liver transplantation *Hepatology.* (2006) 43:1109–17. doi: 10.1002/hep.21152

43. Ekong UD, Melin-Aldana H, Seshadri R, Lokar J, Harris D, Whitington PF, et al. Graft histology characteristics in long-term survivors of pediatric liver transplantation. *Liver Transpl.* (2008) 14:1582–7. doi: 10.1002/lt.21549
44. Hubscher S. What does the long-term liver allograft look like for the pediatric recipient? *Liver Transpl.* (2009) 15(Suppl. 2):S19–24. doi: 10.1002/lt.21902
45. Scheenstra R, Peeters PM, Verkade HJ, Gouw AS. Graft fibrosis after pediatric liver transplantation: ten years of follow-up. *Hepatology.* (2009) 49:880–6. doi: 10.1002/hep.22686
46. Yoshitomi M, Koshiba T, Haga H, Li Y, Zhao X, Cheng D, et al. Requirement of protocol biopsy before and after complete cessation of immunosuppression after liver transplantation. *Transplantation.* (2009) 87:606–14. doi: 10.1097/TP.0b013e318195a7cb
47. Banff Working Group on Liver Allograft P. Importance of liver biopsy findings in immunosuppression management: biopsy monitoring and working criteria for patients with operational tolerance. *Liver Transpl.* (2012) 18:1154–70. doi: 10.1002/lt.23481
48. Miyagawa-Hayashino A, Yoshizawa A, Uchida Y, Egawa H, Yurugi K, Masuda S, et al. Progressive graft fibrosis and donor-specific human leukocyte antigen antibodies in pediatric late liver allografts. *Liver Transpl* (2012) 18:1333–42. doi: 10.1002/lt.23534
49. Briem-Richter A, Ganschow R, Sornsakrin M, Brinkert F, Schirmer J, Schaefer H, et al. Liver allograft pathology in healthy pediatric liver transplant recipients. *Pediatr Transplant.* (2013) 17:543–9. doi: 10.1111/petr.12119
50. Demetris AJ, Isse K. Tissue biopsy monitoring of operational tolerance in liver allograft recipients. *Curr Opin Organ Transplant.* (2013) 18:345–53. doi: 10.1097/MOT.0b013e3283615d48
51. Feng S, Bucuvalas JC, Demetris AJ, Burrell BE, Spain KM, Kanaparthi S, et al. Evidence of chronic allograft injury in liver biopsies from long-term pediatric recipients of liver transplants. *Gastroenterology.* (2018) 155:1838–51 e7. doi: 10.1053/j.gastro.2018.08.023
52. Venturi C, Sempoux C, Quinones JA, Bourdeaux C, Hoyos SP, Sokal E, et al. Dynamics of allograft fibrosis in pediatric liver transplantation. *Am J Transplant.* (2014) 14:1648–56. doi: 10.1111/ajt.12740
53. Londono MC, Souza LN, Lozano JJ, Miquel R, Abraldes JG, Llovet LP, et al. Molecular profiling of subclinical inflammatory lesions in long-term surviving adult liver transplant recipients. *J Hepatol.* (2018) 69:626–34. doi: 10.1016/j.jhep.2018.04.012
54. Owen RD. Immunogenetic consequences of vascular anastomoses between bovine twins. *Science.* (1945) 102:400–1. doi: 10.1126/science.102.2651.400
55. Kashiwagi N, Porter KA, Penn I, Brettschneider L, Starzl TE. Studies of homograft sex and of gamma globulin phenotypes after orthotopic homotransplantation of the human liver. *Surg Forum.* (1969) 20:374–6.
56. Till JE, Mc CE. A direct measurement of the radiation sensitivity of normal mouse bone marrow cells. *Radiat Res.* (1961) 14:213–22.
57. Becker AJ, Mc CE, Till JE. Cytological demonstration of the clonal nature of spleen colonies derived from transplanted mouse marrow cells. *Nature* (1963) 197:452–4. doi: 10.1038/197452a0
58. Seita J, Weissman IL. Hematopoietic stem cell: self-renewal vs. differentiation. *Wiley Interdiscip Rev Syst Biol Med.* (2010) 2:640–53. doi: 10.1002/wsbm.86
59. Starzl TE, Demetris AJ, Trucco M, Murase N, Ricordi C, Ildstad S, et al. Cell migration and chimerism after whole-organ transplantation: the basis of graft acceptance. *Hepatology.* (1993) 17:1127–52. doi: 10.1002/hep.1840170629
60. Sykes M. Hematopoietic cell transplantation for tolerance induction: animal models to clinical trials. *Transplantation.* (2009) 87:309–16. doi: 10.1097/TP.0b013e31819535c2
61. Jenq RR, van den Brink MR. Allogeneic haematopoietic stem cell transplantation: individualized stem cell and immune therapy of cancer. *Nat Rev Cancer.* (2010) 10:213–21. doi: 10.1038/nrc2804
62. Daikeler T, Tichelli A, Passweg J. Complications of autologous hematopoietic stem cell transplantation for patients with autoimmune diseases. *Pediatr Res.* (2012) 71(4 Pt 2):439–44. doi: 10.1038/pr.2011.57
63. Muraro PA, Robins H, Malhotra S, Howell M, Phippard D, Desmarais C, et al. T cell repertoire following autologous stem cell transplantation for multiple sclerosis. *J Clin Invest.* (2014) 124:1168–72. doi: 10.1172/JCI71691
64. Notta F, Doulatov S, Laurenti E, Poeppl A, Jurisica I, Dick JE. Isolation of single human hematopoietic stem cells capable of long-term multilineage engraftment. *Science.* (2011) 333:218–21. doi: 10.1126/science.1201219
65. Pelus LM. Peripheral blood stem cell mobilization: new regimens, new cells, where do we stand. *Curr Opin Hematol.* (2008) 15:285–92. doi: 10.1097/MOH.0b013e328302f43a
66. Khan A, Tomita Y, Sykes M. Thymic dependence of loss of tolerance in mixed allogeneic bone marrow chimeras after depletion of donor antigen. Peripheral mechanisms do not contribute to maintenance of tolerance. *Transplantation.* (1996) 62:380–7. doi: 10.1097/00007890-199608150-00014
67. Elahimehr R, Scheinok AT, McKay DB. Hematopoietic stem cells and solid organ transplantation. *Transplant Rev.* (2016) 30:227–34. doi: 10.1016/j.trre.2016.07.005
68. Wekerle T, Blaha P, Koporc Z, Bigenzahn S, Pusch M, Muehlbacher F. Mechanisms of tolerance induction through the transplantation of donor hematopoietic stem cells: central vs. peripheral tolerance. Transplantation (2003) 75(Suppl. 9):21S-5S. doi: 10.1097/01.TP.0000067947.9 0241.66
69. Mueller DL. Mechanisms maintaining peripheral tolerance. *Nat Immunol.* (2010) 11:21–7. doi: 10.1038/ni.1817
70. Xing Y, Hogquist KA. T-cell tolerance: central and peripheral. *Cold Spring Harb Perspect Biol.* (2012) 4. doi: 10.1101/cshperspect.a006957
71. Salisbury EM, Game DS, Lechler RI. Transplantation tolerance. *Pediatr Nephrol.* (2014) 29:2263–72. doi: 10.1007/s00467-013-2659-5
72. Wood KJ. Passenger leukocytes and microchimerism: what role in tolerance induction? *Transplantation.* (2003) 75(Suppl. 9):17s–20. doi: 10.1097/01.TP.0000067946.90241.2F
73. Szabolcs P, Burlingham WJ, Thomson AW. Tolerance after solid organ and hematopoietic cell transplantation. *Biol Blood Marrow Transplant.* (2012) 18(Suppl. 1):S193–200. doi: 10.1016/j.bbmt.2011.11.005
74. Copelan EA. Hematopoietic stem-cell transplantation. *N Engl J Med.* (2006) 354:1813–26. doi: 10.1056/NEJMra052638
75. Sachs DH, Kawai T, Sykes M. Induction of tolerance through mixed chimerism. *Cold Spring Harb Perspect Med.* (2014) 4:a015529. doi: 10.1101/cshperspect.a015529
76. Fuchs EJ. Transplantation tolerance: from theory to clinic. *Immunol Rev.* (2014) 258:64–79. doi: 10.1111/imr.12154
77. Cobbold SP, Martin G, Qin S, Waldmann H. Monoclonal antibodies to promote marrow engraftment and tissue graft tolerance. *Nature.* (1986) 323:164–6. doi: 10.1038/323164a0
78. Wekerle T, Kurtz J, Ito H, Ronquillo JV, Dong V, Zhao G, et al. Allogeneic bone marrow transplantation with co-stimulatory blockade induces macrochimerism and tolerance without cytoreductive host treatment. *Nat Med.* (2000) 6:464–9. doi: 10.1038/74731
79. Sykes M, Sachs DH. Mixed chimerism. *Philos Trans R Soc Lond B Biol Sci.* (2001) 356:707–26. doi: 10.1098/rstb.2001.0853
80. Kawai T, Cosimi AB, Spitzer TR, Tolkoff-Rubin N, Suthanthiran M, Saidman SL, et al. HLA-mismatched renal transplantation without maintenance immunosuppression. *N Engl J Med.* (2008) 358:353–61. doi: 10.1056/NEJMoa071074
81. Kawai T, Sachs DH, Sykes M, Cosimi AB. HLA-mismatched renal transplantation without maintenance immunosuppression. *N Engl J Med.* (2013) 368:1850–2. doi: 10.1056/NEJMc1213779
82. Leventhal JR, Elliott MJ, Yolcu ES, Bozulic LD, Tollerud DJ, Mathew JM, et al. Immune reconstitution/immunocompetence in recipients of kidney plus hematopoietic stem/facilitating cell transplants. *Transplantation.* (2015) 99:288–98. doi: 10.1097/TP.0000000000000605
83. Scandling JD, Busque S, Shizuru JA, Lowsky R, Hoppe R, Dejbakhsh-Jones S, et al. Chimerism, graft survival, and withdrawal of immunosuppressive drugs in HLA matched and mismatched patients after living donor kidney and hematopoietic cell transplantation. *Am J Transplant.* (2015) 15:695–704. doi: 10.1111/ajt.13091
84. Ringden O, Soderdahl G, Mattsson J, Uzunel M, Remberger M, Hentschke P, et al. Transplantation of autologous and allogeneic bone marrow with liver from a cadaveric donor for primary liver cancer. *Transplantation.* (2000) 69:2043–8. doi: 10.1097/00007890-200005270-00012
85. Donckier V, Troisi R, Toungouz M, Colle I, Van Vlierberghe H, Jacquy C, et al. Donor stem cell infusion after non-myeloablative conditioning for tolerance induction to HLA mismatched adult living-donor liver graft. *Transplant Immunol.* (2004) 13:139–46. doi: 10.1016/j.trim.2004.05.004
86. Donckier V, Troisi R, Le Moine A, Toungouz M, Ricciardi S, Colle

I, et al. Early immunosuppression withdrawal after living donor liver transplantation and donor stem cell infusion. *Liver Transpl.* (2006) 12:1523–8. doi: 10.1002/lt.20872
87. Alexander SI, Smith N, Hu M, Verran D, Shun A, Dorney S, et al. Chimerism and tolerance in a recipient of a deceased-donor liver transplant. *N Engl J Med.* (2008) 358:369–74. doi: 10.1056/NEJMoa0707255
88. Alexander T, Arnold R, Hiepe F, Radbruch A. Resetting the immune system with immunoablation and autologous haematopoietic stem cell transplantation in autoimmune diseases. *Clin Exp Rheumatol.* (2016) 34(4 Suppl. 98):53–7.
89. Arruda LC, Clave E, Moins-Teisserenc H, Douay C, Farge D, Toubert A. Resetting the immune response after autologous hematopoietic stem cell transplantation for autoimmune diseases. *Curr Res Transl Med.* (2016) 64:107–13. doi: 10.1016/j.retram.2016.03.004
90. Snowden JA, Saccardi R, Allez M, Ardizzone S, Arnold R, Cervera R, et al. Haematopoietic SCT in severe autoimmune diseases: updated guidelines of the European Group for Blood and Marrow Transplantation. *Bone Marrow Transplant.* (2012) 47:770–90. doi: 10.1038/bmt.2011.185
91. Sun W, Popat U, Hutton G, Zang YC, Krance R, Carrum G, et al. Characteristics of T-cell receptor repertoire and myelin-reactive T cells reconstituted from autologous haematopoietic stem-cell grafts in multiple sclerosis. *Brain.* (2004) 127(Pt 5):996–1008. doi: 10.1093/brain/awh117
92. Farge D, Henegar C, Carmagnat M, Daneshpouy M, Marjanovic Z, Rabian C, et al. Analysis of immune reconstitution after autologous bone marrow transplantation in systemic sclerosis. *Arthritis Rheum.* (2005) 52:1555–63. doi: 10.1002/art.21036
93. Alexander T, Thiel A, Rosen O, Massenkeil G, Sattler A, Kohler S, et al. Depletion of autoreactive immunologic memory followed by autologous hematopoietic stem cell transplantation in patients with refractory SLE induces long-term remission through de novo generation of a juvenile and tolerant immune system. *Blood.* (2009) 113:214–23. doi: 10.1182/blood-2008-07-168286
94. Dubinsky AN, Burt RK, Martin R, Muraro PA. T-cell clones persisting in the circulation after autologous hematopoietic SCT are undetectable in the peripheral CD34+ selected graft. *Bone Marrow Transplant.* (2010) 45:325–31. doi: 10.1038/bmt.2009.139
95. Malmegrim KCR, Lima-Júnior JR, Arruda LCM, de Azevedo JTC, de Oliveira GLV, Oliveira MC. Autologous hematopoietic stem cell transplantation for autoimmune diseases: from mechanistic insights to biomarkers. *Front Immunol.* (2018) 9:02602. doi: 10.3389/fimmu.2018.02602
96. de Kleer I, Vastert B, Klein M, Teklenburg G, Arkesteijn G, Yung GP, et al. Autologous stem cell transplantation for autoimmunity induces immunologic self-tolerance by reprogramming autoreactive T cells and restoring the CD4+CD25+ immune regulatory network. *Blood.* (2006) 107:1696–702. doi: 10.1182/blood-2005-07-2800
97. Abrahamsson SV, Angelini DF, Dubinsky AN, Morel E, Oh U, Jones JL, et al. Non-myeloablative autologous haematopoietic stem cell transplantation expands regulatory cells and depletes IL-17 producing mucosal-associated invariant T cells in multiple sclerosis. *Brain.* (2013) 136(Pt 9):2888–903. doi: 10.1093/brain/awt182
98. Hendrawan K, Visweswaran M, Ma DDF, Moore JJ. Tolerance regeneration by T regulatory cells in autologous haematopoietic stem cell transplantation for autoimmune diseases. *Bone Marrow Transplant.* (2019) 55:857–66. doi: 10.1038/s41409-019-0710-2
99. Zhang L, Bertucci AM, Ramsey-Goldman R, Burt RK, Datta SK. Regulatory T cell (Treg) subsets return in patients with refractory lupus following stem cell transplantation, and TGF-beta-producing CD8+ Treg cells are associated with immunological remission of lupus. *J Immunol.* (2009) 183:6346–58. doi: 10.4049/jimmunol.0901773
100. Arruda LCM, Oliveira MC, Moraes DA, Covas DT, Voltarelli JC, Malmegrim KCR. THU0501 hematopoietic stem cell transplantation increases naive and regulatory B cells while decreasing memory B cells in systemic sclerosis patients. *Ann Rheum Dis.* (2014) 73:492–509. doi: 10.1136/annrheumdis-2014-eular.4148
101. Snowden JA, Passweg J, Moore JJ, Milliken S, Cannell P, Van Laar J, et al. Autologous hemopoietic stem cell transplantation in severe rheumatoid arthritis: a report from the EBMT and ABMTR. *J Rheumatol.* (2004) 31:482–8.
102. Burt RK, Shah SJ, Dill K, Grant T, Gheorghiade M, Schroeder J, et al. Autologous non-myeloablative haemopoietic stem-cell transplantation compared with pulse cyclophosphamide once per month for systemic sclerosis (ASSIST): an open-label, randomised phase 2 trial. *Lancet.* (2011) 378:498–506. doi: 10.1016/S0140-6736(11)60982-3
103. Hawkey CJ. Hematopoietic stem cell transplantation in crohn's disease: state-of-the-art treatment. *Digest Dis.* (2017) 35:107–14. doi: 10.1159/000449090
104. Leone A, Radin M, Almarzooqi AM, Al-Saleh J, Roccatello D, Sciascia S, et al. Autologous hematopoietic stem cell transplantation in systemic lupus erythematosus and antiphospholipid syndrome: a systematic review. *Autoimmunity Rev.* (2017) 16:469–77. doi: 10.1016/j.autrev.2017.03.008
105. van Megen KM, van 't Wout ET, Forman SJ, Roep BO. A future for autologous hematopoietic stem cell transplantation in type 1 diabetes. *Front Immunol.* (2018) 9:690. doi: 10.3389/fimmu.2018.00690
106. Terai S, Ishikawa T, Omori K, Aoyama K, Marumoto Y, Urata Y, et al. Improved liver function in patients with liver cirrhosis after autologous bone marrow cell infusion therapy. *Stem Cells.* (2006) 24:2292–8. doi: 10.1634/stemcells.2005-0542
107. Pai M, Zacharoulis D, Milicevic MN, Helmy S, Jiao LR, Levicar N, et al. Autologous infusion of expanded mobilized adult bone marrow-derived CD34+ cells into patients with alcoholic liver cirrhosis. *Am J Gastroenterol.* (2008) 103:1952–8. doi: 10.1111/j.1572-0241.2008.01993.x
108. Saito T, Okumoto K, Haga H, Nishise Y, Ishii R, Sato C, et al. Potential therapeutic application of intravenous autologous bone marrow infusion in patients with alcoholic liver cirrhosis. *Stem Cells Dev.* (2011) 20:1503–10. doi: 10.1089/scd.2011.0074
109. Pankaj P, Zhang Q, Bai XL, Liang TB. Autologous bone marrow transplantation in decompensated liver: systematic review and meta-analysis. *World J Gastroenterol.* (2015) 21:8697–710. doi: 10.3748/wjg.v21.i28.8697
110. Gorczynski R, Chen Z, Khatri I, Yu K. Long-term tolerance and skin allograft survival in cd200tg mice after autologous marrow transplantation. *Transplantation.* (2014) 98:1271–8. doi: 10.1097/TP.0000000000000456
111. Gorczynski RM, Sadozai H, Zhu F, Khatri I. Effect of infusion of monoclonal antibodies to tumour necrosis factor-receptor super family 25 on graft rejection in allo-immune mice receiving autologous marrow transplantation. *Immunology.* (2017) 150:418–31. doi: 10.1111/imm.12693
112. Gorczynski RM, Farrokhi K, Gorczynski C, Sadozai H, Zhu F, Khatri I. Importance of B cells to development of regulatory T cells and prolongation of tissue allograft survival in recipients receiving autologous bone marrow transplantation. *Immunology.* (2018) 154:465–75. doi: 10.1111/imm.12895
113. Vaikunthanathan T, Safinia N, Boardman D, Lechler RI, Lombardi G. Regulatory T cells: tolerance induction in solid organ transplantation. *Clin Exp Immunol.* (2017) 189:197–210. doi: 10.1111/cei.12978
114. Vignali DAA, Collison LW, Workman CJ. How regulatory T cells work. *Nat Rev Immunol.* (2008) 8:523–32. doi: 10.1038/nri2343
115. Ten Brinke A, Martinez-Llordella M, Cools N, Hilkens CMU, van Ham SM, Sawitzki B, et al. Ways forward for tolerance-inducing cellular therapies- an AFACTT perspective. *Front Immunol.* (2019) 10:181. doi: 10.3389/fimmu.2019.00181
116. Li W, Zheng XX, Kuhr CS, Perkins JD. CTLA4 engagement is required for induction of murine liver transplant spontaneous tolerance+. *Am J Transpl.* (2005) 5:978–86. doi: 10.1111/j.1600-6143.2005.00823.x
117. Fujiki M, Esquivel CO, Martinez OM, Strober S, Uemoto S, Krams SM. Induced tolerance to rat liver allografts involves the apoptosis of intragraft T cells and the generation of CD4+CD25+FoxP3+T regulatory cells. *Liver Transpl.* (2010) 16:147–54. doi: 10.1002/lt.21963
118. Li Y, Zhao X, Cheng D, Haga H, Tsuruyama T, Wood K, et al. The presence of Foxp3 expressing T cells within grafts of tolerant human liver transplant recipients. *Transplantation.* (2008) 86:1837–43. doi: 10.1097/TP.0b013e31818febc4
119. Pons JA, Revilla-Nuin B, Baroja-Mazo A, Ramirez P, Martinez-Alarcon L, Sanchez-Bueno F, et al. FoxP3 in peripheral blood is associated with operational tolerance in liver transplant patients during immunosuppression withdrawal. *Transplantation.* (2008) 86:1370–8. doi: 10.1097/TP.0b013e318188d3e6
120. Safinia N, Vaikunthanathan T, Fraser H, Thirkell S, Lowe K, Blackmore L, et al. Successful expansion of functional and stable regulatory T cells for immunotherapy in liver transplantation. *Oncotarget.* (2016) 7:7563–77.

doi: 10.18632/oncotarget.6927

121. Todo S, Yamashita K, Goto R, Zaitsu M, Nagatsu A, Oura T, et al. A pilot study of operational tolerance with a regulatory T-cell-based cell therapy in living donor liver transplantation. *Hepatology*. (2016) 64:632–43. doi: 10.1002/hep.28459
122. Gregori S, Passerini L, Roncarolo MG. Clinical outlook for type-1 and FOXP3(+) T regulatory cell-based therapy. *Front Immunol*. (2015) 6:593. doi: 10.3389/fimmu.2015.00593
123. van der Net JB, Bushell A, Wood KJ, Harden PN. Regulatory T cells: first steps of clinical application in solid organ transplantation. *Transpl Int*. (2016) 29:3–11. doi: 10.1111/tri.12608
124. Ellebrecht CT, Bhoj VG, Nace A, Choi EJ, Mao X, Cho MJ, et al. Reengineering chimeric antigen receptor T cells for targeted therapy of autoimmune disease. *Science*. (2016) 353:179–84. doi: 10.1126/science.aaf6756
125. MacDonald KG, Hoeppli RE, Huang Q, Gillies J, Luciani DS, Orban PC, et al. Alloantigen-specific regulatory T cells generated with a chimeric antigen receptor. *J Clin Invest*. (2016) 126:1413–24. doi: 10.1172/JCI 82771
126. Boardman DA, Philippeos C, Fruhwirth GO, Ibrahim MAA, Hannen RF, Cooper D, et al. Expression of a chimeric antigen receptor specific for donor HLA class i enhances the potency of human regulatory t cells in preventing human skin transplant rejection. *Am J Transpl*. (2017) 17:931–43. doi: 10.1111/ajt.14185
127. Noyan F, Zimmermann K, Hardtke-Wolenski M, Knoefel A, Schulde E, Geffers R, et al. Prevention of allograft rejection by use of regulatory T cells with an MHC-specific chimeric antigen receptor. *Am J Transpl*. (2017) 17:917–30. doi: 10.1111/ajt.14175
128. Desreumaux P, Foussat A, Allez M, Beaugerie L, Hebuterne X, Bouhnik Y, et al. Safety and efficacy of antigen-specific regulatory T-cell therapy for patients with refractory Crohn's disease. *Gastroenterology*. (2012) 143:1207–17.e2. doi: 10.1053/j.gastro.2012.07.116
129. Theil A, Tuve S, Oelschlagel U, Maiwald A, Dohler D, Ossmann D, et al. Adoptive transfer of allogeneic regulatory T cells into patients with chronic graft-versus-host disease. *Cytotherapy*. (2015) 17:473–86. doi: 10.1016/j.jcyt.2014.11.005
130. Bayry J, Gautier JF. Regulatory T cell immunotherapy for type 1 diabetes: a step closer to success? *Cell Metab*. (2016) 23:231–3. doi: 10.1016/j.cmet.2016.01.010
131. Thonhoff JR, Beers DR, Zhao W, Pleitez M, Simpson EP, Berry JD, et al. Expanded autologous regulatory T-lymphocyte infusions in ALS. *Neurol Neuroimmunol Neuroinflamm*. (2018) 5:e465. doi: 10.1212/NXI.0000000000000465
132. Chandran S, Tang Q, Sarwal M, Laszik ZG, Putnam AL, Lee K, et al. Polyclonal regulatory T cell therapy for control of inflammation in kidney transplants. *Am J Transplant*. (2017) 17:2945–54. doi: 10.1111/ajt.14415
133. Mathew JM, J HV, LeFever A, Konieczna I, Stratton C, He J, et al. A phase I clinical trial with *ex vivo* expanded recipient regulatory t cells in living donor kidney transplants. *Sci Rep*. (2018) 8:7428. doi: 10.1038/s41598-018-25574-7
134. Fraser H, Safinia N, Grageda N, Thirkell S, Lowe K, Fry LJ, et al. A rapamycin-based GMP-compatible process for the isolation and expansion of regulatory T cells for clinical trials. *Mol Ther Methods Clin Dev*. (2018) 8:198–209. doi: 10.1016/j.omtm.2018.01.006
135. Sanchez-Fueyo A, Whitehouse G, Grageda N, Cramp ME, Lim TY, Romano M, et al. Applicability, safety, and biological activity of regulatory T cell therapy in liver transplantation. *Am J Transplant*. (2019) 20:1125–36. doi: 10.1111/ajt.15700
136. Steinman RM, Cohn ZA. Identification of a novel cell type in peripheral lymphoid organs of mice. I. morphology, quantitation, tissue distribution. *J Exp Med*. (1973) 137:1142–62. doi: 10.1084/jem.137.5.1142
137. Banchereau J, Steinman RM. Dendritic cells and the control of immunity. *Nature*. (1998) 392:245–52. doi: 10.1038/32588
138. Ohnmacht C, Pullner A, King SB, Drexler I, Meier S, Brocker T, et al. Constitutive ablation of dendritic cells breaks self-tolerance of CD4 T cells and results in spontaneous fatal autoimmunity. *J Exp Med*. (2009) 206:549–59. doi: 10.1084/jem.20082394
139. Sato K, Fujita S. Dendritic cells: nature and classification. *Allergol Int*. (2007) 56:183–91. doi: 10.2332/allergolint.R-06-139
140. Steptoe RJ, Thomson AW. Dendritic cells and tolerance induction. *Clin Exp Immunol*. (1996) 105:397–402. doi: 10.1046/j.1365-2249.1996.d01-779.x
141. Takenaka MC, Quintana FJ. Tolerogenic dendritic cells. *Semin Immunopathol*. (2017) 39:113–20. doi: 10.1007/s00281-016-0587-8
142. Sato K, Yamashita N, Baba M, Matsuyama T. Modified myeloid dendritic cells act as regulatory dendritic cells to induce anergic and regulatory T cells. *Blood*. (2003) 101:3581–9. doi: 10.1182/blood-2002-09-2712
143. Sato K, Yamashita N, Yamashita N, Baba M, Matsuyama T. Regulatory dendritic cells protect mice from murine acute graft-versus-host disease and leukemia relapse. *Immunity*. (2003) 18:367–79. doi: 10.1016/S1074-7613(03)00055-4
144. Ezzelarab MB, Zahorchak AF, Lu L, Morelli AE, Chalasani G, Demetris AJ, et al. Regulatory dendritic cell infusion prolongs kidney allograft survival in nonhuman primates. *Am J Transplant*. (2013) 13:1989–2005. doi: 10.1111/ajt.12310
145. Raich-Regue D, Glancy M, Thomson AW. Regulatory dendritic cell therapy: from rodents to clinical application. *Immunol Lett*. (2014) 161:216–21. doi: 10.1016/j.imlet.2013.11.016
146. Thomson AW, Humar A, Lakkis FG, Metes DM. Regulatory dendritic cells for promotion of liver transplant operational tolerance: Rationale for a clinical trial and accompanying mechanistic studies. *Hum Immunol*. (2018) 79:314–21. doi: 10.1016/j.humimm.2017.10.017
147. Thomson AW, Metes DM, Ezzelarab MB, Raïch-Regué D. Regulatory dendritic cells for human organ transplantation. *Transplant Rev*. (2019) 33:130–6. doi: 10.1016/j.trre.2019.05.001
148. Yu H, Tian Y, Wang Y, Mineishi S, Zhang Y. Dendritic cell regulation of graft-vs.-host disease: immunostimulation and tolerance. *Front Immunol*. (2019) 10: 93. doi: 10.3389/fimmu.2019.00093
149. Lutz MB, Suri RM, Niimi M, Ogilvie AL, Kukutsch NA, Rossner S, et al. Immature dendritic cells generated with low doses of GM-CSF in the absence of IL-4 are maturation resistant and prolong allograft survival *in vivo*. *Eur J Immunol*. (2000) 30:1813–22. doi: 10.1002/1521-4141(200007)30:7<1813::AID-IMMU1813>3.0.CO;2-8
150. Thomson AW, Robbins PD. Tolerogenic dendritic cells for autoimmune disease and transplantation. *Ann Rheum Dis*. (2008) 67(Suppl. 3):iii90–6. doi: 10.1136/ard.2008.099176
151. Natarajan S, Thomson AW. Tolerogenic dendritic cells and myeloid-derived suppressor cells: potential for regulation and therapy of liver auto- and alloimmunity. *Immunobiology*. (2010) 215:698–703. doi: 10.1016/j.imbio.2010.05.024
152. Stoop JN, Robinson JH, Hilkens CM. Developing tolerogenic dendritic cell therapy for rheumatoid arthritis: what can we learn from mouse models? *Ann Rheum Dis*. (2011) 70:1526–33. doi: 10.1136/ard.2011.151654
153. Thomson AW, Zahorchak AF, Ezzelarab MB, Butterfield LH, Lakkis FG, Metes DM. Prospective clinical testing of regulatory dendritic cells in organ transplantation. *Front Immunol*. (2016) 7:15. doi: 10.3389/fimmu.2016.00015
154. Ezzelarab MB, Raich-Regue D, Lu L, Zahorchak AF, Perez-Gutierrez A, Humar A, et al. Renal allograft survival in nonhuman primates infused with donor antigen-pulsed autologous regulatory dendritic cells. *Am J Transplant*. (2017) 17:1476–89. doi: 10.1111/ajt.14182
155. Xia MJ, Shan J, Li YP, Zhou YN, Guo YJ, Sun GX, et al. Adoptive transfusion of tolerogenic dendritic cells prolongs the survival of liver allograft: a systematic review. *J Evid Based Med*. (2014) 7:135–46. doi: 10.1111/jebm.12094
156. Raker VK, Domogalla MP, Steinbrink K. Tolerogenic dendritic cells for regulatory T cell induction in man. *Front Immunol*. (2015) 6:569. doi: 10.3389/fimmu.2015.00569
157. Sato K, Uto T, Fukaya T, Takagi H. Regulatory dendritic cells. *Curr Top Microbiol Immunol*. (2017) 410:47–71. doi: 10.1007/82_2017_60
158. Schinnerling K, Garcia-Gonzalez P, Aguillon JC. Gene expression profiling of human monocyte-derived dendritic cells - searching for molecular regulators of tolerogenicity. *Front Immunol*. (2015) 6:528. doi: 10.3389/fimmu.2015.00528
159. Schwartz RH. T cell anergy. *Ann Rev Immunol*. (2003) 21:305–34. doi: 10.1146/annurev.immunol.21.120601.141110

160. Schietinger A, Greenberg PD. Tolerance and exhaustion: defining mechanisms of T cell dysfunction. *Trends Immunol.* (2014) 35:51–60. doi: 10.1016/j.it.2013.10.001
161. Lu L, Qian S, Hershberger PA, Rudert WA, Lynch DH, Thomson AW. Fas ligand (CD95L) and B7 expression on dendritic cells provide counter-regulatory signals for T cell survival and proliferation. *J Immunol.* (1997) 158:5676–84.
162. Mellor AL, Baban B, Chandler P, Marshall B, Jhaver K, Hansen A, et al. Cutting edge: induced indoleamine 2,3 dioxygenase expression in dendritic cell subsets suppresses T cell clonal expansion. *J Immunol.* (2003) 171:1652–5. doi: 10.4049/jimmunol.171.4.1652
163. Huang H, Dawicki W, Zhang X, Town J, Gordon JR. Tolerogenic dendritic cells induce CD4+CD25hiFoxp3+ regulatory T cell differentiation from CD4+CD25-/loFoxp3- effector T cells. *J Immunol.* (2010) 185:5003–10. doi: 10.4049/jimmunol.0903446
164. Hsu SM, Mathew R, Taylor AW, Stein-Streilein J. *Ex-vivo* tolerogenic F4/80(+) antigen-presenting cells (APC) induce efferent CD8(+) regulatory T cell-dependent suppression of experimental autoimmune uveitis. *Clin Exp Immunol.* (2014) 176:37–48. doi: 10.1111/cei.12243
165. Qian L, Qian C, Chen Y, Bai Y, Bao Y, Lu L, et al. Regulatory dendritic cells program B cells to differentiate into CD19hiFcgammaIIbhi regulatory B cells through IFN-beta and CD40L. *Blood.* (2012) 120:581–91. doi: 10.1182/blood-2011-08-377242
166. Hill M, Thebault P, Segovia M, Louvet C, Beriou G, Tilly G, et al. Cell therapy with autologous tolerogenic dendritic cells induces allograft tolerance through interferon-gamma and epstein-barr virus-induced gene 3. *Am J Transplant.* (2011) 11:2036–45. doi: 10.1111/j.1600-6143.2011.03651.x
167. Chauveau C, Remy S, Royer PJ, Hill M, Tanguy-Royer S, Hubert FX, et al. Heme oxygenase-1 expression inhibits dendritic cell maturation and proinflammatory function but conserves IL-10 expression. *Blood.* (2005) 106:1694–702. doi: 10.1182/blood-2005-02-0494
168. Ilarregui JM, Croci DO, Bianco GA, Toscano MA, Salatino M, Vermeulen ME, et al. Tolerogenic signals delivered by dendritic cells to T cells through a galectin-1-driven immunoregulatory circuit involving interleukin 27 and interleukin 10. *Nat Immunol.* (2009) 10:981–91. doi: 10.1038/ni.1772
169. Moreau A, Hill M, Thebault P, Deschamps JY, Chiffoleau E, Chauveau C, et al. Tolerogenic dendritic cells actively inhibit T cells through heme oxygenase-1 in rodents and in nonhuman primates. *FASEB J.* (2009) 23:3070–7. doi: 10.1096/fj.08-128173
170. Remy S, Blancou P, Tesson L, Tardif V, Brion R, Royer PJ, et al. Carbon monoxide inhibits TLR-induced dendritic cell immunogenicity. *J Immunol.* (2009) 182:1877–84. doi: 10.4049/jimmunol.0802436
171. Li H, Shi B. Tolerogenic dendritic cells and their applications in transplantation. *Cell Mol Immunol.* (2015) 12:24–30. doi: 10.1038/cmi.2014.52
172. Ochando J, Ordikhani F, Jordan S, Boros P, Thomson AW. Tolerogenic dendritic cells in organ transplantation. *Transpl Int.* (2020) 33:113–27. doi: 10.1111/tri.13504
173. Liu Q, Rojas-Canales DM, Divito SJ, Shufesky WJ, Stolz DB, Erdos G, et al. Donor dendritic cell-derived exosomes promote allograft-targeting immune response. *J Clin Invest.* (2016) 126:2805–20. doi: 10.1172/JCI84577
174. Song J, Huang J, Chen X, Teng X, Song Z, Xing Y, et al. Donor-derived exosomes induce specific regulatory T cells to suppress immune inflammation in the allograft heart. *Sci Rep.* (2016) 7:20077. doi: 10.1038/srep46389
175. Nestle FO, Banchereau J, Hart D. Dendritic cells: on the move from bench to bedside. *Nat Med.* (2001) 7:761–5. doi: 10.1038/89863
176. Kryczanowsky F, Raker V, Graulich E, Domogalla MP, Steinbrink K. IL-10-modulated human dendritic cells for clinical use: identification of a stable and migratory subset with improved tolerogenic activity. *J Immunol.* (2016) 197:3607–17. doi: 10.4049/jimmunol.1501769
177. Adorini L, Penna G, Giarratana N, Uskokovic M. Tolerogenic dendritic cells induced by vitamin D receptor ligands enhance regulatory T cells inhibiting allograft rejection and autoimmune diseases. *J Cell Biochem.* (2003) 88:227–33. doi: 10.1002/jcb.10340
178. Rutella S, Danese S, Leone G. Tolerogenic dendritic cells: cytokine modulation comes of age. *Blood.* (2006) 108:1435–40. doi: 10.1182/blood-2006-03-006403
179. Morelli AE, Thomson AW. Tolerogenic dendritic cells and the quest for transplant tolerance. *Nat Rev Immunol.* (2007) 7:610–21. doi: 10.1038/nri2132
180. Marin E, Cuturi MC, Moreau A. Tolerogenic dendritic cells in solid organ transplantation: where do we stand? *Front Immunol.* (2018) 9:274. doi: 10.3389/fimmu.2018.00274
181. Fu F, Li Y, Qian S, Lu L, Chambers F, Starzl TE, et al. Costimulatory molecule-deficient dendritic cell progenitors (MHC class II+, CD80dim, CD86-) prolong cardiac allograft survival in nonimmunosuppressed recipients. *Transplantation.* (1996) 62:659–65. doi: 10.1097/00007890-199609150-00021
182. Zhou Y, Shan J, Guo Y, Li S, Long D, Li Y, et al. Effects of adoptive transfer of tolerogenic dendritic cells on allograft survival in organ transplantation models: an overview of systematic reviews. *J Immunol Res.* (2016) 2016:5730674. doi: 10.1155/2016/5730674
183. Stead SO, Kireta S, McInnes SJP, Kette FD, Sivanathan KN, Kim J, et al. Murine and non-human primate dendritic cell targeting nanoparticles for *in vivo* generation of regulatory T-cells. *ACS Nano.* (2018) 12:6637–47. doi: 10.1021/acsnano.8b01625
184. Giannoukakis N, Phillips B, Finegold D, Harnaha J, Trucco M. Phase I (safety) study of autologous tolerogenic dendritic cells in type 1 diabetic patients. *Diabetes Care.* (2011) 34:2026–32. doi: 10.2337/dc11-0472
185. Jauregui-Amezaga A, Cabezon R, Ramirez-Morros A, Espana C, Rimola J, Bru C, et al. Intraperitoneal administration of autologous tolerogenic dendritic cells for refractory crohn's disease: a phase I study. *J Crohns Colitis.* (2015) 9:1071–8. doi: 10.1093/ecco-jcc/jjv144
186. Ten Brinke A, Hilkens CM, Cools N, Geissler EK, Hutchinson JA, Lombardi G, et al. Clinical use of tolerogenic dendritic cells-harmonization approach in european collaborative effort. *Mediators Inflamm.* (2015) 2015:471719. doi: 10.1155/2015/471719
187. Bell GM, Anderson AE, Diboll J, Reece R, Eltherington O, Harry RA, et al. Autologous tolerogenic dendritic cells for rheumatoid and inflammatory arthritis. *Ann Rheum Dis.* (2017) 76:227–34. doi: 10.1136/annrheumdis-2015-208456
188. Willekens B, Presas-Rodriguez S, Mansilla MJ, Derdelinckx J, Lee WP, Nijs G, et al. Tolerogenic dendritic cell-based treatment for multiple sclerosis (MS): a harmonised study protocol for two phase I clinical trials comparing intradermal and intranodal cell administration. *BMJ Open.* (2019) 9:e030309. doi: 10.1136/bmjopen-2019-030309
189. Zahorchak AF, Macedo C, Hamm DE, Butterfield LH, Metes DM, Thomson AW. High PD-L1/CD86 MFI ratio and IL-10 secretion characterize human regulatory dendritic cells generated for clinical testing in organ transplantation. *Cell Immunol.* (2018) 323:9–18. doi: 10.1016/j.cellimm.2017.08.008
190. Obregon C, Kumar R, Pascual MA, Vassalli G, Golshayan D. Update on dendritic cell-induced immunological and clinical tolerance. *Front Immunol.* (2017) 8:1514. doi: 10.3389/fimmu.2017.01514
191. Peche H, Trinite B, Martinet B, Cuturi MC. Prolongation of heart allograft survival by immature dendritic cells generated from recipient type bone marrow progenitors. *Am J Transplant.* (2005) 5:255–67. doi: 10.1111/j.1600-6143.2004.00683.x
192. Moreau A, Alliot-Licht B, Cuturi MC, Blancho G. Tolerogenic dendritic cell therapy in organ transplantation. *Transpl Int.* (2017) 30:754–64. doi: 10.1111/tri.12889

16

The Immunological Basis of Liver Allograft Rejection

Vincenzo Ronca[1,2,3], *Grace Wootton*[2], *Chiara Milani*[1] *and Owen Cain*[4]*

[1] *Division of Gastroenterology and Centre for Autoimmune Liver Diseases, Department of Medicine and Surgery, University of Milan Bicocca, Milan, Italy,* [2] *National Institute of Health Research Liver Biomedical Research Unit Birmingham, Centre for Liver Research, Institute of Immunology and Immunotherapy, University of Birmingham, Birmingham, United Kingdom,* [3] *Liver Unit, University Hospitals Birmingham NHS Foundation Trust, Birmingham, United Kingdom,* [4] *Department of Cellular Pathology, University Hospitals Birmingham NHS Foundation Trust, Birmingham, United Kingdom*

Correspondence:
Owen Cain
owen.cain@nhs.net

Liver allograft rejection remains a significant cause of morbidity and graft failure in liver transplant recipients. Rejection is caused by the recognition of non-self donor alloantigens by recipient T-cells. Antigen recognition results in proliferation and activation of T-cells in lymphoid tissue before migration to the allograft. Activated T-cells have a variety of effector mechanisms including direct T-cell mediated damage to bile ducts, endothelium and hepatocytes and indirect effects through cytokine production and recruitment of tissue-destructive inflammatory cells. These effects explain the histological appearances of typical acute T-cell mediated rejection. In addition, donor specific antibodies, most typically against HLA antigens, may give rise to antibody-mediated rejection causing damage to the allograft primarily through endothelial injury. However, as an immune-privileged site there are several mechanisms in the liver capable of overcoming rejection and promoting tolerance to the graft, particularly in the context of recruitment of regulatory T-cells and promotors of an immunosuppressive environment. Indeed, around 20% of transplant recipients can be successfully weaned from immunosuppression. Hence, the host immunological response to the liver allograft is best regarded as a balance between rejection-promoting and tolerance-promoting factors. Understanding this balance provides insight into potential mechanisms for novel anti-rejection therapies.

Keywords: transplantation, tolerance, immunomodulatory, dendritic cells, regulatory T cell

INTRODUCTION

Liver transplantation is currently the only effective treatment for end-stage liver disease. In the last 40 years the remarkable improvement in the surgical technique and the development of immunosuppressive drugs alongside improved post-transplant medico-surgical management has significantly prolonged transplant recipient survival. The host immunological response to the liver allograft is best regarded as a balance between rejection-promoting and tolerance-promoting

---

Abbreviations: APC, antigen presenting cell; CAR, chimeric antigen receptor; DC, dendritic cell; HLA, human leukocytes antigens; ICAM1, intracellular adhesion molecule 1; IFN-γ, interferon-gamma; KC, Kupffer cell; LSEC, liver sinusoidal endothelial cells; MHC, major histocompatibility system; NK, natural killer; TGF-β, tumor growth factor-beta; Th, T helper cell; Treg, regulatory T cell; VCAM1, vascular adhesion molecule 1.

factors. Whilst the unique features of the liver as an immunoregulatory organ promote an enhanced tolerogenic response in the allograft recipient compared with other organs, immunological rejection remains a significant clinical problem. For this reason the majority of liver transplant recipients require lifelong immunosuppression conferring an increased risk of severe complications such as infection and neoplasia (1–3). Therefore, new therapeutic strategies to induce long-term immune tolerance are required.

The majority of rejection episodes occur within the first month following transplantation and are readily amenable to treatment with high dose steroids. Acute rejection episodes can also occur in the later post-transplant period when the presentation may be less typical (4). Up to 35% of patients may experience at least one episode of acute rejection, although some will have sub-clinical disease (5). Repeated acute episodes may lead to chronic rejection. Whilst historically this was more common and occurred within a few months following transplantation, in the current era of immunosuppressive therapy the incidence of chronic rejection is probably 2–3% at most and may occur several years post-transplant (6, 7). Chronic rejection has a complex and only partly understood etiology probably representing the end stage of a number of different immunological processes (8, 9).

The objective of this review is to provide an overview of the main immunological principles governing rejection and tolerance in the liver allograft and to outline current novel therapeutic approaches aiming to induce long lasting immune tolerance after liver transplantation. Given its low incidence and complex etiology, chronic rejection will not be considered further in this review.

PRESERVATION-REPERFUSION INJURY

A certain degree of ischemic injury to the allograft is an unavoidable consequence of transplantation. This occurs during organ transportation to the transplant center (known as the cold ischemia time because the liver is transported in cold storage) and during organ harvesting and subsequent implantation (known as the warm ischemia time). An additional element of warm ischemia time is unavoidable for donation after circulatory death (DCD) as opposed to donation after brainstem death (DBD) livers because of the time lag between circulatory collapse and organ retrieval.

Ischemia leads to depletion of intracellular adenosine triphosphate particularly in hepatocytes and liver sinusoidal endothelial cells (LSEC), resulting in cell damage and death. Upon reperfusion further damage is elicited by release of reactive oxygen species and pro-inflammatory cytokines such as TNFα, IFN-γ and IL-1 by activated Kupffer cells (10). Within this acute pro-inflammatory environment LSEC are induced to upregulate cellular adhesion molecules including ICAM-1 and VCAM-1, facilitating recruitment of leukocytes to the allograft (11). Thus, the overall effect of transplantation is to induce a pro-inflammatory microenvironment within the liver allograft resulting in tissue damage, a phenomenon termed preservation-reperfusion injury (PRI, also known as ischemia-reperfusion injury) (12).

The method of organ retrieval and the presence of donor-related liver disease influence the extent of PRI related damage. The prolonged warm ischemia time of DCD livers results in exaggerated PRI principally causing additional damage to hepatocytes and resulting in inferior clinical outcomes (13). Steatotic livers are being increasingly utilized for transplantation. Steatosis is associated with increased PRI as measured by molecular markers of inflammation (14) and reflected histologically as increased hepatocyte necrosis (15). Clinically, the sequelae of PRI in DCD livers include an increased risk of primary non-function and ischemic-type biliary lesions and overall reduced graft survival (16).

THE IMMUNOLOGICAL BASIS OF T-CELL MEDIATED REJECTION

T-cell mediated rejection (TCMR, also previously known as "acute cellular rejection") occurs most commonly in the early post-transplant period and is generally amenable to treatment with immunosuppression (17). It typically presents with non-specific clinical symptoms and predominantly cholestatic liver biochemistry. Liver biopsy is required for diagnostic confirmation and shows a dense portal-based mixed inflammatory cell infiltrate with evidence of damage to biliary epithelium, portal and hepatic vein endothelium and hepatocytes (18) (**Figure 1**). Early episodes of TCMR do not impact on long-term outcomes (19) although persistent rejection episodes refractory to standard therapies remain problematic. This section of the review will outline our current understanding of the immunological mechanisms that give rise to TCMR and the mechanisms of allograft damage elicited by the cellular infiltrate.

Major Histocompatibility Complex Antigen Expression

The main antigens responsible for driving rejection are the major histocompatibility complex (MHC) molecules. MHC class I molecules are constitutively expressed by all nucleated cells and present intracellular epitopes to CD8 + cytotoxic T-cells. In contrast, expression of MHC class II molecules is more restricted, presenting epitopes derived from extracellular material to CD4 + helper T-cells. In the normal liver there is strong and diffuse MHC class I expression in all cells whereas MHC class II expression is limited to Kupffer cells and other liver-resident antigen presenting cells. During liver inflammation expression of MHC class I is increased in all cells and MHC class II expression is stimulated in endothelium, biliary epithelium and hepatocytes (20). Thus, liver inflammation upregulates expression of MHC molecules, priming toward a rejection response.

Preservation-Reperfusion Injury

PRI has long been recognized as important factor in skewing the recipient immunological response in favor of rejection (21). Damaged hepatocytes and LSEC release damage-associated molecular pattern molecules (DAMPs): HMGB1, free fatty acids

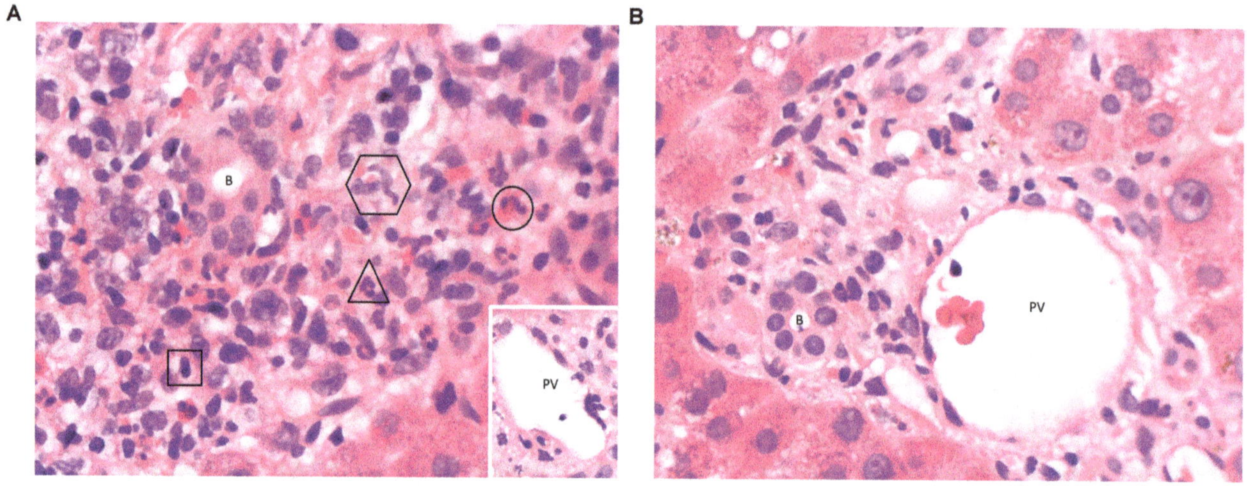

FIGURE 1 | (A) Acute TCMR 6 days post liver transplant. This high-power image (hematoxylin & eosin (H&E), ×600) of a portal tract shows infiltration of a large number of inflammatory cells. Typical examples of a lymphocyte (square), neutrophil (triangle), eosinophil (circle) and two macrophages (hexagon) are highlighted, demonstrating the contribution of cells from both the innate and adaptive immune systems. The majority of the lymphocytes will be T-cells, capable of mediating cell damage through direct cytotoxicity and the release of pro-inflammatory cytokines. There is clustering around the bile duct (B) and portal vein (PV, inset, with damage to endothelium seen at 4 o'clock). Neutrophils and macrophages migrate to the liver in response to pro-inflammatory cytokines, enhanced by Th1 and Th17 responses. Eosinophils are also present in early rejection infiltrates and are more typically associated with a Th2 response. Treatment with high dose pulsed methylprednisolone was able to suppress the rejection episode in this patient and tolerance has since been maintained using a standard immunosuppressive regimen. **(B)** Immune tolerance 8 days post liver transplant. In contrast to **Figure 2A**, a portal tract from this biopsy (H&E, ×600) contains only a small number of lymphocytes, macrophages and neutrophils with no evidence of damage to biliary epithelium (B) or portal vein endothelium (PV). Tolerance to the liver allograft is promoted by multiple factors including the relatively low levels of MHC class II expression on hepatic-resident cells, a tendency toward tolerogenic antigen presentation by the dendritic cells, macrophages, stellate cells and epithelial cells resident in the liver, the dominance of a regulatory T-cell infiltrate and the action of donor-derived NK cells on the recipient immune system. Indeed, a biliary complication of surgery was found to be the reason for liver dysfunction in this patient, and tolerance was maintained on follow-up by means of a standard immunosuppressive regimen without the need for additional therapy.

and heat shock proteins. This activates Kupffer cells via toll-like receptors, stimulating release of pro-inflammatory cytokines such as IL1, TNF, IFN and IL12. Release of CXCL-1, -2 and -3 stimulates neutrophil recruitment to the graft (22). PRI also promotes upregulation of lymphocyte recruitment molecules by LSEC. The end result of PRI is therefore the establishment of a pro-inflammatory microenvironment within the liver.

PRI may promote TCMR by providing the initial stimulus for migration of donor-derived dendritic cells (DC) from the transplanted liver to recipient regional lymph nodes. These professional antigen presenting cells are resident in the liver and upregulate expression of MHC class I and II molecules as a consequence of the inflammatory signals generated by PRI. The chemotactic PRI signals also act as a means of recruiting activated T-cells of the adaptive immune system and to amplify their rejection-mediating effects.

Alloantigen Presentation, T-Cell Activation and Maturation

Alloantigen presentation by DC is a key step in rejection. In the normal liver DC are present in portal tracts and around hepatic veins, and thus significant numbers of donor-derived DC are transferred to the recipient as passengers during transplantation. In response to pro-inflammatory environments such as PRI they become activated, upregulate expression of MHC molecules displaying alloantigens and mobilize to lymphoid tissue (20). Activated donor-derived DC arriving in the lymph node provide a potent immunological stimulus for recipient-derived naïve CD4 + T-cells, which recognize as foreign not only the presented antigen but also the MHC molecule itself, known as the direct pathway of antigen presentation (**Figure 2**). The interaction between the DC and T-cell is dependent on: (1) activation of the T-cell receptor (TCR) by its cognate peptide-MHC complex on the DC, (2) interaction between T-cell integrin adhesion molecules such as LFA-1 and VLA4 interacting with ICAM-1 and VCAM-1 on DC, and (3) co-stimulatory molecule interactions such as CD28 expressed on T-cells interacting with B7 molecules on DC. Since dendritic cells express MHC class I and class II molecules they are able to activate both CD4 + and CD8 + T-cells (23). Successful priming of naïve T-cells leads to activation of the cytoplasmic calcium-dependent phosphatase enzyme calcineurin within T-cells, which in turn activates nuclear transcription factor of activated T-cells (NFAT), upregulating expression of IL-2. This cytokine provides the main stimulus for T-cell proliferation by interacting with the cell surface IL-2 receptor.

The indirect and semi-indirect pathways are more typically associated with later episodes of rejection. These pathways are mediated by recipient (as opposed to donor) DC, which accumulate within the graft over time. The indirect pathway is characterized by alloantigens captured and processed by recipient DC or other antigen presenting cells and then presented upon self-MHC molecules to naïve T-cells (24). The semi-indirect presentation refers to the expression of the intact donor

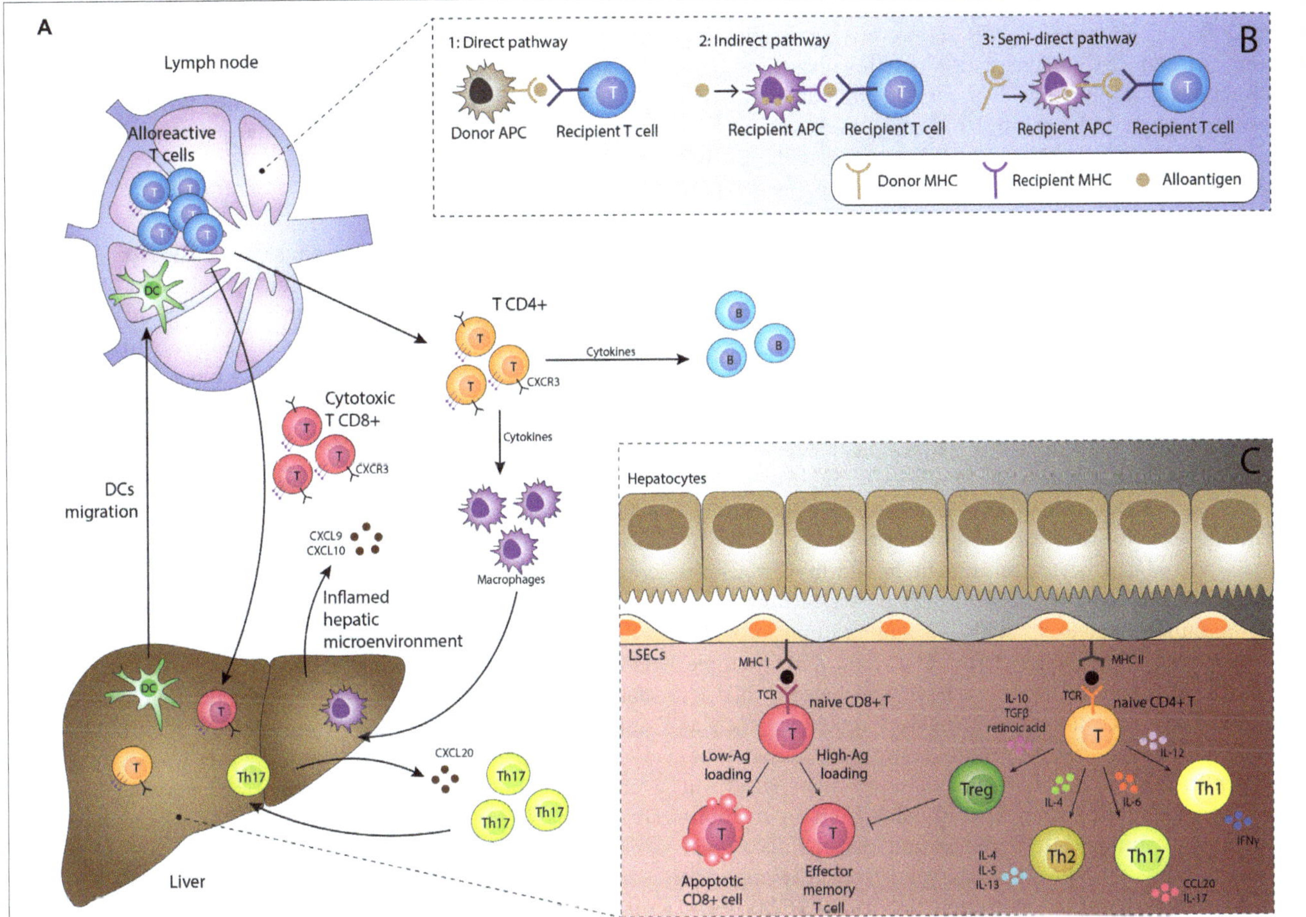

FIGURE 2 | (A) Immunological basis of TCMR. Activated dendritic cells migrate to lymphoid tissue presenting alloantigen on MHC class I and II molecules. Interaction with naïve alloreactive T-cells in the presence of appropriate co-stimulatory molecules and a pro inflammatory cytokine milieu results in proliferation of alloreactive CD4 + and CD8 + effector T-cells and subsequent B-cell proliferation. Migration to the liver is orchestrated by chemokines such as CXCL9 and CXCL10 interacting with the CXCR3 receptor on lymphocytes in addition to complex interactions with the unique immunomodulatory liver sinusoidal endothelial cells. Lymphocyte subsets such as Th17 cells have specific recruitment mechanisms, providing potential therapeutic targets. Cells of the innate immune system including macrophages, neutrophils and eosinophils are recruited to the liver and along with the effector T-cells mediate tissue damage, resulting in the clinical manifestations of TCMR. **(B)** Three pathways for antigen presentation. The strongest alloimmune response is generated by the direct pathway which occurs in the early post-transplant period. Upon activation, donor-derived dendritic cells migrate to the lymph node, displaying non-self donor antigens within non-self donor MHC molecules. This provides potent stimulation for the mounting of a rejection response. The indirect and semi-direct pathways involve recipient-derived dendritic cells displaying self and non-self MHC molecules respectively. Whilst not as potent as the direct pathway, they are still able to sustain ongoing rejection. **(C)** Antigen presentation within the liver generally promotes tolerogenic responses. Antigen is also presented within the allograft by endothelial cells, macrophages, hepatic stellate cells, hepatocytes and biliary epithelium, with increased presentation seen during episodes of inflammation. However, most interactions with naïve lymphocytes within the liver result in tolerance rather than rejection, with apoptosis of effector cells and a skewing of T-cell differentiation toward the regulatory T-cell phenotype through an immunosuppressive cytokine profile.

MHC on the surface of the recipient antigen presenting cells. The semi-indirect pathway is considered to be of particular importance in allograft rejection and is probably the consequence of a cell to cell contact and the fusion of recipient and donor exosomes (25–29). Whilst still capable of initiating a rejection response, the indirect and semi-indirect pathways are less potent than the direct pathway.

Once primed, CD8 + T-cells predominantly differentiate into cytotoxic T-cells (Tc) able to exert direct cell damage on the allograft. CD4 + T-cells have the potential to differentiate into a number of activated subtypes, of which the helper T-cell (Th1, Th2 and Th17) and regulatory T-cell (Treg) subsets are the best characterized. The relative proportion of cells in each subtype is determined by the local inflammatory microenvironment. In acute rejection T-cell differentiation is primarily polarized toward the Th1 response, driven by pro-inflammatory cytokines such as IL-12, TNF-β and particularly IFN-γ. Th1 cells are characterized by secretion of IL-2 and IFN-γ which provide a positive feedback loop stimulating further proliferation of Th1 cells.

Whilst the Th2 response was initially characterized as immunosuppressive, it is now recognized to mediate acute rejection, at least under certain circumstances (30). Differentiation toward the Th2 phenotype is promoted by IL-4; Th2 cells themselves then produce IL-4 and IL-5 providing another example of a positive feedback loop (31). Th17 cells also play a role in acute TCMR. However, the relationship between Th1 and Th17 differentiation remains unclear as Th17 differentiation is inhibited by IFN-γ (32). Th17 differentiation is however, provoked by pro-inflammatory mediators such as Il-1, IL-6, IL-21 and IL-23 and TGF-β, prostaglandin E2 and HMGB-1 (33).

Activated lymphocytes must migrate toward and gain access to the liver in order to carry out their effector functions. A pro-inflammatory microenvironment in the allograft promotes endothelial secretion of IFN-γ inducible chemokines, namely CXCL9 and CXCL10, which facilitate the attraction of circulating leukocytes, including activated T-cells, expressing the chemokine receptor CXCR3 (34). Leukocyte migration across target organ endothelium typically follows a sequential process of (1) tethering, (2) activation mediated by LFA-1/ICAM-1 and VLA-4/VCAM-1 interactions and (3) crawling/transmigration through the endothelium to gain access to the liver (35). However, the main site of leukocyte recruitment in the liver is within the sinusoids, mediated by LSEC, which possess a number of unique immunomodulatory functions resulting in non-classical mechanisms of lymphocyte recruitment (36). For example, whereas CD8 + T-cell recruitment is largely mediated by ICAM-1 (37, 38), Treg recruitment also involves molecules such as stabilin-1 and VAP-1 (39). Neutrophil recruitment across LSEC is independent of the selectin-mediated interactions known to be important at other sites, instead relying on interactions between LSEC-produced hyaluronan and neutrophilic CD44 (40). Furthermore, VAP-1 has been shown to mediate lymphocyte migration across LSEC in an animal model of TCMR (41). Manipulation of the immunological properties of LSEC therefore provides a potential opportunity to shape the immune response to the allograft.

Effector Responses

CD8+ Tc Cells

Primed CD8 + Tc cells are the main effector lymphocytes responsible for mediating tissue damage. This process depends on the binding of the TCR to the non-self donor-derived MHC class I molecules widely expressed on biliary epithelial cells (BEC), endothelium (portal, sinusoidal and centrilobular) and hepatocytes. Activation of cytolytic activity is dependent on interactions of cell adhesion molecules such as LFA1-ICAM1 and CD2-LFA3 as well as the TCR-MHC-peptide complex. The cytolytic activity of Tc cells is mediated through two main pathways: (1) the granzyme/perforin pathway in which the pore-like perforin molecule is released from the T-cell, punctures the cell membrane of the target cells facilitating entry of granzymes to the target cell cytoplasm which initiates apoptosis and (2) the Fas-FasL pathway in which activation of the Fas molecule on the surface of target cells by its ligand FasL on Tc cells leads to activation of the death domain in the cytoplasmic tail of Fas and caspase-dependent apoptosis.

Hepatocytes are relatively resistant to Fas-FasL mediated damage. Instead, other molecules of the TNF superfamily receptors such as CD40, TRAIL and TNFR1-2 which fulfill a similar role appear to be more important. Their expression is upregulated on the surface of BEC and hepatocytes during inflammation, facilitating Tc-mediated cell death (42–44). Interestingly, there is emerging evidence that initial Tc-target cell interactions may occur via cytoplasmic protrusions extending from intra-sinusoidal T-cells (45).

CD4 + Th Cells

The pro-inflammatory Th1 response is considered to be the main driver of acute TCMR. Continued production of IL-2 and IFN-γ by Th1 cells is important for macrophage activation and ongoing stimulation of CD8 + Tc cell subsets, which produces further IFN-γ, acting as a positive feedback loop (33). Th1 subsets also cause allograft damage directly through Fas-FasL mediated cytotoxicity in the same manner as Tc cells (46).

Th1 and Th2 responses have an antagonistic relationship such that production of the Th2 cytokines IL-4 and IL-10 inhibits Th1 differentiation. Indeed, there is some evidence that under certain circumstances a Th2 polarized response is tolerogenic in the liver allograft (47). However, there is also considerable evidence implicating Th2 cells as direct mediators of rejection (30, 48, 49). Mechanisms include interaction between Th2 cells and activated B-cells leading to the production of donor specific antibodies, with proliferation of activated B-cells stimulated by IL-2 production by Th1 cells, illustrating the cross-over between cell- and antibody-mediated rejection. Th2 responses are also important for the recruitment of eosinophils, which are present in abundance in early TCMR.

Th17 cells exert tissue damaging functions by virtue of IL-17 production which acts as a powerful signal for neutrophil recruitment. Th17 cells are able to promote liver allograft rejection in a rat model (50) and high levels of peripheral blood Th17 levels have been associated with impaired tolerance in clinical studies (51). The CXCR3 receptor has been shown to be critical for Th17 cell migration into the inflamed liver; the cells then home to portal tracts with particular tropism toward BEC expressing the CCR6 ligand CCL20 (52). Subsequent work has shown the active role of BEC in maintaining Th17 dominant differentiation via release of IL-6 and IL-1β, and the stimulation of BEC proliferation by Th17 cytokines (53). There appears to be a degree of plasticity between Th17 and Treg differentiation such that the two exist in a state of dynamic equilibrium; this has generated interest in the importance of these divergent populations in skewing the immune response toward rejection or tolerance (see below).

Memory T-Cells

Following initial presentation of a novel antigen, a small number of T-cells differentiate into long-lived memory T-cells rather than effector cells. Memory cells reside in peripheral tissues and are able to respond more rapidly and potently than naïve T-cells on repeat exposure to the antigen. One of the main mechanisms for this enhanced response is the reduced requirement for CD28-B7 co-stimulatory signals.

Counterintuitively, memory T-cells have been shown to play a key role in the initial acute allograft rejection response as well as in later episodes of TCMR despite the fact that the allograft is "new" to the recipient (54). Potentially alloreactive memory T-cells can be demonstrated in the serum of healthy volunteers (55) and higher numbers of alloreactive pre-transplant memory T-cells correlate with an increased risk of post-transplant rejection episodes (56). Potential mechanisms for the generation of immunological memory in the pre-transplant population include:

- Historical direct exposure to alloantigen via pregnancy or blood transfusion.
- Heterologous immunity in which there is cross-reactivity between a previously encountered pathogen-related antigen and allogenic peptides.
- Homeostatic proliferation following lymphodepletion by pharmacological immunosuppression. During this process surviving T cell to undergo homeostatic proliferation and differentiation into "pseudo memory T-cells" despite never having been presented with antigen (57).

Memory T-cells of the CD4 + helper class have the potential to induce antibody mediated rejection via enhanced production of donor specific antibodies by B-cells whereas CD8 + memory T-cells are able to exert direct cytotoxic effects. Memory T-cells are less sensitive to immunosuppressive treatments compared with naïve T-cells and could be one reason why some patients do not fully respond to standard treatments for acute TCMR. As such memory T-cells are a potential barrier to establishing tolerance and their impact on rejection requires further study (58).

B-Cells

B-cells are not generally discussed in the context of TCMR. However, B cell deficiency in mice and humans has been associated with delayed acute rejection (59). Potential mechanisms include the activation of T-cells by B-cells via costimulatory pathways and cytokine release and promoting T-cell differentiation into memory T-cells (60). B-cell presentation of donor antigen is enhanced during liver allograft rejection and may provide a novel target for immunosuppression (61). The main role of B-cells is however, the production of antibody which is of key importance for antibody mediated rejection.

Macrophages

The macrophage response is often conceptualized as being either pro-inflammatory, stimulated by IFN-γ and lipopolysaccharide (the so-called M1 phenotype) or immunosuppressive, stimulated by IL-4 and IL-13 (the M2 phenotype). In acute rejection many macrophages show features of polarization toward an M1 phenotype producing pro-inflammatory cytokines such as IL-1, IL-12, IL-18, IL-6, IL-23, TNF-α and IFN-γ and reactive oxygen and nitrogen species which cause direct cell damage and co-ordinate a pro-inflammatory immune response (62). Recognition of damaged allograft tissue is through the pattern recognition receptors such as the toll-like receptors and macrophages have a major phagocytic role in the clearing of damaged cells (63). As antigen presenting cells intrahepatic macrophages are able to present alloantigens in MHC class II molecules, thus promoting the adaptive immune response. Unsurprisingly an M1 macrophage response has been associated with allograft rejection (64) whereas an immunosuppressive M2 response is associated with tolerance (65). Early M1 macrophages have been shown to differentiate into M2 macrophages following loss of co-stimulatory signals (66). Macrophage polarization is mediated by a number of cytokines and growth factors (67).

The M1/M2 framework for understanding macrophage responses is however, an over-simplification. Whilst different macrophage populations certainly possess divergent functions, understanding macrophage biology is complicated by the replacement of donor derived macrophages in the early post-transplant by recipient derived cells differentiating from circulating monocytes in the later period (68). Furthermore, the phenotypic diversity of macrophage subsets within the liver does not readily permit a binary classification (20). However, attempts at further delineating the pathways involved in producing a more immunosuppressive macrophage response are likely to feed into therapeutic efforts to identify novel anti-rejection therapies.

Neutrophils

Neutrophils are often numerous in acute TCMR and may be recruited to the allograft following PRI and as an early effector response to adaptive alloimmunity, particularly in response to Th17 activation. Neutrophils mediate cell damage via ROS generation, numerous tissue-digesting enzymes such as metalloproteinase-9 and neutrophil elastase (69), and possibly through a unique form of programmed cell death (70). As classical mediators of the acute inflammatory response, neutrophils may also play a role in tipping the immunological balance toward rejection following an episode of infection (71). Intriguingly, neutrophils may also have a role to play in tolerance mechanisms, having been shown to have the capability to inhibit T-cell responses (72) and polarize macrophages toward a M2 phenotype in an animal model (73).

Eosinophils

In contrast to macrophages and neutrophils, which respond primarily to a classical pro-inflammatory Th1 response, eosinophil maturation and migration is orchestrated by Th2 cytokines such as IL-4 and IL-5. Eosinophils have long been recognized as a key feature of TCMR in the liver (74) and peripheral eosinophilia has been associated with rejection (75). Cell damage is mediated by secretion of cytotoxic granules including major basic protein which increases permeability of cell membranes and eosinophil peroxidase. Of interest, eosinophils also have receptors for Th1-associated cytokines such as TNFα (76) and recruitment may therefore not be entirely dependent on Th2 pathways.

NK Cells

Natural kill (NK) cells are lymphocytes that lack expression of CD3, CD20 and other typical T- and B-cell markers, instead expressing CD16 and CD56. NK cells can be stimulated by both activating signals and the loss of inhibitory signals. In the allograft potential activating signals come from molecules such as MIC-A and MIC-B expressed by allograft tissue as a stress response to a pro-inflammatory environment (77). These molecules are recognized by activating receptors on NK cells such as NKG2D. Inhibitory signals come from self MHC class I molecules which normally interact with the inhibitory receptors on NK cells such as killer immunoglobulin-like receptors (KIRs). In rejection it is postulated that the non-self MHC class I molecules present on the cells of the allograft are unable to maintain the inhibitory KIR signal (78). As such solid organ allografts provide multiple mechanisms for activation of recipient NK cells that have migrated to the graft.

NK cells are able to mediate cytotoxicity through production of perforin and granzyme in a similar manner to Tc cells. Activated NK cells and also produce INF-γ and TNF-$^{\alpha}$ promoting early adaptive immune responses and further tissue damage, an effect demonstrated to be of importance in a rat model of liver transplantation (79). NK cells also have the ability to recognize antibody on target cells using Fc receptors, linking the NK response to antibody mediated mechanisms.

However, many of the pathways linking recipient NK cells with rejection remain unclear. A clinical study matching KIR and MHC class I types did not impact upon allograft rejection or clinical outcome (80). Whilst they are most likely of importance, the precise mechanisms of NK-cell mediated rejection requires further clarification.

Further populations of unconventional T-cells such as NK T-cells and gamma delta T-cells may also play a role in rejection and tolerance mechanisms, although at present an understanding of their importance in the allograft is limited (81, 82).

THE IMMUNOLOGICAL BASIS OF ANTIBODY MEDIATED REJECTION

The most severe form of antibody mediated rejection (AMR) is hyperacute rejection which occurs in ABO-incompatible grafts and is vanishingly rare in the liver. It results in acute liver failure within hours to days (83). In contrast to other solid organ transplants, the clinical significance of other forms of AMR in the liver was initially unclear, but it is now generally accepted that antibodies can mediate clinically significant rejection episodes (84). Isolated acute AMR in the liver is rare, has a clinical presentation that overlaps with TCMR and may often quickly evolve into TCMR (85). Furthermore, biopsy findings are not specific and a diagnosis of AMR requires correlation with clinical, serological and immunohistochemical data. The immunological basis of AMR is however, reasonably well characterized, largely based on data from other solid organ transplants, particularly the kidney.

Antibody Production

Donor specific antibodies (DSA) capable of causing AMR may be either pre-formed or arise *de novo* post-transplant. The presence of preformed alloantibodies can be explained by similar mechanisms as those for pre-existing memory T-cells discussed above. *De novo* antibody production occurs when naïve B-cells interact with alloantigens (mainly MHC molecules) via the B-cell receptor following classical adaptive immunological pathways. In the presence of inflammatory signals such as IL-1 this leads to B-cell activation, internalization and degradation of the antigen by the B-cell and re-presentation of antigen fragments by MHC class II molecules. These molecules are able to directly interact with primed Th2 cells in an indirect manner of antigen presentation (86). When co-stimulatory and cell adhesion signals such as CD28-B7, CD40L-CD40, LFA-1-ICAM and CD2-LFA-3 are also activated then B-cell division and differentiation can occur. This process is facilitated by IL-2 production from Th1 cells, in addition to Th2 cytokines such as IL-4 and IL-5. Some activated B-cells differentiate into plasma cells and begin production of DSA. Other cells migrate to lymph nodes forming germinal centers and undergo a process of somatic hypermutation and affinity maturation, refining and amplifying the antibody response. Mature plasma cells are able to produce antibodies indefinitely without T-cell help (87). Memory B-cells are also produced facilitating ongoing episodes of rejection.

Antibody Effector Functions

The main targets of DSA are the non-self class I and II MHC molecules expressed by endothelial cells within the liver allograft, the latter being significantly upregulated by pro-inflammatory signals. Anti-MHC class I antibodies tend to appear earlier, while anti-MHC class II antibodies (particularly anti-HLA-DQ antibodies) develop in the later post-transplant period (88). Interaction between DSA and their target antigen causes activation of the classical pathway of the complement system via the binding of C1q to the Fc regions of bound DSA (**Figure 3A**). This initiates an enzyme cascade producing biologically active complement effector functions. Although the role of these mediators in AMR has not been fully elucidated in the liver, chemotactic signals such as C3a and C5a are potent inflammatory mediators (anaphylatoxins) likely to be important for activating mast cells and basophils and recruiting macrophages and granulocytes including eosinophils, macrophage activation and increasing vascular permeability (89). Production of C3d opsonizes target cells by covalent bonding promoting phagocytosis. C5b forms the membrane attack complex C5b-9 with the potential to cause direct endothelial damage via puncture of the cell membrane with the pore, although expression of CD59 (also known as protectin) may provide endothelial cells with some resistance to this form of injury (90). The non-lytic binding of the C5b-9 complex to the endothelial surface also induces the expression of several pro-inflammatory proteins including IL-6, E-Selectin, and VCAM-1, and upregulates expression of IFN-γ and MHC molecules endothelial cells further amplifying the antibody response (91). Complement also interacts with the adaptive immune system, augmenting T-cell mediated rejection (92).

Immunohistochemical demonstration of C4d deposition on allograft vasculature is used as a marker of complement system activation and AMR. C4d is a product of C4b degradation and is a more sensitive marker of antibody binding than direct measurement of immunoglobulin deposition because C4d shows covalent bonding to the endothelial surface and amplifies the immunoglobulin signal.

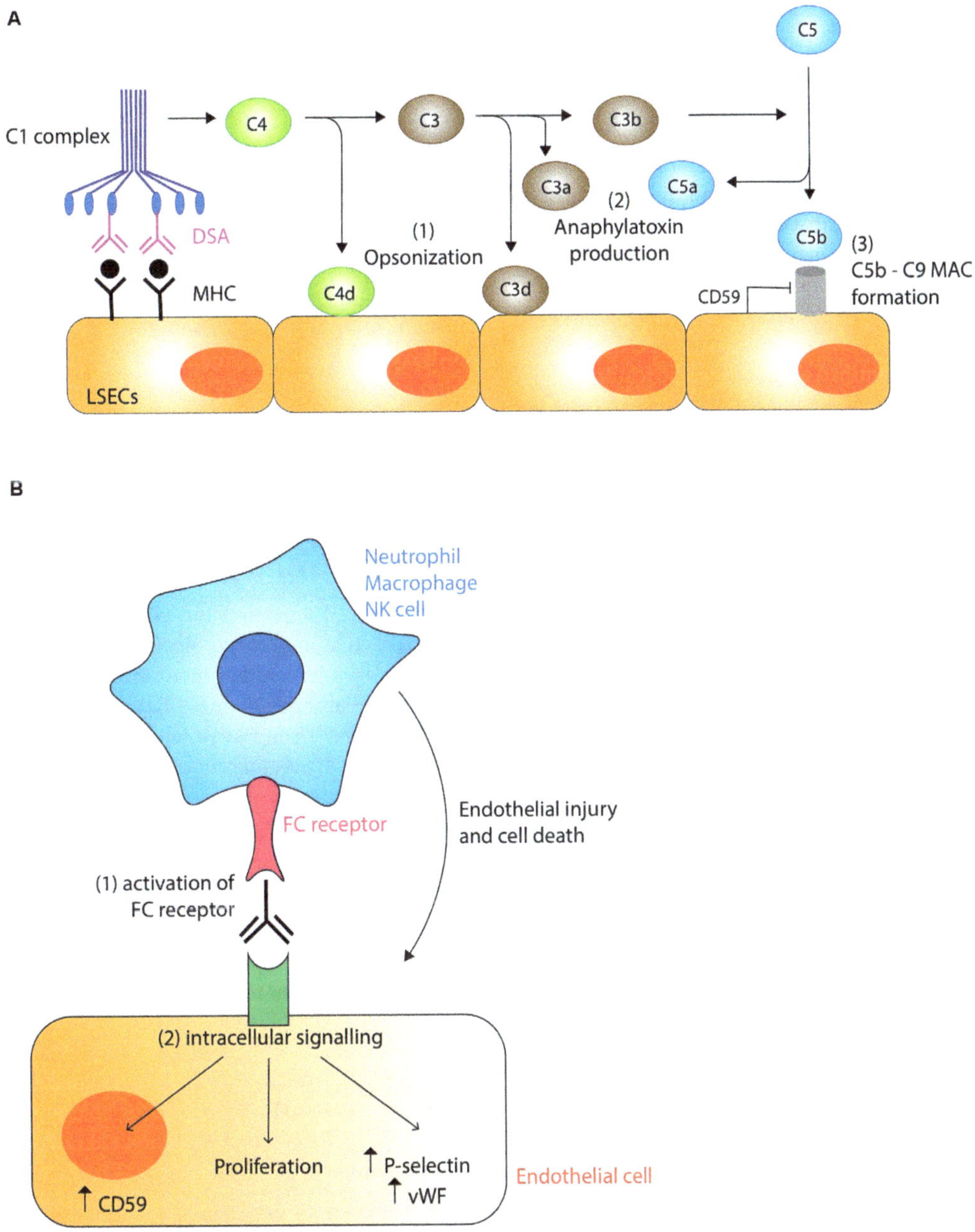

FIGURE 3 | (A) Complement-dependent mechanisms of antibody mediated rejection. Binding of donor specific antibody (DSA) to MHC molecules on the liver allograft causes activation of the classical pathway of complement via binding of the C1 complex. Complement has the potential to damage the graft through three main mechanisms: (1) Opsonization. C4d and C3d covalently bind to target cells marking them for destruction and clearing by cells of the innate immune system. (2) Anaphylatoxin production. C3a and C5a act as potent chemotactic signals recruiting inflammatory cells which cause localized tissue damage. (3) Membrane attack complex (MAC). The C5b-9 MAC has the potential to damage cells by puncturing holes in the membrane, although this action is normally inhibited by endothelial expression of CD59 (protectin). Non-lytic binding of the MAC induces endothelial upregulation of pro-inflammatory, lymphocyte recruitment, and MHC molecules, thus potentiating the rejection response. **(B)** Complement-independent mechanisms of antibody mediated rejection. DSA binding to MHC molecules promotes the recruitment of cells of the innate immune system such as neutrophils, macrophages and NK cells via interactions with the FC receptor. These inflammatory cells are stimulated to cause graft injury via their various effector mechanisms (see text for details). DSA binding also stimulates intracellular signaling pathways.

Although complement appears to be the main mechanism of tissue damage in AMR, it is increasingly recognized that complement-independent pathways are also important (**Figure 3B**). One mechanism involves the binding of Fc receptors on neutrophils, macrophages and NK cells to bound DSAs. The resulting activation of these cells of the innate immune system triggers a cascade of pro-inflammatory pathways leading to endothelial cell damage (90). Another complement-independent mechanism involves the direct activation of intracellular signaling pathways within endothelial cells by the binding of DSA to MHC molecules, resulting in structural changes to cytoskeletal proteins, increased cellular proliferation, increased production of von Willebrand factor and P-selectin and the enhanced expression of CD59 conferring resistance to C5b-9 mediated attack (88, 93).

Thus the end result of DSA binding to allograft endothelium is endothelial damage and swelling, formation of microthrombi, platelet aggregates and inflammation. In acute AMR of the liver these changes generally manifest as portal edema and hemorrhage, bile ductular reaction, and dilatation of portal microvessels (94). Portal eosinophilia, eosinophilic central venulitis and portal microvessel endothelial hypertrophy and "hobnailing" have been identified as more specific features (95).

TOLERANCE MECHANISMS IN THE LIVER ALLOGRAFT

Allograft tolerance is mediated by immunological dampening and inhibition of the rejection response (**Figure 4**). The liver is considered relatively tolerogenic compared with other solid organ transplants, allowing routine transplantation of non-HLA matched organs. "True tolerance" occurs when there is no demonstrable immunological response to the allograft and is a rare event (96). Nonetheless, 20% of adults and up to 65% of pediatric liver allograft recipients can exhibit preserved graft function for at least 1 year after weaning immunosuppression, despite many showing persistent subclinical immunological markers of rejection (97, 98); this is referred to as "operational tolerance."

The explanation for the relative tolerogenicity of the liver is multifactorial: (1) The large size of the organ results in a far greater endothelial surface area over which antibodies are diluted, thus attenuating their effects, (2) The liver has an inherent regenerative capacity such that tissue destruction by episodes of rejection is potentially reversible, (3) Expression of MHC class II molecules on liver cells is variable compared with the constitutive expression seen in kidneys and hearts, (4) cell-specific mechanisms operate to attenuate the rejection response, as discussed below. Enhanced tolerance in the liver has an evolutionary basis since 75% of hepatic blood flow is from the portal vein which collects blood from the gastrointestinal tract enriched with microbial antigens. Thus, the hepatic immune system has evolved to tightly regulate immune reactions to harmless gut-derived micro-organisms in order to avoid inappropriate pro-inflammatory responses. These mechanisms are of importance for allograft tolerance.

Mesenchymal Stromal Cells

Mesenchymal stromal cells (MSCs) are localized in the liver and although they are yet to be fully characterized, their ability to modulate the immune response is well recognized (99). These cells can be found in the perivascular space of virtually all organs (100). It is interesting to compare two highly tolerogenic organs, both extremely vascularized, such liver and placenta. Intriguingly in both the organs MSCs seem to play a decisive role in maintaining tolerance. In a similar manner to the tolerance required in the liver for gut-derived micro-organisms, the placenta needs to maintain a tolerogenic environment to allow the fetus to develop. During pregnancy several immunoregulatory mechanisms ensure the protections of the fetus which expresses paternal antigens, recognized as non-self by maternal immune system. MSCs can interact with APCs to re-program them toward a tolerant phenotype as evident from increased IL-10 secretion. Moreover, they can modulate the co-stimulatory signal on DCs inducing pro-stimulatory functions (99). MSCs can reduce the activity of T-cells using different mechanisms, for example by secretion of indoleamine 2,3-dioxygenase (IDO), an enzyme capable of metabolizing the amino acid tryptophan to kynurenine. T-cells rely on this amino acid to become activated, and the depletion of tryptophan induces apoptosis or inhibiting their proliferation and differentiation by cell to cell contact, a process mediated by PD-L1 (101, 102).

Tolerogenic Antigen Presentation

Successful T-cell activation and differentiation depends upon the presence of co-stimulatory molecules such as CD28-B7 and a pro-inflammatory microenvironment mediated by cytokines such as IL-12. In the absence of these factors alloantigen presentation leads to anergy, a state in which the T-cell is unable to mount an effector response, and cell death.

Whilst DC antigen presentation is a major driver of rejection, a range of tolerogenic DC phenotypes have also been identified in the liver (103, 104). These cells are characterized by low levels of MHC class II and co-stimulatory molecule expression, low levels of IL-12 production, and high levels of IL-10 production; the latter stimulating Treg differentiation and inhibiting production of pro-inflammatory cytokines by macrophages (105, 106). Furthermore, some DC subtypes express PD-L1, which binds to PD-1 on T-cells inhibiting the CD28-B7 co-stimulatory signal and arresting T-cell maturation (107–109). Macrophage colony-stimulating factor (110) and hepatocyte growth factor (111) favor differentiation toward tolerogenic DC whereas FLT3L is associated with an activated alloreactive phenotype (112). Tolerogenic DC have been demonstrated in secondary lymphoid tissue following liver allograft (113) and upregulation of MHC class II and B7 in these cells leads to rejection (114). The possibility of harnessing this mechanism with pre-transplantation infusion of donor-derived tolerogenic DC is now being explored in the clinical setting (115).

Kupffer cells, LSEC, hepatocytes and hepatic stellate cells also have the ability to express MHC class I and II, particularly in pro-inflammatory states, and thus have the potential to activate alloreactive T-cells (103, 116, 117). However, in common with tolerogenic DC, non-professional antigen presentation in the liver tends to lack sufficient co-stimulatory B7 expression, to over-express PD-L1 and PD-L2 and to produce IL-10 and TGF-β, thus favoring tolerogenesis (118, 119). In support of these observations, T-cell activation in lymphoid tissue is generally much more potent than in the liver (120). However, under conditions of high antigen load local hepatic antigen presentation

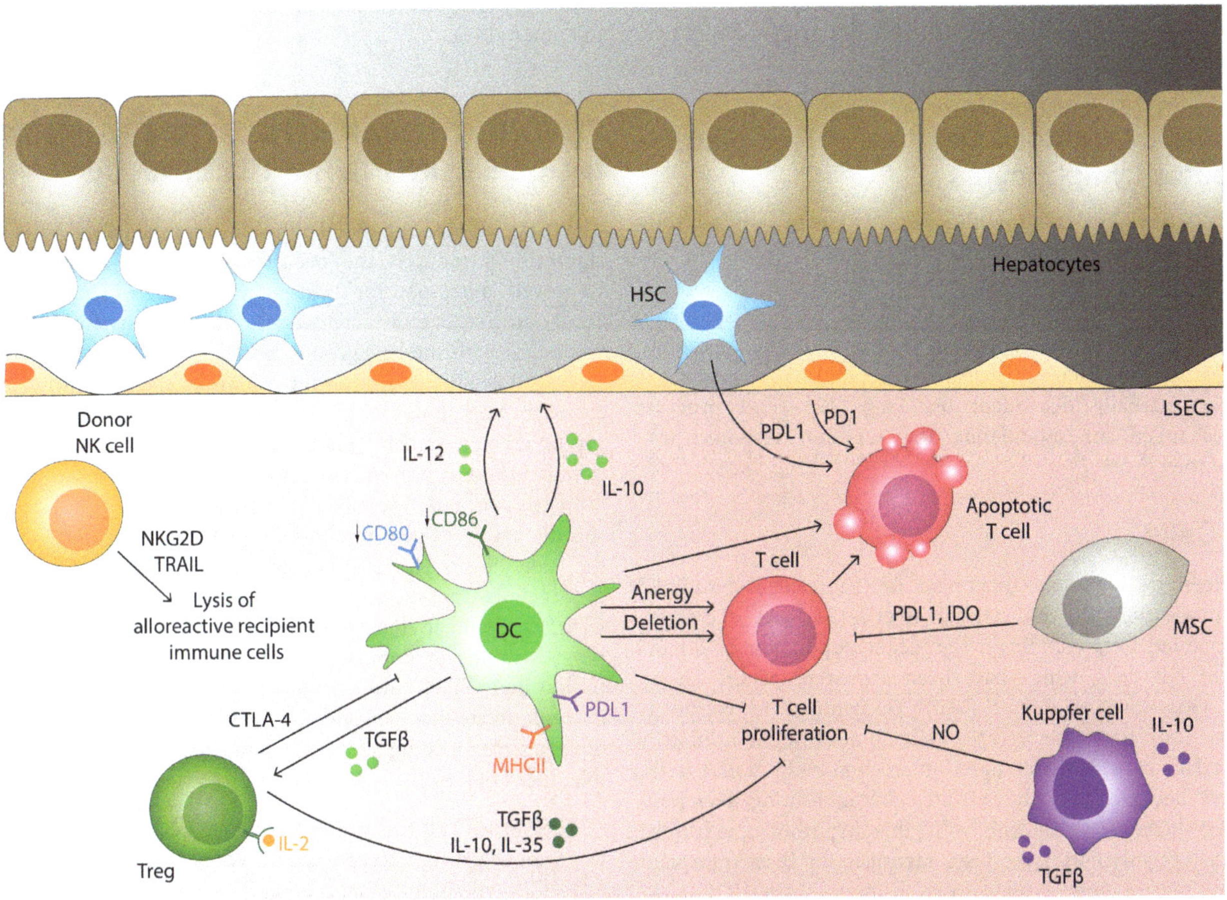

FIGURE 4 | Cellular mechanisms of liver allograft tolerance. A number of cells are able to promote tolerance in the liver allograft. Under normal non-inflamed conditions dendritic cells express low level of co-stimulatory molecules which along with the high expression of PDL1 induces T-cell anergy or deletion of the alloreactive T-cell clone. DCs also promote tolerance by secreting IL-10 and TGF-β which induces the differentiation of Tregs. CTLA4 on Tregs surface binds B7 on DC with a higher affinity than CD28, impairing DC-T-cell interactions. Tregs also contribute to the tolerogenic microenvironment also secreting TGF-β, IL-10 and IL-35, binding IL-2 on CD25 with higher affinity then T effector cells and by direct cytotoxicity through granzyme, perforin and Fas-FasL pathway. In contrast to recipient derived NK cells which tend to mediate rejection, donor derived NK cells transplanted as passenger cells within the liver allograft are able to directly lyse alloreactive recipient immune cells via NKG2D-MIC-A and TRAIL-TRAILR interactions leading to caspase-induced cell death. Mesenchymal stromal cells (MSCs) suppress T-cell proliferation and differentiation through the IDO pathway and cell-cell contact mediated by PDL1. Kupffer cells may be polarized to the M2 phenotype producing IL-10 and TGF-β and thus promoting tolerance. They can also release NO if stimulated by IFN-γ to inhibit T-cell proliferation. LSEC acts as non-professional antigen presenting cells with generally low levels of MHC class II expression; under many conditions induces antigen-specific tolerance. LSEC along with hepatic stellate cells induce T-cell apoptosis through PDL1/PD1 pathway interactions.

is able to overcome tolerogenic barriers and successfully stimulate CD8 + Tc activation (121).

Regulatory T-Cells

Regulatory T-cells (Treg) are a population of T-cells that suppress immune responses and maintain immune homeostasis and self-tolerance. They differentiate either in the thymus or in the periphery and multiple subtypes have been described, of which the CD4 + /CD25 + /FOXP3 + is the prototypical example (122). There is a close reciprocal relationship between Treg and Th17 differentiation: TGF-β in the absence of pro-inflammatory cytokines induces FOXP3 expression and Treg differentiation, whereas if pro-inflammatory cytokines are also present then TGF-β induces Th17 differentiation (123). Treg control effector T-cells via several distinct mechanisms: (1) production of immunosuppressive cytokines such as IL-10, TFG-β and IL-35, (2) consumption of IL-2 via the Treg CD25 receptor, thus depriving activated T-cells of the main driver of proliferation, (3) direct cytotoxicity via granzyme/perforin and Fas-FasL-dependent pathways and (4) constitutive Treg expression of CTLA-4 which acts as an alternative inhibitory ligand for B7 on DC with a higher affinity than the co-stimulatory molecule CD28, thus impairing DC-T-cell interactions (124).

The importance of Treg in liver transplantation has been demonstrated through a liver allograft model in which tolerant mice treated with Treg depleting anti-CD25 antibodies experienced rejection with a reduced Treg/T-effector cell ratio (125). Moreover, animal models have demonstrated Treg stimulated *in vitro* with alloantigens capable of inducing long-term tolerance (126). In clinical studies increased numbers of circulating Treg are associated with tolerance of the allograft liver (127). Treg are also enriched in operationally tolerant liver allograft recipients (128).

Activation-Induced Deletion of Recipient Effector Lymphocytes

The liver retains tolerogenic potential even when tissue destructive alloreactive T-cells have gained access to the parenchyma and begun to mediate tissue damage. Several groups have demonstrated that such alloreactive T-cells undergo cell death either via apoptosis (129, 130) or lysosome-mediated degradation by hepatocytes (131). This process is at least partially dependent on Treg (125) and provides a mechanism for modulating the rejection response into one of tolerance.

NK Cells

NK cells are a major component of the resident lymphoid cell population in the normal liver (132). As such, the transplanted liver contains a significant population of donor-derived NK cells, which have been shown to persist for up to 2 years post-transplant (133). In contrast to recipient-derived cells, donor-derived NK cells do not lose the inhibitory KIR-MHC class I signal upon interaction with donor cells, instead being potentially activated by infiltrating recipient-derived leukocytes. In line with this hypothesis, expanded NK cell populations have been identified in liver transplant patients successfully weaned from immunosuppression (134). Donor-derived NK cells cause direct lysis of alloreactive recipient immune cells via NKG2D-MIC-A and TRAIL-TRAILR interactions leading to caspase-induced cell death (135). Hence, recipient-derived NK cells are likely to mediate rejection whereas donor-derived NK cells are likely to be tolerogenic (135). However, the situation may be complicated by the emergence of tolerogenic recipient-derived NK cell populations, arising through mechanisms such as dysregulation of the IL-12/STAT4 pathway (136).

Chimerism

Chimerism is defined as the presence of donor-derived cells within non-transplanted host organs and has been well documented following liver transplantation (137). This phenomenon has the ability to facilitate tolerance through deletion of alloreactive T-cells within the thymus and through peripheral effects by interactions between recipient- and donor-derived leukocytes. Whilst there are occasional case reports of complete hematopoietic chimerism occurring post-liver transplant (138), persistence of T-cell chimerism beyond the initial few weeks following liver transplantation is considered unusual (139). Furthermore, even patients with high degrees of chimerism continue to exhibit *in vitro* alloimmune responses up to 1 year post-transplant (140) and may still suffer clinically significant rejection episodes (141, 142). Despite these conflicting data, therapeutic options for inducing chimerism such as combined hematopoietic stem cells and solid organ transplant, thymus transplantation and intra-thymic injection of donor alloantigens, remain an exciting avenue for promoting tolerance (143).

FUTURE THERAPEUTIC STRATEGIES TO INDUCE LONG TERM TOLERANCE

The currently recommended immunosuppression regimens have significantly reduced the occurrence of acute rejection and improved outcomes for transplant recipients. However, this comes at the price of increased risk of infections and neoplasia compared with the background population. Currently, patients are treated with a calcineurin inhibitor, either tacrolimus or cyclosporine, along with an antiproliferative drug such as mycophenolate mofetil (**Figure 5**). These drugs target all T-cell populations and prevent the normal activation and function of both effector and regulatory T-cells. Biological drugs targeting specific pathways continue to be tested in an attempt to reduce the side effects. Some biological agents already in clinical use include the monoclonal antibodies alemtuzumab (anti-CD52) and anti-thymocyte globulin. These drugs broadly target most lymphocyte populations, including regulatory subtypes. Interestingly, Treg and regulatory B-cells are among the first to re-populate the peripheral blood in patients treated with these agents, helping to pushing the balance in favor of the tolerance (144, 145).

Treg-based cell therapy is a promising alternative approach to promote allograft acceptance, potentially minimizing reliance on traditional immunosuppression (146–150). An early approach involved infusing donor antigen-specific Treg and allowed seven out of ten patients to successfully wean from immunosuppression by 18 months post-transplantation (151). Recently data from the ONE study have been published, demonstrating that Treg cell therapy in donor kidney transplant recipients is safe, although missing the efficacy endpoint (152). Other transplant centers have ongoing clinical trials mainly focusing on manufacturing alloantigen-specific Treg (**Table 1**). This is based on the evidence that alloantigen specific Treg exhibit a better suppressive function toward the alloreactive T effector cells than polyclonal Treg (153, 154). The *in vitro* expansion of the antigen-specific Treg using antigen presenting cells is inefficient due to the small number of cells in the original polyclonal population. A different solution is to engineer human T-cells with genes encoding for the chimeric antigen receptor (CAR). CAR T-cells were approved for clinical usage in 2017 and have since been proved to be effective in cancer treatment and in preventing allograft rejection (155, 156). The *in vivo* expansion of Treg represents another interesting therapeutic strategy. Treg express a higher affinity for IL-2 thus the usage of a very low dose of this molecule can expand the Treg pool *in vivo* up to eight times without significantly increasing the number of T effector cells (157).

In order to suppress T cell proliferation and activation, MSC-therapy based offers an opportunity to promote the tolerance and reduce the immunosuppressive dose in solid organ transplantation. Although the variation in cell product and the heterogeneity of tissue origin makes interpretation of previous clinical studies challenging, MSC therapy is certainly promising.

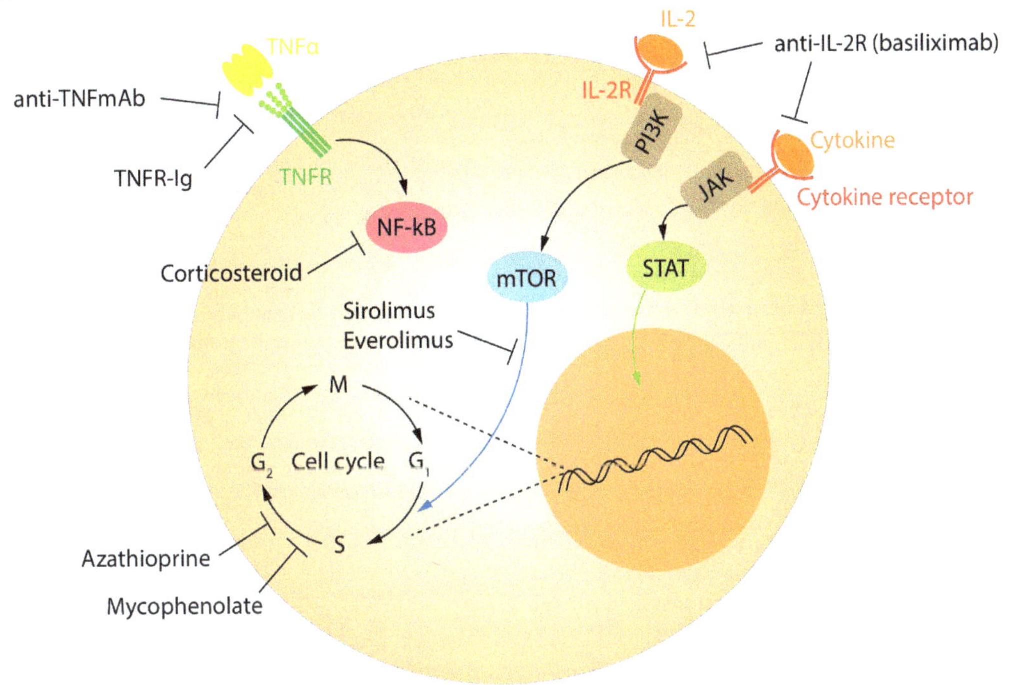

FIGURE 5 | Treatment targets of immunosuppression. The main targets of the immunosuppressive drugs.

TABLE 1 | Registered clinical trials involving regulatory T-cell therapy in liver transplantation.

Trial	Institution	Phase of the study	Primary outcome	Infused Treg clonality	Number of patients enrolled	Status
Todo/Okomura	Hokkaido, Japan	Phase I/IIA	– Safety – IS weaning – Number of Operationally Tolerant participants	Donor specific	10	Data published (140)
ARTEMIS (NCT02474199)	UCSF, United States	Phase I/II	– Safety – Incidence of AR, CR, re-transplantation, and death – Patients Who Are Able to Reduce CNI Dosing and Discontinue a Second IS Drug with stable LFTs	Donor specific	14	Completed
dELTA (NCT02188719)	UCSF, United States	Phase I	– Safety	Donor specific	15	Terminated
LITTMUS-UCSF (NCT03654040)	UCSF, United States	Phase I/II	– Safety – Number of Operationally Tolerant participants	Donor specific	N.A.	Withdrawn
LITTMUS-MGH (NCT03577431)	MGH, United States	Phase I/II	– Safety – Number of Operationally Tolerant participants	Donor specific	9*	Recruiting
ThRIL (NCT02166177)	King's college Hospital, United Kingdom	Phase I/II	– Rate of dose limiting toxicities – Graft Loss	Polyclonal	9	Completed
NCT01624077 (First Trial)	Nanjing, China	Phase I	– Patient and graft survival	Polyclonal	1*	Unknown
NCT01624077 (Second Trial)	Nanjing, China	Phase I	– Patient and graft survival	Donor specific	1*	Unknown

*From Clinicalgrials.gov, last accessed 19/05/2020. Abbreviations: IS, immunosuppression; AR, acute rejection; CR, chronic rejection; LFT, liver function tests. *Estimated.*

Currently the ongoing mYSTEP1 trial is testing safety and efficacy of donor derived bone marrow MSC pediatric living-donor liver transplantation (158).

Another cell therapy-based strategy has been proposed as immunomodulatory treatment using tolerogenic DC with low expression of MHC I and II and costimulatory B7 molecules and increased expression of PD-L1. These cells are readily derived from fresh or cryopreserved bone marrow derived progenitors (159). The infusion of *ex vivo* donor derived DCreg before transplant was shown to be effective in inducing liver transplant tolerance in murine models, inducing T-cell hyporeactivity thus extending liver allograft survival (160). Mesenchymal stromal cells are also being explored as a potential cell based therapy. These are multipotent cells isolated from tissues such as bone marrow, subcutaneous fat, umbilical cord and tooth pulp, with the ability to suppress immune responses via multiple cell to cell interactions and cytokine release (161). Infusion of these cells has been shown to prevent rejection in liver transplant animal models (162, 163).

Novel therapeutic strategies like *ex vivo* perfusion are already augmenting the pool of transplantable organs (164). Organ reconditioning strategies have already been applied in animal models to reduce the ischemia reperfusion injury by the infusion of MSCs or other anti-inflammatory agents (165) or to reduce steatosis using defatting agents before transplantation (166). Organ machine perfusion opens the door to a different approach to try to induce the tolerance by the infusion of tolerogenic molecules or treating the graft by immunomodulatory cells prior to implantation in the donor.

CONCLUSION

Despite major improvements in clinical outcomes following liver transplantation, the majority of patients remain dependent on long term immunosuppressive regimens. This highlights the persistence of alloreactive immunological processes and their tendency to overcome the specific tolerogenic mechanisms of the liver and cause rejection. Further elucidation of the underlying immunology will add to our understanding of this complex phenomenon. Meanwhile, several translational studies, including cell-based therapy approaches, offer the potential of enhancing tolerogenicity whilst avoiding the side effects of current therapeutic strategies.

AUTHOR CONTRIBUTIONS

VR and OC collaborated in writing and editing the manuscript and in developing the figures. CM developed the figures and contributed to manuscript writing. GW contributed to manuscript writing. All authors contributed to the article and approved the submitted version.

REFERENCES

1. Starzl TE, Demetris AJ, Van Thiel D. Liver transplantation (2). *N Engl J Med.* (1989) 321:1092–9. doi: 10.1056/NEJM198910193211606
2. Starzl TE, Demetris AJ, Van Thiel D. Liver transplantation (1). *N Engl J Med.* (1989) 321:1014–22. doi: 10.1056/NEJM198910123211505
3. Starzl TE, Iwatsuki S, Van Thiel DH, Gartner JC, Zitelli BJ, Malatack JJ, et al. Evolution of liver transplantation. *Hepatology.* (1982) 2:614–36. doi: 10.1002/hep.1840020516
4. Thurairajah PH, Carbone M, Bridgestock H, Thomas P, Hebbar S, Gunson BK, et al. Late acute liver allograft rejection; a study of its natural history and graft survival in the current era. *Transplantation.* (2013) 95:955–9. doi: 10.1097/TP.0b013e3182845f6c
5. Bartlett AS, Ramadas R, Furness S, Gane E, McCall JL. The natural history of acute histologic rejection without biochemical graft dysfunction in orthotopic liver transplantation: a systematic review. *Liver Transpl.* (2002) 8:1147–53. doi: 10.1053/jlts.2002.36240
6. Wiesner RH, Ludwig J, van Hoek B, Krom RA. Current concepts in cell-mediated hepatic allograft rejection leading to ductopenia and liver failure. *Hepatology.* (1991) 14(4 Pt 1):721–9. doi: 10.1002/hep.1840140424
7. Blakolmer K, Jain A, Ruppert K, Gray E, Duquesnoy R, Murase N, et al. Chronic liver allograft rejection in a population treated primarily with tacrolimus as baseline immunosuppression: long-term follow-up and evaluation of features for histopathological staging. *Transplantation.* (2000) 69:2330–6. doi: 10.1097/00007890-200006150-00019
8. Demetris AJ, Murase N, Lee RG, Randhawa P, Zeevi A, Pham S, et al. Chronic rejection. A general overview of histopathology and pathophysiology with emphasis on liver, heart and intestinal allografts. *Ann Transplant.* (1997) 2:27–44.
9. Banff Working G, Demetris AJ, Adeyi O, Bellamy CO, Clouston A, Charlotte F, et al. Liver biopsy interpretation for causes of late liver allograft dysfunction. *Hepatology.* (2006) 44:489–501. doi: 10.1002/hep.21280
10. Abu-Amara M, Yang SY, Tapuria N, Fuller B, Davidson B, Seifalian A. Liver ischemia/reperfusion injury: processes in inflammatory networks–a review. *Liver Transpl.* (2010) 16:1016–32. doi: 10.1002/lt.22117
11. Peralta C, Jimenez-Castro MB, Gracia-Sancho J. Hepatic ischemia and reperfusion injury: effects on the liver sinusoidal milieu. *J Hepatol.* (2013) 59:1094–106. doi: 10.1016/j.jhep.2013.06.017
12. Rampes S, Ma D. Hepatic ischemia-reperfusion injury in liver transplant setting: mechanisms and protective strategies. *J Biomed Res.* (2019) 33: 221–34.
13. Hashimoto K. Liver graft from donation after circulatory death donor: real practice to improve graft viability. *Clin Mol Hepatol.* (2020). doi: 10.3350/cmh.2020.0072 [Epub ahead of print].
14. Gehrau RC, Mas VR, Dumur CI, Suh JL, Sharma AK, Cathro HP, et al. Donor hepatic steatosis induce exacerbated ischemia-reperfusion injury through activation of innate immune response molecular pathways. *Transplantation.* (2015) 99:2523–33. doi: 10.1097/TP.0000000000000857
15. Neri AA, Dontas IA, Iliopoulos DC, Karatzas T. Pathophysiological changes during ischemia-reperfusion Injury in rodent hepatic steatosis. *In Vivo.* (2020) 34:953–64. doi: 10.21873/invivo.11863
16. Blok JJ, Detry O, Putter H, Rogiers X, Porte RJ, van Hoek B, et al. Longterm results of liver transplantation from donation after circulatory death. *Liver Transpl.* (2016) 22:1107–14. doi: 10.1002/lt.24449
17. Wang YC, Wu TJ, Wu TH, Lee CF, Chou HS, Chan KM, et al. The risk factors to predict acute rejection in liver transplantation. *Transplant Proc.* (2012) 44:526–8. doi: 10.1016/j.transproceed.2012.01.041
18. Shetty S, Adams DH, Hubscher SG. Post-transplant liver biopsy and the immune response: lessons for the clinician. *Expert Rev Clin Immunol.* (2012) 8:645–61. doi: 10.1586/eci.12.65
19. Dogan N, Husing-Kabar A, Schmidt HH, Cicinnati VR, Beckebaum S, Kabar I. Acute allograft rejection in liver transplant recipients: incidence, risk factors, treatment success, and impact on graft failure. *J Int Med Res.* (2018) 46:3979–90. doi: 10.1177/0300060518785543
20. Demetris AJ, Bellamy CO, Gandhi CR, Prost S, Nakanuma Y, Stolz DB. Functional immune anatomy of the liver-as an allograft. *Am J Transplant.* (2016) 16:1653–80. doi: 10.1111/ajt.13749
21. Howard TK, Klintmalm GB, Cofer JB, Husberg BS, Goldstein RM, Gonwa

TA. The influence of preservation injury on rejection in the hepatic transplant recipient. *Transplantation.* (1990) 49:103–7. doi: 10.1097/00007890-199001000-00023
22. Dar WA, Sullivan E, Bynon JS, Eltzschig H, Ju C. Ischaemia reperfusion injury in liver transplantation: cellular and molecular mechanisms. *Liver Int.* (2019) 39:788–801. doi: 10.1111/liv.14091
23. Sumpter TL, Abe M, Tokita D, Thomson AW. Dendritic cells, the liver, and transplantation. *Hepatology.* (2007) 46:2021–31. doi: 10.1002/hep.21974
24. Lei H, Reinke P, Volk HD, Lv Y, Wu R. Mechanisms of immune tolerance in liver transplantation-crosstalk between Alloreactive T cells and liver cells with therapeutic prospects. *Front Immunol.* (2019) 10:2667. doi: 10.3389/fimmu.2019.02667
25. Brown K, Sacks SH, Wong W. Coexpression of donor peptide/recipient MHC complex and intact donor MHC: evidence for a link between the direct and indirect pathways. *Am J Transplant.* (2011) 11:826–31. doi: 10.1111/j.1600-6143.2011.03437.x
26. Sivaganesh S, Harper SJ, Conlon TM, Callaghan CJ, Saeb-Parsy K, Negus MC, et al. Copresentation of intact and processed MHC alloantigen by recipient dendritic cells enables delivery of linked help to alloreactive CD8 T cells by indirect-pathway CD4 T cells. *J Immunol.* (2013) 190:5829–38. doi: 10.4049/jimmunol.1300458
27. Harper SJ, Ali JM, Wlodek E, Negus MC, Harper IG, Chhabra M, et al. CD8 T-cell recognition of acquired alloantigen promotes acute allograft rejection. *Proc Natl Acad Sci USA.* (2015) 112:12788–93. doi: 10.1073/pnas.1513533112
28. Smyth LA, Lechler RI, Lombardi G. Continuous acquisition of MHC:peptide complexes by recipient cells contributes to the generation of anti-graft CD8(+) T cell immunity. *Am J Transplant.* (2017) 17:60–8. doi: 10.1111/ajt.13996
29. Herrera OB, Golshayan D, Tibbott R, Salcido Ochoa F, James MJ, Marelli-Berg FM, et al. A novel pathway of alloantigen presentation by dendritic cells. *J Immunol.* (2004) 173:4828–37. doi: 10.4049/jimmunol.173.8.4828
30. Barbara JA, Turvey SE, Kingsley CI, Spriewald BM, Hara M, Witzke O, et al. Islet allograft rejection can be mediated by CD4+, alloantigen experienced, direct pathway T cells of TH1 and TH2 cytokine phenotype. *Transplantation.* (2000) 70:1641–9. doi: 10.1097/00007890-200012150-00017
31. Swain SL, McKinstry KK, Strutt TM. Expanding roles for CD4(+) T cells in immunity to viruses. *Nat Rev Immunol.* (2012) 12:136–48. doi: 10.1038/nri3152
32. Heidt S, Segundo DS, Chadha R, Wood KJ. The impact of Th17 cells on transplant rejection and the induction of tolerance. *Curr Opin Organ Transplant.* (2010) 15:456–61. doi: 10.1097/MOT.0b013e32833b9bfb
33. Liu Z, Fan H, Jiang S. CD4(+) T-cell subsets in transplantation. *Immunol Rev.* (2013) 252:183–91. doi: 10.1111/imr.12038
34. Goddard S, Williams A, Morland C, Qin S, Gladue R, Hubscher SG, et al. Differential expression of chemokines and chemokine receptors shapes the inflammatory response in rejecting human liver transplants. *Transplantation.* (2001) 72:1957–67. doi: 10.1097/00007890-200112270-00016
35. Adams DH, Sanchez-Fueyo A, Samuel D. From immunosuppression to tolerance. *J Hepatol.* (2015) 62(1 Suppl):S170–85. doi: 10.1016/j.jhep.2015.02.042
36. Shetty S, Lalor PF, Adams DH. Liver sinusoidal endothelial cells - gatekeepers of hepatic immunity. *Nat Rev Gastroenterol Hepatol.* (2018) 15:555–67. doi: 10.1038/s41575-018-0020-y
37. Bertolino P, Schrage A, Bowen DG, Klugewitz K, Ghani S, Eulenburg K, et al. Early intrahepatic antigen-specific retention of naive CD8+ T cells is predominantly ICAM-1/LFA-1 dependent in mice. *Hepatology.* (2005) 42:1063–71. doi: 10.1002/hep.20885
38. John B, Crispe IN. Passive and active mechanisms trap activated CD8+ T cells in the liver. *J Immunol.* (2004) 172:5222–9. doi: 10.4049/jimmunol.172.9.5222
39. Shetty S, Weston CJ, Oo YH, Westerlund N, Stamataki Z, Youster J, et al. Common lymphatic endothelial and vascular endothelial receptor-1 mediates the transmigration of regulatory T cells across human hepatic sinusoidal endothelium. *J Immunol.* (2011) 186:4147–55. doi: 10.4049/jimmunol.1002961
40. McDonald B, McAvoy EF, Lam F, Gill V, de la Motte C, Savani RC, et al. Interaction of CD44 and hyaluronan is the dominant mechanism for neutrophil sequestration in inflamed liver sinusoids. *J Exp Med.* (2008) 205:915–27. doi: 10.1084/jem.20071765
41. Martelius T, Salaspuro V, Salmi M, Krogerus L, Hockerstedt K, Jalkanen S, et al. Blockade of vascular adhesion protein-1 inhibits lymphocyte infiltration in rat liver allograft rejection. *Am J Pathol.* (2004) 165:1993–2001. doi: 10.1016/S0002-9440(10)63250-6
42. Kahraman A, Barreyro FJ, Bronk SF, Werneburg NW, Mott JL, Akazawa Y, et al. TRAIL mediates liver injury by the innate immune system in the bile duct-ligated mouse. *Hepatology.* (2008) 47:1317–30. doi: 10.1002/hep.22136
43. Eksteen B, Afford SC, Wigmore SJ, Holt AP, Adams DH. Immune-mediated liver injury. *Semin Liver Dis.* (2007) 27:351–66. doi: 10.1055/s-2007-991512
44. Tashiro H, Itamoto T, Ohdan H, Arihiro K, Tateaki Y, Nakahara H, et al. Involvement of tumor necrosis factor-alpha receptor 1 and tumor necrosis factor-related apoptosis-inducing ligand-(TRAIL) receptor-2/DR-5, but not Fas, in graft injury in live-donor liver transplantation. *Transpl Int.* (2004) 17:626–33. doi: 10.1007/s00147-004-0762-z
45. Benechet AP, Iannacone M. Determinants of hepatic effector CD8(+) T cell dynamics. *J Hepatoly.* (2017) 66:228–33. doi: 10.1016/j.jhep.2016.07.011
46. Jiang S, Herrera O, Lechler RI. New spectrum of allorecognition pathways: implications for graft rejection and transplantation tolerance. *Curr Opin Immunol.* (2004) 16:550–7. doi: 10.1016/j.coi.2004.07.011
47. Lin SZ, Chen KJ, Tong HF, Jing H, Li H, Zheng SS. Emodin attenuates acute rejection of liver allografts by inhibiting hepatocellular apoptosis and modulating the Th1/Th2 balance in rats. *Clin Exp Pharmacol Physiol.* (2010) 37:790–4. doi: 10.1111/j.1440-1681.2010.05378.x
48. Chan SY, DeBruyne LA, Goodman RE, Eichwald EJ, Bishop DK. In vivo depletion of CD8+ T cells results in Th2 cytokine production and alternate mechanisms of allograft rejection. *Transplantation.* (1995) 59:1155–61. doi: 10.1097/00007890-199504270-00014
49. Zelenika D, Adams E, Mellor A, Simpson E, Chandler P, Stockinger B, et al. Rejection of H-Y disparate skin grafts by monospecific CD4+ Th1 and Th2 cells: no requirement for CD8+ T cells or B cells. *J Immunol.* (1998) 161:1868–74.
50. Xie XJ, Ye YF, Zhou L, Xie HY, Jiang GP, Feng XW, et al. Th17 promotes acute rejection following liver transplantation in rats. *J Zhejiang Univ Sci B.* (2010) 11:819–27. doi: 10.1631/jzus.B1000030
51. Jhun J, Lee SH, Lee SK, Kim HY, Jung ES, Kim DG, et al. Serial monitoring of immune markers being represented regulatory T cell/T helper 17 cell ratio: indicating tolerance for tapering immunosuppression after liver transplantation. *Front Immunol.* (2018) 9:352. doi: 10.3389/fimmu.2018.00352
52. Oo YH, Banz V, Kavanagh D, Liaskou E, Withers DR, Humphreys E, et al. CXCR3-dependent recruitment and CCR6-mediated positioning of Th-17 cells in the inflamed liver. *J Hepatol.* (2012) 57:1044–51. doi: 10.1016/j.jhep.2012.07.008
53. Jeffery HC, Hunter S, Humphreys EH, Bhogal R, Wawman RE, Birtwistle J, et al. Bidirectional cross-talk between biliary epithelium and Th17 cells promotes local Th17 expansion and bile duct proliferation in biliary liver diseases. *J Immunol.* (2019) 203:1151–9. doi: 10.4049/jimmunol.1800455
54. Hartigan CR, Sun H, Ford ML. Memory T-cell exhaustion and tolerance in transplantation. *Immunol Rev.* (2019) 292:225–42. doi: 10.1111/imr.12824
55. Macedo C, Orkis EA, Popescu I, Elinoff BD, Zeevi A, Shapiro R, et al. Contribution of naive and memory T-cell populations to the human alloimmune response. *Am J Transplant.* (2009) 9:2057–66. doi: 10.1111/j.1600-6143.2009.02742.x
56. Heeger PS, Greenspan NS, Kuhlenschmidt S, Dejelo C, Hricik DE, Schulak JA, et al. Pretransplant frequency of donor-specific. IFN-gamma-producing lymphocytes is a manifestation of immunologic memory and correlates with the risk of posttransplant rejection episodes. *J Immunol.* (1999) 163:2267–75.
57. Cho BK, Rao VP, Ge Q, Eisen HN, Chen J. Homeostasis-stimulated proliferation drives naive T cells to differentiate directly into memory T cells. *J Exp Med.* (2000) 192:549–56. doi: 10.1084/jem.192.4.549
58. Sanchez-Fueyo A, Strom TB. Immunologic basis of graft rejection and tolerance following transplantation of liver or other solid organs. *Gastroenterology.* (2011) 140:51–64. doi: 10.1053/j.gastro.2010.10.059
59. Moreau A, Varey E, Anegon I, Cuturi MC. Effector mechanisms of rejection. *Cold Spring Harb Perspect Med.* (2013) 3:a015461. doi: 10.1101/cshperspect.a015461
60. Ng YH, Oberbarnscheidt MH, Chandramoorthy HC, Hoffman R, Chalasani G. B cells help alloreactive T cells differentiate into memory T cells. *Am J Transplant.* (2010) 10:1970–80. doi: 10.1111/j.1600-6143.2010.03223.x
61. Ningappa M, Ashokkumar C, Higgs BW, Sun Q, Jaffe R, Mazariegos G, et al. Enhanced B cell alloantigen presentation and its epigenetic dysregulation in liver transplant rejection. *Am J Transplant.* (2016) 16:497–508. doi: 10.1111/

ajt.13509
62. Li J, Li C, Zhuang Q, Peng B, Zhu Y, Ye Q, et al. The evolving roles of macrophages in organ transplantation. *J Immunol Res.* (2019) 2019:5763430. doi: 10.1155/2019/5763430
63. Shen XD, Ke B, Zhai Y, Gao F, Busuttil RW, Cheng G, et al. Toll-like receptor and heme oxygenase-1 signaling in hepatic ischemia/reperfusion injury. *Am J Transplantat.* (2005) 5:1793–800. doi: 10.1111/j.1600-6143.2005.00932.x
64. Azad TD, Donato M, Heylen L, Liu AB, Shen-Orr SS, Sweeney TE, et al. Inflammatory macrophage-associated 3-gene signature predicts subclinical allograft injury and graft survival. *JCI Insight.* (2018) 3:e95659. doi: 10.1172/jci.insight.95659
65. Ochando J, Conde P, Bronte V. Monocyte-derived suppressor cells in transplantation. *Curr Transplant Rep.* (2015) 2:176–83. doi: 10.1007/s40472-015-0054-9
66. Conde P, Rodriguez M, van der Touw W, Jimenez A, Burns M, Miller J, et al. DC-SIGN(+) macrophages control the induction of transplantation tolerance. *Immunity.* (2015) 42:1143–58. doi: 10.1016/j.immuni.2015.05.009
67. Martinez FO, Gordon S, Locati M, Mantovani A. Transcriptional profiling of the human monocyte-to-macrophage differentiation and polarization: new molecules and patterns of gene expression. *J Immunol.* (2006) 177:7303–11. doi: 10.4049/jimmunol.177.10.7303
68. Starzl TE, Demetris AJ, Trucco M, Murase N, Ricordi C, Ildstad S, et al. Cell migration and chimerism after whole-organ transplantation: the basis of graft acceptance. *Hepatology.* (1993) 17:1127–52. doi: 10.1002/hep.1840170629
69. Scozzi D, Ibrahim M, Menna C, Krupnick AS, Kreisel D, Gelman AE. The role of neutrophils in transplanted organs. *Am J Transplant.* (2017) 17:328–35. doi: 10.1111/ajt.13940
70. Huang H, Tohme S, Al-Khafaji AB, Tai S, Loughran P, Chen L, et al. Damage-associated molecular pattern-activated neutrophil extracellular trap exacerbates sterile inflammatory liver injury. *Hepatology.* (2015) 62:600–14. doi: 10.1002/hep.27841
71. Chong AS, Alegre ML. Transplantation tolerance and its outcome during infections and inflammation. *Immunol Rev.* (2014) 258:80–101. doi: 10.1111/imr.12147
72. Pillay J, Kamp VM, van Hoffen E, Visser T, Tak T, Lammers JW, et al. A subset of neutrophils in human systemic inflammation inhibits T cell responses through Mac-1. *J Clin Invest.* (2012) 122:327–36. doi: 10.1172/JCI57990
73. Braza MS, Conde P, Garcia M, Cortegano I, Brahmachary M, Pothula V, et al. Neutrophil derived CSF1 induces macrophage polarization and promotes transplantation tolerance. *Am J Transplant.* (2018) 18:1247–55. doi: 10.1111/ajt.14645
74. de Groen PC, Kephart GM, Gleich GJ, Ludwig J. The eosinophil as an effector cell of the immune response during hepatic allograft rejection. *Hepatology.* (1994) 20:654–62. doi: 10.1002/hep.1840200317
75. Rodriguez-Peralvarez M, Germani G, Tsochatzis E, Rolando N, Luong TV, Dhillon AP, et al. Predicting severity and clinical course of acute rejection after liver transplantation using blood eosinophil count. *Transpl Int.* (2012) 25:555–63. doi: 10.1111/j.1432-2277.2012.01457.x
76. Liaskou E, Wilson DV, Oo YH. Innate immune cells in liver inflammation. *Mediators Inflamm.* (2012) 2012:949157. doi: 10.1155/2012/949157
77. Kahraman A, Fingas CD, Syn WK, Gerken G, Canbay A. Role of stress-induced NKG2D ligands in liver diseases. *Liver Int.* (2012) 32:370–82. doi: 10.1111/j.1478-3231.2011.02608.x
78. van der Touw W, Bromberg JS. Natural killer cells and the immune response in solid organ transplantation. *Am J Transplant.* (2010) 10:1354–8. doi: 10.1111/j.1600-6143.2010.03086.x
79. Obara H, Nagasaki K, Hsieh CL, Ogura Y, Esquivel CO, Martinez OM, et al. IFN-gamma, produced by NK cells that infiltrate liver allografts early after transplantation, links the innate and adaptive immune responses. *Am J Transplant.* (2005) 5:2094–103. doi: 10.1111/j.1600-6143.2005.00995.x
80. Moroso V, van der Meer A, Tilanus HW, Kazemier G, van der Laan LJ, Metselaar HJ, et al. Donor and recipient HLA/KIR genotypes do not predict liver transplantation outcome. *Transpl Int.* (2011) 24:932–42. doi: 10.1111/j.1432-2277.2011.01286.x
81. Ware R, Kumar V. Complexity and function of natural killer T cells with potential application to hepatic transplant survival. *Liver Transpl.* (2017) 23:1589–92. doi: 10.1002/lt.24950
82. Rajoriya N, Fergusson JR, Leithead JA, Klenerman P. Gamma delta T-lymphocytes in Hepatitis C and chronic liver disease. *Front Immunol.* (2014) 5:400. doi: 10.3389/fimmu.2014.00400
83. Heidt S, Hester J, Shankar S, Friend PJ, Wood KJ. B cell repopulation after alemtuzumab induction-transient increase in transitional B cells and long-term dominance of naive B cells. *Am J Transplant.* (2012) 12:1784–92. doi: 10.1111/j.1600-6143.2012.04012.x
84. Demetris AJ, Bellamy C, Hubscher SG, O'Leary J, Randhawa PS, Feng S, et al. 2016 Comprehensive update of the banff working group on liver allograft pathology: introduction of antibody-mediated rejection. *Am J Transplant.* (2016) 16:2816–35.
85. O'Leary JG, Kaneku H, Demetris AJ, Marr JD, Shiller SM, Susskind BM, et al. Antibody-mediated rejection as a contributor to previously unexplained early liver allograft loss. *Liver Transpl.* (2014) 20:218–27. doi: 10.1002/lt.23788
86. Chong AS. B cells as antigen-presenting cells in transplantation rejection and tolerance. *Cell Immunol.* (2020) 349:104061. doi: 10.1016/j.cellimm.2020.104061
87. Perry DK, Burns JM, Pollinger HS, Amiot BP, Gloor JM, Gores GJ, et al. Proteasome inhibition causes apoptosis of normal human plasma cells preventing alloantibody production. *Am J Transplant.* (2009) 9:201–9. doi: 10.1111/j.1600-6143.2008.02461.x
88. Valenzuela NM, McNamara JT, Reed EF. Antibody-mediated graft injury: complement-dependent and complement-independent mechanisms. *Curr Opin Organ Transplant.* (2014) 19:33–40. doi: 10.1097/MOT.0000000000000040
89. Grafals M, Thurman JM. The role of complement in organ transplantation. *Front Immunol.* (2019) 10:2380. doi: 10.3389/fimmu.2019.02380
90. Stegall MD, Chedid MF, Cornell LD. The role of complement in antibody-mediated rejection in kidney transplantation. *Nat Rev Nephrol.* (2012) 8:670–8. doi: 10.1038/nrneph.2012.212
91. Jane-Wit D, Manes TD, Yi T, Qin L, Clark P, Kirkiles-Smith NC, et al. Alloantibody and complement promote T cell-mediated cardiac allograft vasculopathy through noncanonical nuclear factor-kappaB signaling in endothelial cells. *Circulation.* (2013) 128:2504–16. doi: 10.1161/CIRCULATIONAHA.113.002972
92. Vieyra M, Leisman S, Raedler H, Kwan WH, Yang M, Strainic MG, et al. Complement regulates CD4 T-cell help to CD8 T cells required for murine allograft rejection. *Am J Pathol.* (2011) 179:766–74. doi: 10.1016/j.ajpath.2011.04.038
93. Stites E, Le Quintrec M, Thurman JM. The complement system and antibody-mediated transplant rejection. *J Immunol.* (2015) 195:5525–31. doi: 10.4049/jimmunol.1501686
94. Demetris AJ, Nakamura K, Yagihashi A, Iwaki Y, Takaya S, Hartman GG, et al. A clinicopathological study of human liver allograft recipients harboring preformed IgG lymphocytotoxic antibodies. *Hepatology.* (1992) 16:671–81. doi: 10.1002/hep.1840160310
95. O'Leary JG, Michelle Shiller S, Bellamy C, Nalesnik MA, Kaneku H, Jennings LW, et al. Acute liver allograft antibody-mediated rejection: an inter-institutional study of significant histopathological features. *Liver Transpl.* (2014) 20:1244–55. doi: 10.1002/lt.23948
96. Feng S, Bucuvalas J. Tolerance after liver transplantation: where are we? *Liver Transpl.* (2017) 23:1601–14. doi: 10.1002/lt.24845
97. Beaudreuil S, Samuel D, Rouas-Freiss N, Durrbach A. New aspect of immunosuppressive treatment in liver transplantation. How could you induce tolerance in liver transplantation? *Transpl Immunol.* (2007) 17:98–107. doi: 10.1016/j.trim.2006.11.007
98. Li L, Wozniak LJ, Rodder S, Heish S, Talisetti A, Wang Q, et al. A common peripheral blood gene set for diagnosis of operational tolerance in pediatric and adult liver transplantation. *Am J Transplant.* (2012) 12:1218–28. doi: 10.1111/j.1600-6143.2011.03928.x
99. Najar M, Raicevic G, Fayyad-Kazan H, Bron D, Toungouz M, Lagneaux L. Mesenchymal stromal cells and immunomodulation: a gathering of regulatory immune cells. *Cytotherapy.* (2016) 18:160–71. doi: 10.1016/j.jcyt.2015.10.011
100. da Silva Meirelles L, Caplan AI, Nardi NB. In search of the in vivo identity of mesenchymal stem cells. *Stem Cells.* (2008) 26:2287–99. doi: 10.1634/stemcells.2007-1122
101. Munn DH, Zhou M, Attwood JT, Bondarev I, Conway SJ, Marshall B, et al. Prevention of allogeneic fetal rejection by tryptophan catabolism. *Science.* (1998) 281:1191–3. doi: 10.1126/science.281.5380.1191
102. Taner T, Abrol N, Park WD, Hansen MJ, Gustafson MP, Lerman LO, et al. Phenotypic transcriptional, and functional analysis of liver mesenchymal stromal cells and their immunomodulatory properties. *Liver Transpl.* (2020) 26:549–63. doi: 10.1002/lt.25718
103. Thomson AW, Knolle PA. Antigen-presenting cell function in the tolerogenic liver environment. *Nat Rev Immunol.* (2010) 10:753–66. doi: 10.1038/nri2858

104. Xia S, Guo Z, Xu X, Yi H, Wang Q, Cao X. Hepatic microenvironment programs hematopoietic progenitor differentiation into regulatory dendritic cells, maintaining liver tolerance. *Blood.* (2008) 112:3175–85. doi: 10.1182/blood-2008-05-159921
105. Rastellini C, Lu L, Ricordi C, Starzl TE, Rao AS, Thomson AW. Granulocyte/macrophage colony-stimulating factor-stimulated hepatic dendritic cell progenitors prolong pancreatic islet allograft survival. *Transplantation.* (1995) 60:1366–70.
106. Thomson AW, Lu L. Are dendritic cells the key to liver transplant tolerance? *Immunol Today.* (1999) 20:27–32. doi: 10.1016/S0167-5699(98)01378-4
107. Liu H, Bakthavatsalam R, Meng Z, Li Z, Li W, Perkins JD, et al. PD-L1 signal on liver dendritic cells is critical for Foxp3(+)CD4(+)CD25(+) Treg and liver tolerance induction in mice. *Transplant Proc.* (2013) 45:1853–5. doi: 10.1016/j.transproceed.2013.03.015
108. Matta BM, Raimondi G, Rosborough BR, Sumpter TL, Thomson AW. IL-27 production and STAT3-dependent upregulation of B7-H1 mediate immune regulatory functions of liver plasmacytoid dendritic cells. *J Immunol.* (2012) 188:5227–37. doi: 10.4049/jimmunol.1103382
109. Mascanfroni ID, Yeste A, Vieira SM, Burns EJ, Patel B, Sloma I, et al. IL-27 acts on DCs to suppress the T cell response and autoimmunity by inducing expression of the immunoregulatory molecule CD39. *Nature Immunol.* (2013) 14:1054–63. doi: 10.1038/ni.2695
110. Li G, Kim YJ, Broxmeyer HE. Macrophage colony-stimulating factor drives cord blood monocyte differentiation into IL-10(high)IL-12absent dendritic cells with tolerogenic potential. *J Immunol.* (2005) 174:4706–17. doi: 10.4049/jimmunol.174.8.4706
111. Rutella S, Bonanno G, Procoli A, Mariotti A, de Ritis DG, Curti A, et al. Hepatocyte growth factor favors monocyte differentiation into regulatory interleukin (IL)-10++IL-12low/neg accessory cells with dendritic-cell features. *Blood.* (2006) 108:218–27. doi: 10.1182/blood-2005-08-3141
112. Kingham TP, Chaudhry UI, Plitas G, Katz SC, Raab J, DeMatteo RP. Murine liver plasmacytoid dendritic cells become potent immunostimulatory cells after Flt-3 ligand expansion. *Hepatology.* (2007) 45:445–54. doi: 10.1002/hep.21457
113. Lu L, Rudert WA, Qian S, McCaslin D, Fu F, Rao AS, et al. Growth of donor-derived dendritic cells from the bone marrow of murine liver allograft recipients in response to granulocyte/macrophage colony-stimulating factor. *J Exp Med.* (1995) 182:379–87. doi: 10.1084/jem.182.2.379
114. Morelli AE, O'Connell PJ, Khanna A, Logar AJ, Lu L, Thomson AW. Preferential induction of Th1 responses by functionally mature hepatic (CD8alpha- and CD8alpha+) dendritic cells: association with conversion from liver transplant tolerance to acute rejection. *Transplantation.* (2000) 69:2647–57. doi: 10.1097/00007890-200006270-00027
115. Thomson AW, Humar A, Lakkis FG, Metes DM. Regulatory dendritic cells for promotion of liver transplant operational tolerance: rationale for a clinical trial and accompanying mechanistic studies. *Hum Immunol.* (2018) 79:314–21. doi: 10.1016/j.humimm.2017.10.017
116. Limmer A, Ohl J, Kurts C, Ljunggren HG, Reiss Y, Groettrup M, et al. Efficient presentation of exogenous antigen by liver endothelial cells to CD8+ T cells results in antigen-specific T-cell tolerance. *Nat Med.* (2000) 6:1348–54. doi: 10.1038/82161
117. Yu MC, Chen CH, Liang X, Wang L, Gandhi CR, Fung JJ, et al. Inhibition of T-cell responses by hepatic stellate cells via B7-H1-mediated T-cell apoptosis in mice. *Hepatology.* (2004) 40:1312–21. doi: 10.1002/hep.20488
118. Diehl L, Schurich A, Grochtmann R, Hegenbarth S, Chen L, Knolle PA. Tolerogenic maturation of liver sinusoidal endothelial cells promotes B7-homolog 1-dependent CD8+ T cell tolerance. *Hepatology.* (2008) 47:296–305. doi: 10.1002/hep.21965
119. Wong YC, Tay SS, McCaughan GW, Bowen DG, Bertolino P. Immune outcomes in the liver: is CD8 T cell fate determined by the environment? *J Hepatol.* (2015) 63:1005–14. doi: 10.1016/j.jhep.2015.05.033
120. Bowen DG, Zen M, Holz L, Davis T, McCaughan GW, Bertolino P. The site of primary T cell activation is a determinant of the balance between intrahepatic tolerance and immunity. *J Clin Invest.* (2004) 114:701–12. doi: 10.1172/JCI200421593
121. Klein I, Crispe IN. Complete differentiation of CD8+ T cells activated locally within the transplanted liver. *J Exp Med.* (2006) 203:437–47. doi: 10.1084/jem.20051775
122. Shalev I, Selzner N, Shyu W, Grant D, Levy G. Role of regulatory T cells in the promotion of transplant tolerance. *Liver Transpl.* (2012) 18:761–70. doi: 10.1002/lt.23458
123. Obermajer N, Popp FC, Soeder Y, Haarer J, Geissler EK, Schlitt HJ, et al. Conversion of Th17 into IL-17A(neg) regulatory T cells: a novel mechanism in prolonged allograft survival promoted by mesenchymal stem cell-supported minimized immunosuppressive therapy. *J Immunol.* (2014) 193:4988–99. doi: 10.4049/jimmunol.1401776
124. Shevach EM. Mechanisms of foxp3+ T regulatory cell-mediated suppression. *Immunity.* (2009) 30:636–45. doi: 10.1016/j.immuni.2009.04.010
125. Li W, Kuhr CS, Zheng XX, Carper K, Thomson AW, Reyes JD, et al. New insights into mechanisms of spontaneous liver transplant tolerance: the role of Foxp3-expressing CD25+CD4+ regulatory T cells. *Am J Transplant.* (2008) 8:1639–51. doi: 10.1111/j.1600-6143.2008.02300.x
126. Joffre O, Santolaria T, Calise D, Al Saati T, Hudrisier D, Romagnoli P, et al. Prevention of acute and chronic allograft rejection with CD4+CD25+Foxp3+ regulatory T lymphocytes. *Nat Med.* (2008) 14:88–92. doi: 10.1038/nm1688
127. Martinez-Llordella M, Puig-Pey I, Orlando G, Ramoni M, Tisone G, Rimola A, et al. Multiparameter immune profiling of operational tolerance in liver transplantation. *Am J Transplant.* (2007) 7:309–19. doi: 10.1111/j.1600-6143.2006.01621.x
128. Taubert R, Danger R, Londono MC, Christakoudi S, Martinez-Picola M, Rimola A, et al. Hepatic infiltrates in operational tolerant patients after liver transplantation show enrichment of regulatory T cells before proinflammatory genes are downregulated. *Am J Transplant.* (2016) 16:1285–93. doi: 10.1111/ajt.13617
129. Sharland A, Yan Y, Wang C, Bowen DG, Sun J, Sheil AG, et al. Evidence that apoptosis of activated T cells occurs in spontaneous tolerance of liver allografts and is blocked by manipulations which break tolerance. *Transplantation.* (1999) 68:1736–45. doi: 10.1097/00007890-199912150-00018
130. Bishop GA, Wang C, Sharland AF, McCaughan G. Spontaneous acceptance of liver transplants in rodents: evidence that liver leucocytes induce recipient T-cell death by neglect. *Immunol Cell Biol.* (2002) 80:93–100. doi: 10.1046/j.1440-1711.2002.01049.x
131. Benseler V, Warren A, Vo M, Holz LE, Tay SS, Le Couteur DG, et al. Hepatocyte entry leads to degradation of autoreactive CD8 T cells. *Proc Natl Acad Sci USA.* (2011) 108:16735–40. doi: 10.1073/pnas.1112251108
132. Lysakova-Devine T, O'Farrelly C. Tissue-specific NK cell populations and their origin. *J Leukoc Biol.* (2014) 96:981–90. doi: 10.1189/jlb.1RU0514-241R
133. Moroso V, Famili F, Papazian N, Cupedo T, van der Laan LJ, Kazemier G, et al. NK cells can generate from precursors in the adult human liver. *Eur J Immunol.* (2011) 41:3340–50. doi: 10.1002/eji.201141760
134. de la Garza RG, Sarobe P, Merino J, Lasarte JJ, D'Avola D, Belsue V, et al. Immune monitoring of immunosuppression withdrawal of liver transplant recipients. *Transpl Immunol.* (2015) 33:110–6. doi: 10.1016/j.trim.2015.07.006
135. Harmon C, Sanchez-Fueyo A, O'Farrelly C, Houlihan DD. Natural killer cells and liver transplantation: orchestrators of rejection or tolerance? *Am J Transplant.* (2016) 16:751–7. doi: 10.1111/ajt.13565
136. Jamil KM, Hydes TJ, Cheent KS, Cassidy SA, Traherne JA, Jayaraman J, et al. STAT4-associated natural killer cell tolerance following liver transplantation. *Gut.* (2017) 66:352–61. doi: 10.1136/gutjnl-2015-309395
137. Kashiwagi N, Porter KA, Penn I, Brettschneider L, Starzl TE. Studies of homograft sex and of gamma globulin phenotypes after orthotopic homotransplantation of the human liver. *Surg Forum.* (1969) 20:374–6.
138. Alexander SI, Smith N, Hu M, Verran D, Shun A, Dorney S, et al. Chimerism and tolerance in a recipient of a deceased-donor liver transplant. *N Engl J Med.* (2008) 358:369–74. doi: 10.1056/NEJMoa0707255
139. Domiati-Saad R, Klintmalm GB, Netto G, Agura, Chinnakotla S, Smith DM. Acute graft versus host disease after liver transplantation: patterns of lymphocyte chimerism. *Am J Transplant.* (2005) 5:2968–73. doi: 10.1111/j.1600-6143.2005.01110.x
140. Bettens F, Tiercy JM, Campanile N, Giostra E, Majno P, Rubbia L, et al. Microchimerism after liver transplantation: absence of rejection without abrogation of anti-donor cytotoxic T-lymphocyte mediated alloreactivity. *Liver Transpl.* (2005) 11:290–7. doi: 10.1002/lt.20360
141. Sivasai KS, Alevy YG, Duffy BF, Brennan DC, Singer GG, Shenoy S, et al. Peripheral blood microchimerism in human liver and renal transplant recipients: rejection despite donor-specific chimerism. *Transplantation.* (1997) 64:427–32. doi: 10.1097/00007890-199708150-00010
142. Schlitt HJ, Hundrieser J, Ringe B, Pichlmayr R. Donor-type microchimerism associated with graft rejection eight years after liver transplantation. *N Engl J*

Med. (1994) 330:646–7. doi: 10.1056/NEJM199403033300919
143. Zuber J, Sykes M. Mechanisms of mixed chimerism-based transplant tolerance. *Trends Immunol.* (2017) 38:829–43. doi: 10.1016/j.it.2017.07.008
144. Braza F, Dugast E, Panov I, Paul C, Vogt K, Pallier A, et al. Central role of CD45RA- Foxp3hi memory regulatory T cells in clinical kidney transplantation tolerance. *J Am Soc Nephrol.* (2015) 26:1795–805. doi: 10.1681/ASN.2014050480
145. Lei H, Kuchenbecker L, Streitz M, Sawitzki B, Vogt K, Landwehr-Kenzel S, et al. Human CD45RA(-) FoxP3(hi) memory-type regulatory T cells show distinct TCR repertoires with conventional T cells and play an important role in controlling early immune activation. *Am J Transplant.* (2015) 15:2625–35. doi: 10.1111/ajt.13315
146. Pons JA, Revilla-Nuin B, Baroja-Mazo A, Ramirez P, Martinez-Alarcon L, Sanchez-Bueno F, et al. FoxP3 in peripheral blood is associated with operational tolerance in liver transplant patients during immunosuppression withdrawal. *Transplantation.* (2008) 86:1370–8. doi: 10.1097/TP.0b013e318188d3e6
147. Savage TM, Shonts BA, Obradovic A, Dewolf S, Lau S, Zuber J, et al. Early expansion of donor-specific Tregs in tolerant kidney transplant recipients. *JCI Insight.* (2018) 3: e124086. doi: 10.1172/jci.insight.124086
148. Todo S, Yamashita K, Goto R, Zaitsu M, Nagatsu A, Oura T, et al. A pilot study of operational tolerance with a regulatory T-cell-based cell therapy in living donor liver transplantation. *Hepatology.* (2016) 64:632–43. doi: 10.1002/hep.28459
149. Landwehr-Kenzel S, Issa F, Luu SH, Schmuck M, Lei H, Zobel A, et al. Novel GMP-compatible protocol employing an allogeneic B cell bank for clonal expansion of allospecific natural regulatory T cells. *Am J Transplant.* (2014) 14:594–606. doi: 10.1111/ajt.12629
150. Landwehr-Kenzel S, Zobel A, Hoffmann H, Landwehr N, Schmueck-Henneresse M, Schachtner T, et al. Ex vivo expanded natural regulatory T cells from patients with end-stage renal disease or kidney transplantation are useful for autologous cell therapy. *Kidney Int.* (2018) 93:1452–64. doi: 10.1016/j.kint.2018.01.021
151. Jain MD, Davila ML. Concise review: emerging principles from the clinical application of chimeric antigen receptor T Cell therapies for B cell malignancies. *Stem Cells.* (2018) 36:36–44. doi: 10.1002/stem.2715
152. Sawitzki B, Harden PN, Reinke P, Moreau A, Hutchinson JA, Game DS, et al. Regulatory cell therapy in kidney transplantation (The ONE Study): a harmonised design and analysis of seven non-randomised, single-arm, phase 1/2A trials. *Lancet.* (2020) 395:1627–39. doi: 10.1016/S0140-6736(20)30167-7
153. Gauthier J, Yakoub-Agha I. Chimeric antigen-receptor T-cell therapy for hematological malignancies and solid tumors: clinical data to date, current limitations and perspectives. *Curr Res Transl Med.* (2017) 65:93–102. doi: 10.1016/j.retram.2017.08.003
154. MacDonald KG, Hoeppli RE, Huang Q, Gillies J, Luciani DS, Orban PC, et al. Alloantigen-specific regulatory T cells generated with a chimeric antigen receptor. *J Clin Invest.* (2016) 126:1413–24. doi: 10.1172/JCI82771
155. Noyan F, Zimmermann K, Hardtke-Wolenski M, Knoefel A, Schulde E, Geffers R, et al. Prevention of allograft rejection by use of regulatory T Cells with an MHC-specific chimeric antigen receptor. *Am J Transplant.* (2017) 17:917–30. doi: 10.1111/ajt.14175
156. Boardman DA, Philippeos C, Fruhwirth GO, Ibrahim MA, Hannen RF, Cooper D, et al. Expression of a chimeric antigen receptor specific for donor HLA Class I enhances the potency of human regulatory T Cells in preventing human skin transplant rejection. *Am J Transplant.* (2017) 17:931–43. doi: 10.1111/ajt.14185
157. Ward NC, Yu A, Moro A, Ban Y, Chen X, Hsiung S, et al. IL-2/CD25: a long-acting fusion protein that promotes immune tolerance by selectively targeting the IL-2 receptor on regulatory T cells. *J Immunol.* (2018) 201:2579–92. doi: 10.4049/jimmunol.1800907
158. Hartleif S, Schumm M, Doring M, Mezger M, Lang P, Dahlke MH, et al. Safety and tolerance of donor-derived mesenchymal stem cells in pediatric living-donor liver transplantation: the MYSTEP1 study. *Stem Cells Int.* (2017) 2017:2352954. doi: 10.1155/2017/2352954
159. Hackstein H, Thomson AW. Dendritic cells: emerging pharmacological targets of immunosuppressive drugs. *Nat Rev Immunol.* (2004) 4:24–34. doi: 10.1038/nri1256
160. Xia MJ, Shan J, Li YP, Zhou YN, Guo YJ, Sun GX, et al. Adoptive transfusion of tolerogenic dendritic cells prolongs the survival of liver allograft: a systematic review. *J Evid Based Med.* (2014) 7:135–46. doi: 10.1111/jebm.12094
161. Hu C, Li L. The immunoregulation of mesenchymal stem cells plays a critical role in improving the prognosis of liver transplantation. *J Transl Med.* (2019) 17:412. doi: 10.1186/s12967-019-02167-0
162. Wang Y, Zhang A, Ye Z, Xie H, Zheng S. Bone marrow-derived mesenchymal stem cells inhibit acute rejection of rat liver allografts in association with regulatory T-cell expansion. *Transplant Proc.* (2009) 41:4352–6. doi: 10.1016/j.transproceed.2009.08.072
163. Tian Y, Wang J, Wang W, Ding Y, Sun Z, Zhang Q, et al. Mesenchymal stem cells improve mouse non-heart-beating liver graft survival by inhibiting Kupffer cell apoptosis via TLR4-ERK1/2-Fas/FasL-caspase3 pathway regulation. *Stem Cell Res Ther.* (2016) 7:157. doi: 10.1186/s13287-016-0416-y
164. Mergental H, Laing RW, Kirkham AJ, Perera M, Boteon YL, Attard J, et al. Transplantation of discarded livers following viability testing with normothermic machine perfusion. *Nat Commun.* (2020) 11:2939. doi: 10.1038/s41467-020-16251-3
165. Verstegen MMA, Mezzanotte L, Ridwan RY, Wang K, de Haan J, Schurink IJ, et al. First report on ex vivo delivery of paracrine active human mesenchymal stromal cells to liver grafts during machine perfusion. *Transplantation.* (2020) 104:e5–7. doi: 10.1097/TP.0000000000002986
166. Boteon YL, Attard J, Boteon A, Wallace L, Reynolds G, Hubscher S, et al. Manipulation of lipid metabolism during normothermic machine perfusion: effect of defatting therapies on donor liver functional recovery. *Liver Transpl.* (2019) 25:1007–22. doi: 10.1002/lt.25439

17

Mesenchymal Stromal Cells, a New Player in Reducing Complications from Liver Transplantation?

Andrew Owen[1,2] *and Philip N. Newsome*[1,3,4*]

[1] National Institute for Health Research Birmingham, Biomedical Research Centre at University Hospitals Birmingham NHS Foundation Trust, University of Birmingham, Birmingham, United Kingdom, [2] Department of Anesthesia and Critical Care, University Hospitals Birmingham NHS Foundation Trust, Birmingham, United Kingdom, [3] Centre for Liver and Gastrointestinal Research, Institute of Immunology and Immunotherapy, University of Birmingham, Birmingham, United Kingdom, [4] Liver Unit, University Hospitals Birmingham NHS Foundation Trust, Birmingham, United Kingdom

***Correspondence:**
Philip N. Newsome
p.n.newsome@bham.ac.uk

In response to the global burden of liver disease there has been a commensurate increase in the demand for liver transplantation. However, due to a paucity of donor organs many centers have moved toward the routine use of marginal allografts, which can be associated with a greater risk of complications and poorer clinical outcomes. Mesenchymal stromal cells (MSC) are a multi-potent progenitor cell population that have been utilized to modulate aberrant immune responses in acute and chronic inflammatory conditions. MSC exert an immunomodulatory effect on innate and adaptive immune systems through the release of both paracrine soluble factors and extracellular vesicles. Through these routes MSC can switch the regulatory function of the immune system through effects on macrophages and T regulatory cells enabling a switch of phenotype from injury to restoration. A key benefit seems to be their ability to tailor their response to the inflammatory environment without compromising the host ability to fight infection. With over 200 clinical trials registered to examine MSC therapy in liver disease and an increasing number of trials of MSC therapy in solid organ transplant recipients, there is increasing consideration for their use in liver transplantation. In this review we critically appraise the potential role of MSC therapy in the context of liver transplantation, including their ability to modulate reperfusion injury, their role in the reduction of medium term complications in the biliary tree and their potential to enhance tolerance in transplanted organs.

Keywords: mesenchymal, stem, stromal, cell therapy, transplantation, liver

INTRODUCTION

Although the global burden of liver pathology is often underestimated due to limitations in mortality recording systems in many countries (1), it is still estimated that over 2 million liver-related deaths occur worldwide (2). Whilst there are many causes of liver disease, end stage liver disease represents a shared final pathway and once reached, the only curative treatment remains liver transplantation (3). With increasing numbers of patients on transplant waiting lists and fewer donor organs there has been a move toward the use of marginal donor organs so as to increase the pool of available organs for transplantation (4). This comes at a clinical cost though, despite improvements in patient selection. Specifically the prolonged warm ischemic time in a donation after cardiac death (DCD) liver transplant results in increased morbidity, mortality, critical care stay, and overall cost (5). The ability to increase the donor pool further by pushing the boundaries of ischemia, as well as reducing the need for toxic immunosuppression could lead to a reduction in complications and an increased number of organs available for transplantation. Mesenchymal stromal cells (MSC) may offer a novel cell therapeutic approach to impact on these negative squeal and potentially allow for expansion of the donor pool.

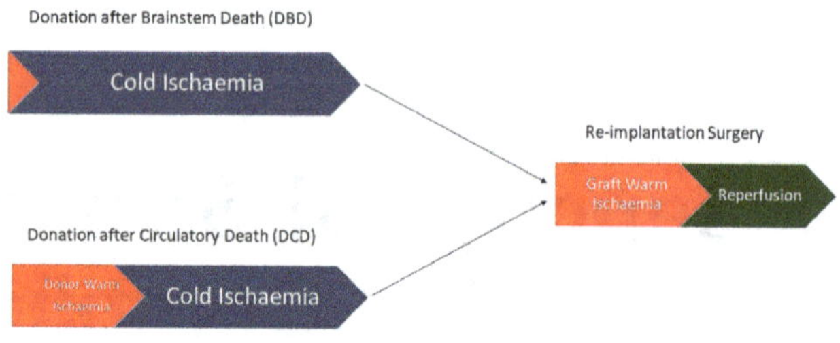

FIGURE 1 | Pathway demonstrating the differences between DBD and DCD liver transplantation with no donor warm ischemic time seen in DBD compared with a variable amount of donor warm ischemia in DCD.

TRANSPLANT RELATED HEPATIC INJURY

The process of liver transplantation includes a combination of both warm ischemia (organ at body temperature) and cold ischemia (organ perfused with cold preservative solution). The relative contribution of these processes during organ retrieval depends principally on the transport duration of the donor organ after cold preservation (6) and the donor liver source (7). Broadly speaking donor livers can come from one of three sources; a living donor, a brainstem dead/heart beating donor (donation after brainstem death, DBD) or a donor undergoing circulatory arrest/non-heart beating donor (donation after circulatory death, DCD). The consequences of the prolonged warm ischemia seen in DCD include greater generation of reactive oxygen species and a delayed adaptive immune response resulting in an injury pattern characterized by hepatocyte loss as opposed to the predominantly endothelial injury seen following DBD (8). Biliary complications are often seen following liver transplantation, however their incidence is different when comparing DCD and DBD with a greater incidence of ischemic cholangiopathy in DCD compared with more strictures and bile duct leaks seen in DBD (9). Liver ischemia and reperfusion injury represent a complex combination of pathologies with a variety of cell types involved and a number of pre-disposing factors related to both the transplant recipient and the donor organ. Ischemia and reperfusion injury are distinct but related pathologies often considered together as ischemia/reperfusion injury (10), with ischemic injury representing the primary damage to cells due to an interruption in organ perfusion and reperfusion injury representing the immunological response to the generation of reactive oxygen species and products of cell death following the re-establishment of organ perfusion.

Ischaemic injury occurs as a result of an inadequate oxygen supply to an organ and one of the first descriptions of liver ischemia was by Pringle in which his eponymous maneuver was shown to reduce bleeding by occluding liver vasculature (11). During liver transplantation warm ischemia can be further subdivided into donor warm ischemic time which is defined as the time from withdrawal of life support to the initiation of cold storage, and graft warm ischemic time which is defined as the time from removal from cold storage until reperfusion has occurred (12). There should be little donor warm ischemic time in living donors or DBD donors, whereas DCD donors will have a longer period of warm ischemia (**Figure 1**). The amount of cellular dysfunction seen following an ischemic insult is related to both the extent and duration of the period of ischemia (13). In humans oxygen is utilized in aerobic respiration in order to generate Adenosine Triphosphate (ATP), an energy source required for metabolic processes (14). Fermentation of glucose (often referred to in human physiology as anaerobic respiration) occurs when there is no oxygen present to act as the terminal electron acceptor leading to the generation of lactate, a less efficient process of energy production leading to the generation of H^+ ions and the subsequent reduction in cellular pH. The subsequent H^+ ion gradient leads to activation of Na^+/H^+ transporters in order to correct the intracellular pH generating an osmotic gradient and leading to cellular edema (15). Depletion of ATP also leads to inactivation of other ion pumps including the ATP dependent Ca^{2+} channels (**Figure 2**). There is also an increase in the breakdown products of ATP including xanthine and hypoxanthine (16). Hepatocytes are particularly vulnerable to warm ischemia (17) and whilst there is some debate over whether necrosis or apoptosis is the predominant factor in hepatocyte death, both modes of cell loss demonstrate mitochondrial dysfunction as a key problem (18–20). Cold ischemia, or preservation related injury, confers similar problems to that of warm ischemia, however there seems to be an increased effect on the sinusoidal endothelial cells whose death at reperfusion has been shown to be related to the duration of cold ischemia through platelet induced apoptosis (21).

Following restoration of blood and oxygen supply to the ischemic liver further damage occurs in the form of reperfusion injury. The generation of reactive oxygen species (ROS) is a key mechanism in this process, initially produced by intracellular xanthine oxidize in combination with resident specialized macrophages (Kupffer cells) and infiltrating polymorphonuclear cells (22). Activated Kupffer cells release pro-inflammatory cytokines which enhance neutrophil recruitment leading to further propagation of ROS release (23, 24). Following reperfusion sinusoidal endothelial cells express a number of adhesion molecules aiding the recruitment of infiltrating immune cells (25). T lymphocyte, in particular $CD4^+$ cells, is a key mechanism of injury following reperfusion (**Figure 2**) and blocking $CD4^+$ recruitment leads to a significant reduction injury (26). Activation of Toll Like Receptors (TLR) in particular TLR4 by damage associated molecular patterns (DAMP) has also been shown to be an important cause of

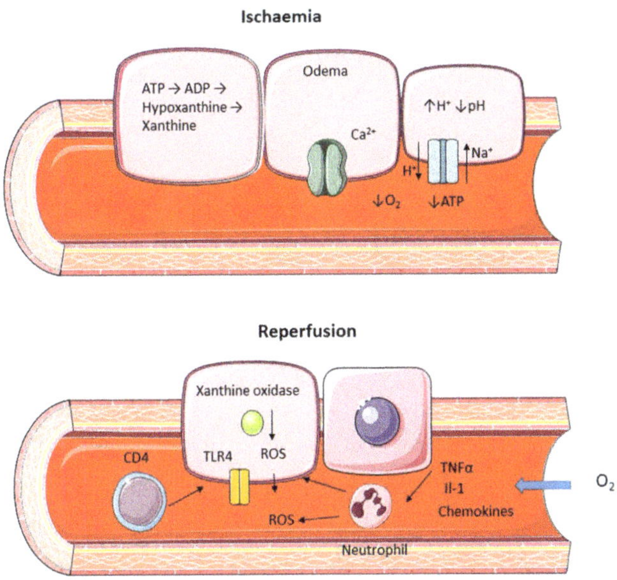

FIGURE 2 | Diagram representing hepatic ischemic and reperfusion injury. Ischemia is characterized by a lack of oxygen supply leading to a depletion of ATP and cellular edema due to increased H^+ leading to activation of the Na^+/H^+ transporter and inactivation of the ATP dependent Ca^{2+} pump. Reperfusion leads to restoration of O_2 supply with ROS generation and recruitment of neutrophils and $CD4^+$ lymphocytes.

reperfusion injury with reduced damage when this pathway is inhibited (27, 28).

MESENCHYMAL STROMAL CELLS

Mesenchymal stromal cells (MSC) are a multi-potent progenitor cell type capable of tri-lineage differentiation and immunomodulation (29). The description of cells in the bone marrow able to perform a supportive role was postulated over a century ago, however more recent work has developed the understanding of the physiological role that MSC play in the bone marrow stem cell niche (30). MSC do not appear to be limited to the bone marrow however, with MSC populations described in umbilical cord (31), placenta (32), adipose tissue 33), dermal tissue (34), and dental pulp (35). Debate still remains in the literature as to what constitutes an MSC and whether they represent true stem cells (36, 37) with the early literature plagued by problems with heterogeneous cells types and isolation techniques. With the advent of cell sorting and the publication of minimal criteria in order to describe MSC some of the problems seen in the earlier literature have improved but comparison between MSC types can still be problematic 29, 38, 39). Whilst the functional role that MSC play is still not fully elicited their ability to modulate the immune system has been well described (40, 41). Variation in human MSC function has been variably ascribed to different batches, donor sources and donor age, however evidence is mixed and there is as yet no standardized source or donor demographic definition to

TABLE 1 | Important cytokines involved in MSC immunosuppression.

Cytokine	Effect
C-C Motif Chemokine Ligand 2 (CCL2)	Suppress the activation and migration of Th17 cells
Haem Oxygenase 1 (HO1)	Suppresses T regulatory cell function
Hepatocyte Growth Factor (HGF)	Inhibits $CD4^+$ and $CD8^+$ T-lymphocyte function
Human Leucocyte Antigen G5 (HLA-G5)	Inhibits Natural Killer (NK) cells
Interleukin 6 (Il-6)	Inhibits neutrophil burst
Inducible Nitric Oxide Synthetase (iNOS)	Inhibits $CD4^+$ T-lymphocyte function
Indolamine 2,3 dioxygenase (IDO)	Inhibits $CD4^+$ and NK cell function
Nerve Growth Factor (NGF)	Binds to P75 on hepatic stellate cells and triggers apoptosis
Prostaglandin E_2 (PGE_2)	Inhibits $CD4^+$ and NK cell function and inhibits differentiation of monocytes into myeloid cells and TNF production by dendritic cells
Transforming Growth Factor β (TGF-β)	Inhibits $CD4^+$ T-lymphocyte function
TNF Stimulated Gene 6 protein (TSG6)	Switches macrophage phenotype to anti-inflammatory

inform cell therapy in clinical trials (42–47). It has also been demonstrated that adipose MSC derived from obese donors have reduced proliferative and differentiation ability (48). MSC tissue source may be important due to differing expression of tissue factor/CD142, as whilst MSC have low levels of MHC Class I and no MHC Class II expression (49), an innate immune response can be triggered following MSC infusion with source and passage being major determinants of tissue factor expression (50). This innate immune response can trigger thrombosis and lead to micro and microvascular complications. This is an important consideration when designing clinical trials as a cell therapy with low tissue factor expression may reduce the potential risks associated with MSC administration or enable steps to be made to mitigate these effects such as co-administration with heparin (51).

There have been a number of mechanisms described by which MSC are able to suppress the immune system with effects on both the innate and adaptive components. A key ability supporting the potential use of MSC in liver transplantation is their ability to suppress T cell activation and proliferation. Bone marrow derived MSC can upregulate the cyclin-dependent kinase inhibitor p27Kip1 and inhibit cyclin D2 leading to early cell cycle arrest in T lymphocytes (52). The effects on cyclin D2 are not limited to T cells however, with evidence that inhibition of B lymphocytes also occurs (53). MSC isolated from bone marrow can also reduce expression of MHC class I and II on dendritic cells, inhibiting their maturation and subsequent immune cell activation (54, 55). Another important ability of MSC is their effects on soluble factors, both secreting themselves and stimulating or inhibiting the secretion from other cells. Whilst many relevant mediators have been shown to be modulated by MSC therapy (**Table 1**;

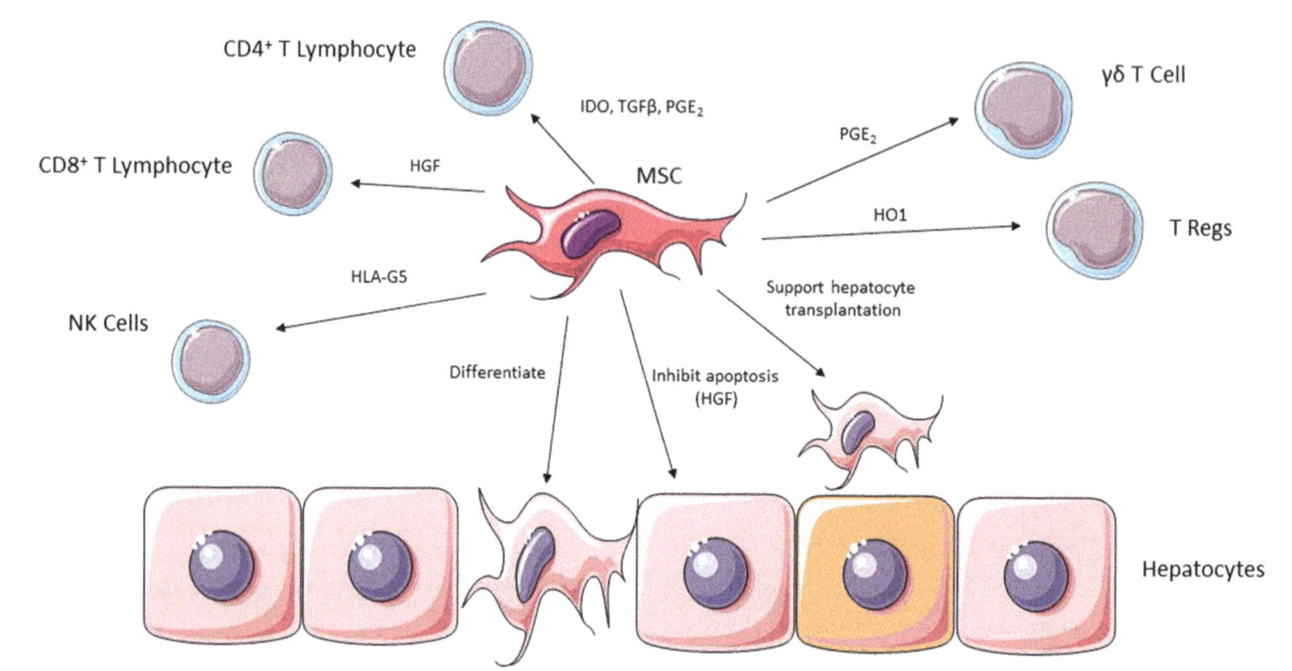

FIGURE 3 | MSC are able to exert their effects in ischemic liver injury via a number of potential effector cells including CD4+ and CD8+ lymphocytes, NK cells, Regulatory T cells and γδT cells. They are also able to support hepatocyte transplantation into injured liver and can undergo differentiation into hepatocytes.

Figure 3), important factors include Il-10, TNFα, IDO, PGE_2, and IFN-γ (56–62).

Given that MSC appear to exert their effect by secreting soluble proteins and extra-cellular vesicles (MSC-EV) administration of the bone marrow MSC secretome may represent a potential therapeutic strategy avoiding some of the potential problems with the use of a cellular therapy (63). In particular, the ability of MSC-EV to transfer non-coding RNA may explain the prolonged effects seen after the rapid clearance of MSC from the systemic circulation (64).

There are a number of potential routes of administration for MSC and extensive research carried out in animal models has not revealed a consensus on the most efficient and effective route of delivery. MSC are relatively large cells compared with immune cells, and as such when administered systemically tend to be filtered by the lungs (65). Both intravenous and intra-arterial routes of administration have been described, however concerns have been raised regarding the potential risk of cerebral ischemia following intra-arterial administration of bone marrow MSC (66), although there are diseases where spread to cerebral tissue may be beneficial such as acute ischemic stroke (67). Subcutaneous administration may represent an alternative as there is evidence in graft versus host disease that bone marrow derived MSC can exert a remote effect when encapsulated (68), however these results have not been reproduced more widely. Intravenous administration is commonly used in clinical and pre-clinical investigation, however this can be problematic due to cells becoming trapped in the lung (69). Human bone marrow derived MSC have been demonstrated to express a number of adhesion molecules on their surface, and whilst many of these are lost in standard culture conditions, expression of CXCR4 is increased in hypoxic culture which may MSC homing to injured tissues (70, 71). Expression of CD44 has also been demonstrated to be involved in MSC engraftment to injured liver tissue *in* vitro suggesting direct administration or routes bypassing the lungs may lead to greater engraftment to the target organ (72). In large animal models of liver injury and liver fibrosis adipose tissue derived MSC have been injected via the intra-portal route directly into the liver vasculature and have demonstrated efficacy without an increase in intra-portal pressure, suggesting that this route is feasible and safe and would be directly accessible during a liver transplantation operation (73). Injection rate and needle gauge has also been shown to be an important consideration when administering MSC with optimum rates in a variety of cell types described *in vitro* (74).

MSC have been successfully used in a variety of different liver pathologies in both pre-clinical and clinical trials with no major safety concerns identified (75), rendering their potential use in liver transplantation a new and exciting prospect.

MSC IN ISCHEMIA/REPERFUSION INJURY

Due to their ability to modulate both innate and adaptive immunity MSC represent an important potential therapy to ameliorate ischemia/reperfusion injury in liver surgery and transplantation. MSC have been shown to reduce ALT and IL-6 when administered systemically in models of hepatic ischemia reperfusion injury, but notably only if given before the ischemic insult (76). There also seems to be a reduction in TUNEL positive hepatocytes indicating less apoptosis in rat models of ischemia reperfusion injury following bone marrow derived MSC therapy (77). An important concern in the context of significant oxidative stress, as seen in both ischemia reperfusion injury and other forms of liver injury such as acute hepatic failure, is the ability of donor cells to survive in such a hostile environment. Bone marrow and adipose derived MSC have been shown to be resistant to oxidative stress and may themselves have antioxidant properties further suggesting a therapeutic role in these types of injury (78, 79).

Immune cell recruitment is a key feature in reperfusion injury with animal studies demonstrating that a reduction in injury can be achieved by blocking recruitment of both neutrophils and lymphocytes (26, 80). MSC derived from bone marrow can also reduce neutrophil recruitment and liver injury by enhancing the intracellular activation of p38 MPK phosphorylation leading to a decrease in the expression of CXCR2 on the surface of neutrophils as well as reducing the production of the neutrophil chemoattractant CXCL2 by inhibiting NK-κB p65 phosphorylation in macrophages (81). MSC-EV have also been shown to reduce liver injury if given systemically prior to an ischemic insult by reducing IL-6, IL10, TNFα, and IFN-γ levels as well as the number of caspase 3 positive apoptotic cells (82).

In larger animal models of ischemia reperfusion injury combined with partial hepatectomy, direct injection of MSC into liver parenchyma following surgery has been shown to reduce the number of apoptotic cells with a downregulation of Fas/Fas ligand and a reduction in enzyme activity of caspase 3, caspase 8 and caspase 9. There was also an increase in the apoptosis regulator protein Bcl2/Bax as well as a reduction in markers of autophagy such as Beclin1, ATG5, and ATG12 (83), suggesting an ability to regulate apoptosis in injured hepatocytes (84). Similar findings have been shown in small animal models of ischemia reperfusion injury (85). Topical application of adipose derived MSC can also augment liver regeneration following reperfusion injury with a reduction in necrotic areas and an increased number of regenerating cells (76) with activation of the notch2 pathway in MSCs (86).

MSC AUGMENT HEPATOCYTE ENGRAFTMENT AS AN ALTERNATIVE TO WHOLE ORGAN TRANSPLANTATION

Hepatic ischemia reperfusion injury can lead to significant hepatocyte loss with a subsequent loss of liver function. Over the last two decades transplantation of human hepatocytes as an alternative to whole organ transplantation has made significant progress with the development of protocols for isolation and storage of hepatocytes along with studies demonstrating early efficacy (87). A major draw-back of hepatocyte transplantation is the poor cell engraftment seen with only 0.1–0.3% hepatocytes remaining in the recipient liver (88). Co-transplantation of hepatocytes with fetal liver derived MSC has been shown to augment engraftment with a greater number of hepatocytes remaining in the recipient liver for a longer time along with improved liver function in animal models (89). This ability may as a result of MSC ability to provide tropic support to hepatocytes (90).

In vitro studies in human pancreatic tissue have shown that human bone marrow derived MSC can increase epithelial cell proliferation and neovascularisation (91) and more recent studies in human pancreatic islet cell transplantation have demonstrated that human bone marrow derived MSC are able to improve survival of transplanted islet cells in animal models (92). The ability of MSC to support transplanted pancreatic tissue via their effects on both vascularisation and endothelial support suggest an additional potential role in hepatocyte transplantation that warrants further study.

As an alternative to hepatocyte transplantation it has been argued that hepatocytes derived from MSC can replace injured cells and improve liver function. Certainly the engraftment and function of these cells appears to show benefit in animal models of bone marrow MSC (93–95), however there are conflicting results from pre-clinical studies rendering this a controversial area still requiring considerable attention before becoming a translatable therapy (96).

THERAPEUTIC STRATEGIES UTILIZING MSC IN LIVER TRANSPLANTATION

Through their ability to reduce injury and cell death in models of ischemia and reperfusion injury it stands to reason that there is a role for MSC therapy in orthotopic liver transplantation (OLT). Coupled with this the ability of MSC to promote liver regeneration and reduce injury could lead to a further benefit in the post-transplant recovery period (75).

Work in small animal models has been encouraging, where adipose tissue derived MSC have been shown to reduce liver injury and TUNEL positive hepatocytes in rat models of liver transplantation (97). MSC derived conditioned media has also shown a beneficial effect in pre-clinical models of liver transplantation with a reduction in injury and an improvement in liver function when 50% reduced size transplantation is undertaken in rats with an increase in VGEF and MMP9 expression (98).

Indeed, a number of early phase clinical trials have been undertaken in this patient cohort with some encouraging results (99). Phase II clinical trials in patients undergoing liver transplantation have shown safety, but were not powered to demonstrate efficacy in patients receiving unrelated bone marrow derived MSC in the first few days following transplantation (100). MSC have also been tested for safety in a pilot study of patients with acute allograft rejection following liver transplantation. In patients treated with MSC in combination with standard immunosuppression protocols for acute rejection there was a significant increase in PGE_2 and TGF-β1, as well as an significant increase in $FoxP3^+$ T regulatory cells isolated from peripheral blood (101). The MYSTEP1 trial currently nearing completion may provide safety information on the use of donor derived bone marrow MSC in pediatric living donor liver transplantation, paving the way for more extensive study in this cohort (102).

Normothermic machine perfusion is rapidly becoming a therapy of interest in the preservation and regeneration of donated livers (103, 104). In contrast to static cold storage, the current gold standard for liver transplantation, normothermic machine perfusion involves cannulation and perfusion of an explanted liver at near physiologic conditions. This technique has advantages over cold storage techniques which tend to be poorly suited to steatotic grafts. With an interest in the use of more marginal grafts to increase the potential pool of donor organs reconditioning and regeneration of donor organs is an area of increasing interest. MSC represent a potential therapy to enhance the regeneration of donor liver tissue. Proof of concept for delivery of MSC during machine perfusion has recently been published paving the way for further study (105). MSC appear to be retained in the perfused liver and are still able to exert paracrine effects on liver tissue, similar findings have been demonstrated in porcine renal perfusion systems (106, 107). In renal perfusion, the effects of perfusion on MSC has been studied in both human and porcine bone marrow cells demonstrating that perfusion amplifies the negative effects of cryopreservation on MSC with lower levels of adhesion and an increase in MSC reactive oxidative species (107). Currently normothermic machine perfusion represents an interesting avenue and in combination with cell therapy may represent a new future standard in liver transplantation.

Another option for transplantation is the use of split liver grafts (108, 109), an accepted technique for pediatric transplantation, although a more mixed experience when splitting a donor liver between two adult recipients. By reducing ischemia/reperfusion injury at the time of surgery and promoting post-operative liver regeneration an increased number of patients could receive a transplantation if grafts were routinely split between 2 recipients. MSC offer a potential therapy to improve the outcomes in this type of liver transplantation surgery with some encouraging animal studies demonstrating reduction in TUNEL positive cells in rat models of partial hepatectomy following MSC treatment and improved survival in rat transplant models (110). MSC are also able to promote regeneration in a 30% partial liver transplant model by increasing the activity of AP-1 and NF-κB as well as demonstrating increased expression of cyclin D1 and proliferating cell nuclear antigen (PCNA) (111). Similar principles could be applied to hepatic resection/partial hepatectomy with improved regeneration allowing for greater resection and therefore increased likelihood of adequate margins in cancer surgery, and faster recovery times. So far animal work has supported this with MSC therapy increasing both hepatocyte and sinusoidal endothelial proliferation and recovery after partial hepatectomy in mouse models (112). MSC conditioned media can also promote liver regeneration in partial hepatectomy models (113). MSC have also been suggested as a rescue therapy for acute liver failure following partial hepatectomy. In rat models, bone marrow MSC are able to improve glucose metabolism and survival following 90% hepatectomy, possibly through modulation of the AKT/GSK-3β/β-catenin pathway (114).

In large animal models of 70% partial hepatectomy, MSC therapy has been shown to improve both liver and renal function, suggesting an initial benefit beyond liver regeneration (115). This improvement was through correction of hemodynamic dysfunction by increasing levels of platelet derived growth factor (PDGF) along with promoting regeneration in the kidneys by increasing pro regenerative cytokines.

MSC AS A THERAPY IN POST-TRANSPLANT CARE

Following orthotopic liver transplantation, as with other organ transplantation, patients are required to take immunosuppressive agents in order to prevent the host immune system rejecting the graft. In most cases this is lifelong therapy which conveys a number of risks including infection and renal failure. Most strategies employ the inhibition of T-cell proliferation. By reducing or even eliminating immunosuppressant agents, morbidity in patients who have received a donor organ would be considerably reduced. MSC may offer an opportunity in these patients due to their ability to suppress T cell proliferation and activation.

Current consensus guidelines recommend the use of calcineurin inhibitors for maintenance immunosuppression in patients who receive a liver transplantation, supplemented with anti-metabolites or m-TOR inhibitors (116). With this in mind it is important to consider the effects of immunosuppressive drugs on MSC as well as the potential additive effect of MSC along with standard immunosuppressive agents used in liver transplantation. In the short term (<7 days) exposure of MSC from a variety of tissues to the calcineurin inhibitor tacrolimus, the anti-metabolite mycophenolate or the m-TOR inhibitor rapamycin, does not appear to lead to any detrimental effects. Prolonged exposure however leads to MSC toxicity in the case of tacrolimus, and reduced MSC proliferation in the case of mycophenolate and rapamycin (117). The combination of drugs seems to be important however with the effects of tacrolimus on MSC being reversed by the combined use of oxytocin (118). Whilst it has been demonstrated that avoidance of corticosteroids in patients following a liver transplantation is likely to be safe and reduce associated complications (119), corticosteroids are still widely used in the setting of liver transplantation, both for induction of immunosuppression and treatment of rejection (120). When combined with dexamethasone in *in* vitro assays the ability of MSC to suppress T cell proliferations seems to be reversed (121), however the ability of MSC to suppress natural killer cell activation seems to be enhanced with dexamethasone augmenting the ability of MSC to IL-2 and IL-12 induced CD69 expression and reduce production of IFNγ (122). This effect appears to be through the blocking of STAT1 in MSC by dexamethasone. MSC ability to suppress mononuclear cells appears to be enhanced by both dexamethasone and budesonide through increased IDO activity (123). In *in vivo* mouse models MSC derived from induced pluripotent cells do not seem to be effected by concomitant administration of dexamethasone (124). It would be challenging to test every combination of drugs that a patients could be taking when MSC therapy is administered, however the potential for both synergy and antagonism of medications with MSC therapy needs careful consideration when designing clinical trials in liver transplantation.

In rat models of orthotopic liver transplantation MSC are able to inhibit acute rejection by increasing expression of FoxP3 T regulatory cells (125), as well as prolonging survival by regulating the expression of TGF-β1 (126). In early phase clinical trials MSC have been shown to be safe in patients undergoing acute rejection following transplantation, as well as demonstrating an ability to increase TGF-β1 and prostaglandin E2 and increase the percentage of T regulatory cells present (101). In small animal models of cardiac and renal transplant allogeneic bone marrow MSC are able to induce organ tolerance by down-regulating T lymphocyte responses through expression of indolamine 2,3-dioxygenase (127, 128). In rats, both recipient and donor derived bone marrow MSC prolonged survival of transplanted livers through induction of FoxP3 T regulatory cells (125). Induction of transplant tolerance is a promising area of research but as yet has not made the transition into clinical studies.

Challenges With MSC Therapy

Whilst MSC appear to show a great deal of promise in liver transplantation there are some challenges that need to be overcome.

Heterogeneity

MSC heterogeneity has long been a problem due to an inability to define and isolate a pure population of cells. The International Society for Cell Therapy (ISCT) defined minimal criteria for describing MSC in an attempt to overcome this but even with these in place the cell populations used still represent a heterogeneous population (29, 129, 130).

Immunogenicity and Haemocompatibility

Although MSC expression of MHC class II low/absent (49), haemocompatibility has still been demonstrated to be an issue, as MSC can upregulate class I and II MHC in response to interferon gamma (131). In mouse models allogeneic bone marrow derived MSC are cleared by the host immune system when transplanted into MHC class I and II mismatched recipients (132), and in graft versus host disease bone marrow derived MSC seem to generate an antibody response in a subset of patients (133). Despite these findings, MSC still seem to illicit a much slower response from the recipient immune system, coining the term "immune evasive" (56). Meta-analysis seems to suggest that whilst bone marrow derived cells appear to be safe, adipose tissue derived and perinatal tissue MSC carry a risk of acute thrombosis due to activation of the innate immune system (134–137). Problems due to haemocompatibility can be mitigated by pre-screening in clinical trials and has been suggested as a pre-requisite to cell therapy (50).

Oncogenesis

MSC have long been studied in oncology where resident MSC have been shown to support the tumor microenvironment and are seen as a therapeutic target to reduce cancer growth (138). It has been suggested that due to their ability to support growth and activation that MSC therapy is at risk of supporting or inducing tumor formation (139). Long term *in vitro* studies of murine bone marrow MSC have demonstrated

TABLE 2 | Ongoing or recently completed clinical trials with MSC in liver transplantation.

References	Study description	Clinical Trial Registration	Patients	Status	MSC Dose	Key Findings
Detry et al. (100)	Phase 1 trial testing MSC therapy in liver transplantation for safety and ability to induce tolerance	NCT01429038	19	Published	1.5-3 × 10^6/kg IV	No side effects seen but tolerance not induced
Remuzzi, G	Test MSC ability to induce tolerance following liver transplantation	NCT02260375	20	Recruiting	1-2 × 10^6/kg IV	Not published
Soeder et al. (143)	First in man case study of MAPC in patients following liver transplant (MiSOT-1)	NCT01841632	1	Published	1.5 × 10^8 MAPC intra-portal	No acute complications seen
Sturm, E	Phase 1 trial to determine the safety of MSC in pediatric liver transplantation (MYSTEP1)	NCT02957552	7	Recruiting	2 doses 1 × 10^6/kg intra-portal then IV	Not published
Walker et al. (144)	Study the peripheral mobilization of MSC following corticosteroid administration in patients following liver transplantation or liver resection	NCT02557724	35	Published	N/A	Reduction in MSC migration following steroid administration
Wang, F	Phase 1 trial of MSC therapy to induce tolerance following liver transplantation	NCT01690247	50	Unknown	IV, details not described	Not published
Yang, Y	To determine if MSC are safe in acute rejection in ABO incompatible liver transplantation (Phase 1/2)	NCT02706132	15	Unknown	6 doses 1 × 10^6/kg IV	Not published

the potential for oncogenic transformation (140), although this has been questioned in more recent studies which suggest there could have been cell line contamination (141). Whilst some small studies have demonstrated this concern may be valid, larger reviews of clinical trials do not support this hypothesis, however vigilance is still required as with all clinical trials (134).

CLINICAL TRIALS

There has been an explosion in the use of MSC in clinical trials since the first study in humans carried out in 1995 (142), with MSC being one of the most clinically studied cell therapies worldwide (39). Due to the types of ischemia and reperfusion injury described earlier MSC represent a promising therapy in many areas liver transplantation and post-transplant care. Despite this, clinical trials in liver transplantation are still early on in their development with very few published trials. There have been few completed trials in patients undergoing liver transplantation but some still ongoing (**Table 2**), all are either phase 1 or phase 2 (145). This first published trials have demonstrated safety of MSC infusion in patients undergoing liver transplantation, but have also failed to demonstrate a benefit (100, 143). The effect of corticosteroids on patient's peripheral MSC populations has also been studied in the context of liver transplantation with a reduction in circulating MSC seen in those receiving corticosteroids (144). The implication of this finding is difficult to put into context though as there are clear differences between native and exogenous transplanted MSC in both number and properties. Interestingly this may be further proof of the pre-clinical studies suggesting that the MSC/HSC niche is controlled in part by the sympathetic nervous system (30). The ongoing MYSTEP1 trial is not only testing safety and efficacy of donor derived bone marrow MSC, but also the intra-portal route of administration in pediatric liver transplantation (102). Due to the inherent complexity and heterogeneity of clinical conditions, coupled with the variation in cell therapeutic products due to differences in donor, batch and cell tissue origin, the conduct and interpretation of clinical trials of MSC is complex and challenging. Whilst trials of MSC therapy in liver transplantation are still in their infancy, given the favorable safety profile demonstrated so far there is more potential work to be done in order to explore the role of MSC therapy in these patients.

CONCLUDING REMARKS

Liver transplantation is a continually evolving field with transplant teams consistently pushing the boundaries to enable the scarce resource of a donor liver to confer greater benefit to increasingly larger numbers of patients. Cell therapy with MSC is an exciting treatment beginning to enter clinical trials that may allow the boundaries to be pushed even further for a greater patient benefit.

AUTHOR CONTRIBUTIONS

All authors listed have made a substantial, direct and intellectual contribution to the work, and approved it for publication.

ACKNOWLEDGMENTS

AO is an NIHR funded clinical lecturer in anesthesia and critical care medicine. PN was supported by the National Institute of Health Research (NIHR) Birmingham Biomedical Research Centre (BRC). The views expressed are those of the authors and not necessarily those of the NHS, the NIHR or the Department of Health. Stock images for figures were provided by Servier medical for use under the Creative Commons Attribution 3.0 Unported License.

REFERENCES

1. Asrani SK, Devarbhavi H, Eaton J, Kamath PS. Burden of liver diseases in the world. *J Hepatol.* (2019) 70:151–71. doi: 10.1016/j.jhep.2018.09.014
2. Mokdad AA, Lopez AD, Shahraz S, Lozano R, Mokdad AH, Stanaway J, et al. Liver cirrhosis mortality in 187 countries between 1980 and 2010: a systematic analysis. *BMC Med.* (2014) 12:145. doi: 10.1186/s12916-014-0145-y
3. Berlakovich GA. Clinical outcome of orthotopic liver transplantation. *Int J Artif Organs.* (2002) 25:935–8. doi: 10.1177/039139880202501007
4. NHSBT. *Annual Report On Liver Transplantation NHSBT.* NHSBT 2018. (2018).
5. Cursio R, Gugenheim J. Ischemia-Reperfusion injury and ischemic-Type biliary lesions following liver transplantation. *J Transpl.* (2012) 2012:1–17. doi: 10.1155/2012/164329
6. DuBay DA, MacLennan PA, Reed RD, Fouad M, Martin M, Meeks CB, et al. The impact of proposed changes in liver allocation policy on cold ischemia times and organ transportation costs. *Am J Transpl.* (2015) 15:541–6. doi: 10.1111/ajt.12981
7. Callaghan CJ, Charman SC, Muiesan P, Powell JJ, Gimson AE, van der Meulen JHP. Outcomes of transplantation of livers from donation after circulatory death donors in the uK: a cohort study. *BMJ Open.* (2013) 3:e003287. doi: 10.1136/bmjopen-2013-003287
8. Zhai Y, Busuttil RW, Kupiec-Weglinski JW. Liver ischemia and reperfusion injury: new insights into mechanisms of innate-adaptive immune-mediated tissue inflammation. *Am J Transpl.* (2011) 11:1563–9. doi: 10.1111/j.1600-6143.2011.03579.x
9. Foley DP, Fernandez LA, Leverson G, Anderson M, Mezrich J, Sollinger HW, et al. Biliary complications after liver transplantation from donation after cardiac death donors: an analysis of risk factors and long-term outcomes from a single center. *Ann Surg.* (2011) 253:817–25. doi: 10.1097/SLA.0b013e3182104784
10. Montalvo-Jave EE, Escalante-Tattersfield T, Ortega-Salgado JA, Pina E, Geller DA. Factors in the pathophysiology of the liver ischemia-reperfusion injury. *J Surg Res.* (2008) 147:153–9. doi: 10.1016/j.jss.2007.06.015
11. Pringle JH. Notes on the arrest of hepatic hemorrhage due to trauma. *Ann Surg.* (1908) 48:541–9. doi: 10.1097/00000658-190810000-00005
12. Hong JC, Yersiz H, Kositamongkol P, Xia VW, Kaldas FM, Petrowsky H, et al. Liver transplantation using organ donation after cardiac death: a clinical predictive index for graft failure-free survival. *Arch Surg.* (2011) 146:1017–23. doi: 10.1001/archsurg.2011.240
13. Kalogeris T, Baines CP, Krenz M, Korthuis RJ. Cell biology of ischemia/reperfusion injury. *Int Rev Cell Mol Biol.* (2012) 298:229–317. doi: 10.1016/B978-0-12-394309-5.00006-7
14. Saraste M. Oxidative phosphorylation at the <em>fin de siècle</em>. *Science.* (1999) 283:1488–93. doi: 10.1126/science.283.5407.1488
15. Pike MM, Luo CS, Clark MD, Kirk KA, Kitakaze M, Madden MC, et al. NMR measurements of na+ and cellular energy in ischemic rat heart: role of na(+)-H+ exchange. *Am J Physiol.* (1993) 265(6 Pt 2):H2017–26. doi: 10.1152/ajpheart.1993.265.6.H2017
16. Peralta C, Bartrons R, Riera L, Manzano A, Xaus C, Gelpi E, et al. Hepatic preconditioning preserves energy metabolism during sustained ischemia. *Am J Physiol.* (2000) 279:G163–71. doi: 10.1152/ajpgi.2000.279.1.G163
17. Gasbarrini A, Borle AB, Farghali H, Bender C, Francavilla A, Van Thiel D. Effect of anoxia on intracellular aTP, na+i, ca2+i, mg2+i, and cytotoxicity in rat hepatocytes. *J Biol Chem.* (1992) 267:6654–63.

18. Gujral JS, Bucci TJ, Farhood A, Jaeschke H. Mechanism of cell death during warm hepatic ischemia-reperfusion in rats: apoptosis or necrosis? *Hepatology.* (2001) 33:397–405. doi: 10.1053/jhep.2001.22002
19. Yang M, Antoine DJ, Weemhoff JL, Jenkins RE, Farhood A, Park BK, et al. Biomarkers distinguish apoptotic and necrotic cell death during hepatic ischemia/reperfusion injury in mice. *Liver Trans.* (2014) 20:1372–82. doi: 10.1002/lt.23958
20. Leist M, Single B, Castoldi AF, Kuhnle S, Nicotera P. Intracellular adenosine triphosphate (ATP) concentration: a switch in the decision between apoptosis and necrosis. *The J Exp Med.* (1997) 185:1481–6. doi: 10.1084/jem.185.8.1481
21. Sindram D, Porte RJ, Hoffman MR, Bentley RC, Clavien PA. Platelets induce sinusoidal endothelial cell apoptosis upon reperfusion of the cold ischemic rat liver. *Gastroenterology.* (2000) 118:183–91. doi: 10.1016/S0016-5085(00)70427-6
22. Jaeschke H. Reactive oxygen and ischemia/reperfusion injury of the liver. *Chemico-Biol Int.* (1991) 79:115–36. doi: 10.1016/0009-2797(91)90077-K
23. Miyashita T, Nakanuma S, Ahmed AK, Makino I, Hayashi H, Oyama K, et al. Ischemia reperfusion-facilitated sinusoidal endothelial cell injury in liver transplantation and the resulting impact of extravasated platelet aggregation. *Eur Surg.* (2016) 48:92–8. doi: 10.1007/s10353-015-0363-3
24. Peralta C, Jimenez-Castro MB, Gracia-Sancho J. Hepatic ischemia and reperfusion injury: effects on the liver sinusoidal milieu. *J Hepatol.* (2013) 59:1094–106. doi: 10.1016/j.jhep.2013.06.017
25. Nakashima H, Ogawa Y, Shono S, Kinoshita M, Nakashima M, Sato A, et al. Activation of cD11b+ kupffer cells/macrophages as a common cause for exacerbation of tNF/Fas-ligand-dependent hepatitis in hypercholesterolemic mice. *PLoS ONE.* (2013) 8:e49339. doi: 10.1371/journal.pone.0049339
26. Shen XD, Ke B, Zhai Y, Amersi F, Gao F, Anselmo DM, et al. CD154-CD40 t-cell costimulation pathway is required in the mechanism of hepatic ischemia/reperfusion injury, and its blockade facilitates and depends on heme oxygenase-1 mediated cytoprotection. *Transplantation.* (2002) 74:315–9. doi: 10.1097/00007890-200208150-00005
27. Zhai Y, Shen XD, O'Connell R, Gao F, Lassman C, Busuttil RW, et al. Cutting edge: tLR4 activation mediates liver ischemia/reperfusion inflammatory response via iFN regulatory factor 3-dependent myD88-independent pathway. *J Immunol.* (2004) 173:7115–9. doi: 10.4049/jimmunol.173.12.7115
28. McDonald KA, Huang H, Tohme S, Loughran P, Ferrero K, Billiar T, et al. Toll-like receptor 4 (TLR4) antagonist eritoran tetrasodium attenuates liver ischemia and reperfusion injury through inhibition of high-mobility group box protein b1 (HMGB1) signaling. *Mol Med.* (2015) 20:639–48. doi: 10.2119/molmed.2014.00076
29. Dominici M, Le Blank K, Mueller I. Minimal criteria for defining multipotent mesenchymal stromal cells. The International Society for Cellular Therapy position statement. *Cytotherapy.* (2006) 8:315–7. doi: 10.1080/14653240600855905
30. Méndez-Ferrer S, Michurina TV, Ferraro F, Mazloom AR, MacArthur BD, Lira SA, et al. Mesenchymal and haematopoietic stem cells form a unique bone marrow niche. *Nature.* (2010) 466:829–34. doi: 10.1038/nature09262
31. Romanov YA, Svintsitskaya VA, Smirnov VN. Searching for alternative sources of postnatal human mesenchymal stem cells: candidate mSC-Like cells from umbilical cord. *Stem Cells.* (2003) 21:105–10. doi: 10.1634/stemcells.21-1-105
32. In 't Anker PS, Scherjon SA, Kleijburg-van der Keur C, de Groot-Swings GM, Claas FH, Fibbe WE, et al. Isolation of mesenchymal stem cells of fetal or maternal origin from human placenta. *Stem Cells.* (2004) 22:1338–45. doi: 10.1634/stemcells.2004-0058
33. Zuk PA, Zhu M, Ashjian P, De Ugarte DA, Huang JI, Mizuno H, et al. Human adipose tissue is a source of multipotent stem cells. *Mol Biol Cell.* (2002) 13:4279–95. doi: 10.1091/mbc.e02-02-0105
34. Toma JG, Akhavan M, Fernandes KJ, Barnabé-Heider F, Sadikot A, Kaplan DR, et al. Isolation of multipotent adult stem cells from the dermis of mammalian skin. *Nat Cell Biol.* (2001) 3:778–84. doi: 10.1038/ncb0901-778
35. Sedgley CM, Botero TM. Dental stem cells and their sources. *Dent Clin.* (2012) 56:549–61. doi: 10.1016/j.cden.2012.05.004
36. Bianco P, Cao X, Frenette PS, Mao JJ, Robey PG, Simmons PJ, et al. The meaning, the sense and the significance: translating the science of mesenchymal stem cells into medicine. *Nat Med.* (2013) 19:35–42. doi: 10.1038/nm.3028
37. Sipp D, Robey PG, Turner L. Clear up this stem-cell mess. *Nature.* (2018) 561:455–7. doi: 10.1038/d41586-018-06756-9
38. Lukomska B, Stanaszek L, Zuba-Surma E, Legosz P, Sarzynska S, Drela K. Challenges and controversies in human mesenchymal stem cell therapy. *Stem Cells Int.* (2019) 2019:9628536. doi: 10.1155/2019/9628536
39. Galipeau J, Sensebe L. Mesenchymal stromal cells: clinical challenges and therapeutic opportunities. *Cell Stem Cell.* (2018) 22:824–33. doi: 10.1016/j.stem.2018.05.004
40. Menaa F, Shahrokhi S, Prasad Shastri V. Impact and challenges of mesenchymal stem cells in medicine: an overview of the current knowledge. *Stem Cells Int.* (2018) 2018:5023925. doi: 10.1155/2018/5023925
41. Gao F, Chiu SM, Motan DAL, Zhang Z, Chen L, Ji HL, et al. Mesenchymal stem cells and immunomodulation: current status and future prospects. *Cell Death Dis.* (2016) 7:e2062–e. doi: 10.1038/cddis.2015.327
42. Hejretová L, Cedíková M. Comparison of the immunomodulatory effect of single mSC batches versus pooled mSC products. *Cell Tissue Bank.* (2020) 21:119–29. doi: 10.1007/s10561-019-09805-3
43. Sammour I, Somashekar S, Huang J, Batlahally S, Breton M, Valasaki K, et al. The effect of gender on mesenchymal stem cell (MSC) efficacy in neonatal hyperoxia-induced lung injury. *PLoS ONE.* (2016) 11:e0164269. doi: 10.1371/journal.pone.0164269
44. Zhu M, Kohan E, Bradley J, Hedrick M, Benhaim P, Zuk P. The effect of age on osteogenic, adipogenic and proliferative potential of female adipose-derived stem cells. *J Tissue Eng Regen Med.* (2009) 3:290–301. doi: 10.1002/term.165
45. Ogawa R, Mizuno H, Hyakusoku H, Watanabe A, Migita M, Shimada T. Chondrogenic and osteogenic differentiation of adipose-derived stem cells isolated from gFP transgenic mice. *J Nippon Med.* (2004) 71:240–1. doi: 10.1272/jnms.71.240
46. Stolzing A, Jones E, McGonagle D, Scutt A. Age-related changes in human bone marrow-derived mesenchymal stem cells: consequences for cell therapies. *Mech Age Dev.* (2008) 129:163–73. doi: 10.1016/j.mad.2007.12.002
47. Gersch RP, Lombardo F, McGovern SC, Hadjiargyrou M. Reactivation of hox gene expression during bone regeneration. *J Orthop Res.* (2005) 23:882–90. doi: 10.1016/j.orthres.2005.02.005
48. Baptista LS, Silva KR, Borojevic R. Obesity and weight loss could alter the properties of adipose stem cells? *World J Stem Cells.* (2015) 7:165–73. doi: 10.4252/wjsc.v7.i1.165
49. Ryan JM, Barry FP, Murphy JM, Mahon BP. Mesenchymal stem cells avoid allogeneic rejection. *J Inflamm.* (2005) 2:8. doi: 10.1186/1476-9255-2-8
50. George MJ, Prabhakara K, Toledano-Furman NE, Wang YW, Gill BS, Wade CE, et al. Clinical cellular therapeutics accelerate clot formation. *Stem Cells Transl Med.* (2018) 7:731–9. doi: 10.1002/sctm.18-0015
51. Gleeson BM, Martin K, Ali MT, Kumar AH, Pillai MG, Kumar SP, et al. Bone marrow-Derived mesenchymal stem cells have innate procoagulant activity and cause microvascular obstruction following intracoronary delivery: amelioration by antithrombin therapy. *Stem Cells.* (2015) 33:2726–37. doi: 10.1002/stem.2050
52. Glennie S, Soeiro I, Dyson PJ, Lam EW, Dazzi F. Bone marrow mesenchymal stem cells induce division arrest anergy of activated t cells. *Blood.* (2005) 105:2821–7. doi: 10.1182/blood-2004-09-3696
53. Zappia E, Casazza S, Pedemonte E, Benvenuto F, Bonanni I, Gerdoni E, et al. Mesenchymal stem cells ameliorate experimental autoimmune encephalomyelitis inducing t-cell anergy. *Blood.* (2005) 106:1755–61. doi: 10.1182/blood-2005-04-1496
54. Chiesa S, Morbelli S, Morando S, Massollo M, Marini C, Bertoni A, et al. Mesenchymal stem cells impair in vivo t-cell priming by dendritic cells. *Proceed Natl Acad Sci USA.* (2011) 108:17384–9. doi: 10.1073/pnas.1103650108
55. Ramasamy R, Fazekasova H, Lam EW, Soeiro I, Lombardi G, Dazzi F. Mesenchymal stem cells inhibit dendritic cell differentiation and function by preventing entry into the cell cycle. *Transplantation.* (2007) 83:71–6. doi: 10.1097/01.tp.0000244572.24780.54
56. Aggarwal S, Pittenger MF. Human mesenchymal stem cells modulate allogeneic immune cell responses. *Blood.* (2005) 105:1815–22. doi: 10.1182/blood-2004-04-1559
57. Min CK, Kim BG, Park G, Cho B, Oh IH. IL-10 transduced bone marrow mesenchymal stem cells can attenuate the severity of acute graft-versus-host disease after experimental allogeneic stem cell transplantation. *Bone Marrow Transpl.* (2007) 39:637–45. doi: 10.1038/sj.bmt.17

05644
58. Le Blanc K, Frassoni F, Ball L, Locatelli F, Roelofs H, Lewis I, et al. Mesenchymal stem cells for treatment of steroid-resistant, severe, acute graft-versus-host disease: a phase iI study. *Lancet.* (2008) 371:1579–86. doi: 10.1016/S0140-6736(08)60690-X
59. Spaggiari GM. Mesenchymal stem cell-natural killer cell interactions: evidence that activated nK cells are capable of killing mSCs, whereas mSCs can inhibit iL-2-induced nK-cell proliferation. *Blood.* (2006) 107:1484–90. doi: 10.1182/blood-2005-07-2775
60. Wang M, Yuan Q, Xie L. Mesenchymal stem cell-Based immunomodulation: properties and clinical application. *Stem Cells Int.* (2018) 2018:3057624. doi: 10.1155/2018/3057624
61. Liu Q, Zheng H, Chen X, Peng Y, Huang W, Li X, et al. Human mesenchymal stromal cells enhance the immunomodulatory function of cD8+CD28– regulatory t cells. *Cell Mol Immunol.* (2015) 12:708–18. doi: 10.1038/cmi.2014.118
62. Ferreira JR, Teixeira GQ, Santos SG, Barbosa MA, Almeida-Porada G, Gonçalves RM. Mesenchymal stromal cell secretome: influencing therapeutic potential by cellular pre-conditioning. *Front Immunol.* (2018) 9:2837. doi: 10.3389/fimmu.2018.02837
63. Driscoll J, Patel T. The mesenchymal stem cell secretome as an acellular regenerative therapy for liver disease. *J Gastroenterol.* (2019) 54:763–73. doi: 10.1007/s00535-019-01599-1
64. Derkus B, Emregul KC, Emregul E. A new approach in stem cell research-Exosomes: their mechanism of action via cellular pathways. *Cell Biol Int.* (2017) 41:466–75. doi: 10.1002/cbin.10742
65. Schrepfer S, Deuse T, Reichenspurner H, Fischbein MP, Robbins RC, Pelletier MP. Stem cell transplantation: the lung barrier. *Transpl Proceed.* (2007) 39:573–6. doi: 10.1016/j.transproceed.2006.12.019
66. Argibay B, Trekker J, Himmelreich U, Beiras A, Topete A, Taboada P, et al. Intraarterial route increases the risk of cerebral lesions after mesenchymal cell administration in animal model of ischemia. *Sci Rep.* (2017) 7:40758. doi: 10.1038/srep40758
67. Watanabe M, Yavagal DR. Intra-arterial delivery of mesenchymal stem cells. *Brain Circul.* (2016) 2:114–7. doi: 10.4103/2394-8108.192522
68. Zanotti L, Sarukhan A, Dander E, Castor M, Cibella J, Soldani C, et al. Encapsulated mesenchymal stem cells for in vivo immunomodulation. *Leukemia.* (2012) 27:500–3. doi: 10.1038/leu.2012.202
69. Tögel F, Yang Y, Zhang P, Hu Z, Westenfelder C. Bioluminescence imaging to monitor the in vivo distribution of administered mesenchymal stem cells in acute kidney injury. *Am J Physiol.* (2008) 295:F315–21. doi: 10.1152/ajprenal.00098.2008
70. Honczarenko M, Le Y, Swierkowski M, Ghiran I, Glodek AM, Silberstein LE. Human bone marrow stromal cells express a distinct set of biologically functional chemokine receptors. *Stem Cells.* (2006) 24:1030–41. doi: 10.1634/stemcells.2005-0319
71. Hung SC, Pochampally RR, Hsu SC, Sanchez C, Chen SC, Spees J, et al. Short-term exposure of multipotent stromal cells to low oxygen increases their expression of cX3CR1 and cXCR4 and their engraftment in vivo. *PLoS ONE.* (2007) 2:e416. doi: 10.1371/journal.pone.0000416
72. Aldridge V, Garg A, Davies N, Bartlett DC, Youster J, Beard H, et al. Human mesenchymal stem cells are recruited to injured liver in a β1-integrin and cD44 dependent manner. *Hepatology.* (2012) 56:1063–73. doi: 10.1002/hep.25716
73. Avritscher R, Abdelsalam ME, Javadi S, Ensor J, Wallace MJ, Alt E, et al. Percutaneous intraportal application of adipose tissue-derived mesenchymal stem cells using a balloon occlusion catheter in a porcine model of liver fibrosis. *J Vasc Interv Radiol.* (2013) 24:1871–8. doi: 10.1016/j.jvir.2013.08.022
74. Amer MH, Rose FR, White LJ, Shakesheff KM. A detailed assessment of varying ejection rate on delivery efficiency of mesenchymal stem cells using narrow-Bore needles. *Stem Cells Transl Med.* (2016) 5:366–78. doi: 10.5966/sctm.2015-0208
75. Owen A, Newsome PN. Mesenchymal stromal cell therapy in liver disease; opportunities and lessons to be learnt? *Am J Physiol Gastro Liver Physiol.* (2015) 2015:ajpgi.00036.2015. doi: 10.1152/ajpgi.00036.2015
76. Saidi RF, Rajeshkumar B, Shariftabrizi A, Bogdanov AA, Zheng S, Dresser K, et al. Human adipose-derived mesenchymal stem cells attenuate liver ischemia-reperfusion injury and promote liver regeneration. *Surgery.* (2014) 156:1225–31. doi: 10.1016/j.surg.2014.05.008
77. Kanazawa H, Fujimoto Y, Teratani T, Iwasaki J, Kasahara N, Negishi K, et al. Bone marrow-derived mesenchymal stem cells ameliorate hepatic ischemia reperfusion injury in a rat model. *PLoS One.* (2011) 6:e19195. doi: 10.1371/journal.pone.0019195
78. Kuo TK, Hung SP, Chuang CH, Chen CT, Shih YRV, Fang SCY, et al. Stem cell therapy for liver disease: parameters governing the success of using bone marrow mesenchymal stem cells. *Gastroenterology.* (2008) 134:2111–21.e3. doi: 10.1053/j.gastro.2008.03.015
79. da Costa Goncalves F, Grings M, Nunes NS, Pinto FO, Garcez TN, Visioli F, et al. Antioxidant properties of mesenchymal stem cells against oxidative stress in a murine model of colitis. *Biotechnol Lett.* (2017) 39:613–22. doi: 10.1007/s10529-016-2272-3
80. Wengner AM, Pitchford SC, Furze RC, Rankin SM. The coordinated action of g-CSF and eLR + cXC chemokines in neutrophil mobilization during acute inflammation. *Blood.* (2008) 111:42–9. doi: 10.1182/blood-2007-07-099648
81. Li S, Zheng X, Li H, Zheng J, Chen X, Liu W, et al. Mesenchymal stem cells ameliorate hepatic ischemia/Reperfusion injury via inhibition of neutrophil recruitment. *J Immunol Res.* (2018) 2018:10. doi: 10.1155/2018/7283703
82. Haga H, Yan IK, Borrelli DA, Matsuda A, Parasramka M, Shukla N, et al. Extracellular vesicles from bone marrow-derived mesenchymal stem cells protect against murine hepatic ischemia/reperfusion injury. *Liver Trans.* (2017) 23:791–803. doi: 10.1002/lt.24770
83. Ge Y, Zhang Q, Jiao Z, Li H, Bai G, Wang H. Adipose-derived stem cells reduce liver oxidative stress and autophagy induced by ischemia-reperfusion and hepatectomy injury in swine. *Life Sci.* (2018) 214:62–9. doi: 10.1016/j.lfs.2018.10.054
84. Ge Y, Zhang Q, Li H, Bai G, Jiao Z, Wang H. Adipose-derived stem cells alleviate liver apoptosis induced by ischemia-reperfusion and laparoscopic hepatectomy in swine. *Sci Rep.* (2018) 8:16878. doi: 10.1038/s41598-018-34939-x
85. Sun CK, Chang CL, Lin YC, Kao YH, Chang LT, Yen CH, et al. Systemic administration of autologous adipose-derived mesenchymal stem cells alleviates hepatic ischemia-reperfusion injury in rats. *Crit Care Med.* (2012) 40:1279–90. doi: 10.1097/CCM.0b013e31823dae23
86. Lam PK, Chong CCN, Lo AWI, Chan AWH, Tong CSW, Chin DWC, et al. Topical application of mesenchymal stromal cells ameliorated liver parenchyma damage after ischemia-Reperfusion injury in an animal model. *Transpl Direct.* (2017) 3:e160. doi: 10.1097/TXD.0000000000000675
87. Iansante V, Mitry RR, Filippi C, Fitzpatrick E, Dhawan A. Human hepatocyte transplantation for liver disease: current status and future perspectives. *Pediat Res.* (2018) 83:232–40. doi: 10.1038/pr.2017.284
88. Wang LJ, Chen YM, George D, Smets F, Sokal EM, Bremer EG, et al. Engraftment assessment in human and mouse liver tissue after sex-mismatched liver cell transplantation by real-time quantitative pCR for y chromosome sequences. *Liver Trans.* (2002) 8:822–8. doi: 10.1053/jlts.2002.34891
89. Joshi M, Patil PB, He Z, Holgersson J, Olausson M, Sumitran-Holgersson S. Fetal liver-derived mesenchymal stromal cells augment engraftment of transplanted hepatocytes. *Cytotherapy.* (2012) 14:657–69. doi: 10.3109/14653249.2012.663526
90. van Poll D, Parekkadan B, Cho CH, Berthiaume F, Nahmias Y, Tilles AW, et al. Mesenchymal stem cell-derived molecules directly modulate hepatocellular death and regeneration in vitro and in vivo. *Hepatology.* (2008) 47:1634–43. doi: 10.1002/hep.22236
91. Johansson U, Rasmusson I, Niclou SP, Forslund N, Gustavsson L, Nilsson B, et al. Formation of composite endothelial cell-mesenchymal stem cell islets: a novel approach to promote islet revascularization. *Diabetes.* (2008) 57:2393–401. doi: 10.2337/db07-0981
92. Fumagalli G, Monfrini M, Donzelli E, Rodriguez-Menendez V, Bonandrini B, Figliuzzi M, et al. Protective effect of human mesenchymal stem cells on the survival of pancreatic islets. *Int J Stem Cells.* (2020) 13:116–26. doi: 10.15283/ijsc19094
93. Oyagi S, Hirose M, Kojima M, Okuyama M, Kawase M, Nakamura T, et al. Therapeutic effect of transplanting hGF-treated bone marrow mesenchymal cells into cCl4-injured rats. *J Hepatol.* (2006) 44:742–8. doi: 10.1016/j.jhep.2005.10.026
94. Abdel Aziz MT, Atta HM, Mahfouz S, Fouad HH, Roshdy NK, Ahmed HH, et al. Therapeutic potential of bone marrow-derived mesenchymal stem cells on experimental liver fibrosis. *Clin Biochem.* (2007) 40:893–9. doi: 10.1016/j.clinbiochem.2007.04.017

95. Luo X, Gupta K, Ananthanarayanan A, Wang Z, Xia L, Li A, et al. Directed differentiation of adult liver derived mesenchymal like stem cells into functional hepatocytes. *Sci Rep.* (2018) 8:2818. doi: 10.1038/s41598-018-20304-5
96. Christ B, Stock P. Mesenchymal stem cell-Derived hepatocytes for functional liver replacement. *Front Immunol.* (2012) 3:168. doi: 10.3389/fimmu.2012.00168
97. Wan CD, Cheng R, Wang HB, Liu T. Immunomodulatory effects of mesenchymal stem cells derived from adipose tissues in a rat orthotopic liver transplantation model. *Hepatobil Pancr Dis Int.* (2008) 7:29–33.
98. Du Z, Wei C, Cheng K, Han B, Yan J, Zhang M, et al. Mesenchymal stem cell-conditioned medium reduces liver injury and enhances regeneration in reduced-size rat liver transplantation. *J Surg Res.* (2013) 183:907–15. doi: 10.1016/j.jss.2013.02.009
99. Haldar D, Henderson NC, Hirschfield G, Newsome PN. Mesenchymal stromal cells and liver fibrosis: a complicated relationship. *FASEB J.* (2016) 30:3905–28. doi: 10.1096/fj.201600433R
100. Detry O, Vandermeulen M, Delbouille MH, Somja J, Bletard N, Briquet A, et al. Infusion of mesenchymal stromal cells after deceased liver transplantation: a phase i-II, open-label, clinical study. *J Hepatol.* (2017) 67:47–55. doi: 10.1016/j.jhep.2017.03.001
101. Shi M, Liu Z, Wang Y, Xu R, Sun Y, Zhang M, et al. A pilot study of mesenchymal stem cell therapy for acute liver allograft rejection. *Stem Cells Trans Med.* (2017) 6:2053–61. doi: 10.1002/sctm.17-0134
102. Hartleif S, Schumm M, Doring M, Mezger M. Safety and tolerance of donor-derived mesenchymal stem cells in pediatric living-donor liver transplantation: the mYSTEP1 study. *Stem Cells Int.* (2017) 2017:2352954. doi: 10.1155/2017/2352954
103. Op den Dries S, Karimian N, Porte RJ. Normothermic machine perfusion of discarded liver grafts. *Am J Trans.* (2013) 13:2504. doi: 10.1111/ajt.12374
104. Ceresa CDL, Nasralla D, Coussios CC, Friend PJ. The case for normothermic machine perfusion in liver transplantation. *Liver Trans.* (2018) 24:269–75. doi: 10.1002/lt.25000
105. Verstegen MMA, Mezzanotte L, Ridwan RY, Wang K, de Haan J, Schurink IJ, et al. First report on ex vivo delivery of paracrine active human mesenchymal stromal cells to liver grafts during machine perfusion. *Transplantation.* (2020) 104:2986. doi: 10.1097/TP.0000000000002986
106. Pool M, Eertman T, Sierra Parraga J. Infusing mesenchymal stromal cells into porcine kidneys during normothermic machine perfusion: intact mSCs can be traced and localised to glomeruli. *Int J Mol Sci.* (2019) 20:14. doi: 10.3390/ijms20143607
107. Sierra-Parraga JM, Munk A, Andersen C, Lohmann S, Moers C, Baan CC, et al. Mesenchymal stromal cells are retained in the porcine renal cortex independently of their metabolic state after renal intra-Arterial infusion. *Stem Cells Dev.* (2019) 28:1224–35. doi: 10.1089/scd.2019.0105
108. Pichlmayr R, Ringe B, Gubernatis G, Hauss J, Bunzendahl H. [Transplantation of a donor liver to 2 recipients (splitting transplantation)–a new method in the further development of segmental liver transplantation]. *Langenbecks Arch Chir.* (1988) 373:127–30. doi: 10.1007/BF01262776
109. Bismuth H, Morino M, Castaing D, Gillon MC, Declere AD, Saliba F, et al. Emergency orthotopic liver transplantation in two patients using one donor liver. *Br J Surg.* (1989) 76:722–4. doi: 10.1002/bjs.1800760723
110. Uemoto S, Fujimoto Y, Teratani T, Kanazawa H, Iwasaki J, Xiangdong Z, et al. editors. *Introduction of Mesenchymal Stem Cells for Liver Surgery (Hepatectomy and Transplantation) 2015.* Tokyo: Springer Japan. doi: 10.1007/978-4-431-55651-0_23
111. Wang W, Du Z, Yan J, Ma D, Shi M, Zhang M, et al. Mesenchymal stem cells promote liver regeneration and prolong survival in small-For-Size liver grafts: involvement of c-Jun n-Terminal kinase, cyclin d1, and nF-κB. *PLoS ONE.* (2014) 9:e112532. doi: 10.1371/journal.pone.0112532
112. Wabitsch S, Benzing C, Krenzien F, Splith K, Haber PK, Arnold A, et al. Human stem cells promote liver regeneration after partial hepatectomy in bALB/C nude mice. *J Surg Res.* (2019) 239:191–200. doi: 10.1016/j.jss.2019.02.010
113. Fouraschen SM, Pan Q, de Ruiter PE, Farid WR, Kazemier G, Kwekkeboom J, et al. Secreted factors of human liver-derived mesenchymal stem cells promote liver regeneration early after partial hepatectomy. *Stem Cells Dev.* (2012) 21:2410–9. doi: 10.1089/scd.2011.0560
114. Ding H, Wang J, Tang Z, Wang Y, Zhou G, Liu Y, et al. Mesenchymal stem cells improve glycometabolism and liver regeneration in the treatment of post-hepatectomy liver failure. *Front Physiol.* (2019) 10:412. doi: 10.3389/fphys.2019.00412
115. Tautenhahn H-M, Brückner S, Uder C, Erler S, Hempel M, von Bergen M, et al. Mesenchymal stem cells correct haemodynamic dysfunction associated with liver injury after extended resection in a pig model. *Sci Rep.* (2017) 7:2617. doi: 10.1038/s41598-017-02670-8
116. Charlton M, Levitsky J, Aqel B, O'Grady J, Hemibach J, Rinella M, et al. International liver transplantation society consensus statement on immunosuppression in liver transplant recipients. *Transplantation.* (2018) 102:727–43. doi: 10.1097/TP.0000000000002147
117. Hoogduijn MJ, Crop MJ, Korevaar SS, Peeters AMA, Eijken M, Maat LPWM, et al. Susceptibility of human mesenchymal stem cells to tacrolimus, mycophenolic acid, and rapamycin. *Transplantation.* (2008) 86:1283–91. doi: 10.1097/TP.0b013e31818aa536
118. Sir G, Goker Bagca B, Yigitturk G, Cavusoglu T, Biray Avci C, Gunduz C, et al. Antagonistic effect of oxytocin and tacrolimus combination on adipose tissue - derived mesenchymal stem cells: antagonistic effect of oxytocin and tacrolimus. *Biomed Pharmacother.* (2018) 97:1173–81. doi: 10.1016/j.biopha.2017.10.076
119. Fairfield C, Penninga L, Powell J, Harrison EM, Wigmore SJ. Glucocorticosteroid-free versus glucocorticosteroid-containing immunosuppression for liver transplanted patients. *Cochr Datab Syst Rev.* (2015) 2015:Cd007606. doi: 10.1002/14651858.CD007606.pub3
120. Hussaini T, Turgeon RD, Partovi N, Erb SR, Scudamore CH, Yoshida EM. Immunosuppression practices in liver transplantation: a Survey of north american centers. *Exp Clin Transpl.* (2018) 16:550–3. doi: 10.6002/ect.2017.0096
121. Chen X, Gan Y, Li W, Su J, Zhang Y, Huang Y, et al. The interaction between mesenchymal stem cells and steroids during inflammation. *Cell Death Dis.* (2014) 5:e1009–e. doi: 10.1038/cddis.2013.537
122. Michelo CM, Fasse E, van Cranenbroek B, Linda K, van der Meer A, Abdelrazik H, et al. Added effects of dexamethasone and mesenchymal stem cells on early natural killer cell activation. *Trans Immunol.* (2016) 37:1–9. doi: 10.1016/j.trim.2016.04.008
123. Ankrum JA, Dastidar RG, Ong JF, Levy O, Karp JM. Performance-enhanced mesenchymal stem cells via intracellular delivery of steroids. *Sci Rep.* (2014) 4:4645. doi: 10.1038/srep04645
124. Wang D, Sun Y-Q, Gao W-X, Fan X-L, Shi J-B, Fu Q-L. An *in vitro* and *in vivo* study of the effect of dexamethasone on immunoinhibitory function of induced pluripotent stem cell-Derived mesenchymal stem cells. *Cell Trans.* (2018) 27:1340–51. doi: 10.1177/0963689718780194
125. Wang Y, Zhang A, Ye Z, Xie H, Zheng S. Bone marrow-derived mesenchymal stem cells inhibit acute rejection of rat liver allografts in association with regulatory t-cell expansion. *Transplant Proc.* (2009) 41:4352–6. doi: 10.1016/j.transproceed.2009.08.072
126. Niu J, Wang Y, Liu B, Yao Y. Mesenchymal stem cells prolong the survival of orthotopic liver transplants by regulating the expression of tGF-β1. *Turk J Gastroenterol.* (2018) 29:601–9. doi: 10.5152/tjg.2018.17395
127. Ge W, Jiang J, Arp J, Liu W, Garcia B, Wang H. Regulatory t-cell generation and kidney allograft tolerance induced by mesenchymal stem cells associated with indoleamine 2,3-dioxygenase expression. *Transplantation.* (2010) 90:1312–20. doi: 10.1097/TP.0b013e3181fed001
128. Zhou HP, Yi DH, Yu SQ, Sun GC, Cui Q, Zhu HL, et al. Administration of donor-derived mesenchymal stem cells can prolong the survival of rat cardiac allograft. *Transplant Proc.* (2006) 38:3046–51. doi: 10.1016/j.transproceed.2006.10.002
129. Horwitz EM, Le Blanc K, Dominici M, Mueller I, Slaper-Cortenbach I, Marini FC, et al. Clarification of the nomenclature for mSC: the international society for cellular therapy position statement. *Cytotherapy.* (2005) 7:393–5. doi: 10.1080/14653240500319234
130. Viswanathan S, Shi Y, Galipeau J, Krampera M, Leblanc K, Martin I, et al. Mesenchymal stem versus stromal cells: international society for cell & gene therapy (ISCT®) mesenchymal stromal cell committee position statement on nomenclature. *Cytotherapy.* (2019) 21:1019–24. doi: 10.1016/j.jcyt.2019.08.002
131. Le Blanc K, Tammik C, Rosendahl K, Zetterberg E, Ringdén O. HLA expression and immunologic properties of differentiated and undifferentiated mesenchymal stem cells. *Exp Hematol.* (2003) 31:890–6. doi: 10.1016/S0301-472X(03)00110-3

132. Eliopoulos N, Stagg J, Lejeune L, Pommey S, Galipeau J. Allogeneic marrow stromal cells are immune rejected by mHC class i- and class iI-mismatched recipient mice. *Blood.* (2005) 106:4057–65. doi: 10.1182/blood-2005-03-1004
133. Hare JM, Fishman JE, Gerstenblith G, DiFede Velazquez DL, Zambrano JP, Suncion VY, et al. Comparison of allogeneic vs autologous bone marrow-derived mesenchymal stem cells delivered by transendocardial injection in patients with ischemic cardiomyopathy: the pOSEIDON randomized trial. *JAMA.* (2012) 308:2369–79. doi: 10.1001/jama.2012.25321
134. Lalu MM, McIntyre L, Pugliese C, Fergusson D, Winston BW, Marshall JC, et al. Safety of cell therapy with mesenchymal stromal cells (SafeCell): a systematic review and meta-analysis of clinical trials. *PLoS ONE.* (2012) 7:e47559. doi: 10.1371/journal.pone.0047559
135. Jung JW, Kwon M, Choi JC, Shin JW, Park IW, Choi BW, et al. Familial occurrence of pulmonary embolism after intravenous, adipose tissue-derived stem cell therapy. *Yonsei Med J.* (2013) 54:1293–6. doi: 10.3349/ymj.2013.54.5.1293
136. Tatsumi K, Ohashi K, Matsubara Y, Kohori A, Ohno T, Kakidachi H, et al. Tissue factor triggers procoagulation in transplanted mesenchymal stem cells leading to thromboembolism. *Biochem Biophys Res Commun.* (2013) 431:203–9. doi: 10.1016/j.bbrc.2012.12.134
137. Moll G, Ankrum JA, Kamhieh-Milz J, Bieback K, Ringdén O, Volk H-D, et al. Intravascular mesenchymal stromal/Stem cell therapy product diversification: time for new clinical guidelines. *Trends Mol Med.* (2019) 25:149–63. doi: 10.1016/j.molmed.2018.12.006
138. D'Souza N, Burns JS, Grisendi G, Candini O, Veronesi E, Piccinno S, et al. MSC and tumors: homing, differentiation, and secretion influence therapeutic potential. *Adv Biochem Eng Biotechnol.* (2013) 130:209–66. doi: 10.1007/10_2012_150
139. Prockop DJ, Brenner M, Fibbe WE, Horwitz E, Le Blanc K, Phinney DG, et al. Defining the risks of mesenchymal stromal cell therapy. *Cytotherapy.* (2010) 12:576–8. doi: 10.3109/14653249.2010.507330
140. Miura M, Miura Y, Padilla-Nash HM, Molinolo AA, Fu B, Patel V, et al. Accumulated chromosomal instability in murine bone marrow mesenchymal stem cells leads to malignant transformation. *Stem Cells.* (2006) 24:1095–103. doi: 10.1634/stemcells.2005-0403
141. Tolar J, Nauta AJ, Osborn MJ, Panoskaltsis Mortari A, McElmurry RT, Bell S, et al. Sarcoma derived from cultured mesenchymal stem cells. *Stem Cells.* (2007) 25:371–9. doi: 10.1634/stemcells.2005-0620
142. Lazarus HM, Haynesworth SE, Gerson SL, Rosenthal NS, Caplan AI. Ex vivo expansion and subsequent infusion of human bone marrow-derived stromal progenitor cells (mesenchymal progenitor cells): implications for therapeutic use. *Bone Marrow Trans.* (1995) 16:557–64.
143. Soeder Y, Loss M, Johnson CL, Hutchinson JA, Haarer J, Ahrens N, et al. First-in-Human case study: multipotent adult progenitor cells for immunomodulation after liver transplantation. *Stem Cells Transl Med.* (2015) 4:899–904. doi: 10.5966/sctm.2015-0002
144. Walker ND, Mourad Y, Liu K, Buxhoeveden M, Schoenberg C, Eloy JD, et al. Steroid-Mediated decrease in blood mesenchymal stem cells in liver transplant could impact long-Term recovery. *Stem Cell Rev Rep.* (2017) 13:644–58. doi: 10.1007/s12015-017-9751-3
145. *NIH. ClinicalTrials.gov.* Available online at: https://clinicaltrials.gov

18

The Next Frontier of Regulatory T Cells: Promising Immunotherapy for Autoimmune Diseases and Organ Transplantations

Lauren V. Terry[1*] *and Ye Htun Oo*[1,2,3*]

[1] Centre for Liver and Gastrointestinal Research, National Institute for Health Research Birmingham Biomedical Research Council, Institute of Immunology and Immunotherapy, University of Birmingham, Birmingham, United Kingdom, [2] European Reference Network (ERN) Centre—Rare Liver, Queen Elizabeth Hospital, Birmingham, United Kingdom, [3] Liver Transplant Unit, University Hospital of Birmingham National Health Service Foundation Trust, Birmingham, United Kingdom

***Correspondence:**
Lauren V. Terry
lvterry95@gmail.com
Ye Htun Oo
y.h.oo@bham.ac.uk

Regulatory T cells (Tregs) are crucial in maintaining tolerance. Hence, Treg immunotherapy is an attractive therapeutic option in autoimmune diseases and organ transplantations. Currently, autoimmune diseases do not have a curative treatment and transplant recipients require life-long immunosuppression to prevent graft rejection. There has been significant progress in understanding polyclonal and antigen-specific Treg biology over the last decade. Clinical trials with good manufacturing practice (GMP) Treg cells have demonstrated safety and early efficacy of Treg therapy. GMP Treg cells can also be tracked following infusion. In order to improve efficacy of Tregs immunotherapy, it is necessary that Tregs migrate, survive and function at the specific target tissue. Application of antigen specific Tregs and maintaining cells' suppressive function and survival with low dose interleukin-2 (IL-2) will enhance the efficacy and longevity of infused GMP-grade Tregs. Notably, stability of Tregs in the local tissue can be manipulated by understanding the microenvironment. With the recent advances in GMP-grade Tregs isolation and antigen-specific chimeric antigen receptor (CAR)-Tregs development will allow functionally superior cells to migrate to the target organ. Thus, Tregs immunotherapy may be a promising option for patients with autoimmune diseases and organ transplantations in near future.

Keywords: regulatory T cell, liver transplant, autoimmune liver diseases, antigen specific, recruitment, tolerance, polyclonal

BACKGROUND OF REGULATORY T CELLS

Naturally occurring $CD4^{+}CD25^{high}$ regulatory T (Treg) cells maintain peripheral self-tolerance in rodents and humans (1, 2). In 1995, Sakaguchi and colleagues demonstrated that adoptive transfer of a subset of $CD4^{+}$ T cells expressing the IL-2 receptor α-chain (CD25) prevented autoimmunity (1). $CD4^{+}CD25^{high}$ T cells constitute 5 to 10% of $CD4^{+}$ T cells in the blood (3) and they are able to maintain immunologic self-tolerance and transplantation tolerance by actively suppressing self-reactive, alloantigen-reactive lymphocytes. Treg cells prevent activation and expansion of auto-reactive T cells that escape clonal deletion in the thymus.

Treg cell development and function is controlled by the transcription factor Foxp3, however defects can lead to autoimmune and inflammatory syndromes in humans and mice (4).

Immunodysregulation, polyendocrinopathy, X-linked (IPEX) syndrome, a rare X-linked recessive disorder, was first described in 1982 in which mutations in the Foxp3 gene caused defective development of $CD4^+CD25^{high}$ Treg cells (5). Similarly, lymphoproliferation and multi-organ autoimmunity in scurfy mutant mice was caused by mutations in Foxp3 (6). Further to this, expression of the IL-7 receptor, CD127, correlated inversely with Foxp3 expression and Treg cell suppressive function; hence Treg cells are currently defined as $CD4^+CD25^{high}CD127^{low}Foxp3^+$ cells (7, 8).

Treg cells main function is to control auto-reactive T cells via multiple mechanisms. Treg cells express CTLA-4 and suppress effector T cells, via endocytosis of CD80/CD86 molecules expressed on antigen presenting dendritic cells (9). They can also secrete immunosuppressive cytokines (interleukin-10), cytotoxic granzymes and immunomodulatory molecule, kynurenine. Treg cells can generate the immunosuppressive molecule, adenosine, via CD39 expressed on the cell surface (8). By continuously surveying and controlling self-reactive T effector cells, Treg cells are crucial in restoring tolerance in both autoimmunity and transplantation.

TYPES OF REGULATORY T CELLS

$CD4^+CD25^{high}$ $Foxp3^+$ Treg cells are a heterogeneous population, often categorized into two main subtypes, which include thymic-derived natural Treg (tTreg) cells and peripheral-derived Treg (pTreg) cells (10, 11). Both subtypes act in a complementary manner to maintain peripheral tolerance. tTreg cells express Foxp3, however Foxp3 is transiently induced in pTreg cells; they may not have high levels of Treg specific demethylated region (TSDR), a conserved region within the Foxp3 gene (12). pTreg cells recognize non-self-antigens, such as those encountered in the gut and airways, in addition to providing maternal-fotal tolerance and commensal micro-biota tolerance (13–15). pTreg cells develop from conventional T cells once they have been exposed to non-self-antigens and transforming growth factor-β (16, 17). Although tTreg cells and pTreg cells can be distinguished by using epigenetics markers, phenotypically they share the same surface markers, which poses difficulty in specifically isolating tTreg cells for subsequent therapeutic purposes.

INTERLEUKIN-2

Treg cell survival and function is dependent on the cytokine, interleukin-2 (IL-2) (18), which is required for maintaining effective levels of functional Treg cells in autoimmune disease (AID) (19–21). The cell surface receptor for IL-2 (IL-2R) is composed of three subunits, alpha (IL-2RA, CD25), beta (IL-2RB, CD122), and gamma (IL-2RG, CD132). Treg cells constitutively express IL-2RA. IL-2RA is required for high-affinity IL-2 binding, whilst IL-2RB and IL-2RG transduce the IL-2 signal (22). Owing to their high levels of high-affinity CD25, Treg cells competitively consume IL-2, thereby maintaining their survival and function, whilst suppressing bystander effector cells (23, 24). Where IL-2 availability is low, such as in the inflamed hepatic microenvironment, Treg cell function may be compromised and be inadequate to counteract the activated immune infiltrate (25). At tissue level, Treg cell suppression is via IL-2 and CTLA-4 dependent mechanisms, yet tissue Treg cells, such as intrahepatic Treg cells, constitutively express CTLA-4 (25, 26). CTLA-4 can capture its ligands, CD80 and CD86, from antigen presenting cells (APCs) by trans-endocytosis, there by acting as an effector molecule to inhibit CD28 co-stimulation by the cell-extrinsic depletion of ligands (9).

AUTOIMMUNE DISEASES

The pathogenesis of AID is attributed by genetic susceptibilities, environmental factors, and gut micro-biota (27). The majority of organs and tissues in humans are susceptible to AIDs; such as in solid organs (liver–autoimmune liver diseases and kidneys–autoimmune glomerulonephritis), brain (multiple sclerosis), lung (autoimmune idiopathic lung fibrosis), gut (Coeliac disease, pernicious anemia, inflammatory bowel diseases), skin (psoriasis, pemphigus, erythema nodosum), endocrine (autoimmune thyroiditis, diabetes, Addison's disease), and multi-organ involvement, for example, systemic lupus erythematosus (SLE) (**Figure 1**).

Autoimmune liver diseases (AILDs) include autoimmune hepatitis (AIH), primary biliary cholangitis (PBC) and primary sclerosing cholangitis (PSC) (28, 29). Both AIDs and AILDs are immune mediated diseases of unknown etiology, and occur as a result of a breakdown in immune homeostasis (30). Immunological homeostasis in humans is maintained between a balance of effector T cells and Treg cells. It is now accepted that there is a lack of control of self-reactive T effectors cells by Treg cells in AIDs (31). Most AIDs co-exist with other autoimmune conditions in the same individual (**Figure 1**), therefore, restoring the tolerance in one autoimmune condition may also alleviate other AIDs, if the origin of initial pathology stems from the same tissue.

Therapies targeting AIDs, often aim to inhibit pro-inflammatory immune responses by preventing activation of immune cells in the target organ or diminishing tissue specific T cell populations (32). Treg cells play a role in restoring multiple human liver autoimmune conditions, however, Treg-directed therapies could potentially inhibit protective immune responses and lead to a higher risk of susceptibility to infection (31). As Treg cells have significant immune-homeostatic properties to prevent autoimmunity in mice and human, Treg-based cellular therapies have gained extensive interest in the past decade. Yet, most approaches to suppress autoimmunity currently use polyclonal Treg cells due to their success in animal models.

Polyclonal Treg cells have several limitations, such as the possibility of inducing global immunosuppression and predisposing patients to infection. These limitations may be overcome by using auto-antigen specific Treg cells. Most investigators are currently focusing on the suppression of auto-reactive T cells in an antigen-specific manner (33, 34). The use of T cell receptor (TCR) transgenic mice confirmed that

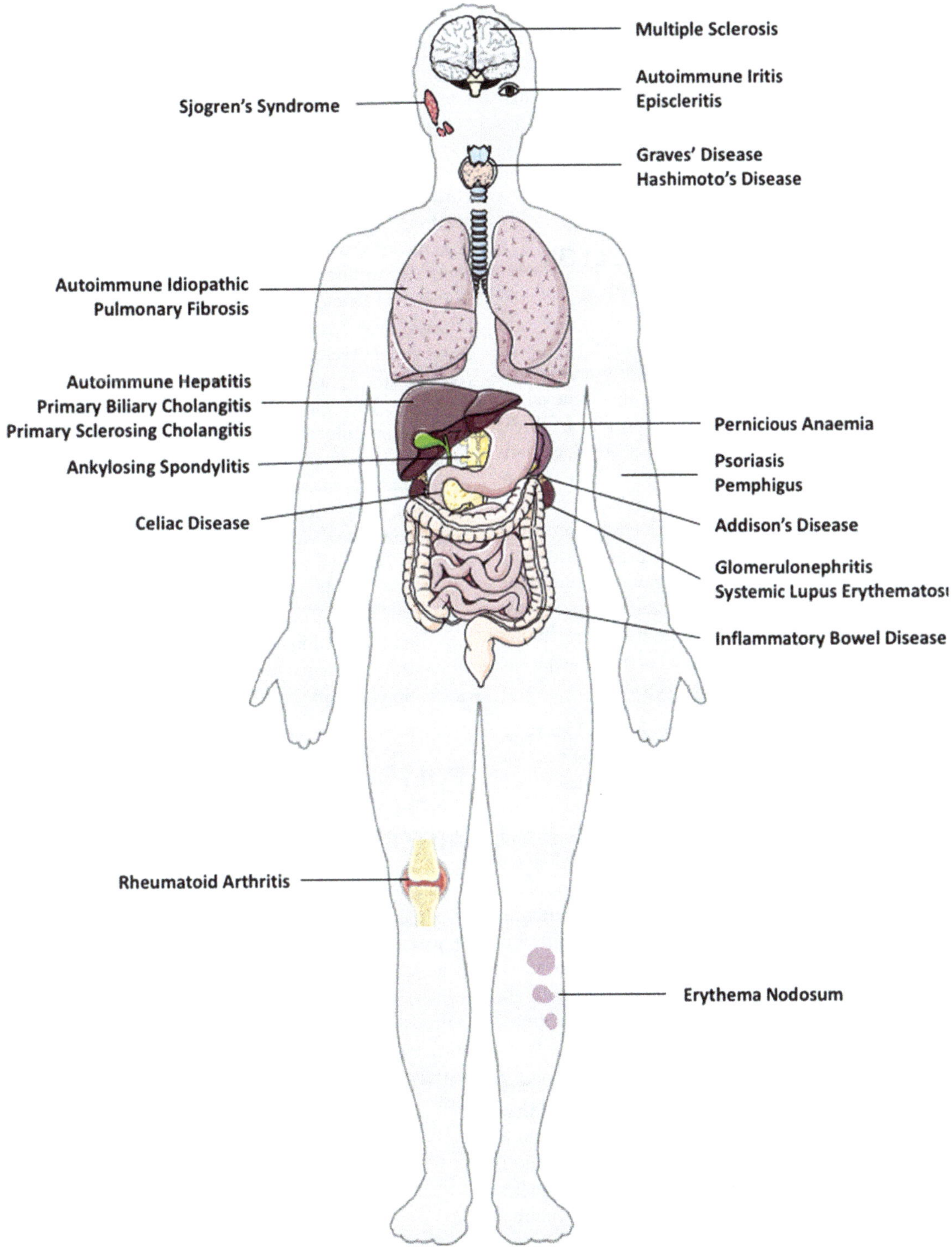

FIGURE 1 | Autoimmune diseases in multiple organs in humans. e.g. autoimmune diseases that can co-exist in multiple tissues are: brain (multiple sclerosis), eye (autoimmune iritis and episcleritis), lung (autoimmune idiopathic pulmonary fibrosis), gut (Coeliac disease, pernicious anemia, inflammatory bowel disease), liver—autoimmune liver diseases (autoimmune hepatitis, primary biliary cholangitis, primary sclerosing cholangitis), kidneys (autoimmune glomerulonephritis), skin (psoriasis, pemphiqus), endocrine (autoimmune thyroid disease such as Hashimoto thyroiditis, Graves' disease, type 1 diabetes, Addison's disease), and multi-organ involvement, such as systemic lupus erythematosus.

antigen-specific Treg cells are more potent and efficacious in autoimmune diabetes (35). Although antigen-specific Treg cells provide a new direction for Treg cellular therapy, the challenges remain in isolating and expanding antigen-specific Treg cells, in addition to a lack of understanding of their mechanism of suppression, survival and plasticity. These aspects require addressing before embarking on organ-specific Treg cellular therapy.

POLYCLONAL REGULATORY T CELLS AND LOW DOSE IL-2 THERAPY IN AUTOIMMUNE DISEASE

In healthy individuals, antigens can be efficiently eliminated without damaging their own tissue, due to the removal or inactivation of self-reactive cells, without posing a threat to the individual (36). Yet, when there is a breakdown in peripheral tolerance, the control of self-reactive cells can become dysregulated and aberrant immune responses can lead to harmful effects in their own tissue, which may lead to the development of AID (8). Reduction in the frequency of Treg cells or a decline in their function has been reported in various autoimmune condition settings (37). Failure of Treg cells to suppress effector cells is a typical feature of autoimmunity and has led to studies exploring the use of either polyclonal (38, 39) or antigen-specific Treg cells (40–42) as cellular therapies for AIDs (43).

AIDs can affect specific organs of the body (**Figure 1**). Multiple sclerosis is a debilitating and known AID of the nervous system. As mentioned, AILD includes AIH, PBC, and PSC. Autoimmune endocrine diseases include autoimmune thyroiditis (both Hashimoto and Grave's disease) Sjogren's syndrome, and type-1 diabetes mellitus. Autoimmune musculo-skeletal diseases are ankylosing spondylitis, rheumatoid arthritis, pemphigus and psoriasis. Further to this, gastrointestinal autoimmune conditions comprise of coeliac disease, pernicious anemia, and inflammatory bowel diseases (**Figure 1**). AIDs can also affect multiple organs and tissues in the same patient, for example, autoimmune PBC patients often have associated Sjogren's syndrome and autoimmune thyroid disease (28).

Adoptive Treg cell therapy has been applied in SLE patients with active skin disease (44). The study demonstrated that Treg cell accumulation in the skin was associated with a marked attenuation of the interferon-γ pathway and a reciprocal augmentation of the interleukin-17 pathway (44). Additionally, good manufacturing practice (GMP) Treg cell therapy in children with another autoimmune condition, *Type 1 diabetes mellitus* demonstrated that Treg therapy was safe without any serious side effects, at a Treg cell dose ranging from 10–20 millions/Kg. Children were followed up for a year and the trial revealed that there was a lower insulin requirement and higher C peptides compared to the control patient group (39, 45). A recent trial from UCSF on adult patients with diabetes that utilized GMP polyclonal Treg cells ranging from 5 million to 2.6 billion showed that Treg cell therapy is safe and that there was stable C peptide levels and insulin for 2 years after GMP Treg cell therapy. Cells were labeled with Deuterium and could be traced in the circulation for up to 12 months (38). In addition, $CD4^{+}CD25^{+}CD127^{low}CD45RA^{+}$ Treg cells have been suggested as the most suitable subset for GMP Treg cell trial in *inflammatory bowel disease* (46). Thus, there are many investigators attempting to restore tolerance in AIDs with direct application of Treg cells to patients.

In addition to GMP-Treg cell infusion, Treg cell enhancing therapy with very low dose IL-2, has also been applied in various AIDs. In *HCV induced vasculitis* (47), this therapy has been shown to be safe and led to Treg cell recovery with concomitant clinical improvements in patients who had cutaneous vasculitis. Additionally, a randomized double blind clinical trial using subcutaneous low dose IL-2 on alternate days for 2 weeks, followed by a 2-week break at a dose of 1 million IU or placebo, in patients with active SLE, suggested that low dose IL-2 was again safe and may be an effective therapy (48). Immunological and clinical efficacy of low dose IL-2 was assessed in a recent open-label, phase I-IIa study of 46 patients with *multiple autoimmune conditions*: including rheumatoid arthritis, ankylosing spondylitis, SLE, psoriasis, Behcet's disease, granulomatosis with polyangiitis, Takayasu's disease, Crohn's disease, ulcerative colitis, AIH or PSC. All patients received low dose IL-2 (1 million IU/day) for 5 days, followed by fortnightly injections for 6 months. The results suggested that low dose IL-2 was well tolerated in all AIDs, in addition to observing Treg cell expansion and activation in all patients, without effector T cell activation (49, 50).

POLYCLONAL REGULATORY T CELLS AND LOW DOSE IL-2 THERAPY IN AUTOIMMUNE LIVER DISEASE

As previously mentioned, AILDs include AIH, which affects hepatocytes, PBC and PSC, which affects bile ducts. Functional impairment or quantitative deficiency of Treg cells has been described in AILD (25, 51, 52). In AIH, hepatocytes, which constitute around 70% of liver cells, are mainly damaged by auto-reactive T cells (51, 53–55). PBC affects the intrahepatic bile ducts and PSC affects both the intra- and extrahepatic bile ducts and is associated with inflammatory bowel disease. Current therapies for AILD are non-curative, provide unsatisfactory control of hepatic and biliary inflammation and require long-term immunosuppressive medications that carry unfavorable side effects. Thus, autologous Treg cell therapy is an attractive option for the treatment of AILD, which could provide long-term immune-regulation without requiring global immunosuppression.

To work effectively, adoptively transferred Treg cells must migrate to and mediate suppression of auto-reactive T cells at the targeted tissue. Chemokines direct the trafficking and positioning of leukocytes within the tissue by attracting T cells, which express the corresponding chemokine receptors (56, 57). Deficiency of chemokine receptor, CXCR3, which drives recruitment of T cells across hepatic sinusoids (25, 58) has been associated with the exacerbation of liver disease and abrogation of tolerance in mouse models of immune-mediated hepatitis (59). A recent report by Oo and colleagues described that around 22–44% of infused GMP Treg cells migrate to the human autoimmune liver via utilizing CXCR3 (60). There is also another registered Phase 1 clinical trial to treat AIH patients with Treg cells (NCT02704338) yet the result is still awaited.

The stability of Treg cells at the site of hepatic inflammation is crucial. Our group has previously demonstrated that Treg cells expressing Treg Th1 phenotype are more common in an inflamed liver microenvironment (25). In addition, our recent data suggested that the human liver has low levels of IL-2 that may not support Treg cell survival (26). Based on this data, low dose IL-2 was administered in two patients with refractory AIH and an increase in the frequency of Treg cells in the peripheral circulation was observed (61).

ORGAN TRANSPLANTATIONS

Transplantation provides the best chance of survival in organ failure or cancer and has become a routine clinical treatment option for many patients. Bone marrow, heart, liver, and kidney transplantations are performed in many countries however, recently the transplantation field has progressed to islet cell and multi-visceral transplantations in some centers (**Figures 2, 3**). Due to the current demand of organ donors exceeding the number of transplantable organs, live donation (liver and kidneys), and split graft transplants (liver) have become a vital option (62).

In the early period following transplantation, both direct and indirect pathways of antigen presentation by donor and recipient dendritic cells play a role in graft rejection (63). Transplant recipients are required to take long term immunosuppression to prevent graft loss. Graft rejection is driven by an imbalance in the adaptive T and B immune cells: mainly a decline in the frequency of Treg cells or impairment in Treg cell function, which controls alloantigen specific T cells. To prevent graft rejection in both live and cadaveric transplantation, switching the immune balance toward the regulatory arm with Treg cellular therapy has become an exciting therapeutic option. Two main aims of Treg immunotherapy are 1) to restore immune tolerance and 2) to avoid life-long immunosuppression following transplantation. The side effects of immunosuppression range from sepsis, hypertension, diabetes, and renal dysfunction, to, the long term-effects of malignancies and post-transplant lymphoproliferative disorder (PTLD).

In the context of living-related liver and kidney transplantation, Treg cell infusion could be planned in advance. For example, recipient Treg cells could be isolated several weeks prior to the organ transplant and expanded with donor-derived APCs (dendritic cells, monocytes or B cells). This would allow sufficient numbers to be obtained in order to infuse them back into the organ recipient within the first few days post-transplant when immunosuppression and microenvironment milieu is optimized (**Figures 2** and **3**). Recipient Treg generation could be 1) polyclonal (if recipient Treg cells are expended with CD3, CD28 beads, IL-2 and Rapamycin) or 2) antigen-specific (if recipient Treg cells are expanded with donor APCs primed with the donor antigen) (**Figure 2**). Thus, autologous, polyclonal or antigen-specific Treg cell therapy can be administered to the liver or kidney organ transplant recipient immediately following transplantation. This could potentially lead to prevention of early graft rejection with a potential withdrawal of life-long immunosuppression.

Multiple clinical trials are registered for polyclonal Treg cell immunotherapy or low dose IL-2 cytokine therapy, in autoimmune conditions and organ transplantations (clinicalTrials.gov) (**Table 1**). These trials are currently being carried out or completed with $CD4^+CD25^{high}$ or $CD4^+CD25^{high}CD127^{low}$ populations, which are GMP cell-sorted and expanded with TCR stimulation, or subcutaneous administration of low dose IL-2 (Aldesleukin). So far, there is no clinical trial completed with antigen-specific Treg cell immunotherapy.

POLYCLONAL REGULATORY T CELLS AND LOW DOSE IL-2 THERAPY IN HUMAN TRANSPLANTATIONS

Polyclonal Treg cells have been applied in bone marrow and solid organ transplantations with a view to either reduce immunosuppression or achieve transplant tolerance without requiring immunosuppression. Treg cells mediate suppression of anti-donor immune responses, thus Treg cell enrichment following bone marrow, liver, and kidney transplantation could potentially lead to immunosuppression-free operational tolerance.

Treg cells can be isolated and expanded in large scale from the peripheral blood and the umbilical cord blood, which have been infused back to patients and proved to be safe in graft vs. host disease (GvHD) clinical trials (64, 65). Additionally, Treg cells have been applied in renal transplantation clinical trials. In the context of bone marrow transplantation, adoptive Treg cell therapy has been applied to control GVHD by utilizing freshly isolated or *ex vivo* expanded $CD4^+CD25^+$ Treg cells (65–67).

The TRACT trial infused $500–5000 \times 10^6$ $CD4^+$ $CD25^+$ Treg cells (>80% $Foxp3^+$) to nine patients, 2 months after live donor renal transplantation (68). The immunosuppression regimens included Alemtuzumab, followed by mycophenolate mofetil (MMF) and Tacrolimus. During this trial, there were no reported cases of opportunistic infections or graft rejection. In addition, the UCSF team applied polyclonal Treg cells into renal allograft subclinical inflammation. This type of low-grade inflammation can lead to late graft rejection, thus it demonstrated the application of Treg cells in this context (69). The team recruited three patients with biopsy-proven inflammation and administered a dose of 320 million $CD4^+$ $CD25^+$ $CD127^{low}$ Treg (>93% $Foxp3^+$) cells. Patients were on MMF, tacrolimus, and prednisolone immunosuppression. Following infusion, deuterated glucose was applied into the culture media to track infused Treg cells in the circulation. There were no side effects noted after infusion, however deuterated cells were not detected at the site of renal inflammation.

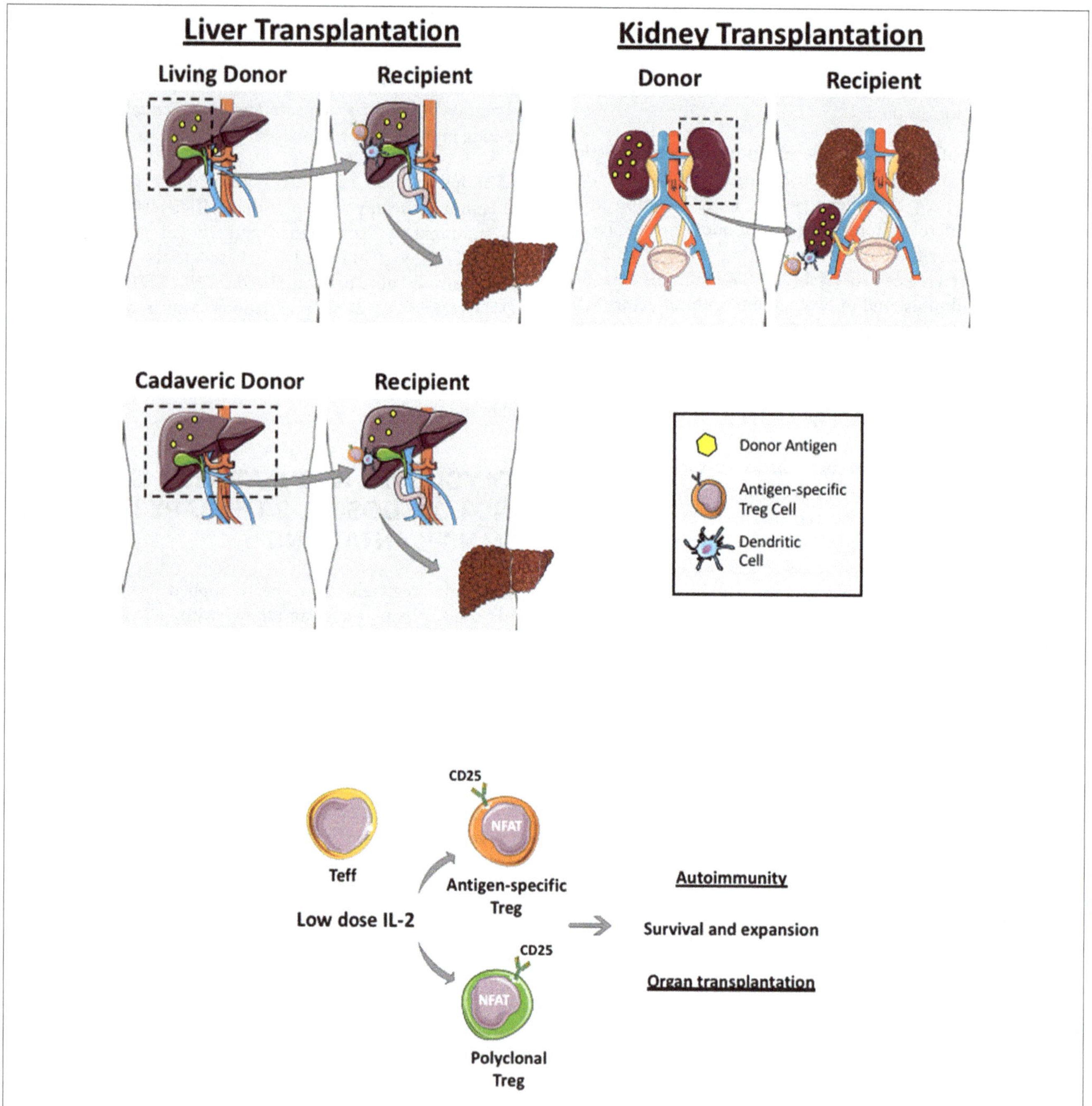

FIGURE 2 | Regulatory T cells in live and cadaveric liver transplant. Liver transplantation can be a living-related (right lobe graft- upper figure) or a cadaveric transplant (whole liver transplant—lower figure). Renal transplantation can also be cadaveric or a live donor allograft. If it is a living donor transplantation, antigen-specific Treg cells can be generated and expanded before transplantation whereby recipient Treg cells are co-cultured with donor dendritic cells, which are primed with donor antigens (yellow dots). Both polyclonal and antigen-specific Treg cells proliferate and function via utilizing interleukin-2 as Treg highly express IL-2 receptor, CD25. These generated Treg cells are applied in both autoimmune disease and transplantation clinical trials.

More recently, the application of Treg cells in renal transplantation was studied in the ONE study (in press, Vol 395 May 23, 2020, Lancet). The ONE Study consisted of seven investigator-led, single-arm trials done internationally at eight hospitals in France, Germany, Italy, the UK, and the USA (60 week follow-up). Included patients were living-donor kidney transplant recipients aged 18 years and older. The reference group trial (RGT) was a standard-of-care group given basiliximab, tapered steroids, MMF, and tacrolimus. The trial has just been completed and investigators concluded that regulatory cell therapy is achievable and safe in living-donor kidney transplant recipients, and is associated with fewer infectious complications, but similar rejection rates in the first year. Therefore, immune cell therapy is a potentially useful therapeutic

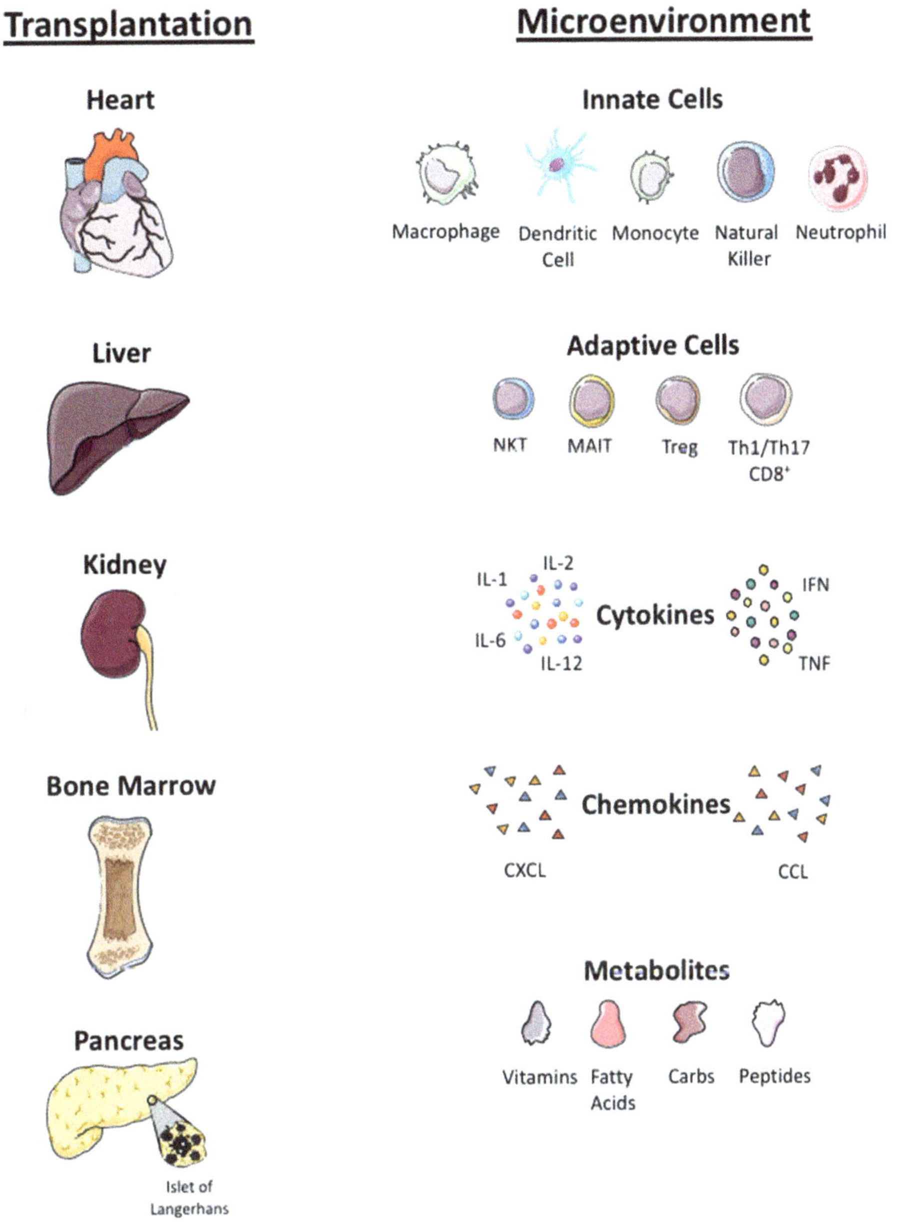

FIGURE 3 | Microenvironmental factors in different organs. Local tissue microenvironmental factors in organ (heart, liver, kidney, bone marrow, islet cells) transplantation. Infused Treg cells arrive to local tissue where they crosstalk with innate immune cells (macrophage, dendritic cells, monocyte, natural killer cells, neutrophils) and adaptive immune cells (NKT, Mucosa associated invariant T cells, Treg, Th1, Th17 cells) in the local tissue. Treg cells localize in tissue with pro-inflammatory cytokines (interleukin 1, 6 and 12, tumor necrosis factor (TNF) and interferon (IFN)), chemokines (CXCL and CCL) and local metabolites (carbohydrate, fatty acid, peptides and vitamins). Infused Treg cell plasticity and their function in the local tissue microenvironment is dependent on these factors.

approach in recipients of kidney transplant to minimize the burden of general immunosuppression.

POLYCLONAL REGULATORY T CELLS AND LOW DOSE IL-2 THERAPY IN LIVER TRANSPLANTATION

Liver transplantation has now become a standard therapeutic option for patients with acute liver failure or end-stage chronic liver disease. The ideal situation would be to achieve operational tolerance, which is defined as successful withdrawal of immunosuppression and to maintain a stable, preserved graft function following transplantation (31, 70). However, less than 20% of liver transplant recipients will achieve operational tolerance (71). The majority of patients will require life-long immunosuppression in order to control recipient immune responses toward allogeneic major histocompatibility complex (MHC) antigens from the donor liver graft and to reduce the risk of graft rejection and graft loss (72). Whilst immunosuppression

TABLE 1 | Table summarizing clinical applications of Treg cells in liver and autoimmune diseases in current clinical trials.

	Trial ID/ Name	Lead institution	Expansion: donor-specific or polyclonal	Application dose	Mechanism of recovery	Status of trial
LIVER TRANSPLANTATIONS						
Liver transplant (live donor) (2–6 years post-Tx)	NCT02474199 Donor Alloantigen Reactive Tregs (darTregs) for Calcineurin Inhibitor (CNI) Reduction (ARTEMIS)	University of California (UCSF), USA	Donor-specific	300–500 × 10^6 cells intravenous infusion	Cell sorting of $CD4^+$, $CD25^{++}$, $CD127^{low}$ Treg	Completed results awaiting
Liver transplant	NCT02188719 Donor-Alloantigen-Reactive Regulatory T Cell (darTregs) in Liver Transplantation (deLTa) dELTA	UCSF, USA	Donor-specific	4 cohorts dose escalation 25-960 × 10^6 cells	Cell sorting of $CD4^+$, $CD25^{++}$, $CD127^{low}$ Treg	Terminated
Liver transplant	NCT03654040 LITTMUS-UCSF	UCSF, USA	Donor-specific alloantigen-specific T regulatory cells (arTreg)	Target dose: 100-500 × 10^6 cells	Cell sorting of $CD4^+$, $CD25^{++}$, $CD127^{low}$ Treg	Not yet recruiting
Liver	NCT01624077 1st Trial	Nanjing, China	Polyclonal	1 × 10^6/kg at intervals	Unknown	Unknown
Liver	NCT01624077 2nd Trial	Nanjing, China	Donor-specific (MHC peptides)	1 × 10^6/kg at intervals	Unknown	Unknown
Liver	NCT02166177 ThRIL	King's College Hospital, UK	Polyclonal	0.5–6.5 × 10^6/kg	CliniMACS $CD4^+$ $CD25^{high}$ Treg	Completed Safe, well tolerated
Liver Live-donor transplant	Todo Okumura	Hokkaido, Japan	Donor-specific and co-stimulation blockade	0.23–6.37 × 10^6/kg $CD4^+$ $CD25^+$ $Foxp3^+$ Treg cells		Completed Safe, immunosuppression withdrawal achieved in 7/10 patients
AUTOIMMUNE DISEASES						
Type 1 diabetes mellitus	NCT01210664	UCSF	Polyclonal Treg	5-2,600 × 10^6 cells/kg		Safe, c peptide improved, insulin requirement decline, cell can be tracked for 12 months
Type 1 diabetes mellitus	NCT02772679	UCSF, USA	Polyclonal Tregs + IL-2 (TILT)	3–20 × 10^6 cells and two 5-day courses of IL-2 (1 × 106 IU daily)	Cell sorting of $CD4^+$, $CD25^{++}$, $CD127^{low}$ Treg	Active, not recruited yet
Type 1 diabetes mellitus	ISRCTN06128462	Medical University of Gdansk, Poland	Polyclonal	10–20 × 10^6 cells/kg	Cell sorting of $CD4^+$, $CD25^{++}$, $CD127^{low}$ Treg	Safe, well tolerated
Autoimmune hepatitis	AUTUMN	University of Birmingham, UK	Polyclonal	8.9–86 × 10^6 cells	GMP $CD4^+$ $CD25^{high}$ CliniMACS isolation	Completed 22–44% of Treg home to autoimmune livers
Pemphigus Vulgaris	NCT03239470	UCSF	Polyclonal	1–2.5 × 10^8 cells	Cell sorting of $CD4^+$, $CD25^{++}$, $CD127^{low}$ Treg	Recruiting

TABLE 2 | Immunosuppressive medications applied in autoimmunity and transplantation with their mechanisms, and impact on immune systems.

Medications	Effect on immune cells, cytokines	Mechanism	Clinical applications
Steroid (Prednisolone/ Budesonide)	Broad suppression of pro-inflammatory cytokines (74, 75)	Bind their cytosolic glucocorticoid receptor, translocate to the nucleus, and inhibit NF-κB-mediated transcription	Organ transplants Autoimmune diseases
Mycophenolate mofetil (MMF)	Purine is required for proliferation of T cells and B cells	Block enzyme IMPDH resulting in inhibition of *de novo* purine synthesis (76) Down-regulate co-stimulatory molecules on dendritic cells (77)	Organ transplants Autoimmune diseases
Calcineurin inhibitors (Tacrolimus/FK506) Cyclosporine A	IL-2 is crucial cytokines for Treg and T effectors survival and function (25)	Inhibit intracellular phosphatase calcineurin thus impair IL-2 production (78, 79)	Organ transplants
JAK3 inhibitor (Tofacitinib)	JAK3 signaling is critical to normal homeostasis and function of T cells, B cells, and NK cells; SCID in JAK3 mutations	JAK3 transduces signals downstream of CD132, which is the common gamma chain	Autoimmune diseases (80–83)
mTOR inhibitors Sirolimus (more effective for mTORC1), Everolimus	T cells differentiation (84, 85) Selective Treg expansion compared to T conventional cell in cell culture (86)	Inhibit downstream of PI3K and Akt via mTORC1 and mTORC2 mTORC1 is required for Treg activation (87)	Organ transplants
Anti-TNF Infliximab	Promote activation of innate and adaptive immunity	Pro-inflammatory cytokine	Rheumatoid arthritis Autoimmune hepatitis
Anti-IL6 R Tocilizumab	IL-6 leads to conventional T cells resistant to Treg suppression, Destabilizes Treg by inhibiting Foxp3 expression (88)	Pro-inflammatory cytokine promotes B and T cell proliferation and differentiation	Rheumatoid arthritis
Chemokine Receptor e.g. CXCR3	Both Treg and T effector cells express CXCR3 (58, 89)	Migrate to inflamed tissue where expression of CXCL9, (9, 10)	Autoimmune diseases
Anti-CD25 Basiliximab Daclizumab	Suppress immune response by targeting recently activated effector T cells that express CD25	Block the IL-2-binding site of CD25 (90)	Organ transplants
Rituximab	Depletes B cells	Anti-CD20 mAb	Antibody-mediated rejection, ABO-incompatible kidney transplants (91) Autoimmune hepatitis (92) GVHD (93) SLE

Inosine monophosphate dehydrogenase (IMPDH), phosphatidylinositol 3-kinase (PI3K), Akt. mTOR complex 1 (mTORC1) and mTOR complex 2 (mTORC2), Janus associated kinase 3 (JAK3).

has drastically improved survival rates over the last five decades, there are detrimental side effects that impose substantial risks to transplant recipients, such as: opportunistic infections, increased susceptibility to sepsis, renal dysfunction, and an increased risk of *de novo* malignancy (73). Immunosuppressive medications generally used are steroids, MMF, Tacrolimus, and Sirolimus. These medications have different impacts on different immune cell subset, which has been described in detail, in **Table 2.**

If transplant tolerance is to be achieved, it is essential that early inflammatory responses to allograft tissue must be regulated (94). In comparison to other organ transplantations, the liver is uniquely tolerant, which was first evidenced in 1969 by Sir Roy Calne, who demonstrated that liver allografts were accepted across MHC mismatch in pigs without immunosuppression (95). $CD4^{+}CD25^{+}Foxp3^{+}$ Treg cells function by maintaining immunological self-tolerance of the allograft, immune homeostasis, and suppression of immune responses in order to reduce the destruction of tissue and support the allograft (96). Within a transplanted liver and hepatic draining lymph nodes, there is highly complex immune cells interplay between effector T cells, Treg cells, and antigen presenting dendritic cells (69). Dysregulation of effector T cell response to transplanted antigens and failure of Treg cells to suppress donor antigen-specific T effector cells leads to transplant rejection.

Todo and colleagues first described the application of Treg cells in liver transplantation. They infused autologous Treg-enriched cell populations (Treg cell frequency range from 2.6–16.9% of cell population) to ten living donor liver transplant recipients 2 weeks following transplantation. Treg cells from recipient lymphocytes are amplified by co-culture with irradiated donor cells in the presence of anti-CD80/CD86 monoclonal antibodies *in vitro* for 2 weeks. Additionally, liver recipients underwent splenectomy. Liver transplant patients received MMF, cyclosporine and tacrolimus during the post-transplant period. The study showed that seven out of ten patients were successfully withdrawn from immunosuppression, ranging from 6 to 18 months post-transplantation (97).

Furthermore, in a recent phase I clinical trial using $CD4^{+}CD25^{+}Foxp3^{+}$ GMP-Treg cells, it was revealed that

Treg cell administration was safe in liver transplantation. Peripheral blood Treg cells were isolated by leukapheresis and expanded under GMP conditions with IL-2 and rapamycin and subsequently administered to post-liver transplant patients at either 0.5–1 million/Kg or 3–4.5 million/kg. A total of nine patients (three patients less than 6 months after transplantation and six patients more than 6 months post-transplantation) received the GMP-Treg cells. The study showed that Treg cell therapy was safe and increased the pool of circulating Treg cells (98).

In addition to GMP-Treg cellular therapy, IL-2 has also been applied in liver transplant recipients to enhance Treg cell frequency and function. Treg cells constitutively express the high affinity IL-2 receptor, which makes them exquisitely sensitive to very low-doses of IL-2. A clinical trial to test the capacity of low-dose IL-2 in order to promote the selective expansion of endogenous Treg cells in liver transplant recipients is still on-going and results are awaited (LITE trial, NCT02949492).

IMMUNOSUPPRESSIVE MEDICATIONS AND REGULATORY T CELLS

Either single or combination of immunosuppressive medications is normally applied in both AIDs and following organ transplantations. Calcineurin inhibitors (Tacrolimus and cyclosporine), mycophenolate mofetil (MMF or myfortif), Sirolimus, and corticosteroids are commonly used immunosuppressive drugs in both contexts. Rituximab, B cells depleting therapy, is also widely used in SLE and recently in difficult-to-treat AIH. Anti-cytokine therapy (anti-TNF and anti-IL-6) and JAK inhibitors have been applied in AIDs. **Table 2** describes the types of immunosuppressive medications, their impact on immune cells and their mechanisms of action (99).

DEVELOPMENT OVER LAST DECADE

Target Tissue Homing and Tracking of Tregs

In order for Treg cells to exert their suppressive ability to tissue damaging effector T cells, cellular migration to the target tissue is essential. A recent study by our laboratory demonstrated that 22–44% of indium labeled GMP clinical grade Treg cells could be detected in the inflamed human liver by SPECT CT scan (60). These GMP Treg cells had high levels of CXCR3 expression. CXCR3 ligands (CXCL9, CXCL10, CXCL11) are expressed on the sinusoids, hepatocytes, and bile ducts in the inflamed liver (60, 100). Thus, up-regulating chemokine receptors on the Treg cells or enhancing chemokine expression at the target tissue site would be an option to achieve homing of Treg cells in both organ specific AID and transplantation. Labeling of GMP Treg cells with deuterium can track the infused cells in the peripheral circulation (38) and hence can be applied to track cells for longitudinal phenotyping. Labeling of GMP Treg cells with indium and tracking the cells in real time with SPECT-CT scan would be an alternative way to reassure that cells that express tissue specific chemokine receptors migrate to the target tissue (60).

Current Treg cell manufacturing technologies are only available for large-scale polyclonal Treg cell production. Polyclonal Treg cells can be expanded using anti-CD3 and anti-CD28-coated beads and subsequent supplementation with IL-2 (101). The use of large numbers of polyclonal Treg cells with unknown antigen specificities has led to unwanted effects, such as systemic immunosuppression, which can be avoided via utilization of antigen-specific Treg cells.

Antigen Specificity and Chimeric Antigenic Receptor Tregs

Antigen-specific chimeric antigen receptor (CAR)-Treg cells have an advantage compared to polyclonal Treg cells due to their ability to migrate to the target organ, which express a specific antigen. Antigen-specific Treg cells have been shown to be functionally superior to polyclonal Treg cells in animal models, for example, Tang and colleagues isolated and expanded Treg cells derived from a transgenic mice that expressed islet cell specific TCR (102). In addition, antigen-specific CAR-Treg cells migrate specifically to the site of the antigen, thus has the advantage of less global immunosuppression compared to polyclonal Treg cells. CAR Treg cells could be developed to redirect Tregs toward a specific donor leucocyte antigen (HLA) class I molecule (HLA-A2) that is expressed in grafts.

Autologous or allogenic choice of Treg cell will influence the timing of administration for cell therapy. Donor-derived or third-party cells, such as umbilical cord blood derived Treg cells, may be used to generate CAR-Treg cells rapidly in batch production, however they could be immunogenic. Yet, autologous CAR-Treg cells, although not immunogenic, are produced individually, which is time-consuming (31). Other major challenges of Treg cell immunotherapy is the manufacturing of a large number of Treg cells to provide timely delivery of therapy, the efficacious dose of cells, the frequency of administration and recently, a major question being, what role does the low dose of IL-2 play in enhancing survival and function of polyclonal and antigen-specific Treg cells (28).

There are different approaches to obtain antigen-specific Treg cells and these include conferring antigen expression via CARs or engineering Treg cells with TCRs, specificity via transfection of viral vectors encoding specific TCRs. Both types of cells are promising given that they preferentially migrate to target sites and exert more potent and specific immunosuppression than polyclonal Treg cells. Engineering Treg cells with TCRs is a promising approach but limitations occur due to MHC-restrictions. Alloantigen-reactive Treg cells can be expanded through donor APCs, such as dendritic cells, PBMCs, and B cells (103). Compared to Treg cells engineered with TCRs (TCR-Treg), CAR-modified Treg (CAR-Treg) cells engineered in a non-MHC restricted manner have the advantage of widespread application. Additionally, CAR-Treg cells are less dependent on IL-2 than TCR-Treg cells.

Large Scale Treg Cell Production

Many investigators now have a GMP cell production facility and apply large scale Treg cell isolation and expansion. Cells are then frozen in GMP condition and thaw before infusing back to patients (**Figure 4**).

The quality of Treg cell function can be assessed before infusion by phenotyping isolated Treg cells to make sure that the purity is more than 95% ($CD4^{+}$ $CD25^{high}$ and $CD127^{low}$), with a high level of transcription factor Foxp3 expression. Flow cytometry analysis can also be applied to assess functional markers of Treg (CD39, CTLA-4, IL-10) on the isolated and expanded Treg cells. In addition, quality of Treg cells can be assessed by epigenetic testing of isolated and expanded GMP Treg cells with analysis of Treg specific demethylated region (TSDR) with epigenetic analysis.

Treg therapeutic effect could be predicted by clinical readouts. For example, in the context of liver disease to assess whether Treg cell infusion could improve liver function tests (liver enzymes—alanine transaminase and aspartate transaminase, bilirubin) and in the context of diabetes (insulin requirement and c-peptide level improvement). Also, Treg therapeutic effect can be monitored with immunological readouts (e.g., decline in effector Th1 or CD8+ T cell frequency in the blood and assessing the

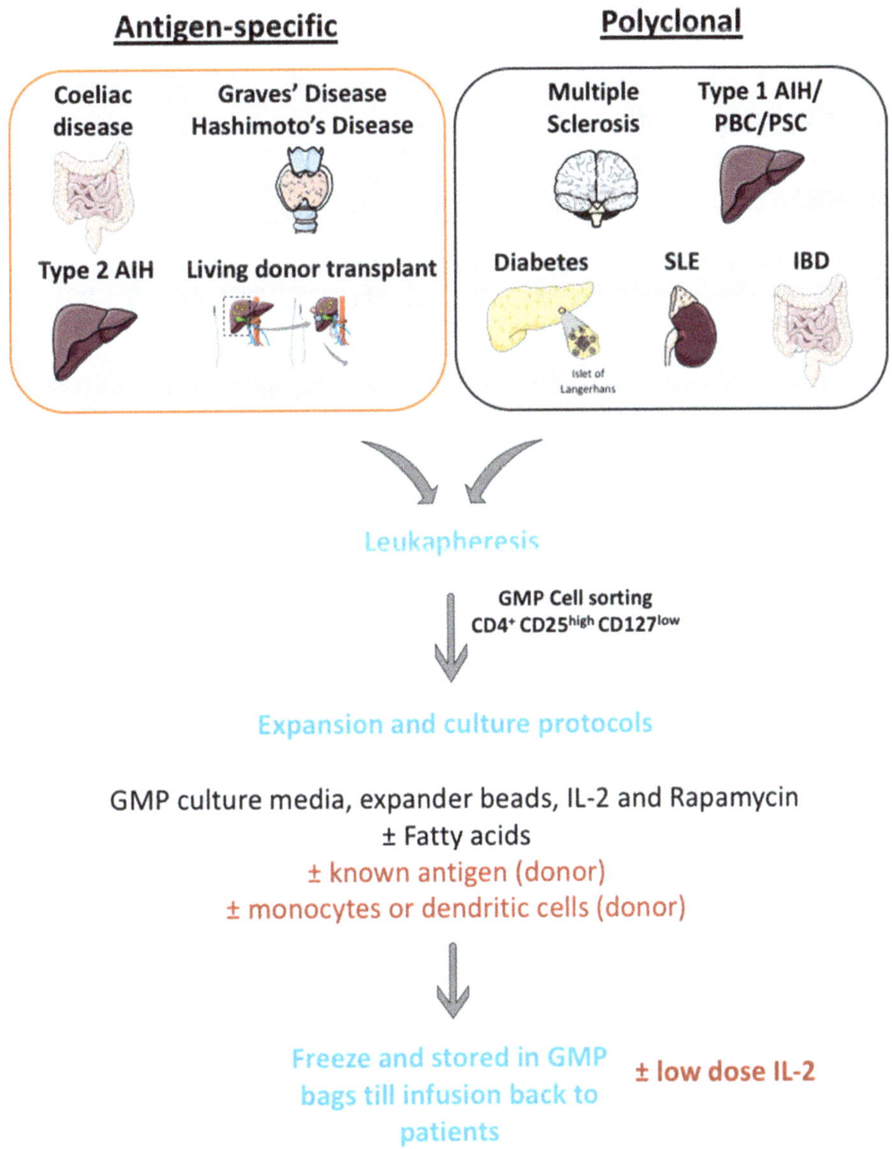

FIGURE 4 | Schematic illustration of large scale GMP Treg production. Leukapharesis procedures are performed to those patients with either autoimmune diseases or those who will undergo transplantations. GMP Treg will be cell sorted using surface markers to obtain highly pure $CD4^{+}$ $CD25^{high}$ $CD127^{low}$ cells population. Then, cells will be expanded in GMP culture media with GMP-grade IL-2 cytokines, GMP-grade rapamycin (to prevent effector T cells outgrowth) and GMP-grade CD3, CD28 Treg expander beads (with or without known antigen). These cells will then undergo quality assessment process and will be frozen until infusion back to patients.

frequency of cells in the tissue before and after infusion of cells with liver biopsy).

It is crucial to monitor the persistence of Treg cells when deciding the timing and frequency of Treg cells infusion. Treg cells can be monitored in both peripheral circulation and at tissue level. A recent study by our group showed Indium tropolonate labeling (60) and Deuterium labeling (38) can be applied to investigate the persistence of Treg cells in the circulation. Furthermore, persistence of infused Treg cells can sometimes be assessed in the tissue by performing a biopsy if it is ethically feasible and approved by the local team.

Treg cell function after infusion can be assessed directly by tracing the infused GMP Treg cells and conducting suppressive assays with autologous effector T cells, or indirectly by longitudinal phenotyping of effector T cells to investigate the decline in the frequency of these cells.

REGULATORY T CELLS IN CLINICAL TRIALS IN LIVER TRANSPLANTATION AND AUTOIMMUNE DISEASES

Current Treg cell therapy use autologous cells. The drawback of using autologous cells is the time-delay to administer Treg cells from taking peripheral blood to obtaining sufficient numbers of cells. To achieve the Treg cell infusion at the time of transplantation, allogeneic Treg cells produced by umbilical cord blood would be a potential option. In addition, live donor transplantations (liver and kidney) would also allow the investigator to obtain sufficient numbers of functional Treg cells before the day of organ transplantation. It is crucial to obtain tissue biopsies following Treg infusion to access the localization of infused cells. A recent study focusing on skin biopsies of lupus lesions following Treg cell infusion suggested that there was a shift in Th1 to Th17 gene signature (44). In addition, the choice of immunosuppression in patients with Treg cell therapy is crucial, for example, rapamycin has been shown to enhance Treg cell frequency (104). To achieve efficacious and successful Treg therapy, it is necessary to continue on immunosuppression that is favorable to Treg cell survival and proliferation.

Application of CAR-Treg cells is an exciting option, in both transplantation and AID, where there is a known antigen. However, there are still major hurdles that must be overcome before CAR-Treg cells can be used in clinic. Antibodies specific for self- or alloantigen must be characterized to construct antigen-specific CAR-Treg cells. Additionally, it is crucial to achieve homing of CAR-Treg cells to the exact target site. Treatments with anti-tumor CAR-T cells cause side effects such as a cytokine "storm" and neuronal cytotoxicity (105). Yet, exhaustion of CAR Treg cells may limit their efficacy in immunosuppression. Therefore, more work is required to administer CAR-Treg cells effectively and safely to restore tolerance in transplantations and AIDs.

Plasticity of polyclonal or CAR-Treg cells in an inflamed microenvironment is still an unknown factor and concern to most investigators. Some data suggested that the plasticity and instability of cells in inflamed tissue and Treg cells could convert into pathogenic effector T cells (106, 107). The inflamed microenvironment enriched with pro-inflammatory cytokines can either lead to a reduction in the potency of Treg cells or resistance of T effector cells to Treg cell suppression (25). There are also questions to be addressed regarding the long-term proliferative potential and survival of polyclonal or antigen-specific Treg cells in the tissue microenvironment, which is enriched with cytokines, metabolites, low oxygen levels, and microbial peptides (in the context of liver) (107, 108). Additionally, metabolites and microbes from the portal vein toward the liver can have an impact on metabolism, phenotype, and function of intrahepatic Treg cells. These microenvironmental factors will determine the biology of GMP Treg cells at the specific tissue locations. Treg cells co-localize not only with effector $CD4^+$ and $CD8^+$ T cells but also with other immune cells, including antigen presenting dendritic cells, microbes-primed MAIT cells, phagocytic macrophages, innate NK cells, and neutrophils (109). The cross talk of Treg cells with other immune cells and microenvironmental factors will shape the phenotype and function of Treg cells; thus it is worth considering these factors for each tissue when designing Treg cell clinical trials (**Figure 3**).

EXTRACELLULAR VESICLES

Recently, it has been reported that intracellular communication of Treg cells can occur through extracellular vesicles (EVs), which include exosomes, apoptotic vesicles, and macrovesicles (110) Importantly, they appear to be involved in alloimmunity, thus, EVs may be an alternative therapeutic approach. EVs were identified in $CD4^+CD25^+$ Treg cells isolated from rodents, which were found to be produced after TCR activation. Smyth and colleagues identified that CD73 was present on Treg-derived EVs, which was essential for Treg cell mediated suppression. To support this, Yu and colleagues reported that in an *in vitro* kidney transplantation mouse model, Treg-derived EVs effectively suppressed T cell proliferation in a dose-dependent manner (111). Patients with relapsing-remitting multiple sclerosis had Treg-derived exosomes with impaired suppressive function (112, 113). It has been previously shown that in an autoimmune colitis model, Treg exosomes suppressed inflammatory T cell immunity, thereby preventing systemic inflammation, through transfer of IFN-γ suppressing miRNA to T helper cells (114). Tung and colleagues identified that human Treg-derived EVs may be immune regulators and could be a potential treatment of transplant rejection (115). They also reported that TCR-activation of human Treg cells resulted in a release of EVs that efficiently suppressed T cell proliferation. Additionally, they identified that EVs had the ability to alter their cytokine profile to favor IL-10 and IL-4 secretion, whilst reducing expression of IL-6, IL-2, and IFN-γ simultaneously (116). In line with this evidence, the group demonstrated that in a humanized mouse skin transplant model, human Treg-derived EVs were capable of protecting human skin grafts from alloimmune-mediated damage, through reducing immune cell infiltrate, thus supporting that EVs may be immune regulators, and thus an important therapeutic alternative. It is noteworthy that EVs derived from dendritic cells have previously been utilized in phase 2 clinical trials for non-small cell lung cancer therapy and were identified to be efficacious (116). This suggests that EVs may be a promising therapeutic option, however there are many limitations that would be necessary to address prior to EVs being utilized in a clinical setting, including, but not limiting to, the dose regimen, optimization of *ex vivo* isolation of GMP-grade Treg-derived EV protocols, and identification of *in vivo* targets.

FUTURE DIRECTION OF REGULATORY T CELLS IN TRANSPLANTATION AND AUTOIMMUNITY

Treg cells have proved to be a major breakthrough as an exciting immunotherapy option in the last two decades. Early phase clinical trials demonstrated safety, feasibility, and early efficacy with GMP Tregs therapy in both autoimmune diseases and organ transplantation. Achieving successful Treg immunotherapy would lead to an immunosuppression-free period for patients. Development of antigen-specific Treg cells and CAR-Treg cells would lead to exciting new frontiers in the cell therapy field as these cells are more efficacious and lesser numbers of cells will be required due to their target tissue homing affinity. Over the last decade, manufacturing processes and culture media has been optimized. In addition, cytokines, such as IL-2, can support infused Treg cell survival and they would play as an adjuvant therapy in GMP Treg trials. Additionally, enhanced understanding of the patient's OMICs profile with new technologies will also allow us to apply personalized Treg cell immunotherapy. Although there are challenges, the future is exciting for the cell therapy community to collaborate closely in order to achieve a potentially effective immunotherapy and replace immunosuppression in both autoimmune disease and transplantation.

AUTHOR CONTRIBUTIONS

LT and YO conceptualize, wrote, edit, and approve the manuscript. All authors contributed to the article and approved the submitted version.

ACKNOWLEDGMENTS

All figures were created using ServierMedical Art templates.

REFERENCES

1. Sakaguchi S, Sakaguchi N, Asano M, Itoh M, Toda M. Immunologic self-tolerance maintained by activated T cells expressing IL-2 receptor alpha-chains (CD25). Breakdown of a single mechanism of self-tolerance causes various autoimmune diseases. *J Immunol.* (1995) 155:1151–64.
2. Liu W, Putnam A, Xu-Yu Z, Szot G, Lee M, Zhu S, et al. CD127 expression inversely correlates with FoxP3 and suppressive function of human CD4+ T reg cells. *J Exp Med.* (2006) 203:1701–11. doi: 10.1084/jem.20060772
3. Itoh M, Takahashi T, Sakaguchi N, Kuniyasu Y, Shimizu J, Otsuka F, et al. Thymus and autoimmunity: production of CD25+CD4+ naturally anergic and suppressive T cells as a key function of the thymus in maintaining immunologic self-tolerance. *J Immunol.* (1999) 162:5317–26.
4. Hori S, Nomura T, Sakaguchi S. Control of regulatory T cell development by the transcription factor Foxp3. *Science.* (2003) 299:1057–61. doi: 10.1126/science.1079490
5. Vandenbark AA, Offner H. Critical evaluation of regulatory T cells in autoimmunity: are the most potent regulatory specificities being ignored? *Immunology.* (2008) 125:1–13. doi: 10.1111/j.1365-2567.2008.02900.x
6. Lyon M, Peters J, Glenister P, Ball S, Wright E. The scurfy mouse mutant has previously unrecognized hematological abnormalities and resembles Wiskott-Aldrich syndrome. *Proc Natl Acad Sci USA.* (1990) 87:2433–7. doi: 10.1073/pnas.87.7.2433
7. Seddiki N, Santner-Nanan B, Martinson J, Zaunders J, Sasson S, Landay A, et al. Expression of interleukin (IL)-2 and IL-7 receptors discriminates between human regulatory and activated T cells. *J.Exp.Med.* (2006) 203:1693–700. doi: 10.1084/jem.20060468
8. Sakaguchi S, Yamaguchi T, Nomura T, Ono M. Regulatory T cells and immune tolerance. *Cell.* (2008) 133:775–87. doi: 10.1016/j.cell.2008.05.009
9. Qureshi O, Zheng Y, Nakamura K, Attridge K, Manzotti C, Schmidt E, et al. Trans-endocytosis of CD80 and CD86: a molecular basis for the cell-extrinsic function of CTLA-4. *Science.* (2011) 332:600–3. doi: 10.1126/science.1202947
10. Gratz I, Truong H, Yang S, Maurano M, Lee K, Abbas AK, et al. Cutting edge: memory regulatory t cells require IL-7 and not IL-2 for their maintenance in peripheral tissues. *J Immunol.* (2013) 190:4483–7. doi: 10.4049/jimmunol.1300212
11. Abbas A, Benoist C, Bluestone J, Campbell D, Ghosh S, Hori S, et al. Regulatory T cells: recommendations to simplify the nomenclature. *Nat Immunol.* (2013) 14:307–8. doi: 10.1038/ni.2554
12. Polansky J, Kretschmer K, Freyer J, Floess S, Garbe A, Baron U, et al. DNA methylation controls Foxp3 gene expression. *Eur J Immunol.* (2008) 38:1654–63. doi: 10.1002/eji.200838105
13. Curotto de Lafaille MA, Lafaille JJ. Natural and adaptive foxp3+ regulatory T cells: more of the same or a division of labor? *Immunity.* (2009) 30:626–35. doi: 10.1016/j.immuni.2009.05.002
14. Kim K, Hong S, Han D, Yi J, Jung J, Yang B, et al. Dietary antigens limit mucosal immunity by inducing regulatory T cells in the small intestine. *Science.* (2016) 351:858–63. doi: 10.1126/science.aac5560
15. Steinman L, Merrill J, McInnes I, Peakman M. Optimization of current and future therapy for autoimmune diseases. *Nat Med.* (2012) 18:59–65. doi: 10.1038/nm.2625
16. Chen W, Jin W, Hardegen N, Lei K, Li L, Marinos N, et al. Conversion of peripheral CD4+CD25- naive T cells to CD4+CD25+ regulatory T cells by TGF-beta induction of transcription factor Foxp3. *J Exp Med.* (2003) 198:1875–86. doi: 10.1084/jem.20030152
17. Kretschmer K, Apostolou I, Hawiger D, Khazaie K, Nussenzweig M, von Boehmer H. Inducing and expanding regulatory T cell populations by foreign antigen. *Nat Immunol.* (2005) 6:1219–27. doi: 10.1038/ni1265
18. Wing K, Sakaguchi S. Regulatory T cells exert checks and balances on self tolerance and autoimmunity. *Nat Immunol.* (2010) 11:7–13. doi: 10.1038/ni.1818
19. Hartemann A, Bensimon G, Payan C, Jacqueminet S, Bourron O, Nicolas N, et al. Low-dose interleukin 2 in patients with type 1 diabetes: a phase 1/2 randomised, double-blind, placebo-controlled trial. *Lancet Diabetes Endocrinol.* (2013) 1:295–305. doi: 10.1016/S2213-8587(13)70113-X
20. Yang J, Sherry R, Steinberg S, Topalian S, Schwartzentruber D, Hwu P, et al. Randomized study of high-dose and low-dose interleukin-2 in patients with metastatic renal cancer. *J Clin Oncol.* (2003) 21:3127–32. doi: 10.1200/JCO.2003.02.122
21. Klatzmann D, Abbas AK. The promise of low-dose interleukin-2 therapy for autoimmune and inflammatory diseases. *Nat Rev Immunol.* (2015) 15:283–94. doi: 10.1038/nri3823
22. Taniguchi T, Miyazaki T, Minami Y, Kawahara A, Fujii H, Nakagawa Y, et al. IL-2 signaling involves recruitment and activation of multiple protein tyrosine kinases by the IL-2 receptor. *Ann N Y Acad Sci.* (1995) 766:235–44. doi: 10.1111/j.1749-6632.1995.tb26671.x

23. Hofer T, Krichevsky O, Altan-Bonnet G. Competition for IL-2 between regulatory and effector T cells to Chisel immune responses. *Front Immunol.* (2012) 3:268. doi: 10.3389/fimmu.2012.00268
24. Busse D, de la Rosa M, Hobiger K, Thurley K, Flossdorf M, Scheffold A, et al. Competing feedback loops shape IL-2 signaling between helper and regulatory T lymphocytes in cellular microenvironments. *Proc Natl Acad Sci USA.* (2010) 107:3058–63. doi: 10.1073/pnas.0812851107
25. Chen Y, Jeffery H, Hunter S, Bhogal R, Birtwistle J, Braitch M, et al. Human intrahepatic regulatory T cells are functional, require IL-2 from effector cells for survival, and are susceptible to Fas ligand-mediated apoptosis. *Hepatology.* (2016) 64:138–50. doi: 10.1002/hep.28517
26. Jeffery H, Jeffery L, Lutz P, Corrigan M, Webb G, Hirschfield G, et al. Low-dose interleukin-2 promotes STAT-5 phosphorylation, Treg survival and CTLA-4-dependent function in autoimmune liver diseases. *Clin Exp Immunol.* (2017) 188:394–411. doi: 10.1111/cei.12940
27. Oo YH, Hubscher SG, Adams DH. Autoimmune hepatitis: new paradigms in the pathogenesis, diagnosis, and management. *Hepatol Int.* (2010) 4:475–93. doi: 10.1007/s12072-010-9183-5
28. Than NN, Jeffery HC, Oo YH. Autoimmune hepatitis: progress from global immunosuppression to personalised regulatory T cell therapy. *Can J Gastroenterol Hepatol.* (2016) 2016:7181685. doi: 10.1155/2016/7181685
29. Oo YH, Neuberger J. Options for treatment of primary biliary cirrhosis. *Drugs.* (2004) 64:2261–71. doi: 10.2165/00003495-200464200-00001
30. Miyara M, Sakaguchi S. Human FoxP3(+)CD4(+) regulatory T cells: their knowns and unknowns. *Immunol Cell Biol.* (2011) 89:346–51. doi: 10.1038/icb.2010.137
31. Oo YH, Sakaguchi S. Regulatory T-cell directed therapies in liver diseases. *J Hepatol.* (2013) 59:1127–34. doi: 10.1016/j.jhep.2013.05.034
32. Jeffery H, Braitch M, Brown S, Oo Y. Clinical potential of regulatory T cell therapy in liver siseases: an overview and current perspectives. *Front Immunol.* (2016) 7:334. doi: 10.3389/fimmu.2016.00334
33. Ronca V, Mancuso C, Milani C, Carbone, M, Oo Y, Invernizzi, P. Immune system and cholangiocytes: a puzzling affair in primary biliary cholangitis. *J Leukoc Biol.* (2020) 108:659–71. doi: 10.1002/JLB.5MR0320-200R
34. Atif M, Warner S, Oo YH. Linking the gut and liver: crosstalk between regulatory T cells and mucosa-associated invariant T cells. *Hepatol Int.* (2018) 12:305–14. doi: 10.1007/s12072-018-9882-x
35. Herman A, Freeman G, Mathis D, Benoist C. CD4+CD25+ T regulatory cells dependent on ICOS promote regulation of effector cells in the prediabetic lesion. *J Exp Med.* (2004) 199:1479–89. doi: 10.1084/jem.20040179
36. Walker LS, Abbas AK. The enemy within: keeping self-reactive T cells at bay in the periphery. *Nat Rev Immunol.* (2002) 2:11–9. doi: 10.1038/nri701
37. Miyara M, Gorochov G, Ehrenstein M, Musset L, Sakaguchi S, Amoura Z. Human FoxP3+ regulatory T cells in systemic autoimmune diseases. *Autoimmun Rev.* (2011) 10:744–55. doi: 10.1016/j.autrev.2011.05.004
38. Bluestone J, Buckner J, Fitch M, Gitelman S, Gupta S, Hellerstein M, et al. Type 1 diabetes immunotherapy using polyclonal regulatory T cells. *Sci Transl Med.* (2015) 7:315ra189. doi: 10.1126/scitranslmed.aad4134
39. Marek-Trzonkowska N, Mysliwiec M, Dobyszuk A, Grabowska M, Techmanska I, Juscinska J, et al. Administration of CD4+CD25highCD127-regulatory T cells preserves beta-cell function in type 1 diabetes in children. *Diabetes Care.* (2012) 35:1817–20. doi: 10.2337/dc12-0038
40. MacDonald K, Hoeppli R, Huang Q, Gillies J, Luciani D, Orban P, et al. Alloantigen-specific regulatory T cells generated with a chimeric antigen receptor. *J Clin Invest.* (2016) 126:1413–24. doi: 10.1172/JCI82771
41. Boardman D, Philippeos C, Fruhwirth G, Ibrahim M, Hannen R, Cooper D, et al. Expression of a chimeric antigen receptor specific for donor HLA class I enhances the potency of human regulatory T cells in preventing human skin transplant rejection. *Am J Transplant.* (2017) 17:931–43. doi: 10.1111/ajt.14185
42. Noyan F, Zimmermann K, Hardtke-Wolenski M, Knoefel A, Schulde E, Geffers R, et al. Prevention of allograft rejection by use of regulatory T cells with an MHC-specific Chimeric antigen receptor. *Am J Transplant.* (2017) 17:917–30. doi: 10.1111/ajt.14175
43. Esensten J, Muller Y, Bluestone J, Tang Q. Regulatory T-cell therapy for autoimmune and autoinflammatory diseases: the next frontier. *J Allergy Clin Immunol.* (2018) 142:1710–18. doi: 10.1016/j.jaci.2018.10.015
44. Dall'Era M, Pauli M, Remedios K, Taravati K, Sandova P, Putnam A, et al. Adoptive treg cell therapy in a patient with systemic lupus erythematosus. *Arthritis Rheumatol.* (2019) 71:431–40. doi: 10.1002/art.40737
45. Marek-Trzonkowska N, Mysliwiec M, Dobyszuk A, Grabowska M, Derkowska I, Juścińska J, et al. Therapy of type 1 diabetes with CD4(+)CD25(high)CD127-regulatory T cells prolongs survival of pancreatic islets—results of one year follow-up. *Clin Immunol.* (2014) 153:23–30. doi: 10.1016/j.clim.2014.03.016
46. Canavan J, Scotta C, Vossenkamper A, Goldberg R, Elder M, Shoval I, et al. Developing in vitro expanded CD45RA+ regulatory T cells as an adoptive cell therapy for Crohn's disease. *Gut.* (2016) 65:584–94. doi: 10.1136/gutjnl-2014-306919
47. Saadoun D, Rosenzwajg M, Joly F, Six A, Carrat F, Thibault V, et al. Regulatory T-cell responses to low-dose interleukin-2 in HCV-induced vasculitis. *N Engl J Med.* (2011) 365:2067–77. doi: 10.1056/NEJMoa1105143
48. He J, Zhang R, Shao M, Zhao X, Miao M, Chen J, et al. Efficacy and safety of low-dose IL-2 in the treatment of systemic lupus erythematosus: a randomised, double-blind, placebo-controlled trial. *Ann Rheum Dis.* (2020) 79:141–9. doi: 10.1136/annrheumdis-2019-215396
49. Rosenzwajg M, Lorenzon R, Cacoub P, Pham H, Pitoiset F, Soufi K, et al. Immunological and clinical effects of low-dose interleukin-2 across 11 autoimmune diseases in a single, open clinical trial. *Ann Rheum Dis.* (2019) 78:209–17. doi: 10.1136/annrheumdis-2018-214229
50. Todd J, Evangelou M, Cutler A, Pekalski M, Walker N, Stevens H, et al. Regulatory T cell responses in participants with Type 1 diabetes after a single dose of interleukin-2: a non-randomised, open label, adaptive dose-finding trial. *PLoS Med.* (2016) 13:e1002139. doi: 10.1371/journal.pmed.1002139
51. Sebode M, Peiseler M, Franke B, Schwinge D, Schoknecht T, Wortmann F, et al. Reduced FOXP3(+) regulatory T cells in patients with primary sclerosing cholangitis are associated with IL2RA gene polymorphisms. *J Hepatol.* (2014) 60:1010–6. doi: 10.1016/j.jhep.2013.12.027
52. Beuers U, Gershwin M, Gish R, Invernizzi P, Jones D, Lindor K, et al. Changing nomenclature for PBC: From 'cirrhosis' to 'cholangitis'. *Hepatology.* (2015) 62:1620–2. doi: 10.1016/j.clinre.2015.08.001
53. Oo YH, Adams DH. Regulatory T cells and autoimmune hepatitis: defective cells or a hostile environment? *J Hepatol.* (2012) 57:6–8. doi: 10.1016/j.jhep.2012.04.005
54. Oo YH, Adams DH. Regulatory T cells and autoimmune hepatitis: what happens in the liver stays in the liver. *J Hepatol.* (2014) 61:973–5. doi: 10.1016/j.jhep.2014.08.005
55. Longhi M, Hussain M, Mitry R, Arora S, Mieli-Vergani G, Vergani D, et al. Functional study of CD4+CD25+ regulatory T cells in health and autoimmune hepatitis. *J.Immunol.* (2006) 176:4484–91. doi: 10.4049/jimmunol.176.7.4484
56. Oo YH, Adams DH. The role of chemokines in the recruitment of lymphocytes to the liver. *J Autoimmun.* (2010) 34:45–54. doi: 10.1016/j.jaut.2009.07.011
57. Adams DH, Lloyd AR. Chemokines: leucocyte recruitment and activation cytokines. *Lancet.* (1997) 349:490–5.
58. Oo Y, Weston C, Lalor P, Curbishley S, Withers D, Reynolds G, et al. Distinct roles for CCR4 and CXCR3 in the recruitment and positioning of regulatory T cells in the inflamed human liver. *J Immunol.* (2010) 184:2886–98. doi: 10.4049/jimmunol.0901216
59. Erhardt A, Wegscheid C, Claass B, Carambia A, Herkel J, Mittrücker H, et al. CXCR3 deficiency exacerbates liver disease and abrogates tolerance in a mouse model of immune-mediated hepatitis. J Immunol. (2011) 186:5284–93. doi: 10.4049/jimmunol.1003750
60. Oo Y, Ackrill S, Cole R, Jenkins L, Anderson P, Jeffery H, et al. Liver homing of clinical grade Tregs after therapeutic infusion in patients with autoimmune hepatitis. *JHEP Rep.* (2019) 1:286–96. doi: 10.1016/j.jhepr.2019.08.001
61. Lim T, Martinez-Llordella M, Kodela E, Gray E, Heneghan M, Sanchez-Fueyo A. Low-dose interleukin-2 for refractory autoimmune hepatitis. *Hepatology.* (2018) 68:1649–52. doi: 10.1002/hep.30059
62. Battula N, Platto M, Anbarasan R, Perera M, Ong E, Roll G, et al. Intention to split policy: a successful strategy in a combined pediatric and adult liver transplant center. *Ann Surg.* (2017) 265:1009–15. doi: 10.1097/SLA.0000000000001816
63. Hornick P, Lechler R. Direct and indirect pathways of alloantigen recognition: relevance to acute and chronic allograft rejection. *Nephrol Dial Transplant.* (1997) 12:1806–10.
64. Brunstein C, Miller J, McKenna D, Hippen K, DeFor T, Sumstad D, et al. Umbilical cord blood-derived T regulatory cells to prevent GVHD:

kinetics, toxicity profile, and clinical effect. *Blood.* (2016) 127:1044–51. doi: 10.1182/blood-2015-06-653667
65. Brunstein C, Miller J, Cao Q, McKenna D, Hippen K, Curtsinger J, et al. Infusion of ex vivo expanded T regulatory cells in adults transplanted with umbilical cord blood: safety profile and detection kinetics. *Blood.* (2011) 117:1061–70. doi: 10.1182/blood-2010-07-293795
66. Edinger M, Hoffmann P, Ermann J, Drago K, Fathman C, Strober S, et al. CD4+CD25+ regulatory T cells preserve graft-versus-tumor activity while inhibiting graft-versus-host disease after bone marrow transplantation. *Nat Med.* (2003) 9:1144–50. doi: 10.1038/nm915
67. Martelli M, Di Ianni M, Ruggeri L, Falzetti F, Carotti A, Terenzi A, et al. HLA-haploidentical transplantation with regulatory and conventional T-cell adoptive immunotherapy prevents acute leukemia relapse. *Blood.* (2014) 124:638–44. doi: 10.1182/blood-2014-03-564401
68. Mathew J, H-Voss J, LeFever A, Konieczna I, Stratton C, He J, et al. A phase I clinical trial with ex vivo expanded recipient regulatory T cells in living donor kidney transplants. *Sci Rep.* (2018) 8:7428. doi: 10.1038/s41598-018-25574-7
69. Chandran S, Tang Q, Sarwal M, Laszik Z, Putnam A, Lee K, et al. Polyclonal regulatory T cell therapy for control of inflammation in kidney transplants. *Am J Transplant.* (2017) 17:2945–54. doi: 10.1111/ajt.14415
70. Feng S, Ekong U, Lobritto S, Demetris A, Roberts J, Rosenthal P, et al. Complete immunosuppression withdrawal and subsequent allograft function among pediatric recipients of parental living donor liver transplants. *JAMA.* (2012) 307:283–93. doi: 10.1001/jama.2011.2014
71. Ramos H, Reyes J, Abu-Elmagd K, Zeevi A, Reinsmoen N, Tzakis A, et al. Weaning of immunosuppression in long-term liver transplant recipients. *Transplantation.* (1995) 59:212–7.
72. Sagoo P, Ali N, Garg G, Nestle F, Lechler R, Lombardi G. Human regulatory T cells with alloantigen specificity are more potent inhibitors of alloimmune skin graft damage than polyclonal regulatory T cells. *Sci Transl Med.* (2011) 3:83ra42. doi: 10.1126/scitranslmed.3002076
73. Tang Q, Bluestone JA. Regulatory T-cell therapy in transplantation: moving to the clinic. *Cold Spring Harb Perspect Med.* (2013) 3:a015552. doi: 10.1101/cshperspect.a015552
74. Vandevyver S, Dejager L, Tuckermann J, Libert C. New insights into the anti-inflammatory mechanisms of glucocorticoids: an emerging role for glucocorticoid-receptor-mediated transactivation. *Endocrinology.* (2013) 154:993–1007. doi: 10.1210/en.2012-2045
75. McKay LI, Cidlowski JA. Molecular control of immune/inflammatory responses: interactions between nuclear factor-kappa B and steroid receptor-signaling pathways. *Endocr Rev.* (1999) 20:435–59. doi: 10.1210/edrv.20.4.0375
76. Silverman Kitchin J, Pomeranz M, Pak G, Washenik K, Shupack J. Rediscovering mycophenolic acid: a review of its mechanism, side effects, and potential uses. *J Am Acad Dermatol.* (1997) 37:445–9. doi: 10.1016/s0190-9622(97)70147-6
77. Mehling A, Grabbe S, Voskort M, Schwarz T, Luger T, Beissert S. Mycophenolate mofetil impairs the maturation and function of murine dendritic cells. *J Immunol.* (2000) 165:2374–81. doi: 10.4049/jimmunol.165.5.2374
78. Moes A, Hesselink D, Zietse R, van Schaik R, van Gelder T, Hoorn E. Calcineurin inhibitors and hypertension: a role for pharmacogenetics? *Pharmacogenomics.* (2014) 15:1243–51. doi: 10.2217/pgs.14.87
79. Giese T, Zeier M, Schemmer P, Uhl W, Schoels M, Dengler T, et al. Monitoring of NFAT-regulated gene expression in the peripheral blood of allograft recipients: a novel perspective toward individually optimized drug doses of cyclosporine A. *Transplantation.* (2004) 77:339–44. doi: 10.1097/01.TP.0000109260.00094.01
80. Xing L, Dai Z, Jabbari A, Cerise J, Higgins C, Gong W, et al. Alopecia areata is driven by cytotoxic T lymphocytes and is reversed by JAK inhibition. *Nat Med.* (2014) 20:1043–9. doi: 10.1038/nm.3645
81. Tavakolpour S. Tofacitinib as the potent treatment for refractory pemphigus: a possible alternative treatment for pemphigus. *Dermatol Ther.* (2018) 31:e12696. doi: 10.1111/dth.12696
82. Kennedy Crispin M, Ko J, Craiglow B, Li S, Shankar G, Urban J, et al. Safety and efficacy of the JAK inhibitor tofacitinib citrate in patients with alopecia areata. *JCI Insight.* (2016) 1:e89776. doi: 10.1172/jci.insight.89776
83. Hodge JA, Kawabata TT, Krishnaswami S, Clark JD, Telliez JB, Dowty ME, et al. The mechanism of action of tofacitinib—an oral Janus kinase inhibitor for the treatment of rheumatoid arthritis. *Clin Exp Rheumatol.* (2016) 34:318–28.
84. Delgoffe G, Pollizzi K, Waickman A, Heikamp E, Meyers D, Horton M. The kinase mTOR regulates the differentiation of helper T cells through the selective activation of signaling by mTORC1 and mTORC2. *Nat Immunol.* (2011) 12:295–303. doi: 10.1038/ni.2005
85. Araki K, Turner A, Shaffer V, Gangappa S, Keller S, Bachmann M, et al. mTOR regulates memory CD8 T-cell differentiation. *Nature.* (2009) 460:108–12. doi: 10.1038/nature08155
86. Hippen K, Merkel S, Schirm D, Sieben C, Sumstad D, Kadidlo D, et al. Massive ex vivo expansion of human natural regulatory T cells (T(regs)) with minimal loss of in vivo functional activity. *Sci Transl Med.* (2011) 3:83ra41. doi: 10.1126/scitranslmed.3001809
87. Zeng H, Yang K, Cloer C, Neale G, Vogel P, Chi H. mTORC1 couples immune signals and metabolic programming to establish T(reg)-cell function. *Nature.* (2013) 499:485–90. doi: 10.1038/nature12297
88. Samanta A, Li B, Song X, Bembas K, Zhang G, Katsumata M, et al. TGF-beta and IL-6 signals modulate chromatin binding and promoter occupancy by acetylated FOXP3. *Proc Natl Acad Sci USA.* (2008) 105:14023–7. doi: 10.1073/pnas.0806726105
89. Oo Y, Banz V, Kavanagh D, Liaskou E, Withers D, Humphreys E, et al. CXCR3-dependent recruitment and CCR6-mediated positioning of Th-17 cells in the inflamed liver. *J Hepatol.* (2012) 57:1044–51. doi: 10.1016/j.jhep.2012.07.008
90. Pascual J, Marcen R, Ortuno J. Anti-interleukin-2 receptor antibodies: basiliximab and daclizumab. *Nephrol Dial Transplant.* (2001) 16:1756–60. doi: 10.1093/ndt/16.9.1756
91. Clatworthy MR. Targeting B cells and antibody in transplantation. *Am J Transplant.* (2011) 11:1359–67. doi: 10.1111/j.1600-6143.2011.03554.x
92. Than N, Hodson J, Schmidt-Martin D, Taubert R, Wawman R, Botter M, et al. Efficacy of rituximab in difficult-to-manage autoimmune hepatitis: results from the International Autoimmune Hepatitis Group. *JHEP Rep.* (2019) 1:437–45. doi: 10.1016/j.jhepr.2019.10.005
93. Kim S, Lee J, Jung C, Min C, Cho B, Shin H, et al. Weekly rituximab followed by monthly rituximab treatment for steroid-refractory chronic graft-versus-host disease: results from a prospective, multicenter, phase II study. *Haematologica.* (2010) 95:1935–42. doi: 10.3324/haematol.2010.026104
94. Salisbury EM, Game DS, Lechler RI. Transplantation tolerance. *Pediatr Nephrol.* (2014) 29:2263–72. doi: 10.1007/s00467-013-2659-5
95. Calne R, Sells R, Pena J, Davis D, Millard P, Herbertson B, et al. Induction of immunological tolerance by porcine liver allografts. *Nature.* (1969) 223:472–6. doi: 10.1038/223472a0
96. Tang Q, Bluestone JA. The Foxp3+ regulatory T cell: a jack of all trades, master of regulation. *Nat Immunol.* (2008) 9:239–44. doi: 10.1038/ni1572
97. Todo S, Yamashita K, Goto R, Zaitsu M, Nagatsu A, Oura T, et al. A pilot study of operational tolerance with a regulatory T-cell-based cell therapy in living donor liver transplantation. *Hepatology.* (2016) 64:632–43. doi: 10.1002/hep.28459
98. Sanchez-Fueyo A, Whitehouse G, Grageda N, Cramp M, Lim T, Romano M, et al. Applicability, safety, and biological activity of regulatory T cell therapy in liver transplantation. *Am J Transplant.* (2020) 20:1125–36. doi: 10.1111/ajt.15700
99. Furukawa A, Wisel SA, Tang Q. Impact of immune-modulatory drugs on regulatory T cell. *Transplantation.* (2016) 100:2288–300. doi: 10.1097/TP.0000000000001379
100. Curbishley S, Eksteen B, Gladue R, Lalor P, Adams D. CXCR 3 activation promotes lymphocyte transendothelial migration across human hepatic endothelium under fluid flow. *Am J Pathol.* (2005) 167:887–99. doi: 10.1016/S0002-9440(10)62060-3
101. Putnam A, Brusko T, Lee M, Liu W, Szot G, Ghosh T, et al. Expansion of human regulatory T-cells from patients with type 1 diabetes. *Diabetes.* (2009) 58:652–62. doi: 10.2337/db08-1168
102. Spence A, Purtha W, Tam J, Dong S, Kim Y, Ju C, et al. Revealing the specificity of regulatory T cells in murine autoimmune diabetes. *Proc Natl Acad Sci USA.* (2018) 115:5265–70. doi: 10.1073/pnas.1715590115
103. Duggleby R, Danby R, Madrigal J, Saudemont A. Clinical grade regulatory CD4(+) T cells (Tregs): moving toward cellular-based immunomodulatory therapies. *Front Immunol.* (2018) 9:252. doi: 10.3389/fimmu.2018.00252
104. Battaglia M, Stabilini A, Roncarolo MG. Rapamycin selectively expands CD4+CD25+FoxP3+ regulatory T cells. *Blood.* (2005) 105:4743–8.

doi: 10.1182/blood-2004-10-3932
105. Cao J, Wang H, Gao W, You J, Wu L, Wang Z. The incidence of cytokine release syndrome and neurotoxicity of CD19 chimeric antigen receptor-T cell therapy in the patient with acute lymphoblastic leukemia and lymphoma. *Cytotherapy.* (2020) 22:214–26. doi: 10.1016/j.jcyt.2020.01.015
106. Itoh S, Kimura N, Axtell R, Velotta J, Gong Y, Wang X, et al. Interleukin-17 accelerates allograft rejection by suppressing regulatory T cell expansion. *Circulation.* (2011) 124:S187–96. doi: 10.1161/CIRCULATIONAHA.110.014852
107. Jeffery H, Hunter S, Humphreys E, Bhogal R, Wawman R, Birtwistle J, et al. Bidirectional cross-talk between biliary epithelium and Th17 cells promotes local Th17 expansion and bile duct proliferation in biliary liver diseases. *J Immunol.* (2019) 203:1151–9. doi: 10.4049/jimmunol.1800455
108. Wawman RE, Bartlett H, Oo YH. Regulatory T cell metabolism in the hepatic microenvironment. *Front Immunol.* (2017) 8:1889. doi: 10.3389/fimmu.2017.01889
109. Jeffery H, van Wilgenburg B, Kurioka A, Parekh K, Stirling K, Roberts S, et al. Biliary epithelium and liver B cells exposed to bacteria activate intrahepatic MAIT cells through MR1. *J Hepatol.* (2016) 64:1118–27. doi: 10.1016/j.jhep.2015.12.017
110. Samir EL Andaloussi, Mäger I, Breakefield XO, Matthew JA Wood. Extracellular vesicles: biology and emerging therapeutic opportunities. *Nat Rev Drug Discov.* (2013) 12:347–57. doi: 10.1038/nrd397
111. Smyth L, Ratnasothy K, Tsang J, Boardman D, Warley A, Lechler R, et al. CD73 expression on extracellular vesicles derived from CD4+ CD25+ Foxp3+ T cells contributes to their regulatory function. *Eur J Immunol.* (2013) 43:2430–40. doi: 10.1002/eji.201242909
112. Yu X, Huang C, Song B, Xiao Y, Fang M, Feng J, et al. CD4+CD25+ regulatory T cells-derived exosomes prolonged kidney allograft survival in a rat model. *Cell Immunol.* (2013) 285:62–8. doi: 10.1016/j.cellimm.2013.06.010
113. Azimi M, Ghabaee M, Moghadasi AN, Noorbakhsh F, Izad M. Immunomodulatory function of Treg-derived exosomes is impaired in patients with relapsing-remitting multiple sclerosis. *Immunol Res.* (2018) 66:513–20. doi: 10.1007/s12026-018-9008-5
114. Okoye I, Coomes S, Pelly V, Czieso S, Papayannopoulos V, Tolmachova T, et al. MicroRNA-containing T-regulatory-cell-derived exosomes suppress pathogenic T helper 1 cells. *Immunity.* (2014) 41:89–103. doi: 10.1016/j.immuni.2014.05.019
115. Tung S, Fanelli G, Matthews R, Bazoer J, Letizia M, Vizcay-Barrena G, et al. Regulatory T cell extracellular vesicles modify t-effector cell cytokine production and protect against human skin allograft damage. *Front Cell Dev Biol.* (2020) 8:317. doi: 10.3389/fcell.2020.00317
116. Besse B, Charrier M, Lapierre V, Dansin E, Lantz O, Planchard D, et al. Dendritic cell-derived exosomes as maintenance immunotherapy after first line chemotherapy in NSCLC. *Oncoimmunology.* (2015) 5:e1071008. doi: 10.1080/2162402X.2015.1071008

Permissions

All chapters in this book were first published Frontiers; hereby published with permission under the Creative Commons Attribution License or equivalent. Every chapter published in this book has been scrutinized by our experts. Their significance has been extensively debated. The topics covered herein carry significant findings which will fuel the growth of the discipline. They may even be implemented as practical applications or may be referred to as a beginning point for another development.

The contributors of this book come from diverse backgrounds, making this book a truly international effort. This book will bring forth new frontiers with its revolutionizing research information and detailed analysis of the nascent developments around the world.

We would like to thank all the contributing authors for lending their expertise to make the book truly unique. They have played a crucial role in the development of this book. Without their invaluable contributions this book wouldn't have been possible. They have made vital efforts to compile up to date information on the varied aspects of this subject to make this book a valuable addition to the collection of many professionals and students.

This book was conceptualized with the vision of imparting up-to-date information and advanced data in this field. To ensure the same, a matchless editorial board was set up. Every individual on the board went through rigorous rounds of assessment to prove their worth. After which they invested a large part of their time researching and compiling the most relevant data for our readers.

The editorial board has been involved in producing this book since its inception. They have spent rigorous hours researching and exploring the diverse topics which have resulted in the successful publishing of this book. They have passed on their knowledge of decades through this book. To expedite this challenging task, the publisher supported the team at every step. A small team of assistant editors was also appointed to further simplify the editing procedure and attain best results for the readers.

Apart from the editorial board, the designing team has also invested a significant amount of their time in understanding the subject and creating the most relevant covers. They scrutinized every image to scout for the most suitable representation of the subject and create an appropriate cover for the book.

The publishing team has been an ardent support to the editorial, designing and production team. Their endless efforts to recruit the best for this project, has resulted in the accomplishment of this book. They are a veteran in the field of academics and their pool of knowledge is as vast as their experience in printing. Their expertise and guidance has proved useful at every step. Their uncompromising quality standards have made this book an exceptional effort. Their encouragement from time to time has been an inspiration for everyone.

The publisher and the editorial board hope that this book will prove to be a valuable piece of knowledge for researchers, students, practitioners and scholars across the globe.

List of Contributors

Lorraine Wallace and Gary M. Reynolds
NIHR Liver Biomedical Research Unit, Centre for Liver Research, College of Medical and Dental Sciences, Institute of Immunology and Immunotherapy, University of Birmingham, Birmingham, United Kingdom

Richard W. Laing, Ricky H. Bhogal, Yuri L. Boteon, Darius F. Mirza, Philip N. Newsome, Hynek Mergental and Simon C. Afford
NIHR Liver Biomedical Research Unit, Centre for Liver Research, College of Medical and Dental Sciences, Institute of Immunology and Immunotherapy, University of Birmingham, Birmingham, United Kingdom
Liver Unit, Queen Elizabeth Hospital, University Hospitals Birmingham NHS Foundation Trust, Birmingham, United Kingdom

Andrea Schlegel
Liver Unit, Queen Elizabeth Hospital, University Hospitals Birmingham NHS Foundation Trust, Birmingham, United Kingdom

Samantha Stubblefield and Anthony E. Ting
Athersys Inc., Cleveland, OH, United States

Valerie D. Roobrouck
ReGenesys BVBA, Leuven, Belgium

Geoffrey W. McCaughan
Liver Injury and Cancer Program, The Centenary Institute, University of Sydney and Royal Prince Alfred Hospital, Sydney, NSW, Australia
AW Morrow Gastroenterology and Liver Centre, University of Sydney and Royal Prince Alfred Hospital, Sydney, NSW, Australia

David G. Bowen and Patrick J. Bertolino
AW Morrow Gastroenterology and Liver Centre, University of Sydney and Royal Prince Alfred Hospital, Sydney, NSW, Australia
Liver Immunology Program, The Centenary Institute, University of Sydney and Royal Prince Alfred Hospital, Sydney, NSW, Australia

Yasmin R. Mohseni, Sim L. Tung, Caroline Dudreuilh, Robert I. Lechler and Giovanna Lombardi
Peter Gorer Department of Immunobiology, MRC Centre for Transplantation, School of Immunology and Microbial Science, King's College London (KCL), Guy's Hospital, London, United Kingdom

Gilbert O. Fruhwirth
Imaging Therapies and Cancer Group, Department of Imaging Chemistry and Biology, School of Biomedical Engineering and Imaging Sciences, King's College London, London, United Kingdom

Weitao Que and Xiao-Kang Li
Division of Transplantation Immunology, National Research Institute for Child Health and Development, Tokyo, Japan

Yanzhi Jiang
Division of Transplantation Immunology, National Research Institute for Child Health and Development, Tokyo, Japan
Guangdong Cardiovascular Institute, Guangdong Provincial People's Hospital, Guangdong Academy of Medical Sciences, Guangzhou, China

Ping Zhu
Guangdong Cardiovascular Institute, Guangdong Provincial People's Hospital, Guangdong Academy of Medical Sciences, Guangzhou, China

Xuhao Ni, Qi Wang, Jian Gu and Ling Lu
Jiangsu Cancer Hospital, Jiangsu Institute of Cancer Research, Nanjing Medical University Affiliated Cancer Hospital, Nanjing, China
Hepatobiliary Center, The First Affiliated Hospital of Nanjing Medical University, Nanjing, China
Research Unit of Liver Transplantation and Transplant Immunology, Chinese Academy of Medical Sciences, Nanjing, China
Key Laboratory of Liver Transplantation, Chinese Academy of Medical Sciences, NHC Key Laboratory of Living Donor Liver Transplantation, Nanjing, China

Pusen Wang, Zhongyi Jiang, Chunguang Wang, Xueni Liu, Hao Li and Lin Zhong
Department of General Surgery, Shanghai General Hospital, Shanghai Jiao Tong University School of Medicine, Shanghai

Dingyin Xu
Department of Hepatobiliary Surgery, Ruian People's Hospital, Ruian, China

Angus Hann
The Liver Unit, Queen Elizabeth Hospital Birmingham, Birmingham, United Kingdom
Institute of Immunology and Immunotherapy, University of Birmingham, Birmingham, United Kingdom

Desley A. H. Neil
Institute of Immunology and Immunotherapy, University of Birmingham, Birmingham, United Kingdom
Department of Cellular Pathology, University Hospitals Birmingham NHS Foundation Trust, Birmingham, United Kingdom

Suz Warner
Institute of Immunology and Immunotherapy, University of Birmingham, Birmingham, United Kingdom
The Liver Unit, Birmingham Children's Hospital, Birmingham, United Kingdom

M. Thamara P. R. Perera
The Liver Unit, Queen Elizabeth Hospital Birmingham, Birmingham, United Kingdom
The Liver Unit, Birmingham Children's Hospital, Birmingham, United Kingdom

Alessandro Parente and M. Thamara P. R. Perera
Liver Unit, Queen Elizabeth Hospital, University Hospitals Birmingham NHS Foundation Trust, Birmingham, United Kingdom

Daniel-Clement Osei-Bordom and Vincenzo Ronca
Institute of Immunology and Immunotherapy, University of Birmingham, Birmingham, United Kingdom
Liver Unit, Queen Elizabeth Hospital, University Hospitals Birmingham NHS Foundation Trust, Birmingham, United Kingdom
Centre for Liver and Gastrointestinal Research, Institute of Immunology and Immunotherapy, University of Birmingham, Birmingham, United Kingdom
National Institute for Health Research Birmingham Liver Biomedical Research Centre, University Hospitals Birmingham National Health Service Foundation Trust, Birmingham, United Kingdom
Division of Gastroenterology and Centre for Autoimmune Liver Diseases, Department of Medicine and Surgery, University of Milan Bicocca, Milan, Italy

Darius Mirza
Liver Unit, Queen Elizabeth Hospital, University Hospitals Birmingham NHS Foundation Trust, Birmingham, United Kingdom
Centre for Liver and Gastrointestinal Research, Institute of Immunology and Immunotherapy, University of Birmingham, Birmingham, United Kingdom

Naomi Richardson, Sky T. H. Ng and David C. Wraith
Institute of Immunology and Immunotherapy, College of Medical and Dental Sciences, University of Birmingham, Birmingham, United Kingdom

Olivier Scatton
Unité de Transplantation Hépatique, Hôpital Pitié-Salpêtrière, AP-HP, Paris, France

Audrey Mohr, Guy Gorochov and Makoto Miyara
Inserm U1135, Centre d'Immunologie et des Maladies Infectieuses (CIMI-Paris), Hôpital Pitié Salpêtrière, AP-HP, Sorbonne Université, Paris, France

Filomena Conti
Inserm U1135, Centre d'Immunologie et des Maladies Infectieuses (CIMI-Paris), Hôpital Pitié Salpêtrière, AP-HP, Sorbonne Université, Paris, France
Unité de Transplantation Hépatique, Hôpital Pitié-Salpêtrière, AP-HP, Paris, France

Mo Atif
Inserm U1135, Centre d'Immunologie et des Maladies Infectieuses (CIMI-Paris), Hôpital Pitié Salpêtrière, AP-HP, Sorbonne Université, Paris, France
Unité de Transplantation Hépatique, Hôpital Pitié-Salpêtrière, AP-HP, Paris, France
Centre for Liver and Gastrointestinal Research, NIHR Birmingham Biomedical Research Centre, University of Birmingham, Birmingham, United Kingdom

Liping Ye, Xinli Mao, Yu Zhang, Yue Cai and Shaowei Li
Department of Gastroenterology, Taizhou Hospital of Zhejiang Province Affiliated to Wenzhou Medical University, Linhai, China

Saiqin He
Department of Gastroenterology, Taizhou Hospital of Zhejiang Province Affiliated to Wenzhou Medical University, Linhai, China
Endoscopy Center, Taizhou Hospital of Zhejiang Province Affiliated to Wenzhou Medical University, Linhai, China

Mingjie Ding, Shuijun Zhang, Xiaoxiao Du, Wenzhi Guo and Shuijun Zhang
Henan Key Laboratory of Digestive Organ Transplantation, Open and Key Laboratory of Hepatobiliary & Pancreatic Surgery and Digestive Organ Transplantation at Henan Universities, ZhengZhou Key Laboratory of Hepatobiliary & Pancreatic Diseases and Organ Transplantation, Department of Hepatobiliary and Pancreatic Surgery, The First Affiliated Hospital of Zhengzhou University, Zhengzhou, China
Department of Hepatobiliary and Pancreatic Surgery, The First Affiliated Hospital of Zhengzhou University, Zhengzhou, China
Open and Key Laboratory of Hepatobiliary & Pancreatic Surgery and Digestive Organ Transplantation at Henan Universities, Zhengzhou, China
Zhengzhou Key Laboratory of Hepatobiliary & Pancreatic Diseases and Organ Transplantation Medicine, Zhengzhou, China

Yuting He
Department of Hepatobiliary and Pancreatic Surgery, The First Affiliated Hospital of Zhengzhou University, Zhengzhou, China
Open and Key Laboratory of Hepatobiliary & Pancreatic Surgery and Digestive Organ Transplantation at Henan Universities, Zhengzhou, China

Helong Dai
Department of Kidney Transplantation, The Second Xiangya Hospital of Central South University, Changsha, China
Clinical Research Center for Organ Transplantation in Hunan Province, Changsha, China
Clinical Immunology Center, Central South University, Changsha, China

Yawen Zheng
Department of Kidney Transplantation, The Second Xiangya Hospital of Central South University, Changsha, China
Clinical Research Center for Organ Transplantation in Hunan Province, Changsha, China
Clinical Immunology Center, Central South University, Changsha, China
Department of Surgery, Thomas E. Starzl Transplantation Institute, University of Pittsburgh School of Medicine, Pittsburgh, PA, United States

Angus W. Thomson
Department of Surgery, Thomas E. Starzl Transplantation Institute, University of Pittsburgh School of Medicine, Pittsburgh, PA, United States
Department of Immunology, University of Pittsburgh School of Medicine, Pittsburgh, PA, United States

Natasha M. Rogers
Department of Surgery, Thomas E. Starzl Transplantation Institute, University of Pittsburgh School of Medicine, Pittsburgh, PA, United States
Center for Transplant and Renal Research, Westmead Institute for Medical Research, Westmead, NSW, Australia
Renal Division, Westmead Hospital, Westmead, NSW, Australia
Westmead Clinical School, University of Sydney, Westmead, NSW, Australia

Naoki Tanimine, Hiroyuki Tahara, Kentaro Ide, Yuka Tanaka and Hideki Ohdan
Department of Gastroenterological and Transplant Surgery, Graduate School of Biomedical and Health Sciences, Hiroshima University, Hiroshima, Japan

Masahiro Ohira
Department of Gastroenterological and Transplant Surgery, Graduate School of Biomedical and Health Sciences, Hiroshima University, Hiroshima, Japan
Medical Center for Translational and Clinical Research Hiroshima University Hospital, Hiroshima, Japan

Takashi Onoe
Department of Gastroenterological and Transplant Surgery, Graduate School of Biomedical and Health Sciences, Hiroshima University, Hiroshima, Japan
Kure Medical Center and Chugoku Cancer Center, National Hospital Organization, Kure, Japan

Sheng Chang and Zhonghua Klaus Chen
Key Laboratory of Organ Transplantation, Institute of Organ Transplantation, Tongji Hospital, Tongji Medical College, Huazhong University of Science and Technology, Ministry of Education, NHC Key Laboratory of Organ Transplantation, Key Laboratory of Organ Transplantation, Chinese Academy of Medical Sciences, Wuhan, China

Chiara Milani
Division of Gastroenterology and Centre for Autoimmune Liver Diseases, Department of Medicine and Surgery, University of Milan Bicocca, Milan, Italy

Grace Wootton
National Institute of Health Research Liver Biomedical Research Unit Birmingham, Centre for Liver Research, Institute of Immunology and Immunotherapy, University of Birmingham, Birmingham, United Kingdom

Owen Cain
Department of Cellular Pathology, University Hospitals Birmingham NHS Foundation Trust, Birmingham, United Kingdom

Andrew Owen
National Institute for Health Research Birmingham, Biomedical Research Centre at University Hospitals Birmingham NHS Foundation Trust, University of Birmingham, Birmingham, United Kingdom
Department of Anesthesia and Critical Care, University Hospitals Birmingham NHS Foundation Trust, Birmingham, United Kingdom

Philip N. Newsome
National Institute for Health Research Birmingham, Biomedical Research Centre at University Hospitals Birmingham NHS Foundation Trust, University of Birmingham, Birmingham, United Kingdom
Centre for Liver and Gastrointestinal Research, Institute of Immunology and Immunotherapy, University of Birmingham, Birmingham, United Kingdom

Liver Unit, University Hospitals Birmingham NHS Foundation Trust, Birmingham, United Kingdom

Lauren V. Terry
Centre for Liver and Gastrointestinal Research, National Institute for Health Research Birmingham Biomedical Research Council, Institute of Immunology and Immunotherapy, University of Birmingham, Birmingham, United Kingdom

Ye Htun Oo
Centre for Liver and Gastrointestinal Research, National Institute for Health Research Birmingham Biomedical Research Council, Institute of Immunology and Immunotherapy, University of Birmingham, Birmingham, United Kingdom
European Reference Network (ERN) Centre—Rare Liver, Queen Elizabeth Hospital, Birmingham, United Kingdom
Liver Transplant Unit, University Hospital of Birmingham National Health Service Foundation Trust, Birmingham, United Kingdom

Index

www.ingramcontent.com/pod-product-compliance
Lightning Source LLC
LaVergne TN
LVHW082206200926
848484LV00008B/2221